RICKETTSIOSES

FROM GENOME TO PROTEOME, PATHOBIOLOGY, AND RICKETTSIAE AS AN INTERNATIONAL THREAT

ANNALS OF THE NEW YORK ACADEMY OF SCIENCES

Volume 1063

RICKETTSIOSES

FROM GENOME TO PROTEOME, PATHOBIOLOGY, AND RICKETTSIAE AS AN INTERNATIONAL THREAT

Edited by Karim E. Hechemy, José A. Oteo, Didier A. Raoult, David J. Silverman, and José R. Blanco

The New York Academy of Sciences
New York, New York
2005

♾ *The paper used in this publication meets the minimum requirements of the American National Standard for Information Sciences—Permanence of Paper for Printed Library Materials, ANSI Z39.48-1984.*

Library of Congress Cataloging-in-Publication Data

International Conference on Rickettsiae and Rickettsial Diseases (4th : 2005 : Logroño, Spain)
Rickettsioses : from genome to proteome, pathobiology, and rickettsiae as an international threat / edited by Karim E. Hechemy … [et al.].
p. ; cm. — (Annals of the New York Academy of Sciences, ISSN 0077-8923 ; v. 1063)
"Result of a conference entitled 4th International Conference on Rickettsiae and Rickettsial Diseases, June 18–21, 2005, Logroño, Spain"— Contents p.
Includes bibliographical references and index.
ISBN 1-57331-600-8 (cloth : alk. paper) — ISBN 1-57331-601-6 (pbk. : alk. paper)
1. Rickettsial diseases—Congresses. 2. Rickettsias—Congresses. I. Hechemy, Karim E. II. New York Academy of Sciences. III. Title. IV. Series.
[DNLM: 1. Rickettsia Infections--Congresses. 2. Rickettsia--Congresses. W1 AN626YL v.1063 2005 / WC 600 I608r 2005]
Q11.N5 vol. 1063
[RC114.5]
500 s—dc22
[614.5'26]

2005035059

GYAT / PCP

Printed in the United States of America
ISBN 1-57331-600-8 (cloth)
ISBN 1-57331-601-6 (paper)
ISSN 0077-8923

ANNALS OF THE NEW YORK ACADEMY OF SCIENCES

Volume 1063
December 2005

RICKETTSIOSES

FROM GENOME TO PROTEOME, PATHOBIOLOGY, AND RICKETTSIAE AS AN INTERNATIONAL THREAT

Editors

KARIM A. HECHEMY, JOSÉ A. OTEO, DIDIER A. RAOULT, DAVID J. SILVERMAN, AND JOSÉ R. BLANCO

Conference Organizers

JOSÉ A. OTEO, JOSÉ R. BLANCO, DIDIER A. RAOULT, PEDRO ANDA, BURT ANDERSON, FATIMA BACELLAR, PHILIPPE BROUQUI, AGUSTÍN ESTRADA-PEÑA, ANTONIO GUERRERO ESPEJO, VALVANERA IBARRA, SANTOS JIMÉNEZ, VÍCTOR MARTÍNEZ DE ARTOLA, FRANCISCO J. MÁRQUEZ, MIGUEL ANGEL MUNIAÍN, ARÁZAZU PORTILLO, DAVID J. SILVERMAN, IRINA TARASEVICH, AND DAVID H. WALKER

Scientific Advisory Board

RICHARD BIRTLES, WEI-MEI CHING, J. STEPHEN DUMLER, PIERRE EDOUARD FOURNIER, MÁRCIO A.M. GALVÃO, STEPHEN GRAVES, KARIM E. HECHEMY, HISASHI INOKUMA, MOGENS JENSENIUS, AMEL LETAÏEF, MIKE MINNICK, GUY PALMER MIROSLAV PETROVEC, SANJEEV K. SAHNI, FERRÁN SEGURA, ZUZANA SEKEYOVÁ

This volume is the result of the **4th International Conference on Rickettsiae and Rickettsial Diseases**, held June 18 –21, 2005, in Logroño (La Rioja), Spain.

CONTENTS

Part I. Genomics and Proteomics

Part II. Pathobiology of Q Fever Infection

Part III. Pathobiology of Rickettsial Infection, Antibiotic Resistance, and Vaccines

Part IV. *Bartonella*

Part V. New Rickettsiae or Rickettsiae Not Previously or Recently Known to Cause Human Infection

Part VI. Pathobiology of *Ehrlichia* and *Anaplasma* Infections

Part VII. Ricketsiae Agents of Bioterrorism

Financial assistance was received from:

General Sponsors

- Gobierno de la Rioja, Fundacíon Rioja Salud
- European Society of Clinical Microbiology and Infectious Diseases (ESCMID)
- American Society For Rickettsiology (ASR)

Supporters

- National Institutes of Health, USA
- Fundacíon Logroño Turismo. Ayuntamiento de Logroño
- Consejo Regulador DOC Rioja
- Asociación para Estudio de Patógenos Especiales
- Sociedad Española de Enfermedades Infecciosas y Microbiología Clínica (SEIMC)

Corporate Supporters

- Abbott
- Böehringer Ingelheim
- Bristol-Myers-Squibb
- Focus Diagnostics
- Gilead
- GlaxoSmithKline
- Ibercaja
- Merck
- Pfizer
- Sanofi-Aventis
- Schering-Plough
- Vircell
- Vitro
- Wyeth

New Insights into Rickettsioses: Genomics, Proteomics, Pathobiology, and the International Threat of Rickettsial Diseases

Introduction

KARIM E. HECHEMY,[a] JOSÉ A. OTEO,[b] DIDIER RAOULT,[c] DAVID J. SILVERMAN,[d] AND JOSÉ RAMÓN BLANCO[b]

[a]*Division of Infectious Disease, Wadsworth Center, New York State Department of Health, Albany, New York 12208, USA*

[b]*Area de Enfermedades Infecciosas. Complejo Hospitalario San Millan, San Pedro de La Rioja, Hospital de La Rioja. 26001 Logroño (La Rioja), Spain*

[c] *Université de la Mediterranée, Faculté de Médecine, Unité des Rickettsies, CNRS UMR 6020, 13385 Marseille Cedex 05, France*

[d]*University of Maryland School of Medicine, Dept. of Microbiology/Immunology, Baltimore, Maryland 21201, USA*

THE 4th INTERNATIONAL CONFERENCE ON RICKETTSIAE AND RICKETTSIAL DISEASES: VOLUME 1

The 4th International Conference on Rickettsiae and Rickettsial Diseases was held in Logroño, capital of the region of La Rioja in Spain, June 18–21, 2005. The autonomous region of La Rioja lies in the north of Spain. It borders the Basque Country and Navarre in the north, Aragon in the east, and Castile and Leon in the south and east.

Scientists from 36 countries attended the meeting. The Conference presentations described new findings and significant advances that have occurred in the discipline of rickettsiology since 2003, when the New York Academy of Sciences published the presentations of the International Conference on Rickettsiae and Rickettsial Diseases held in Slovenia in 2002.[e] The scope of the program reflected the high level of current international research on rickettsiae and associated organisms that were formerly in the Order Rickettsiales, namely, *Coxiella burnetii* and the genus *Bartonella*. *C. burnetii* is now a member of the Order Legionelalles, and the *Bartonella* species are members of the Order Rhizobiales.

The Conference's program and the number of presentations on the various subdisciplines of rickettsiology were so extensive that the decision was made to publish

Addresses for correspondence: Karim E. Hechemy, khechemy@nycap.rr.com, José A. Oteo, jaoteo@riojasalud.es, Didier Raoult, Didier.raoult@medecine.univ-mrs.fr, David J. Silverman, dsilverm@umaryland.edu, José Ramón Blanco, jrblanco@riojasalud.es

[e]Rickettsiology: Present and Future Directions, edited by Karim E. Hechemy, Tatjana Avšič-Županc, James E. Childs, Eds. 2003. Ann. N.Y. Acad. Sci. **990**.

Ann. N.Y. Acad. Sci. 1063: xiii–xx (2005). © 2005 New York Academy of Sciences.
doi: 10.1196/annals.1355.200

the presentations in two volumes of the *Annals*. The scope of this first volume encompasses several subdisciplines of Rickettsiology: the advances made in the fields of genomics and proteomics; a suggested protocol for the naming of newly isolated rickettsiae, whose numbers are continually increasing; the pathobiology of Q(query) fever caused by *C. burnetii,* a potential agent for illegitimate (bioterrorism) use; a minisymposium on bioterrorism; the pathobiology of rickettsial infections, as well as the possible appearance of antibiotic resistance of rickettsiae and the resulting need for the development of effective vaccines; the discoveries of new rickettsiae and the discoveries that other known rickettsiae can produce infections in humans; the increase in importance of infections in humans by *Ehrlichiae* and *Anaplasma*, due to the morbidity and mortality induced by these organisms in certain instances, especially when the patient's immune system is compromised; and, finally, the persistence of *Bartonella*-associated disease in certain regions of the world and in their association with other diseases such as AIDS.

The second volume will focus on the epidemiology of rickettsial diseases worldwide; known vectors and vectors previously not known to transmit a given rickettsial species; and clinical presentations that are atypical or previously not seen, but have been shown by molecular studies to be due to known rickettsiae. The latter type of study indicates that there is more heterogeneity in clinical presentations than had been previously identified. Advances in laboratory diagnoses and in cell culturing will be described. In addition, a section will be devoted to Veterinary Rickettsiology, a field of scientific and economic significance that has long been neglected. Volume 2 will feature a contribution on the molecular biology of rickettsiae that are of veterinary importance in nonhuman vertebrates and invertebrates.

In Volume 1, state-of-the-art contributions in genomics and proteomics illustrate the fact that over the last 20 years, advances in molecular techniques have greatly facilitated the reclassification of previously known members of the Order Rickettsiales. For example, in *Orientia tsutsugamushi*, the aggregate characteristics of tandem repeat sequences differ significantly from those members of the Genus *Rickettsia.* These sequences share no significant synteny with sequences from those of members of the Genus *Rickettsia* or members of the Family Anaplasmatacea. This heterology supports the naming of a new Genus *Orientia* to include *O. tsutsugamushi*. This organism also contains several ankyrin gene repeats. It is proposed that exploitation of host factors by ankyrin-repeat proteins of *O. tsutsugamushi* plays a critical role in the organism's pathogenesis.

As a result of epidemiologic and ecologic investigation of rickettsial vectors, numerous new species and diseases have been identified and classified. Naming and classification of these many new isolates constitute a daunting task, given the many shared characteristics that connect a given organism to family and/or genus. It is, e.g., claimed that *sca2* gene sequences be used as a valuable tool for phylogenic classification of *Rickettsia* species. Until additional scientific tools applicable to taxonomic studies are established, these sequences could provide a flexible system for classification, provided that a consensus among rickettsiologists is reached. Progress in rickettsial genome analyses and comparative genomic studies of virulent low-laboratory-passage strains and "relatively avirulent/attenuated" high-passage strains may reveal critical aspects of rickettsial virulence factors. These have eluded scientists since the first rickettsia; *Rickettsia rickettsii*, was isolated a century ago. Thus, the sequencing of the genomes of low-and high-passage rickettsial isolates should have a high priority. Studies also reveal strong similarities among rickettsial genomes, signifying that those rickettsiae that are placed in the same genus and are closely related comprise fewer distinct species than the present abundance of names suggests. The genomic sequence of a relatively new rickettsia, *Rickettsia felis,* shows that this organism's chromosome is larger than that of any other previously sequenced rickettsia. An interesting point is that, microscopically, this rickettsia exhibits two forms of pili. One form is suggested to play a role in conjugation and the other a role in pathogenicity. The presence of a plasmid in *R. felis* is also described. The plasmid may have been present in ancestors of some rickettsiae such as *Rickettsia akari* that later was lost in this latter species. Complete genome sequencing is an effective tool to identify previously unrecognized phenotypic traits and genes associated with rickettsial pathogenicity. Debate continues on whether a correlation exists between gene content and pathogenic potential of *C. burnetii* isolates. Early studies on a limited number of isolates showed that isolates from human chronic-disease patients, such as K and G, differ genetically from acute-disease isolates. This presumed association became less firm with the analysis of more isolates. Comparison of the complete genome sequences of the Nine Mile, K, and G isolates may improve our understanding of the unique virulence properties of *C. burnetii*, and may provide important insights into the genome architecture and genetic diversity of this pathogen. DNA repair genes that promote survival of microorganisms like *C. burnetii* indicate the existence/operation of an effective and functional DNA repair system that uses a minimum set of genes to sustain genome stability under conditions of oxidative stress. In another contribution, rickettsial survival is shown to relate to a strong capability or capacity to adapt to varying rigorous environmental conditions. It is hypothesized that multiple copies of genes in bacteria with reduced genomes account for such a process. In addition, the promiscuity of the genome in *Ehrlichia ruminantium*, and the genomes stability after transfer of the genes are described. These findings have implications for the formulation of vaccines for use in agriculture.

Genomic and proteomic studies on the epidemic typhus organism *Rickettsia prowazekii* are presented. A genetic approach was applied to isolate rickettsial mutants that can potentially be used, e.g., in pathogenicity studies. It is now possible to generate both random and gene-specific mutations in rickettsiae, e.g., *R. prowazekii*, thereby opening the door to the genetic analysis techniques that have been so successful in dissecting and deciphering gene function in free-living bacteria. However, because of the obligate intracellular nature of the rickettsiae, investigators will need to correlate gene identification with actual function via surrogate hosts, until techniques are developed. The field of proteomics holds great promise for the analysis of rickettsial gene expression. For example, examination of rickettsial gene expression through characterization of the rickettsial proteome has allowed the identification of an extensive number of proteins in a complex rickettsial protein sample representing 71% of *R. prowazekii's* coding genes. Another proteomic contribution describes a comparative analysis of two rickettsiae, one from the spotted fever group (SFG) and one from the typhus group (TG) that revealed proteins to be either unique, or held in by the two strains. Together, the genomic and proteomic approaches will help in characterization of rickettsial intracellular growth and the functional analysis (either qualitative or quantitative) of differentially expressed proteins. Another proteomic application described is the detection of immunodominant antigens of *C. burnetii* with patient sera, followed by cloning and expression of the selected antigens.

C. burnetii, the agent for Q fever, has gained in importance because of its potential for illegitimate use to induce harm in humans and in domestic animals. It thus has a human and economic impact, if misused. This organism occupied an important niche at the conference; a general review of *C. burnetii* was given in one of the lecture series. An interesting contribution to this volume is the description of activities in Australia where Q fever was first observed. Other contributions deal with various aspects of this microorganism, including proteomics. In common with the rickettsiae, a significant number of proteins have been identified by mass spectrometry and tandem mass spectrometry; these proteins can be analyzed to elucidate *C. burnetii* pathobiology. Another study shows the importance of cholesterol in the large parasitophorous vacuole where the organism resides and multiplies. Recombinant outer membrane protein P1 (OmpP1)- heat shock protein HspB shows, potential as a vaccine candidate since it elicits protective humoral and cellular immunity to *C. burnetii* in mice. In the same vein, another contribution proposes the use of multiple recombinant proteins from *C. burnetii* as a potential vaccine. The results may not however, be as clear as is hoped by the authors. Structural and functional characterizations of the glycan antigens of *C. burnetii* indicated that certain subclasses of glycan may be involved in the immunobiology of Q fever. Data in another study show that lipopolysaccharide chemotype is not a determinant of cytokine production in dendritic cells in the host, in response to *C. burnetii* infection. This lack of chemotype specificity results in persistent infection of an otherwise immunocompetent host. In contrast, it is shown by another group that that Toll-like receptor TLR2 is required for inflammatory and immune responses to *C. burnetii. In vivo* studies in severely immunodefficient mice are also presented, using phase I (the highly virulent phase) and phase II (the avirulent variant) of *C. burnetii* to examine the differences in host response to infection between the two phase variants. Others have developed a real-time quantitative polymerase chain reaction (PCR) for evaluation of the immunoprotectivity against Q fever in a mouse model.

Advances in the understanding of rickettsial pathogenesis have been dramatic with the development of powerful research tools. These are reviewed in one of the lecture series, which discusses the multifactorial effects of rickettsial infection on interendothelial junctions, leading to increased microvascular permeability—the hallmark of the rickettsioses. Another contribution presents potential roles for the regulatory oxygenases as inducible antioxidants, in maintaining the integrity of endothelial cells. Data are also presented to support the notion that nitric oxide produced by infected endothelial cells contributes to the changes in vascular permeability that occur during acute rickettsioses. Other studies show that SFG and TG rickettsiae use apparently similar signaling mechanisms for endothelial activation; however, the intensity and kinetics of host cell responses exhibit distinct variations depending on intracytoplasmic characteristics.

Pathogenicity of the rickettsia has also been studied from a different perspective, that of the cell types permissive for rickettsial growth. Dependence of the rickettsial growth on the type of host cell for growth is seen for the SFG rickettsiae, which did not grow on all cell types, unlike the TG rickettsiae. This lack of growth of the SFG rickettsiae was despite their ability to adhere and invade these cells that did not sustain their growth. The mechanism responsible for this difference remains to be determined. The presence of eschars on patients in certain rickettsioses, for example Israeli spotted fever and Mediterranean spotted fever, was not statistically different in the geographic study site. As previous studies have shown for other rickettsiae, early treatment for DEBONEL/TIBOLA is recommended before laboratory test results become available.

The study of molecular mechanisms of resistance to antibiotics in rickettsiae is essential, especially now because of the potential for induction of antibiotic resistance in rickettsiae, which may be a valuable trait for its use as a potential weapon. It is suggested that whole genome sequence analyses can help to predict phenotypic characteristics relating to resistance to antibiotics in these obligate intracellular bacteria, for which transformation assays are usually not suitable. Also, real-time quantitative PCR assays appear to be more sensitive than is the evaluation of antibiotic susceptibility in cell cultures. The documented resistance of *C. burnetii* to standard treatment with tetracycline is likely to become more widespread and could therefore be a major problem if the bacterium is used for illegitimate purposes. Clinical trials are suggested to be warranted for macrolide antibiotics like telithromycin, which, at least for now, appears to be effective against *C. burnetii* in *in vitro* experiments.

The development of new vaccines focuses on cloning and sequencing analyses to determine the most appropriate antigens to use in formulating a vaccine. In this way, the side effects are minimized that could prevent the vaccine's potential use. Examples of such vaccine-development efforts include the cloning and sequence analysis of the 22-kDa antigen genes of several strains of *O. tsutsugamushi*, and the analysis of 51-kDa antigenic protein of *Neorickettsia risticii*. In another study, antigen-specific immune responses to a DNA vaccine from scrub typhus p47Kp have been found to be still observable 6 months following immunization, suggesting that memory lymphocytes are generated by this vaccine candidate. Such findings will facilitate the selection of antigens to be formulated in a multivalent vaccine.

Results using truncated outer membrane protein A (OmpA) of *Rickettsia heilongjiangii* and SFG rickettsia isolated in China show humoral and cell-mediated immune responses against homologous and heterologous species in the SFG rickettsiae. Also, biochemical analyses of the LPS from *Rickettsia typhi*, a strong immunogen, show that LPS does not contain heptose, which is a common sugar constituent of the core regions of enterobacterial LPSs.

Another of the lecture series reviews members of the Family Bartonellaceae, which are hemotropic organisms. The low prevalence of clinical manifestations in the host induced by these species, as compared to the high prevalence of infection in animals, underscores the important fact that these parasites exploit rather than kill their hosts. A high incidence of *Bartonella* infection was observed in small rodents in the Russian Far East, using molecular analysis. Studies of *Bartonella*'s parasitism will continue to yield significant insights, allowing the bacterial attributes that mediate this parasitism to be unraveled, and also offering possible clarification of the mediator molecules. The development of mutants of *Bartonella* that have lost the ability to adhere to, to invade, or to multiply in erythrocytes will provide important tools for the study of this organism's biological attributes. In one contribution, it is shown that the rate of *Bartonella* infection among immunocompromised patients (e.g., HIV-infected patients) is much greater than among the healthy population, within the particular geographic area studied. The authors further suggest that *Bartonella* infection be considered in the differential diagnosis for other infections in patients with HIV. It has been shown in a patient co-infected with HIV and *Bartonella quintana* that no new bacillary angiomatosis lesions are evident after three months of antibiotic treatment.

In contrast, tropical bartonellosis caused by *Bartonella bacilliformis* (not formerly in the Order Rickettsiales) is a highly fatal disease of the Andes Mountains in South America. The production of recombinant protein, and the application of this recombinant protein in an ELISA handheld rapid assay for the diagnosis of *B. bacilliformis*, are described. Studies on the effect of GroEL released by *B. bacilliformis* during intracellular infection illustrate another potential strategy for regulation of human vascular endothelial host cell growth.

Over the past two decades, the discovery that rickettsiae previously not considered pathogenic in humans are able to cause disease has opened new avenues in rickettsial research from the molecular, clinical and epidemiologic perspectives. An example of a rickettsia previously not considered to be pathogenic is *Rickettsia parkeri*, which has been detected in a patient. It is to be hoped that the recognition of *R. parkeri* as a cause of disease in humans will encourage a closer examination for specific etiologies of tick-borne SFG rickettsioses worldwide. The *Amblyomma* tick, a vector for *R. parkeri,* has also been found to be a vector for *R. prowazekii* in Mexico. The known vector is the louse and hence the disease has been termed louse-borne typhus. "*Candidatus* Rickettsia andeanae," a novel agent, has been molecularly detected, although not cultured from two different ticks collected from horses in two separate locations in northern Peru. A *Dermacentor* tick has been described containing mainly the pathogenic *Rickettsia slovaca*, but also other *Rickettsia* species, as indicated by PCR and sequencing. The roles of these species of rickettsia in disease causation have yet to be determined. *Rickettsia aeschlimanii,* which has recently been found as a human pathogen, is considered to be of low risk in Northern Spain, because of its low prevalence in the vector and the apparent low transmission of the rickettsia after a tick bite on humans with the rickettsia-infected ticks.

The presence of the newly discovered "nonpathogenic" AP-Variant of *A. phagocytophilum* may in part explain the low prevalence of disease caused by *A. phagocytophilum*, owing to the competitive nature of the parasitism of the bacterium in the vector. In addition, it was shown that the tick *Am. americanum*, a vector for ehrlichial antigen, does carry *Rickettsia amblyommi* sp. nov. The spread of rickettsiae worldwide is much broader than previously appreciated and the notion of geographic compartmentalization has been disproved by the new molecular techniques. For example, the presence of species of ehrlichiae and rickettsiae other than the agent of Brazilian spotted fever has been noted in an area of Brazil not previously known to harbor these organisms. Another newly recognized human pathogen is *E. ruminantium*. Specimens from three fatally (presumably) infected children had molecular evidence indicating the presence of this organism.

The conference included a minisymposium on the potential illegitimate use of *Rickettsiae* and associated organisms, e.g., the use of *C. burnetii*, a Category B biodefense organism as a potential bioweapon because of this organism's ease of transmission via aerosol and its survival under unfavorable environmental conditions. Through history, rickettsial species have been pathogens significant in the field of military medicine, mainly through epidemic typhus outbreaks during military expeditions. From a public health and biodefense perspective, exposures of humans/population to different strains, natural, or the result of the illegitimate release, are likely to have differing outcomes. This volume includes presentations from a group dedicated to the creation of a comprehensive database of information on selected CDC Category A, B, C pathogens, as well as other organisms that cause emerging and re-emerging human diseases. The approach and strategies devised/used for biological data annotation/curation for the rickettsial research as well as others should lead to a better understanding of the management and prevention of rickettsial diseases. A contribution from the minisymposium suggests that, when extensive genomic-level information is available from diverse strains, investigators will be able to determine effective drug and vaccine targets and design methods to accurately type *Coxiella* and other organisms, based on a subset of genes. This ability would pave the way for cost-effective targeted PCR- or antibody-based tests. Another study has shown the differing abilities of various genomic groups of *C. burnetii* to induce pathologic changes in the liver. *C. burnetii* Group IV isolates produce consistently larger and more numerous hepatic granulomas than do isolates from other groups. A probabilistic model has been devised to assess the potential for low concentrations of *C. burnetii* in aerosol form to infect humans. Another contribution describes the patient and laboratory management as well as the political effects and media implications that are involved in a mock-attack scenario using rickettsiae or associated organisms.

Human and animal infections by members of the Family Anaplasmataceae are increasingly recognized as important and potentially fatal arthropod-transmitted diseases. One of the lecture series in the present volume reviews the current knowledge on this family, which belongs to the Order Rickettsiales. The incidence of infections has linearly increased, and the old members of this family and new members are continually being discovered worldwide. An understanding of the diseases their pathophysiology, pathogenesis, control, and management is crucial since most data now suggest that alterations in host neutrophil function, and protection from innate and adaptive immunity, contribute to disease manifestations. One contribution deals with the roles of innate and adaptive immune responses in mice in terms of protection from severe monocytic ehrlichiosis; the functions of these responses in immunopathology are discussed. Another paper, describes the role of cellular immunity in monocytic ehrlichiosis by analyzing a model of mice infected with *Ixodes ovatus* ehrlichia (IOE). Another paper shows that the genetic sequence of the *Ehrlichia muris p*28s gene loci was completed. The authors asserted that this will enable the study of the roles of these loci in a mouse model of persistent infection. Cytokine responses in *Ehrlichia canis*–infected dogs have also been studied. Persistent expression of IFN-γ and TNF-α mRNA starting on day 2 or 8 and continuing to day 56 post-inoculation was found in all infected dogs. Molecular characterization of the genes/sequences encoding *E. canis* gp36 and *E. chaffeensis* gp47 tandem repeats among isolates from different geographic locations showed complete conservation of tandem repeats between strains of *E. canis* around the world and only a limited divergence of *E. chaffeensis*. This conservation could have positive implications for future vaccine and diagnostic use of these proteins. Sustained-release doxycycline formulation has been shown to be efficacious in preventing tick-transmitted *A. phagocytophilum* infection in a mouse model.

A study using *A. phagocytophilum* has shown that in mice, an endothelial reservoir of this bacterium offers opportunities for ongoing, direct cell-to-cell infection of neutrophil granulocytes, and through avoidance of host immune effectors. Also, completion of the bacterium life cycle, by infection of circulating leukocytes available for transfer to blood-feeding ticks, occurs. Innate and/or adaptive T cell immune responses are shown to be critical in studies on the mechanisms of immunologic control of *A. phagocytophilum* in mice. It is postulated in another paper that the elucidation of mechanisms leading to perturbation of neutrophil phagocytosis will enable the spectrum of abnormalities to be defined, and will assist in identification of host cell targets important in *A. phagocytophilum* pathogenesis. An *in vitro* model used to assess alterations in platelet function failed to show direct stimulation of human platelet aggregation by *A. phagocytophilum.* Another study shows that tissue injury, in the murine model of granulocytic anaplasmosis, relates to host innate immune response, and not to the pathogen load. A human study has shown that in a patient with febrile illness occurring after a tick bite, the concentration of C-reactive protein and the level of serum procalcitonin were both elevated, perhaps implicating an acute infection of human granulocytic ehrlichiosis, rather than tick-borne encephalitis.

In this Introduction, we have attempted to present an overview of all of the papers contained in Volume 1 of the two volumes emerging from the conference. Of course, we have merely scratched the surface. The aim of these two volumes is to present to rickettsiologists and to scientists outside our field a snapshot of the range of the work that is being carried out in rickettsiology worldwide. It is our hope that established scientists interested in intracellular bacteria would consider moving into the field of rickettsiology, and that young scientists who are looking for an interesting and demanding field will consider rickettsiology as a career. The Editors here wish to thank all the contributors to this volume. We also thank the reviewers of the manuscripts who have generously given their time to assist the editors in the reviewing process. Lastly, we thank The New York Academy of Sciences for providing the *Annals* as a venue for publication of the presentations at the Conference. We extend our special thanks to the staff of the *Annals*, Linda Mehta, Joyce Hitchcock, and Justine Cullinan.

Naming of Rickettsiae and Rickettsial Diseases

DIDIER RAOULT,[a] PIERRE-EDOUARD FOURNIER,[a] MARINA EREMEEVA,[b] STEPHEN GRAVES,[c] PATRICK J. KELLY,[d] JOSÉ A. OTEO,[e] ZUZANA SEKEYOVA,[f] AKIRA TAMURA,[g] IRINA TARASEVICH,[h] AND LIJUAN ZHANG[i]

[a]*Unité des Rickettsies, IFR 48, CNRS UMR 6020, Faculté de Médecine, Université de la Méditerranée, 13385 Marseille Cedex 05, France*

[b]*Viral and Rickettsial Zoonoses Branch, Centers for Disease Control and Prevention, Atlanta, Georgia, USA*

[c]*Department of Microbiology, Geelong Hospital, Geelong, Victoria, Australia*

[d]*Ross University School of Veterinary Medicine, West Farm, Basseterre, St. Kitts, West Indies*

[e]*Area de Gestión Clínica en Enfermedades Infecciosas, Hospital de La Rioja, Logroño, Spain*

[f]*Institute of Virology, Slovak Academy of Sciences, Bratislava, Slovakia*

[g]*Niigata University of Pharmacy and Applied Life Sciences, Niigata, Japan*

[h]*Laboratory of Rickettsial Ecology, Russian Academy of Medical Science, Gamaleya Institute for Epidemiology and Microbiology, Moscow, Russia*

[i]*Chinese Center for Diseases Control and Prevention, Beijing, China*

ABSTRACT: Over the last 20 years, advances in molecular techniques have greatly facilitated the identification of the members of the *Rickettsiales*, and numerous new species and diseases have been described. In this paper, we review taxonomic rules and appropriate approaches to valid naming of rickettsial species and the diseases they cause.

KEYWORDS: *Rickettsia*; taxonomy; genus; species; rickettsiosis; name

BACKGROUND

The *Rickettsia* are gram-negative obligate intracellular bacteria that have invertebrate hosts as vectors or reservoir hosts. Da Rocha Lima named the first species, *Rickettsia prowazekii*, which is the agent of epidemic typhus, in honor of Ricketts and von Prowazek, who both died of typhus while studying the disease.[1] The role of lice as vectors of *R. prowazekii* was demonstrated by Nicolle, who also described the first experimental infections with the organism and received the Nobel Prize for this work.[1] Wilson and Chowning first identified the role of ticks and tick bites in the

Address for correspondence: Didier Roault, Unité des Rickettsies, IFR 48, CNRS UMR 6020, Faculté de Médecine, Université de la Méditerranée, 27 Boulevard Jean Moulin, 13385 Marseille Cedex 05, France. Voice: +33-04-91-38-55-17; fax: +33-04-91-83-03-90.
didier.raoult@medecine.univ-mrs.fr

Ann. N.Y. Acad. Sci. 1063: 1–12 (2005).
doi: 10.1196/annals.1355.002

transmission of Rocky Mountain spotted fever in their report in the *Lancet* in 1902,[2] and this suggestion was confirmed by Ricketts in his later publication in 1906.[3] Subsequently, Ricketts obtained the first isolate of *R. rickettsii* in guinea pigs and noted the similarity of *R. rickettsii* and the agent of epidemic typhus.[3] Wolbach was the first to clearly identify the intracellular nature of *Rickettsia* spp. in 1919.[4] In this paper, we review the contemporary taxonomic rules and appropriate approaches to valid naming of species of *Rickettsia* and the diseases they cause.

IDENTIFICATION OF BACTERIA

The first step in the identification of a bacterium is the assignment of the organism to a genus. Ideally, a bacterial genus consists of a group of species exhibiting similar genetic and phenotypic characteristics. It has been suggested that a genus includes bacterial species with DNA-DNA hybridization levels of 25 to 60%, degrees of 16S rDNA sequence similarity of > 90%, and G+C contents not diverging by more than 10%. The only real necessity for creating a new genus is when there is phylogenetic incongruence in these traits.[5]

A bacterial species reflects the sum of the biological information on a group of closely related strains isolated in pure culture. This information should include their taxonomic affinities, morphology, distribution, ecology, and pathogenicity. Initially, the identification of bacterial species was based on combinations of phenotypic criteria. The first genomic parameter used for taxonomic purposes was the G+C content; strains within a species should not have differences in G+C content of more than 5%.[6] Later, DNA-DNA hybridization techniques were introduced and a bacterial species included strains with DNA-DNA relatedness of ≥70 % and a ΔTm of ≤5%.[7] The latter method became the standard arbiter for the designation of genomospecies. The extensive use of 16S rDNA sequencing for identification of bacteria in environmental and clinical specimens has led to a dramatic increase in the number of potential new species.[8,9] It is currently considered that strains with more than 3% divergence belong to different species.[10]

Specific rules for recognizing, naming, and classifying species have been established which avoid redundant descriptions and the use of the same name for more than one species. Several prerequisites must be met before a new bacterial species is validated[11] (TABLE 1). Also, all information available should be included in its de-

TABLE 1. Prerequisites for the validation of bacterial species or subspecies

A. The species concept only applies to bacteria which have been isolated in **pure culture**.

B. To be as accurate as possible, the species description should be based on a minimum of **five isolates** for environmental bacteria.

C. The new species should exhibit **both genomic and phenotypic discriminative** characteristics.

D. A type strain should be identified for each new species, and should be made available to the scientific community through **two independent** official culture collections.

E. The new bacterial name should appear in the **approved lists** of bacterial names.

scription, such as the structure, metabolic and reproductive features, and the biology of the organism. Bacterial isolates not meeting all the prerequisites should be referred to in quotation marks.

A subspecies is the lowest taxonomic rank that is recognized officially.[7] It contains closely related strains that have distinct phenotypic traits, but do not meet the genomic criteria required for classification as a distinct species.[7] The official validation of a subspecies is comparable to that of species.

NAMING OF BACTERIA

Scientists use taxonomic names when they communicate with one other. A species name is proposed by the first publication which meets the current requirement for designation of a species. The description of a new bacterial species should be based on well-characterized isolates, but there have been exceptions for organisms that are difficult to isolate in artificial culture, such as *Mycobacterium leprae*.

The current nomenclature for bacteria is based on the binomial naming system introduced by Linnaeus in the eighteenth century. Genus names begin with a capital letter and are written in italics. They are substantives or adjectives treated as substantives and are Latin or Latinized names. New genus names are followed by "gen. nov." Species names are composed of a binary combination of the genus name followed by an epithet indicating the species. The epithet begins with a small letter and is Latin or Latinized. The epithet may be derived from a person's name, a geographical location, or from any origin. It also may be composed of a combination of two or more names (e.g., *B. thetaiotaomicron*). For names derived from a geographical location, the Latin name should be used whenever possible or the modern name should be Latinized. The specific epithet must be treated as an adjective that must agree with the gender of the generic name (e.g., *Staphylococcus aureus*), as a substantive in apposition in the nominative case (e.g., *Desulfovibrio gigas*), or as a substantive in the genitive case (e.g., *Escherichia coli*). Species names are written in italics. New species names are followed by "sp. nov." Subspecies names are composed of a combination of the species name followed by "subsp." and an epithet indicating the subspecies. The subspecific epithet should be treated as specific epithets. Subspecies names are written in italics. New subspecies names are followed by "subsp. nov." Bacteria which cannot be cultivated but which fullfill genomic criteria to be classified as a species may provisionally be classified as *Candidatus*.[12] *Candidatus* names are derived in the same manner as species names but they are written in quotation marks instead of italics, and follow the word *Candidatus* in italics. For a more detailed description of the etymological guidelines used in naming a genus, species, or subspecies, we recommend readers to the exhaustive review by H.G. Trüper.[12]

RICKETTSIAE

The taxonomic classification of rickettsiae has long been a matter of controversy, and remains currently debated for some taxa. Taxonomic classification of members of the order *Rickettsiales* was originally based on relatively few phenotypic criteria.[13]

These bacteria are described as small, rod-shaped, Gram-negative, obligate intracellular organisms that retain basic fuschin when stained by the method of Gimenez.[13] They divide by binary fission, can be cultivated in living tissues, and are associated with invertebrate hosts that act as vectors and/or reservoirs. Initially, most bacteria with an obligate association with eukaryotic cells were included in the order *Rickettsiales* because they could not be classified with the phenotypic methods applied to bacteria that grew readily on artificial media. With the advent of 16S rDNA sequencing, several bacteria in the order *Rickettsiales* were reclassified. These included *Coxiella burnetii* and *Rickettsiella grylli*, which moved to the *Legionellaceae,*[14] *Eperythrozoon* sp. and *Haemobartonella* sp. to the *Mycoplasmataceae*,[15,16] *Wolbachia persica* to the γ-subdivision of *Proteobacteria* close to *Francisella* sp., and *Wolbachia melophagito* (Birtles and Molyneux, GenBank accession number X89110), *Bartonella* sp., *Rochalimaea* sp., and *Grahamella* sp. to the *Bartonellaceae.*[17] With the recent organization of the ehrlichiae,[18] the order *Rickettsia*les now comprises the family Anaplasmataceae which includes *Anaplasma*, *Ehrlichia*, *Neorickettsia*, and *Wolbachia*, and the family Rickettsiaceae which includes *Orientia*, *Rickettsia*.

Members of the *Rickettsia* are closely related phylogenetically and have a high degree of 16S rDNA nucleotide sequence similarity.[19,20] Historically, cross-reactions of patient's sera with somatic antigens of strains of *Proteus* OX19, OX2, and OXK were used to classify rickettsial isolates into 3 groups, respectively: spotted fever group, typhus group (TG), and scrub typhus group (STG). Subsequently, the only scrub typhus species, *R. tsutsugamushi*, was reclassified within the genus *Orientia.*[21] Other phenotypic criteria that have been used to describe *Rickettsia* species include the geographical distribution of the strain, the arthropod vector, pathogenicity in humans, mice, and guinea pigs, optimal culture temperature, time for plaque formation, size of plaques, growth in embryonated chicken eggs, and hemolytic activity.[22] However, the immunofluorescent antibody assay with acute phase sera of Swiss Webster mice developed by Philip in 1978 became the reference method for the identification of new SFG rickettsiae.[23] With this method, a rickettsial isolate is regarded as a new species if it has a specificity difference of ≥ 3 with all the other SFG rickettsia species. Thus, a species corresponds to a serotype. Since its introduction, this method has been considered a useful guide to speciation. However, opinions divide as to whether this holds true for all rickettsial strains. In addition, although useful, the method has several drawbacks including lack of reproducibility and the need to compare each new isolate with all previously described species.

With the advent of molecular classification, many of the currently accepted *Rickettsia* species were identified genetically before they were cultured in the laboratory. As is the case with other bacteria, *Rickettsia* can be given *Candidatus* status if they fulfill the genomic criteria but have yet to be cultured. Of the molecular classification techniques available, the DNA G+C content (32–33% for the SFG and 29% for the TG) and DNA-DNA re-association[7] are not easily applied to rickettsiae. Gene sequencing has become the most widely used method to identify rickettsial isolates.[19,24–27] However, no official rules have been adopted to classify these bacteria, in particular the boundaries of the genus and species status were confusing. This prompted an attempt to revise taxonomic rules applied to rickettsiae in order to clarify the status of all currently known rickettsiae, and to propose guidelines for the classification and denomination of rickettsial isolates. In particular, it was proposed to apply to rickettsial isolates gene sequence–based methods that are used for other

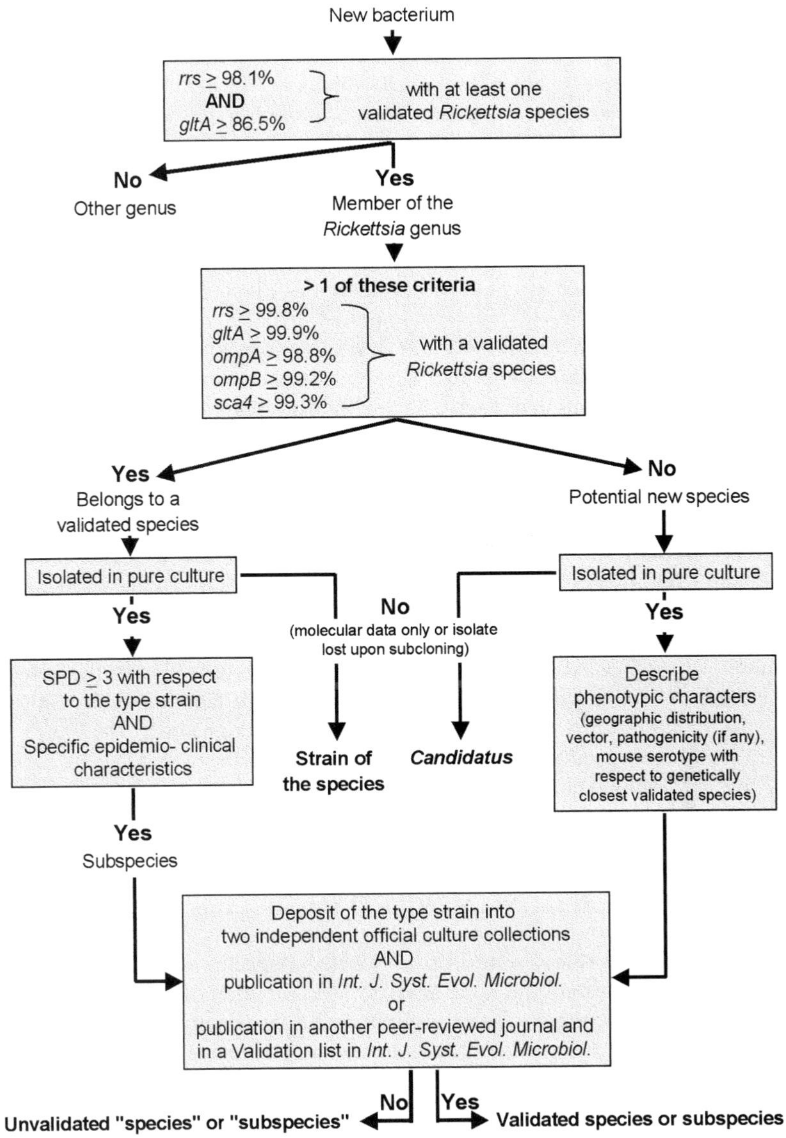

FIGURE 1. Taxonomic scheme for classification of rickettsiae at the genus and species levels. Genes: *rrs* encodes the 16S rRNA; *gltA* encodes the citrate synthase; *ompA* encodes the rOmpA; *ompB* encodes the rOmpB; *sca4* (gene D) encodes the PS-120. SPD = specificity difference in mouse serotyping.

bacteria. First,a method was proposed based on sequencing several genes, derived from the multi-locus sequence typing officially accepted as a taxonomic tool for other bacteria,[28] to provide genetic criteria to classify isolates at the group and species levels within the *Rickettsia* genus[29] (FIG. 1). The method was validated using 20 *Rickettsia* species that were uncontested and identified by serotyping with mouse antisera. The technique has enabled the demonstration that mouse serotyping does not always identify species that are genetically distinct.[29] In particular, it was demonstrated that rickettsiae closely related to *R. conorii* within the "*R. conorii* complex," and for which some authors disagreed as to whether these bacteria were distinct species or not,[30–32] belonged to the *R. conorii* species. However, as confusion persisted regarding the exact taxonomic status of these bacteria within the *R. conorii* species, a rule of the *ad hoc* committee on reconciliation of approaches to bacterial systematics[7] was used. This rule states that, even if related genetically, bacterial isolates within a given species could be considered as distinct subspecies if they differed phenotypically. When this rule was applied to the "*R. conorii* complex," it was observed that, although genetically homogeneous, rickettsial isolates within the *R. conorii* species had distinct genotypic, serotypic, and epidemio-clinical characteristics. Therefore, the creation of four *R. conorii* subspecies was proposed: "*R. conorii* subsp. *conorii*", "*R. conorii* subsp. *indica*", "*R. conorii* subsp. *caspia*" and "*R. conorii* subsp. *israelensis*".[33] With the use of similar criteria, the creation of two subspecies will soon be proposed within the *R. sibirica* species: "*R. sibirica* subsp. *sibirica*" and "*R. sibirica* subsp. *mongolitimonae*."[34]

To be officially validated as a new species or subspecies, a rickettsia should fulfill the same requirements as other bacteria (TABLE 1). Also, sustained cell culture–adapted strains must be deposited in two collections from two different countries officially recognized by the World Data Centre for Microorganisms before they can be officially named. The American Type Culture Collection (ATCC) was the only official culture collection that accepted rickettsiae until our laboratory, the Unité des Rickettsies, was recently recognized as an official collection site by the World Data Centre for Microorganisms. The official description of uncultured species, such as *R. peacockii*,[35] should no longer be possible. Such rickettsiae should be classified as *Candidatus* "Rickettsia sp."

NAMING A *RICKETTSIA* SPECIES

The etymological rules used to name rickettsial species and subspecies and to give *Candidatus* status are the same as those used for other bacteria (see above). It is important to follow these rules carefully to avoid incorrectly Latinized names, as was the case with *R. canadensis* and *R. montanensis* (previously *R. canada* and *R. montana*). To date, 21 *Rickettsia* species have been officially validated (the Approved Lists of Bacterial Names is available online at <http://www.bacterio.cict.fr/>) (TABLE 2). The names of some species were derived from their geographical origin, mainly *R. africae*, *R. australis*, *R. canadensis*, *R. helvetica*, *R. japonica*, *R. massiliae*, *R. montanensis*, *R. sibirica*, and *R. slovaca.* The names of others were derived from the names of investigators who contributed significantly to the current knowledge on rickettsiae and rickettsial diseases. These include *R. aeschlimannii* (A. Aeschlimann), *R. belli* (E.J. Bell), *R. conorii* (A. Conor), *R. honei* (F.S. Hone), *R.*

TABLE 2. Validated species and subspecies of the genus *Rickettsia* and *Orientia*

Name	Former or Other names	Source of the Name	Investigators
R. prowazekii	R. prowazeki	Investigators	Ricketts and von Prowazek
R. typhi	R. mooseri	Clinical situation (typhos)	
R. rickettsii	Dermatocentro-xenus rickettsi	Investigator	Ricketts
R. conorii	D. conorii	Investigator	Conor
R. conorii subsp. conorii		Investigator	Conor
R. conorii subsp.indica	Indian tick typhus rickettsia	India	
R. conorii subsp.israe-lensis	Israeli spotted fever rickettsia, *R. sharoni*	Israel	
R. conorii subsp. caspia	Astrakhan fever rickettsia	Caspian Sea	
R. akari		Greek name of the mite vector	
R. africae		Africa	
R. japonica		Japan	
R. massiliae		Latin name of Marseille	
R. montanensis	R. montana	Montana	
R. canadensis	R. canada	Canada	
R. helvetica		Latin name of Switzerland	
R. sibirica		Siberia	
R. slovaca		Slovakia	
R. aeschlimanii		Investigator	Aeschlimann
R. parkeri		Investigator	Parker
R. bellii		Investigator	Bell
R. honei		Investigator	Hone
R. peacockii		Investigator	Peacock
R. rhipicephali		Tick vector	
R. felis	R. ctenocephali	Latin name of the cat, host of the flea vector	
R. heilongjiangensis	R. heilongjiangi	Heilongjiang (Chinese area)	
R. monacensis		Latin name of Munich	
R. australis		Australia	
Orientia tsutsuga-mushi	R. tsutsugamushi, R. orientalis	Orient, and Japanese name of the mite vector	

parkeri (R.R. Parker), *R. peacockii* (M.G. Peacock), *R. prowazekii* (S. von Prowazek) and *R. rickettsii* (H.T. Ricketts). Some species were named after their vectors, mainly *R. akari* ("akari" is Greek for mite) and *R. rhipicephali* (*Rhipicephalus sanguineus*). The agent of flea-borne spotted fever may have been first described as *R. ctenocephali* in 1918,[36] but is now called *R. felis* after the domestic cat (*Felis domesticus*), which is the host of *Ctenocephalides felis*, its flea vector. *R. typhi* was derived from the Greek term for "stupor" (*tuphos*), a symptom of typhus. The genus name of *Orientia tsutsugamushi*[21] (formerly *R. tsutsugamushi*), a bacterial species closely related to *Rickettsia* species within the family *Rickettsiaceae*, was derived from the Orient, where it was discovered and the species name was derived from the common name of the disease in Japanese ("tsutsugamushi," the mite disease). In addition to the validated species, as-yet unofficial species names have been published, mainly "*R. amblyommii*" [37] (also referred to as strain 85-1034, WB-8-2, or MOAa), named for its vector, *Amblyomma americanum*; "*R. monacensis*," [38] derived from the Latin name for Munich, Germany; "*R. heilongjiangensis*," [29] derived from the Heilongjiang province of China; "*R. texiana*," [39] derived from Texas; "*R. hulinii*," [40] derived from the Hulin province of China; and "*R. thailandii*," [41] derived from Thailand. It should be noted that the latter two species names have been incorrectly Latinized and should be "*R. hulinensis*" and "*R. thailandensis*," respectively.

Of the four *R. conorii* subspecies that have recently been proposed, "*R. conorii* subsp. *conorii*" is named for an early rickettsiologist (A. Conor), while "*R. conorii* subsp. *indica*," "*R. conorii* subsp. *caspia*," and "*R. conorii* subsp. *israelensis*" are named for their geographic location. The two *R. sibirica* subspecies that will soon be proposed have also been named for their geographic locations; "*R. sibirica* subsp. *sibirica*" and "*R. sibirica* subsp. *mongolitimonae*."

Although many new rickettsiae have been described on the basis of genomic criteria only, to date there are only two rickettsiae with recognized *Candidatus* status. The one is "*Candidatus* R. tarasevichiae,"[42] named in honor of I.V. Tarasevich, and the other is "*Candidatus* R. andeanae."[43]

Other rickettsial strains or amplicons that have been designated by strain names include *Rickettsia* sp. genotype cooleyi,[44] named after R.A. Cooley, and *Rickettsia* sp. strain cooperi,[45] named for its vector, *Amblyomma cooperi*. A number have been named according to their laboratory identification: *Rickettsia* sp. strain AT1;[46] *Rickettsia* sp. strain 364-D;[47] *Rickettsia* sp. strains RDa420 and RD1a440;[48] *Rickettsia* sp. strains ATT, HOT1 and HOT2;[49] *Rickettsia* sp. strain RpA4, DnS14 and DnS28;[50] *Rickettsia* sp. strain R300;[51] *Rickettsia* sp. strains IRS3 and IRS4;[52] and *Rickettsia* sp. strain AaR/SoCarolina (Kurtti *et al.*, unpublished material).

NAMING OF RICKETTSIAL DISEASES

To date, there have been no concrete rules for naming of diseases. A rickettsiosis is usually named by the first publication that describes its distinctive epidemiologic and clinical characteristics. It is not necessary for the causative agent to be identified, but a new disease may not be named with a description of a single patient, a clinical description only, or with only serological evidence. In general, a specific name has been given to the disease caused by each rickettsial species. Most commonly, rickettsioses have been named for their geographical distribution and also their vector and/or clinical features: African tick-bite fever, Astrakhan fever, Flinders Island spotted fever, Indian tick typhus, Israeli spotted fever, Japanese spotted fever, Mediterranean spotted fever, North Asian tick typhus, Queensland tick typhus, and Rocky Mountain spotted fever. It is of note that the names of some of these rickettsioses do not reflect the position of their etiological agents in the typhus or spotted fever groups. Other rickettsioses have been named for their epidemiological features: epidemic typhus, endemic typhus, tick-borne lymphadenopathy (TIBOLA), flea-borne spotted fever, murine typhus, and scrub typhus. A few rickettsioses have been named for only their clinical appearance: lymphangitis-associated rickettsiosis (LAR)[53] and rickettsialpox.

To avoid confusion, it is preferable for each disease to have only a single name. Unfortunately, several names exist for older rickettsioses. North Asian tick typhus has also been named Siberian tick typhus, Mediterranean spotted fever has been named Marseilles fever or Boutonneuse fever, epidemic typhus has been named louse-borne typhus, and murine typhus has also been named endemic typhus. Although improvements in diagnostic and reporting methods should have prevented the situation, there are also recently described rickettsioses with several names: TIBOLA and *Dermacentor*-borne-necrosis-erythema lymphadenopathy (DEBONEL)[54] in Spain; Flinders Island spotted fever goes by the name Thai tick typhus in Thailand; Japanese spotted fever, and Oriental spotted fever.

In some cases, newly generated information has led to the name of a disease becoming inaccurate. Rocky Mountain spotted fever was initially described in the Rocky Mountains, but is now known to occur from Canada to South America; African tick-bite fever was initially described in sub-Saharan Africa but was subsequently identified in the West Indies. In these cases the original name of the disease has been maintained.

In conclusion, naming bacteria and their diseases is not only a matter of science and rules, but also a question of agreement among specialists in the field. The current proposal for initial name generation reflects the state of the art of the scientific tools applicable to these organisms. It is not a rigid system but a flexible model that will be developed upon the time as scientific knowledge is evolving.

[*Conflict of interest statement*: The authors of this research declare that they have no conflict of interest.]

REFERENCES

1. RAOULT, D., T. WOODWARD & J.S. DUMLER. 2004. The history of epidemic typhus Infect. Dis. Clin. N. Amer. **18:** 127–140.
2. WILSON, L.B. & W.M. CHOWNING. 1904. Studies in *Pyroplasmosis hominis* ("Spotted Fever" or "Tick Fever" of the Rocky Mountains). J. Infect. Dis. **1:** 37–57.
3. RICKETTS, H.T. & R.M. WILDER. 1910. The etiology of the typhus fever (*tabardillo*) of Mexico City. JAMA **54:** 463–467.
4. WOLBACH, S.B., J.L. TODD & F.W. PALFREY. 1922. The Etiology and Pathology of typhus. Harvard University Press. Cambridge, MA.
5. MURRAY, R.G.E., D.J. BRENNER, R.R. COLWELL, *et al.* 1990. Report of the ad hoc committee on approaches to taxonomy within the proteobacteria. Int. J. Syst. Bacteriol. **40:** 213–215.
6. ROSSELLO-MORA, R. & R. AMANN. 2001. The species concept for prokaryotes. FEMS Microbiol. Rev. **25:** 39–67.

7. WAYNE, L.G., D.J. BRENNER, R.R. COLWELL, *et al.* 1987. Report of the Ad Hoc committee on reconciliation of approaches to bacterial systematics. Int. J. Syst. Bact. **37:** 463–464.
8. CLARRIDGE, J.E., III. 2004. Impact of 16S rRNA gene sequence analysis for identification of bacteria on clinical microbiology and infectious diseases. Clin. Microbiol. Rev. **17:** 840–862.
9. DRANCOURT, M., P. BERGER & D. RAOULT. 2004. Systematic 16S rRNA gene sequencing of atypical clinical isolates identified 27 new bacterial species associated with humans. J. Clin. Microbiol. **42:** 2197–2202.
10. CAVALIER-SMITH, T. 1993. Kingdom protozoa and its 18 phyla. Microbiol. Rev. **57:** 953–994.
11. ROSSELLO-MORA, R. & R. AMANN. 2001. The species concept for prokaryotes. FEMS Microbiol. Rev. **25:** 39–67.
12. TRÜPER, H.G. 1999. How to name a prokaryote: etymological considerations, proposals and practical advice in prokaryote nomenclature. FEMS Microbiol. Rev. **23:** 231–249.
13. RAOULT, D. & V. ROUX. 1997. Rickettsioses as paradigms of new or emerging infectious diseases. Clin. Microbiol. Rev. **10:** 694–719.
14. ROUX, V., M. BERGOIN, N. LAMAZE & D. RAOULT. 1997. Reassessment of the taxonomic position of *Rickettsiella grylli.* Int. J. Syst. Bacteriol. **47:** 1255–1257.
15. NEIMARK, H., K.-E. JOHANSSON, Y. RIKHISA & J.G. TULLY. 2001. Proposal to transfer some members of the genera *Haemobartonella* and *Erythrozoon* to genus *Mycoplasma* with descriptions of "*Candidatus Mycoplasma haemofelis,*" "*Candidatus Mycoplasma haemomuris,*" "*Candidatus Mycoplasma haemousuis*" and "*Candidatus Mycoplasma wenyonii.*" Int. J. Syst. Evol. Microbiol. **51:** 891–899.
16. RAOULT, D. 2005. Rickettsioses and Ehrlichioses. *In* Principles and Practice of Infectious Diseases, Vol. 2. G.L. Mandell, *et al.*, Eds.: 2284–2287. Elsevier, Churchill Livingstone. Philadelphia.
17. BIRTLES, R.J., T.G. HARRISON, N.A. SAUNDERS & D.H. MOLYNEUX. 1995. Proposals to unify the genera G*rahamella* and *Bartonella*, with descriptions of *Bartonella talpae* comb.nov., *Bartonella peromysci* comb. nov., and three new species, *Bartonella grahamii* sp. nov., *Bartonella taylorii* sp. nov., and *Bartonella doshiae* sp. nov. Int. J. Syst. Bacteriol. **45:** 1–8.
18. DUMLER, J.S., A. F. BARBET, C.P.J. BEKKER, *et al.* 2001. Reorganisation of genera in the families *Rickettsiaceae* and *Anaplasmataceae* in the order *Rickettsiales*: unification of some species of *Ehrlichia* with *Anaplasma, Cowdria* with *Ehrlichia* and *Ehrlichia* with *Neorickettsia*, descriptions of six new species combinations and designation of *Ehrlichia equi* and "HGE agent" as subjective synonyms of *Ehrlichia phagocytophila.* Int. J. Syst. Evol. Microbiol. **51:** 2145–2165.
19. ROUX, V. & D. RAOULT. 1995. Phylogenetic analysis of the genus Rickettsia by 16S rDNA sequencing. Res. Microbiol. **146:** 385–396.
20. STOTHARD, D.R. & P.A. FUERST. 1995. Evolutionary analysis of the spotted fever and typhus groups of *Rickettsia* using 16S rRNA gene sequences. Syst. Appl. Microbiol. **18:** 52–61.
21. TAMURA, A., N. OHASHI, H. URAKAMI & S. MIYAMURA. 1995. Classification of *Rickettsia tsutsugamushi* in a new genus, *Orientia* gen nov, as *Orientia tsutsugamushi* comb. nov. Int. J. Syst. Bacteriol. **45:** 589–591.
22. WEISS, E. & J.W. MOULDER. 1984. Order I, *Rickettsiales* Gieszczkiewicz 1939, 25AL. *In* Bergey's Manual of Systematic Bacteriology, Vol. 1. N.R. Krieg & J.G.Holt, Eds.: 687–701. Williams and Wilkins. Baltimore.
23. PHILIP, R.N., E.A. CASPER, W. BURGDORFER, *et al.* 1978. Serologic typing of rickettsiae of the spotted fever group by microimmunofluoresence J. Immunol. **121:** 1961–1968.
24. ROUX, V., E. RYDKINA, M. EREMEEVA & D. RAOULT. 1997. Citrate synthase gene comparison, a new tool for phylogenetic analysis, and its application for the rickettsiae. Int. J. Syst. Bact. **47:** 252–261.
25. FOURNIER, P.E., V. ROUX & D. RAOULT. 1998. Phylogenetic analysis of spotted fever group rickettsiae by study of the outer surface protein rOmpA. Int. J. Syst. Bacteriol. **48:** 839–849.

26. ROUX, V. & D. RAOULT. 2000. Phylogenetic analysis of members of the genus *Rickettsia* using the gene encoding the outer-membrane protein rOmpB (ompB). Int. J. Syst. Evol. Microbiol. **50:** 1449–1455.
27. SEKEYOVA, Z., V. ROUX & D. RAOULT. 2001. Phylogeny of Rickettsia spp. inferred by comparing sequences of "gene D," which encodes an intracytoplasmic protein. Int. J. Syst. Evol. Microbiol. **51:** 1353–1360.
28. MAIDEN, M.C.J., J.A. BYGRAVES, E. FEIL, *et al.* 1998. Multilocus sequence typing: a portable approach to the identification of clones within populations of pathogenic microorganisms. Proc. Natl. Acad . Sci. USA **95:** 3140–3145.
29. FOURNIER, P.E., J.S. DUMLER, G. GREUB, *et al.* 2003. Gene sequence-based criteria for the identification of new *Rickettsia* isolates and description of *Rickettsia heilongjiangensis* sp. nov. J. Clin. Microbiol. **41:** 5456–5465.
30. WALKER, D.H., H.M. FENG, J.I. SAADA, *et al.* 1995. Comparative antigenic analysis of spotted fever group rickettsiae from Israel and other closely related organisms. Am. J. Trop. Med. Hyg. **52:** 569–576.
31. DASCH, G.A. & L.M. JACKSON. 1998. Genetic analysis of isolates of the spotted fever group of rickettsiae belonging to the *R. conorii* complex Ann. N.Y. Acad. Sci. **849:** 11–20.
32. EREMEEVA, M., L. BEATI, V.A. MAKAROVA, *et al.* 1994. Astrakhan fever rickettsiae: antigenic and genotypic analysis of isolates obtained from human and *Rhipicephalus pumilio* ticks. Am. J. Trop. Med. Hyg. **51:** 697–706.
33. ZHU, Y., P.E. FOURNIER, M. EREMEEVA & D. RAOULT. 2005. Proposal to create subspecies of *Rickettsia conorii* based on multi-locus sequence typing and an emended description of *Rickettsia conorii.* BMC Microbiol **5:** 11.
34. FOURNIER, P.E., F. GOURIET, P. BROUQUI, *et al.* 2005. Lymphangitis-associated rickettsiosis, a new rickettsiosis caused by *Rickettsia sibirica* mongolotimonae: seven new cases and review of the literature. Clin. Infect. Dis **40:** 1435–1444.
35. NIEBYLSKI, M.L., M.E. SCHRUMPF, W. BURGDORFER, *et al.* 1997. *Rickettsia peacockii* sp.nov., a new species infecting wood ticks, *Dermacentor andersoni,* in Western Montana. Int. J. Syst. Bacteriol. 446–452.
36. WOLBACH, S.B. 1919. Studies on rocky mountain spotted fever. J. Med. Res. **41:** 1–70.
37. BURGDORFER, W., S.F. HAYES, L.A. THOMAS & J.L. LANCASTER. 1981. A new spotted fever group rickettsia form the lone star tick, *Amblyomma americanum. In* Rickettsiae and Rickettsial Diseases. W. Burgdorfer & R.L. Anacker, Eds.: 595–602. Academic Press. New York.
38. SIMSER, J.A., A.T. PALMER, V. FINGERLE, *et al.* 2002. *Rickettsia monacensis* sp. nov., a spotted fever group Rickettsia, from ticks (*Ixodes ricinus*) collected in a European city park. Appl. Environ. Microbiol. **68:** 4559–4566.
39. ANIGSTEIN, L. & D. ANIGSTEIN. 1975. A review of the evidence in retrospect for a rickettsial etiology in Bullis fever. Tex. Rep. Biol. Med. **33:** 201–211.
40. ZHANG, J.Z., M.Y. FAN, Y.M. WU, *et al.*. 2000. Genetic classification of *Rickettsia heilongjiangii* and *Rickettsia hulinii* two chinese spotted fever group rickettsiae. J. Clin. Microbiol. **38:** 3498–3501.
41. KOLLARS, T.M., B. TIPPAYACHAI & D. BODHIDATTA. 2001. Thai tick typhus, *Rickettsia honei*, and a unique rickettsia detected in *Ixodes granulatus* (*Ixodidae : Acari*). Am. J. Trop. Med. Hyg. **65:** 535–537.
42. SHPYNOV, S., P.E. FOURNIER, N. RUDAKOV & D. RAOULT. 2003. "*Candidatus Rickettsia tarasevichiae*" in *Ixodes persulcatus* ticks collected in Russia. Ann. N.Y. Acad. Sci. **990:** 162–172.
43. BLAIR, P.J., J. JIANG, G.B. SCHOELER, *et al.*. 2004. Characterization of spotted fever group rickettsiae in flea and tick specimens from northern Peru. J. Clin. Microbiol. **42:** 4961–4967.
44. BILLINGS, A.N., G.J. TELTOW, S.C. WEAVER & D.H. WALKER. 1998. Molecular characterization of a novel Rickettsia species from *Ixodes scapularis* in Texas. Emerg. Infect. Dis. **4:** 305–309.
45. LABRUNA, M.B., T. WHITWORTH, M.C. HORTA, *et al.* 2004. Rickettsia species infecting *Amblyomma cooperi* ticks from an area in the state of Sao Paulo, Brazil, where Brazilian spotted fever is endemic. J. Clin. Microbiol. **42:** 90–98.

46. FOURNIER, P.E., H. FUJITA, N. TAKADA & D. RAOULT. 2002. Genetic identification of rickettsiae isolated from ticks in Japan. J. Clin. Microbiol. **40:** 2176–2181.
47. LANE, R.S., R.W. EMMONS, D.V. DONDERO & B.C. NELSON. 1981. Ecology of tick borne agents in California: further observations on rickettsiae. *In* Rickettsiae and Rickettsial Diseases. W. Burgdorfer & R.L. Anacker, Eds.: 575–584. Academic Press. New York.
48. PAROLA, P., J.P. CORNET, Y.O. SANOGO, *et al.* 2003. Detection of Ehrlichia spp., Anaplasma spp., Rickettsia spp., and other eubacteria in ticks from the Thai-Myanmar border and Vietnam. J. Clin. Microbiol. **41:** 1600–1608.
49. HIRUNKANOKPUN, S., P. KITTAYAPONG, J.P. CORNET & J.P. GONZALEZ. 2003. Molecular evidence for novel tick-associated spotted fever group rickettsiae from Thailand. J. Med. Entomol. **40:** 230–237.
50. RYDKINA, E., V. ROUX, N. FETISOVA, *et al.* 1999. New rickettsiae in ticks collected in territories of the former Soviet Union. Emerg. Infect. Dis. **5:** 811–814.
51. LABRUNA, M.B., L.M. CAMARGO, E.P. CAMARGO & D.H. WALKER. 2005. Detection of a spotted fever group Rickettsia in the tick Haemaphysalis juxtakochi in Rondonia, Brazil. Vet. Parasitol. **127:** 169–174.
52. SEKEYOVA, Z., P.E. FOURNIER, J. REHACEK & D. RAOULT. 2000. Characterization of a new spotted fever group Rickettsia detected in *Ixodes ricinus* (Acari: Ixodidae) collected in Slovakia. J. Med. Entomol. **37:** 707–713.
53. RAOULT,D., P. BROUQUI & V. ROUX. 1996. A new spotted-fever-group rickettsiosis. Lancet **348:** 412.
54. OTEO, J.A., V. IBARRA, J.R. BLANCO, *et al.* 2004. *Dermacentor*-borne necrosis erythema and lymphadenopathy: clinical and epidemiological features of a new tick-borne disease. Clin. Microbiol. Infect. **10:** 327–331.

Progress in Rickettsial Genome Analysis from Pioneering of *Rickettsia prowazekii* to the Recent *Rickettsia typhi*

DAVID H. WALKER AND XUE-JIE YU

Department of Pathology, University of Texas Medical Branch–Galveston, Galveston, Texas 77555, USA

ABSTRACT: Three rickettsial genomes have been sequenced and annotated. *Rickettsia prowazekii* and *R. typhi* have similar gene order and content. The few differences between *R. prowazekii* and *R. typhi* include a 12-kb insertion in *R. prowazekii*, a large inversion close to the origin of replication in *R. typhi*, and loss of the complete cytochrome *c* oxidase system by *R. typhi*. *R. prowazekii*, *R. typhi*, and *R. conorii* have 13, 24, and 560 unique genes, respectively, and share 775 genes, most likely their essential genes. The small genomes contain many pseudogenes and much noncoding DNA, reflecting the process of genome decay. *R. typhi* contains the largest number of pseudogenes (41), and *R. conorii* the fewest, in accordance with its larger number of genes and smaller proportion of noncoding DNA. Conversely, typhus rickettsiae contain fewer repetitive sequences. These genomes portray the key themes of rickettsial intracellular survival: lack of enzymes for sugar metabolism, lipid biosynthesis, nucleotide synthesis, and amino acid metabolism, suggesting that rickettsiae depend on the host for nutrition and building blocks; enzymes for the complete TCA cycle and several copies of ATP/ADP translocase genes, suggesting independent synthesis of ATP and acquisition of host ATP; and type IV secretion system. All rickettsiae share two outer membrane proteins (OmpB and Sca 4) and LPS biosynthesis machinery. RickA, unique to spotted fever rickettsiae, plays a role in induction of actin polymerization in *R. conorii*, but not in *R. prowazekii* or *R. typhi*. The genome of *R. typhi* contains four potentially membranolytic genes (*tlyA*, *tlyC*, *pldA*, and *pat-1*) and five autotransporter genes, *sca 1*, *sca 2*, *sca 3*, *ompA*, and *ompB*. The presence of six 50-amino acid repeat units in Sca 2 suggests function as an adhesin. The high laboratory passage of the sequenced strains raises the issue of the occurrence of laboratory mutations in genes not required for growth in cell culture or eggs. Resequencing revealed that eight annotated pseudogenes of E strain are actually intact genes. Comparative genomics of virulent and avirulent strains of rickettsial species may reveal their virulence factors.

KEYWORDS: Rickettsia; genome reduction; ATP/ADP translocase; autotransporter; type IV secretion

Address for correspondence: David H. Walker, M.D., University of Texas Medical Branch–Galveston, 301 University Blvd., Keiller Bldg., University of Texas Medical Branch Galveston, TX 77555-0609. Voice: 409-772-3989; fax: 409-772-1850.

dwalker@utmb.edu

Ann. N.Y. Acad. Sci. 1063: 13–25 (2005). © 2005 New York Academy of Sciences.
doi: 10.1196/annals.1355.003

INTRODUCTION

Because of their small genome sizes, *Rickettsia* were attractive subjects of early bacterial sequencing projects. The isolated intracellular location, where there is little opportunity for horizontal transfer of prokaryotic genes, offers a special opportunity to analyze natural selection and evolution. The constraints of genetic fitness in both arthropod and vertebrate hosts remain important facets to elucidate, and genome analysis offers approaches to determine the critical elements.

RICKETTSIAL GENOME STRUCTURES

Seven rickettsial genomes have been sequenced, and three of them have been annotated. The annotated rickettsial genomes, including *Rickettsia prowazekii*, *R. typhi*, and *R. conorii*, indicate that they are similar in gene order and gene content.[1–3] The rickettsial genomes are small with low G+C content (TABLE 1).[2] *R. conorii* has 1412 genes; *R. prowazekii*, 835; and *R. typhi*, 838. There are 776 genes in common among the three species of rickettsiae and 24 unique genes for *R. typhi*, 13 unique genes for *R. prowazekii*, and 560 unique genes for *R. conorii* (FIG. 1). Comparative genomic analysis indicates a few inversion/translocation rearrangements of the rickettsial genomes. A region of the chromosome is inverted in typhus group rickettsiae, which

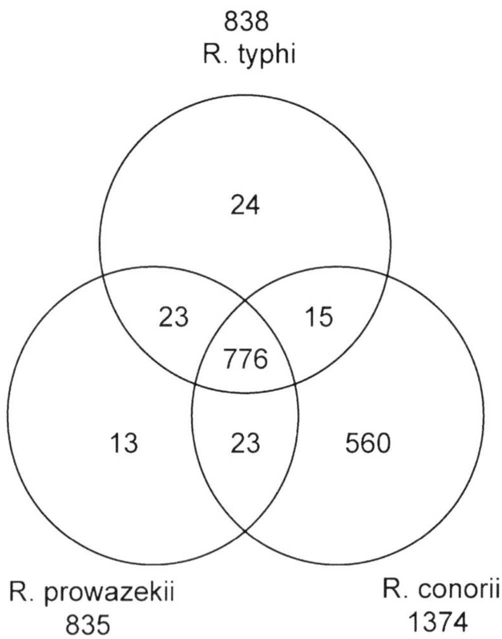

FIGURE 1. Shared proteins among *R. typhi*, *R. prowazekii*, and *R. conorii* and proteins unique to each organism: 23 are shared only between *R. typhi* and *R. prowazekii*, 23 are present only in *R. prowazekii* and *R. conorii*, and 15 are found only in *R. typhi* and *R. conorii*.

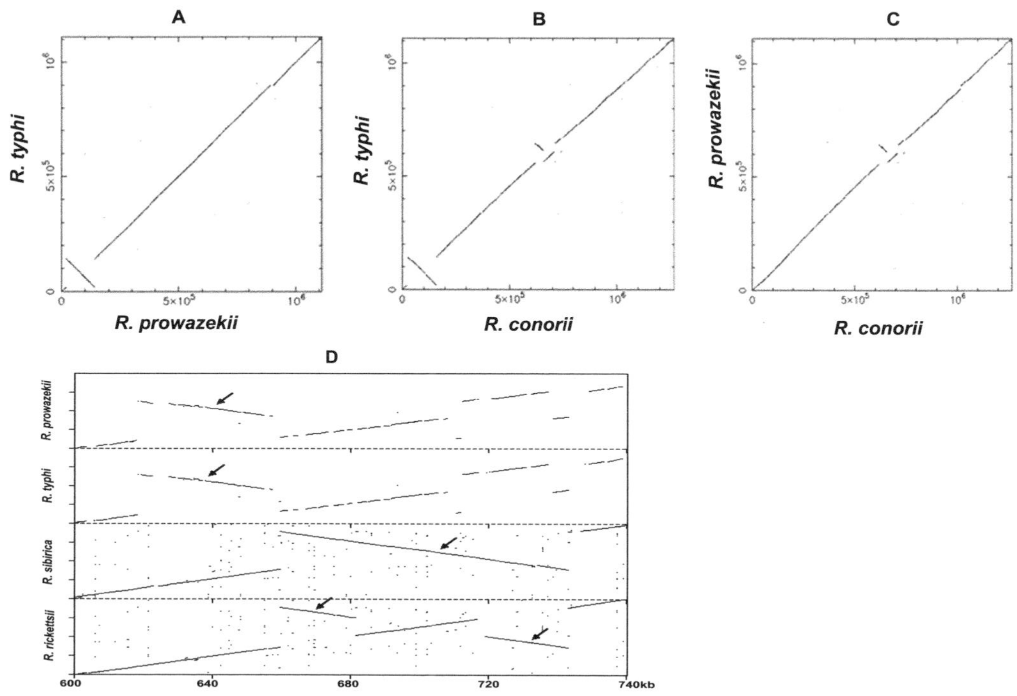

FIGURE 2. Nucleotide alignment among *R. typhi*, *R. prowazekii*, *R. conorii*, *R. sibirica*, and *R. rickettsii*. Each line represents an alignment obtained by BLASTN (E $\leq 11e^{-10}$). (**A**) Nucleotide alignment between *R. typhi* and *R. prowazekii* genomes; (**B**) nucleotide alignment between *R. typhi* and *R. conorii* genomes; (**C**) nucleotide alignment between *R. prowazekii* and *R. conorii* genomes; (**D**) nucleotide alignment of the region from 600 to 740 kb of *R. conorii* with the corresponding regions of *R. prowazekii*, *R. typhi*, *R. sibirica*, and *R. rickettsii*. Inversions are indicated by *arrows*.

corresponds to the region from 612 to 644 kb in *R. typhi*. This region is similar in typhus group (TG) rickettsiae but differs from the spotted fever group (SFG) rickettsiae, suggesting that the rearrangement of the region occurred after the divergence of TG and SFG rickettsiae, but before the divergence of *R. typhi* and *R. prowazekii*. Another region from 19 to 142 kb in the *R. typhi* genome is inverted, but the region is not inverted in *R. prowazekii* compared to *R. conorii*, *R. rickettsii*, and *R. sibirica* (FIG. 2). Thus, the inversion occurred in *R. typhi* after the divergence of *R. typhi* and *R. prowazekii*. Further comparison of the rickettsial genomes reveals that a 12-kb DNA segment from nt 890649 to 902874 in *R. prowazekii* is missing in *R. typhi* and all SFG rickettsiae. This unique *R. prowazekii* DNA segment contains three pseudogenes (RP701, RP711, and PR717) and five genes (RP709, RP712, RP713, RP714, and RP716). All three pseudogenes and one gene (RP709) share similarity with transposons, and two genes (RP714 and RP716) share homology with human Ankyrin B. It is most likely that *R. prowazekii* acquired this DNA fragment by horizontal transfer since it contains pseudogenes similar to transposons.[2]

GENOME IN DECAY

The coding content of rickettsial genomes ranges from 76% to 81%, which is substantially lower than that of other bacterial genomes, in which the coding sequences range from 87% to 94%.[1] Thus, the rickettsial genomes are considered to be in decay. Recent complete genome sequence of *Ehrlichia ruminantium* further supports the hypothesis that the rickettsial genome is in decay. Only 62% of the *E. ruminantium* genome is coding sequence.[4] Rickettsial genomes contain not only many noncoding sequences and pseudogenes, but also many split genes. A split gene is a gene that is intact in one rickettsial species but is interrupted into two or more open reading frames by internal stop(s) in another species.[3] Sixteen split genes have been annotated in the *R. prowazekii* genome. We sequenced all the apparent split genes in *R. prowazekii* and found that 8 of the 16 split genes in the reported genome sequence were not true split genes but were sequence errors. Thus, *R. prowazekii* has 10 split genes compared to *R. typhi* and *R. conorii*. Transcriptional expression has been detected in some of the split genes.[3] Thus, some of the split genes may be still functional. There are 41 pseudogenes in *R. typhi*, 36 of them have functional homologues in *R. conorii,* and 16 of them have functional homologues in *R. prowazekii*.[2] Among the 575 genes that are present in *R. conorii*, but not in *R. prowazekii*, 229 have remnant sequences in the *R. prowazekii* genome.[3] Thus, the genomes of the TG rickettsiae have decayed faster than those of the SFG rickettsiae.

RICKETTSIA AND MITOCHONDRION EVOLUTION

There is a general consensus in the evolutionary biology literature that mitochondria evolved from bacteria in the α-subgroup of the Proteobacteria phylum.[5] Comparative genomics of mitochondria and rickettsiae strongly support this hypothesis. Phylogenetic analyses based on ribosomal proteins and NADH dehydrogenase indicate that there is a close evolutionary relationship between *R. prowazekii* and mitochondria.[1] However, the exact position of the mitochondria within the α-

TABLE 1. Comparison of genome statistics between *R. typhi*, *R. prowazekii*, *R. conorii*, *R. sibirica*, and *R. ricketsii*

Organism	Genome statistics
R. typhi	
Genome size (bp)	1,111,496
Number of genes	877
Coding region of genome[a]	76.27
%G+C[b] for the:	
Genome	28.92
Coding regions	30.56
Noncoding regions	23.55
First codon position	41.11
Second codon position	31.69
Third codon position	18.39
R. prowazekii	
Genome size (bp)	1,111,523
Number of genes	872
Coding region of genome[a]	76.24
%G+C[b] for the:	
Genome	29.00
Coding regions	30.59
Noncoding regions	23.61
First codon position	41.07
Second codon position	31.75
Third codon position	18.44
R. conorii	
Genome size (bp)	1,268,755
Number of genes	1,412
Coding region of genome[a]	81.45
%G+C[b] for the:	
Genome	32.44
Coding regions	32.98
Noncoding regions	30.05
First codon position	42.53
Second codon position	32.42
Third codon position	23.58
R. sibirica[c]	
Genome size (bp)	1,250,021
Number of genes	1,234
Coding region of genome[a]	77.76

TABLE 1. ***(continued)*** **Comparison of genome statistics between *R. typhi*, *R. prowazekii*, *R. conorii*, *R. sibirica*, and *R. ricketsii***

Organism	Genome statistics
%G+C[b] for the:	
Genome	32.47
Coding regions	32.90
Noncoding regions	39.94
First codon position	42.85
Second codon position	32.50
Third codon position	23.35
***R. rickettsii*[d]**	
Genome size (bp)	1,257,710
Number of genes	NA
Coding region of genome[a]	NA
%G+C[b] for the:	NA
Genome	32.47
Coding regions	NA
Noncoding regions	NA
First codon position	NA
Second codon position	NA
Third codon position	NA

[a]The coding regions include ORFs for proteins, rRNAs, tRNAs and ncRNAs except for *R. sibirica.*

[b]The G+C content for the first, second, and third codon positions was calculated from protein-encoding ORFs.

[c]The numbers calculated for *R. sibirica* are based on available protein-encoding ORFs (accession no. NZ_AABW01000001) only. They do not include ORFs for rRNA, tRNA, or snRNA, which are not available.

[d]The annotations for *R. rickettsii* (accession no. AADJ01000001) are not available (NA) in GenBank.

Proteobacteria is uncertain. Some studies have suggested that mitochondria are a sister taxon to the *Rickettsia* genus within the family *Rickettsiaceae* and mitochondria are more closely related to *Rickettsia* spp. than to species in the family *Anaplasmataceae* such as *Wolbachia* (reviewed by Wu *et al.*[5]). Recent sequencing of the complete genome of *Wolbachia pipientis* wMel supports a grouping of *Wolbachia* and *Rickettsia* to the exclusion of the mitochondria, but not placing the mitochondria within the order Rickettsiales.[5]

PATHOGENESIS

Little is known about the genetic determinants of rickettsial pathogenesis. Comparative genomics identifies 42 genes that may be involved in virulence (TABLE 2).

TABLE 2. Rickettsial genes effecting pathogenesis

Adhesins: *ompA*, *ompB*
Phagosomal escape: *pld*, *thyC*
Actin-based mobility: *rickA*
Other potential membranolytic activity: *tlyA*, *pat-1*
Autotransporters: *ompA*, *ompB*, and three *sca* proteins
Type IV secretion system: *virB* and *virD* genes
invA and others such as *sodB* (superoxide dismutase)
Lipopolysaccharide synthesis genes

These include enzymes that allow intracellular survival and membranolytic enzymes that permit escape of the organism from the phagolysosome and hypothetically from the cell.[2]

Actin-Based Mobility

Many intracytoplasmic bacteria can spread from the primary infected cell into neighboring cells by polymerizing cellular actin at one pole of the bacterial cell.[6] SFG rickettsiae also move inside the host cells by actin-based mobility.[7] The bacterial proteins stimulating polymerization of actin are different among bacteria, including ActA in *L. monocytogenes* and IcsA (VirG) in *S. flexneri*.[8] Ogata *et al.* identified a protein in *R. conorii* (RC0909) that has a domain similar to ActA, and they hypothesized that this protein might play a role in rickettsial actin tail formation.[3] Further work showed that this rickettsial protein, now called RickA, can activate Arp2/3 and induce actin polymerization.[9] *Rickettsia typhi* forms very short actin tails, and its movement is circular.[7] It is interesting that *rickA* does not exist in typhus group rickettsiae.[2] The absence of the *rickA* gene in TG rickettsiae may explain the failure of these rickettsiae to polymerize actin.[9] The *rickA* gene of *R. peacockii*, a spotted fever group rickettsia, which also lacks actin-based mobility, is disrupted by a naturally occurring transposon.[10,11]

Membranolytic Activity

Rickettsia spp. quickly escape from the phagosome into the host cell cytoplasm after entering the cell. After multiplying into a large population, TG rickettsiae lyse the host cell membrane and are released. SFG rickettsiae escape continuously into adjacent cells or the extracellular space via filopodia associated with actin-based mobility. The host cell membrane at the tip of the filopodium is also lysed, enabling spread and release. Phospholipase A2 activity has been hypothesized to mediate the lysis of host cell membranes. Phospholipase A2 activity has been observed in rickettsia-infected cells, and the phospholipase A2 activity was believed to be of rickettsial origin.[12–15] However, the only phospholipase A gene that has been identified in the genome of any rickettsia including *R. typhi,* which has hemolytic activity, is *pat-1*.[2] A phospholipase D has been detected in rickettsiae.[16] This enzyme or other potentially membranolytic genes such as *pat-1* might account for the activity previously attributed to phospholipase A2.

TABLE 3. Autotransporters in *R. prozekii*, *R. typhi*, and *R. conorii*

	OmpA	OmpB	Sca1	Sca2	Sca3
R. prowazekii	–	+	Split to 3 ORFs	Split to 4 ORFs	+
R. typhi	–	+	+	+	+
R. conorii	+	+	+	+	Split to 2 ORFs

NOTE: – = the genome does not have the gene; + = the genome contains the intact gene.

Autotransporters

Autotransporters are proteins that are responsible for their own secretion across the inner membrane and the outer membrane of gram-negative bacteria.[17] An autotransporter protein consists of three functional domains: the amino-terminal leader sequence, the secreted mature (α) protein and a carboxy-terminal (β) domain. The signal peptide inserts itself into the inner membrane directing the export of the precursor molecule by action of the general secretion pathway into the periplasm. The precursor is cleaved by a signal peptidase to release the mature polypeptide into the periplasm. Once in the periplasm, the β-domain of the protein is inserted into the outer membrane to form a β-barrel pore, and the passenger-domain is translocated to the cell surface through the pore.[17,18] A striking feature of the rickettsial outer membrane is that many rickettsial outer membrane proteins belong to the autotransporter family (TABLE 3). These proteins include OmpA, OmpB (RT0699, RP704), and three open reading frames (ORFs) encoding the hypothetical proteins, Sca1 (RT0015, RP018), Sca2 (Rt0052, RP081), and Sca3 (RT0438, RP451).[1,2,19] The precursor of OmpB is a 168-kDa protein that is post-translationally processed to the 135-kDa mature OmpB by cleavage of a 32-kDa β-peptide.[20] The amino acid sequences of the β-peptides of all five rickettsial autotransporters are highly homologous and share homology with autotransporters of distantly related bacteria.[17] The diversity among the passenger domains that are coupled with the conserved β-domain suggests that the autotransporters are either derived originally from a single gene or resulted from recombination of unrelated proteins with the β-domains.[17]

Except for *ompB*, the genes for other autotransporters are either deleted or mutated in at least one rickettsial species. *ompA* exists in SFG rickettsiae but not in typhus rickettsiae. *ompA* of *R. conorii* is located between the cell division protein gene *ftsK* and a hypothetical ORF (RC1272).[3] *R. prowazekii* possesses the orthologs for *ftsK* and ORF RC1272, but not *ompA*. The intergenic sequence between the *R. prowazekii* orthlogs has significant similarity to the *ompA* gene, suggesting that *ompA* became a pseudogene in TG rickettsiae.[3] *Sca1* and *Sca2* have been split into three and four ORFs, respectively, in *R. prowazekii* owing to deletion/insertion of nucleotides in the genes.[1,2] Sca3 sequences are found in two different ORFs in *R. conorii* (RC0630 and RC0631).[2] Sca3 and OmpA share homology not only in the β-peptide but also in the passenger domain. Thus, it seems that the genes for these Sca proteins originated from a single ancestor gene. After duplication of the gene, the Sca proteins were redundant in function initially and diverged into different proteins or were deleted from the genome such as OmpA in typhus rickettsiae.

Some autotransporters have adhesin or protease activities, and thus the autotransporters could play a role in rickettsial virulence. Both OmpA and OmpB have been demonstrated as adhesins in SFG rickettsiae.[21,22] The presence of six 50–amino acid repeat units in Sca2 suggests that it may also function as an adhesin.

Type IV Secretion System

The type IV secretion systems use a complex of membrane proteins and a pilus to export protein or DNA substrates across bacterial and eukaryotic cell membranes and into the cytosol of eukaryotic host cells.[23–26] Type IV secretion systems have been found in *Agrobacterium tumefaciens*,[27,28] *Brucella abortus*,[29] *E. coli*,[26,30] *Bordetella pertussis*,[25,31] *Legionella pneumophila*,[32–34] *Helicobacter pylori*,[24] *E. chaffeensis*, *A. phagocytophilum*,[35] and *Wolbachia*.[5,36] In the facultative intracellular bacteria *L. pneumophila* and *B. abortus*, the type IV secretion systems are essential for intracellular multiplication.[29,32] The *Legionella pneumophila icm* mutant is deficient in its ability to cause lysis of the host cell.

Several ORFs related to the type IV proteins are present in *R. typhi*, *R. prowazekii*, and *R. conorii*. Fifteen ORFs related to the *Agrobacterium tumefaciens* VirB type IV secretion system are found in *R. typhi*. These include orthlogs of the inner membrane components VirB4 (RT0033 and RT0771) and VirB11 (RT0283). In *A. tumefaciens*, VirB4 binds to the DNA substrate, which is translocated across the membrane;[37] the presence of two VirB4 proteins in *R. typhi* may indicate versatility in substrate selection. The substrate-binding protein VirD4[37] is also present (RT0283). The periplasmic components VirB6, VirB8, and VirB10 (RT0282) have also been identified. These include two ORFs resembling VirB8 (RT0278 and RT0280) in addition to five different ORFs with similarity to VirB6 (RT0028, RT0029, RT0030, RT0031, and RT0032). VirB6 functions in the stabilization of VirB5 and VirB7,[38] neither of which has been identified in *R. typhi*. VirB6 also stabilizes VirB3,[38] which is present in *R. typhi* (RT0034). Multiple VirB6-like ORFs may be the result of inactivation of one or more genes or the development of new functions not yet described. Outer membrane components VirB3 and VirB9 (RT0277 and RT0281) were also found, but an orthlog of VirB7, which bridges the pilus to the transmembrane complex, was not.[38] Neither VirB2 nor VirB5, the major and minor pilus components, were identified.[37] Because *R. typhi* lives within the host cell cytoplasm, there may be no need to secrete substrates across a eukaryotic host cell membrane, and hence the lack of pilus components.

A potential protein substrate for a type IV secretion system has also been found. *R. typhi* has a Sec7 domain–containing protein (RT0362) that is similar to RalF in *Legionella pneumophila*. RalF is secreted by the *L. pneumophila dot/icm* type IV secretion system.[39] Along with a *R. prowazekii* ortholog, there are only three known examples of Sec7 family proteins in bacteria.[39] Sec7 proteins, named for *Saccharomyces cerevisiae* Sec7p, are guanine-nucleotide exchange factors and cofactors for ADP-ribosylation factors (ARFs), which function in the regulation of membrane traffic and organelle structure in eukaryotic cells.[40,41] The similarity to the *L. pneumophila* RalF protein suggests that RT0362 may be secreted by the *R. typhi* type IV system. In *Legionella*, the function of RalF is related to recruiting host ARFs to bacterium-containing phagosomes,[39] but since rickettsiae do not live in phagosomes, the role of the RalF-like protein in *R. typhi* is unknown.

METABOLIC PATHWAYS

Energy Production

Genes encoding all enzymes in the tricarboxylic acid (TCA) cycle are present in the rickettsial genomes, suggesting that rickettsiae can synthesize their own ATP. However, rickettsiae are deficient in enzymes to metabolize sugar to generate energy.[1–3] Genome sequence analyses reveal that enzymes for sugar metabolism such as the glycolytic and Entner-Doudoroff pathways are absent in the rickettsial genomes.[1,42] Thus, rickettsiae do not produce pyruvate, as the final product of glycolysis. However, pyruvate is a key intermediate in the TCA cycle to produce ATP, and rickettsiae possess enzymes for metabolism of pyruvate such as pyruvate dehydrogenase, suggesting that rickettsiae metabolize pyruvate. Like mitochondria, rickettsiae may acquire pyruvate directly from the host cell cytoplasm and convert it into acetyl-CoA by pyruvate dehydrogenase.[1,42]

ATP/ADP translocases catalyze the highly specific transport of ATP across a membrane in an exchange mode with ADP. Such unique transport proteins are employed by plant plastids and among the prokaryotes so far have only been identified in few obligately intracellular bacteria belonging to the *Chlamydiales* and the *Rickettsiales*. Phylogenetic analysis of all known ATP/ADP translocases indicate that the genes encoding ATP/ADP translocases originated from a chlamydial ancestor and were, after an ancient gene duplication, transferred horizontally to rickettsiae and plants.[43] *R. conorii*, *R. prowazekii*, and *R. typhi* each have five copies of ATP/ADP translocase genes.[1–3] Rickettsiae are hypothesized to transport ATP from the host cell cytosol into rickettsiae using the ATP/ADP translocases during the early infection, when ATP is sufficient in the host cytosol, and to synthesize ATP through the TCA cycle, when the host cytosol ATP is exhausted.

Amino Acid Metabolism

Genes for synthesis and conversion of most amino acids are generally absent in rickettsial genomes. Rickettsiae have a few genes for some amino acid biogenesis pathways, but these pathways are usually incomplete. The serine hydroxymethyltransferase gene (*glyA*) is present in all sequenced rickettsial genomes. Serine hydroxymethyltransferase catalyses the conversion of serine and tetrahydrofolate into glycine and methylenetetrahydrofolate. Genes (*lysC* and *asd*) associated with lysine biosynthesis are also present in all sequenced rickettsial genomes. However, the lysine pathway is incomplete because the downstream gene *lysA* for lysine biosynthesis is missing from the rickettsial genomes.[1]

Nucleotide Biosynthesis

Rickettsial genomes contain all genes encoding enzymes required for the interconversion of nucleotide monophosphates into all of the other required nucleotides. However, rickettsial genomes have no genes encoding enzymes for *de novo* syntheses of nucleotides. Thus, the nucleoside monophosphates are probably imported from the host cell.[1]

In the stringent response to conditions of stress such as starvation, bacteria increase their intracellular concentration of GDP 3′-diphosphate and GTP 3′-diphosphate, or (p)ppGpp, resulting in downregulation of transcription and translation. In *E. coli*, the (p)ppGpp level is regulated by two enzymes RelA and SpotT. No intact ORF with similarity to either complete RelA or SpoT proteins is found in *R. conorii*, *R prowazekii*, or *R. typhi,* although 4–5 small ORFs with significant similarity to SpoT are present. The *R. typhi* SpoTa and SpoTb ORFs align to the catalytic domain of the (p)ppGpp hydrolases of the SpoT, and the *R. typhi* SpoTc and SpoTd correspond to the (p)ppGpp synthetase domain. Thus, these proteins may not function singly, but instead may form active complexes. Further support of SpoT functionality is the high level of conservation of the genes among the *Rickettsia* species and their differential transcription under different environmental conditions.[2,44]

CONCLUSIONS

Comparative genomics indicate that all rickettsiae have lost genes encoding enzymes for sugar metabolism, lipid biosynthesis, nucleotide synthesis and amino acid synthesis. Thus, rickettsiae have to depend on the host for nutrition and building blocks, which may explain why rickettsiae have not yet been cultivated outside of eukaryotic cells. The strong similarities of the genomes suggest that these closely related organisms comprise fewer distinct species than the current overabundance of names that to date has only confused other microbiologists and physicians and repelled them from attempting to comprehend these bacteria.

The extensive laboratory passages of the organisms that have been sequenced is very likely to have resulted in deletion of genes owing to the absence of critical environmental selective genetic fitness pressures that are important in nature, such as prolonged survival in an arthropod host and avoidance of host innate immunity. Thus, the sequencing of the genomes of low-passage rickettsial isolates should have a high priority.

Possession of several rickettsial genome sequences offers immense opportunities, but much creative effort will be required for experimental demonstration of the physiologic function of the genes, especially the genus-specific genes of unknown function. The questions of the functionality of split genes and the selective advantage, if any, of the repetitive sequences remain to be answered.

Of greatest importance are the determination of the critical virulence mechanisms and the rational development of attenuated vaccines.

[*Conflict of interest statement*: The authors of this research declare that they have no conflict of interest.]

NOTE ADDED IN PRODUCTION: During the revision of this paper, a fourth rickettsial genome, that of *Rickettsia felis*, was annotated. The genome of *R. felis* (1,485,148 bp) is the largest among all sequenced rickettsial genomes. *R. felis* contrasts with previously sequenced *Rickettsia* in many features, including a number of transposases, several chromosomal toxin-antitoxin genes, many more *spoT* genes, and a very large number of ankyrin- and tetratricopeptide-motif–containing genes, and plasmids (OGATA, H. *et al*., PLoS Biol. 2005 Aug;3(8): e248. e-pub 2005 Jul 5).

REFERENCES

1. Andersson, S.G., A. Zomorodipour, J.O. Andersson, *et al.* 1998. The genome sequence of *Rickettsia prowazekii* and the origin of mitochondria. Nature **396:** 133–140.
2. McLeod, M.P., X. Qin, S.E. Karpathy, *et al.* 2004. Complete genome sequence of *Rickettsia typhi* and comparison with sequences of other rickettsiae. J. Bacteriol. **186:** 5842–5855.
3. Ogata, H., S. Audic, P. Renesto-Audiffren, *et al.* 2001. Mechanisms of evolution in *Rickettsia conorii* and *R. prowazekii.* Science **293:** 2093–2098.
4. Collins, N.E., J. Liebenberg, E.P. de Villiers, *et al.* 2005. The genome of the heart-water agent *Ehrlichia ruminantium* contains multiple tandem repeats of actively variable copy number. Proc. Natl. Acad. Sci. USA **102:** 838–843.
5. Wu, M., L.V. Sun, J. Vamathevan, *et al.* 2004. Phylogenomics of the reproductive parasite *Wolbachia pipientis* wMel: a streamlined genome overrun by mobile genetic elements. PLoS. Biol **2:** E69.
6. Gouin, E., H. Gantelet, C. Egile, *et al.* 1999. A comparative study of the actin-based motilities of the pathogenic bacteria *Listeria monocytogenes, Shigella flexneri* and *Rickettsia conorii.* J. Cell Sci. **112:** 1697–1708.
7. Teysseire, N., C. Chiche-Portiche & D. Raoult. 1992. Intracellular movements of *Rickettsia conorii* and *R. typhi* based on actin polymerization. Res. Microbiol. **143:** 821–829.
8. Domann, E., J. Wehland, M. Rohde, *et al.* 1992. A novel bacterial virulence gene in *Listeria monocytogenes* required for host cell microfilament interaction with homology to the proline-rich region of vinculin. EMBO J. **11:** 1981–1990.
9. Gouin, E., C. Egile, P. Dehoux, *et al.* 2004. The RickA protein of *Rickettsia conorii* activates the Arp2/3 complex. Nature **427:** 457–461.
10. Baldridge, G.D., N.Y. Burkhardt, J.A. Simser, *et al.* 2004. Sequence and expression analysis of the *ompA* gene of *Rickettsia peacockii*, an endosymbiont of the Rocky Mountain wood tick, *Dermacentor andersoni.* Appl. Environ. Microbiol. **70:** 6628–6636.
11. Simser, J.A., M.S. Rahman, S.M. Dreher-Lesnick, *et al.* 2005. A novel and naturally occurring transposon, ISRpe1, in the *Rickettsia peacockii* genome disrupting the *rickA* gene involved in actin-based motility. Mol. Microbiol. **58:** 71–79.
12. Ojcius, D.M., M. Thibon, C. Mounier, *et al.* 1995. pH and calcium dependence of hemolysis due to *Rickettsia prowazekii*: comparison with phospholipase activity. Infect. Immun. **63:** 3069–3072.
13. Walker, D.H., H.M. Feng & V.L. Popov. 2001. Rickettsial phospholipase A2 as a pathogenic mechanism in a model of cell injury by typhus and spotted fever group rickettsiae. Am. J. Trop. Med. Hyg. **65:** 936–942.
14. Winkler, H.H. & R.M. Daugherty. 1989. Phospholipase A activity associated with the growth of *Rickettsia prowazekii* in L929 cells. Infect. Immun. **57:** 36–40.
15. Winkler, H.H. & E.T. Miller. 1980. Phospholipase A activity in the hemolysis of sheep and human erythrocytes by *Rickettsia prowazeki.* Infect. Immun. **29:** 316–321.
16. Renesto, P., P. Dehoux, E. Gouin, *et al.* 2003. Identification and characterization of a phospholipase D-superfamily gene in rickettsiae. J. Infect.. Dis. **188:** 1276–1283.
17. Henderson, I.R., F. Navarro-Garcia & J.P. Nataro. 1998. The great escape: structure and function of the autotransporter proteins. Trends Microbiol. **6:** 370–378.
18. Blanc, G., M. Ngwamidiba, H. Ogata, *et al.* 2005. Molecular evolution of *Rickettsia* surface antigens: evidence of positive selection. Mol. Biol. Evol. **22:** 2073–2083.
19. Bouyer, D.H., J. Stenos, P. Crocquet-Valdes, *et al.* 2001. *Rickettsia felis*: molecular characterization of a new member of the spotted fever group. Int. J. Syst. Evol. Microbiol. **51:** 339–347.
20. Hackstadt, T., R. Messer, W. Cieplak, *et al.* 1992. Evidence for proteolytic cleavage of the 120-kilodalton outer membrane protein of rickettsiae: identification of an avirulent mutant deficient in processing. Infect. Immun. 60: 159–165.
21. Li, H. & D.H. Walker. 1998. rOmpA is a critical protein for the adhesion of *Rickettsia rickettsii* to host cells. Microb. Pathogen. **24:** 289–298.
22. Uchiyama, T. 1999. Role of major surface antigens of *Rickettsia japonica* in the attachment to host cells. *In* Rickettsiae and Rickettsial Diseases at the Turn of the Third Millennium. P. Brouqui and R. Raoult, Eds.: 182–188. Elsevier. Paris.

23. Christie, P.J. 1997. *Agrobacterium tumefaciens* T-complex transport apparatus: a paradigm for a new family of multifunctional transporters in eubacteria. J. Bacteriol. **179:** 3085–3094.
24. Covacci, A., J.L. Telford, G. Del Giudice, *et al.* 1999. *Helicobacter pylori* virulence and genetic geography. Science **284:** 1328–1333.
25. Weiss, A.A., F.D. Johnson & D.L. Burns. 1993. Molecular characterization of an operon required for pertussis toxin secretion. Proc. Natl. Acad. Sci. USA **90:** 2970–2974.
26. Winans, S.C. & G.C. Walker. 1985. Conjugal transfer system of the IncN plasmid pKM101. J. Bacteriol. **161:** 402–410.
27. Kuldau, G.A., G. De Vos, J. Owen, *et al.* 1990. The virB operon of *Agrobacterium tumefaciens* pTiC58 encodes 11 open reading frames. Mol. Gen. Genet. **221:** 256–266.
28. Stachel, S.E. & E.W. Nester. 1986. The genetic and transcriptional organization of the vir region of the A6 Ti plasmid of *Agrobacterium tumefaciens*. EMBO J. **5:** 1445–1454.
29. Sieira, R., D.J. Comerci, D.O. Sanchez, *et al.* 2000. A homologue of an operon required for DNA transfer in *Agrobacterium* is required in *Brucella abortus* for virulence and intracellular multiplication. J. Bacteriol. **182:** 4849–4855.
30. Pohlman, R.F., H.D. Genetti & S.C. Winans. 1994. Common ancestry between IncN conjugal transfer genes and macromolecular export systems of plant and animal pathogens. Mol. Microbiol. **14:** 655–668.
31. Kotob, S.I., S.Z. Hausman & D.L. Burns. 1995. Localization of the promoter for the ptl genes of *Bordetella pertussis*, which encode proteins essential for secretion of pertussis toxin. Infect. Immun. **63:** 3227–3230.
32. Brand, B.C., A.B. Sadosky & H.A. Shuman. 1994. The *Legionella pneumophila icm* locus: a set of genes required for intracellular multiplication in human macrophages. Mol. Microbiol. **14:** 797–808.
33. Segal, G., J.J. Russo & H.A. Shuman. 1999. Relationships between a new type IV secretion system and the icm/dot virulence system of *Legionella pneumophila*. Mol. Microbiol. **34:** 799–809.
34. Segal, G. & H.A. Shuman. 1997. Characterization of a new region required for macrophage killing by *Legionella pneumophila*. Infect. Immun. **65:** 5057–5066.
35. Ohashi, N., N. Zhi, Q. Lin & Y. Rikihisa. 2002. Characterization and transcriptional analysis of gene clusters for a type IV secretion machinery in human granulocytic and monocytic ehrlichiosis agents. Infect. Immun. **70:** 2128–2138.
36. Masui, S., T. Sasaki & H. Ishikawa. 2000. Genes for the type IV secretion system in an intracellular symbiont, *Wolbachia*, a causative agent of various sexual alterations in arthropods. J. Bacteriol. **182:** 6529–6531.
37. Burns, D.L. 2003. Type IV transporters of pathogenic bacteria. Curr. Opin. Microbiol. **6:** 29–34.
38. Hapfelmeier, S., N. Domke, P. C. Zambryski, *et al.* 2000. VirB6 is required for stabilization of VirB5 and VirB3 and formation of VirB7 homodimers in *Agrobacterium tumefaciens*. J. Bacteriol. **182:** 4505–4511.
39. Nagai, H., J. C. Kagan, X. Zhu, *et al.* 2002. A bacterial guanine nucleotide exchange factor activates ARF on *Legionella* phagosomes. Science **295:** 679–682.
40. Donaldson, J.G. & C.L. Jackson. 2000. Regulators and effectors of the ARF GTPases. Curr. Opin. Cell Biol. **12:** 475–482.
41. Jackson, C.. L. & J.. E. Casanova. 2000. Turning on ARF: the Sec7 family of guanine-nucleotide-exchange factors. Trends Cell Biol. **10:** 60–67.
42. Renesto, P., H. Ogata, S. Audic, *et al.* 2005. Some lessons from *Rickettsia* genomics. FEMS Microbiol. Rev. **29:** 99–117.
43. Schmitz-Essner, S., N. Linka, A. Collingro, *et al.* 2004. ATP/ADP translocases: a common feature of obligate intracellular amoebal symbionts related to chlamydiae and rickettsiae. J. Bacteriol. **186:** 683–691.
44. Rovery, C., P. Renesto, N. Crapoulet, *et al.* 2005. Transcriptional response of *Rickettsia conorii* exposed to temperature variation and stress starvation. Res. Microbiol. **156:** 211–218.

Rickettsia felis, from Culture to Genome Sequencing

H. OGATA,[a] C. ROBERT,[b] S. AUDIC,[a] S. ROBINEAU,[b] G. BLANC,[a]
P.E. FOURNIER,[a] P. RENESTO,[b] J. M. CLAVERIE,[a] AND D. RAOULT[b]

[a]*CNRSIBSM, Information Génomique et Structurale, 13402 Marseille Cedex 20, France*

[b]*Université de la Méditerranée, CNRS UMR 6020, Faculté de Médecine, Unité des Rickettsies, 13385 Marseille, France*

ABSTRACT: *Rickettsia felis* has been recently cultured in XTC2 cells. This allows production of enough bacteria to create a genomic bank and to sequence it. The chromosome of *R. felis* is longer than that of previously sequenced rickettsiae and it possess 2 plasmids. Microscopically, this bacterium exhibits two forms of pili: one resembles a conjugative pilus and another forms hair-like projections that may play a role in pathogenicity. *R. felis* also exhibits several copies of ankyrin-repeat genes and tetratricopeptide encoding gene that are specifically linked to pathogenic host-associated bacteria. It also contains toxin–antitoxin system encoding genes that are extremely rare in intracellular bacteria and may be linked to plasmid maintenance.

KEYWORDS: *Rickettsia felis*; pili; gene; genome sequencing; plasmid

INTRODUCTION

Rickettsiae are fastidious intracellular bacteria. Their first definition by Wolbach emphasized both these specifications since they were uncultivable on usual medium and seen with specific staining within cells.[1] *Rickettsiae* were first propagated in animals (apes, monkeys, guinea pigs), then in embryonnated eggs, and finally in cell cultures.[2] The first description of a *Rickettsia* in the cat flea *Ctenocephalides felis* was provided by Sikora in Germany in 1918.[1,3] It was named *R. ctenocephali* and its transovarial transmission observed in the flea host. This work was largely ignored until now.

In 1990, when *C. felis* were examined in California as potential vectors of *R. typhi*, the agent of murine typhus, a new rickettsia was observed by electronic microscopy and named the ELB agent.[4] By genomic sequence comparison, based on the 17-kDa protein gene sequencing, this organism was considered to be a rickettsia.[5] It was lately detected by PCR in other fleas such as *Pulex irritans* in the USA[6] and *C. felis* and *C. canis* worldwide. *R. felis* is found in Africa,[7] in Oceania,[8] in Europe,[7] in America[5] and in Asia.[9] *R. felis* is a common intracellular parasite of a very common pet flea and as many as 15% of *C. felis* may be infected.[10]

Address for correspondence: Didier Raoult, Université de la Méditerranée, CNRS UMR 6020, Faculté de Médecine, Unité des Rickettsies, 27 Bd Jean Moulin, 13385 Marseille, France. Voice: +33 4 91 38 55 17; fax: +33 4 91 38 77 72.
didier.raoult@medecine.univ-mrs.fr

**Ann. N.Y. Acad. Sci. 1063: 26–34 (2005). © 2005 New York Academy of Sciences.
doi: 10.1196/annals.1355.004**

Cases of human infections were described first by using PCR amplification. The first case was detected in the blood of a patient from Texas when investigating possible cases of murine typhus in 1994.[11] Since then, cases were found from France,[7] Brazil,[7] Mexico,[12] Germany,[13] Canary Islands and Tunisia (unpublished). The incidence of *R. felis* infection in patients is unknown.

CULTURE OF *RICKETTSIA FELIS*

R. felis culture was a challenge. It was first reported that it grows in cell culture at 37°C in 1995.[14,15] Surprisingly, the authors found that the protein and immunogenic profiles of *R. felis* were identical to that of *R. typhi.*[6] The phylogenic position of *R. felis*, obtained by the 17-kDa protein-encoding gene, showed that it is clustered in the spotted fever group rickettsiae. Lately the same group reported, in an *erratum,* that at some point their cultures were contaminated.[16] Their work was never reproduced, and when we began working with *R. felis* we were unable to grow it following

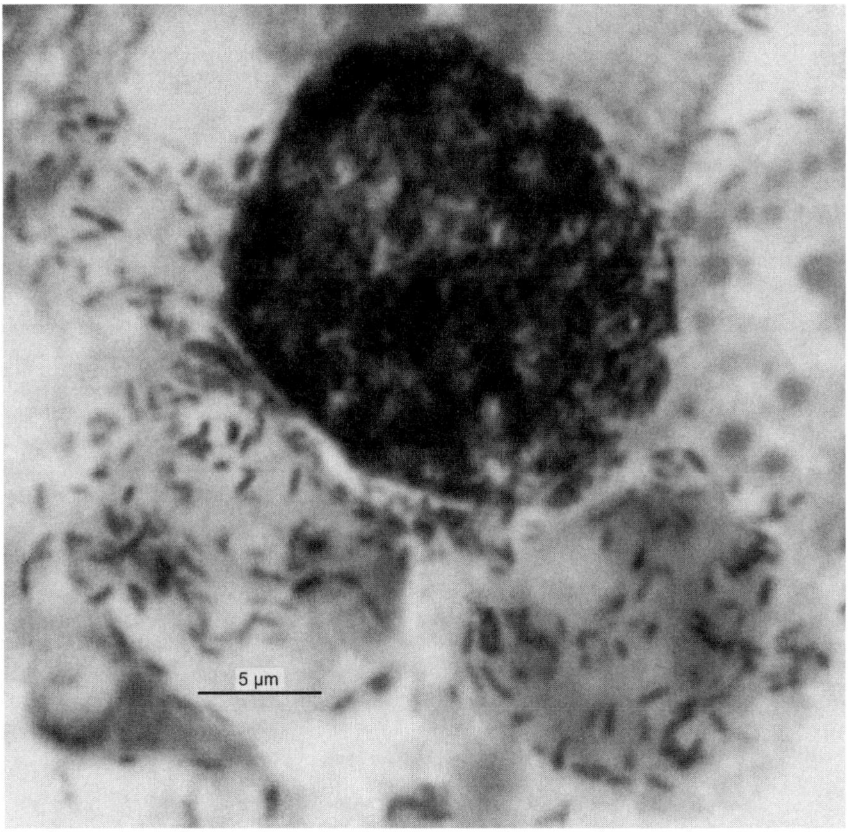

FIGURE 1. *R. felis* growing in XTC2 cells. (**a**) Gimenez staining magnification ×1000 (note the multiplication within the nucleus).

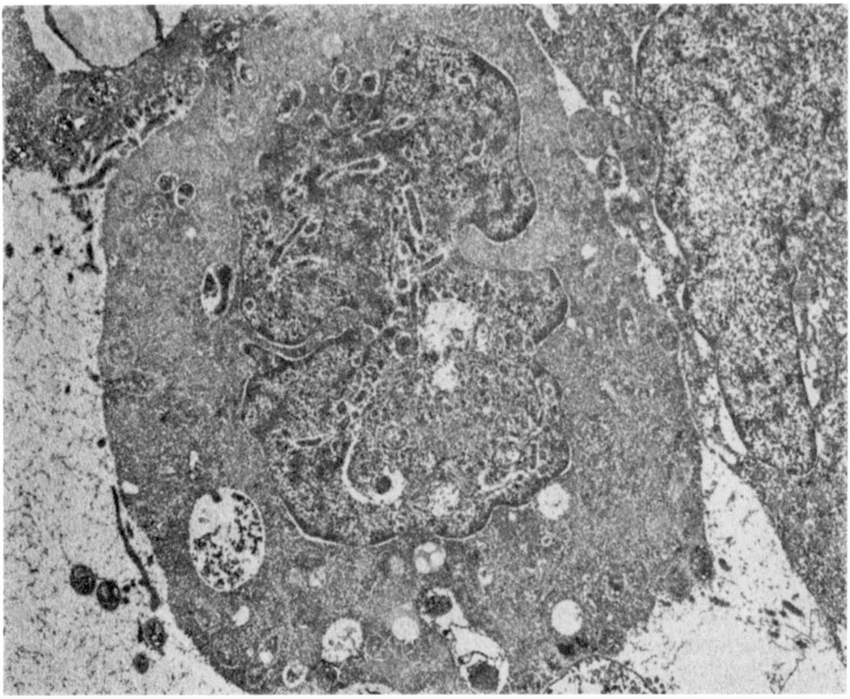

FIGURE 1—*continued.* (**b**) Electronic microscopy showing bacteria in the eukaryotic nucleus.

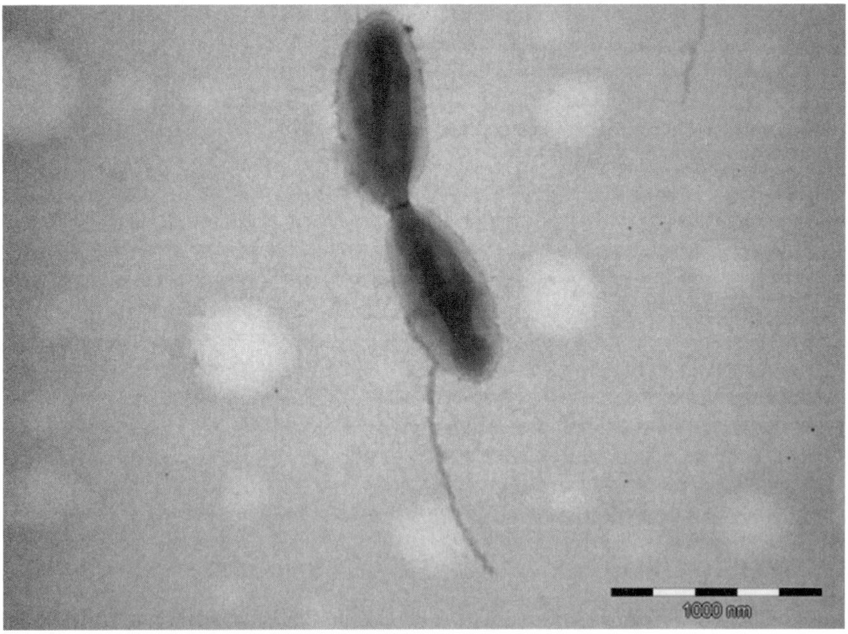

FIGURE 1—*continued.* (**c**) Identification of pili on *R. felis* by transmission electronic microscopy (negative staining).

their report. Our conclusion was that the previous report of culture of *R. felis* may have resulted from a contamination by *R. typhi* from the very beginning.

We decided to use XTC2 cells to grow *R. felis.*[7] These cells, taken from *Xenopus*, grow at 28°C and are used for *Arbovirus* cultures. We were able, using this cell line, to grow, identify, and characterize *R. felis*[17] (FIG. 1). This culture system allowed us to produce large amounts of rickettsiae and therefore to purify the bacteria in order to clone and sequence its genome.

GENOME SEQUENCING

The sequence of *R. felis* genome was surprising. We identified early the presence of a plasmid that was apparently 63 kb long.[18] However, we have had problems in closing our putative plasmid molecule based on the various clones generated by our bank. Finally, we tested the hypothesis that in fact 2 plasmids were present (one, being of 39 kb is a deleted form of the longer) (see FIG. 2). This was confirmed by PCR, and by pulse field gel electrophoresis coupled to hybridization. Moreover, we found them in all the *R. felis*–positive fleas by PCR.[18] The longer plasmid apparently contains the equipment to allow conjugative plasmd transfer. This is the first rickettsia harboring a plasmid. Moreover, this potential conjugative capability has been reported only once in an intracellular bacterium. Greub *et al.* reported that *Parachlamydia acanthamoebae* have an integron harboring the essential gene for conjugation.[19]

The size of the chromosome is longer (1,485 kb) than other previously sequenced rickettsiae (i.e., *R. prowazekii*, *R. conorii*, *R. sibirica*, *R. rickettsii*, *R. akari*, and *R. typhi*). It is colinear with the other rickettsiae but some inversions and transloca-

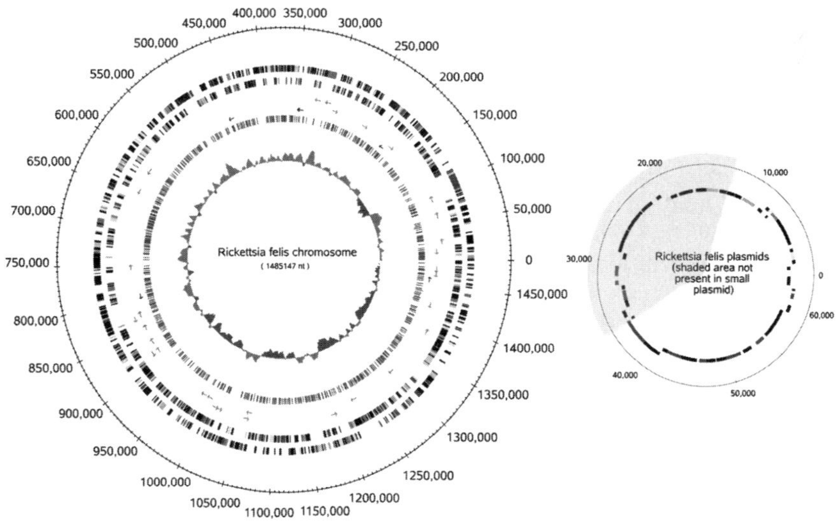

FIGURE 2. Circular representation of *R. felis* chromosome and plasmids.

tions were found. They were associated with genes encoding transposases. We identified 530 *R. felis*–specific genes compared to other published genomes (*R. prowazekii, R. typhi, R. conorii, R. sibirica*). *R. felis* have more paralogs in several identified gene families and unidentified gene families than other rickettsiae.

These families comprise 82 transposases, *tnp,* 22 ankyrin repeat-containing genes, *ank*, 13 surface cell antigens, *sca* (9 complete and 4 split), 11 tetratricopeptide repeat-containing protein genes, *tpr*, 14 s*po*T genes, and 5 families of toxin-antitoxin (TAT) system genes (16 toxins and 14 antitoxin genes). These specific features may be associated with the higher genome plasticity oberved in *R. felis* and with specific protein interactions mediated by *ank* and *tpr.*

R. FELIS SPECIFIC GENES

R. felis have 22 ankyrin repeats which is more than any prokaryotes sequenced so far. Ankyrin repeats are protein-protein interaction motifs involved in many steps of cell division. It is found mainly in eukaryotic cells, but also has been identified in pathogenic bacteria and in viruses.[20] Tetratricopeptide are also associated with protein interactions. Eleven copies were found in *R. felis*, and only host-associated bacteria exhibit such high number of copies such as *Legionella pneumophila*, *Treponema*, and *Leptospira.*[21]

As for TAT and *spoT* a recent review showed that TAT cassettes are abundant in prokaryotes including many pathogenic organisms.[22] During starvation, bacteria downregulate RNA synthesis by upregulating the secretion of the alarmones P_4G (ppGpp and pppGpp) under the control of two genes *relA* and *spoT.* P_4G inhibits stable RNA promoters specifically involving stable RNA promoters with short half-life. The consequence is to increase cell survival during nutritional stress. Toxins of the TAT have been identified first as gene killers present in plasmids to stabilize plasmid in bacteria. A long-time toxin is secreted along with a short-life antitoxin. If the TAT loci disappear, the toxin may destroy the bacteria as the antitoxin is no longer transcribed. A comparable system uses antisense RNAs. This system is also known as the plasmid-addiction system. There are 8 families of TAT loci.[22] Interestingly before our findings in *R. felis* the TAT system was considered exceptionel in intracellular organisms. As a matter of fact *R. felis* have 16 genes encoding for toxin and 14 for antitoxins of 5 of these TAT loci. The fact that *rel* BE (found in *R. felis*) has been demonstrated to stabilize plasmid efficiently even when it is chromosomal may indicate its role in *R. felis* plasmid maintenance. In general, chromosomally located TAT loci may help to stabilize mobile genetic elements including integron. Its presence in *R. felis* may indicate that it is associated with plasmid as other sequenced rickettsiae have no plasmid and few TAT copies.[23] Moreover, *R. felis* exhibits 14 paralogs. This gene is also critical in controlling the duplication rate.

SURFACE APPENDAGES OF *R. FELIS*

Two types of surface appendages can be recognized on certain bacterial species: the flagella that provide cell motility and pili, also known as fimbriae. While flagella occur on both gram-positive and gram-negative bacteria, pili are found almost exclusively on gram-negative bacteria with only a few gram-positive exceptions.[24,25] Analysis of the complete genome sequence of *R. felis* has revealed that this microorganism has genes susceptible of involvement in pili biogenesis. To determine whether pili were expressed or not on the *R. felis* surface, an electron microscopy study was carefully performed to avoid disruption of such appendages. *R. felis* cultivated in *Xenopus laevis* XTC-2 cells for 48 hours at 28°C were collected and centrifuged (400 × *g*, 10 min) before fixation for 1 hour at 4°C in glutaraldehyde (2.5% in PBS). Cells were then washed in PBS and placed on a carbon-formvar-coated 400-mesh copper grid (Electron Microscopy Sciences) for 15 min then negatively stained with 2% phosphotungstic acid for 10 s before analysis by electron microscopy (Philips Morgagni 268D). These experiments allowed the existence of two types of pili to be confirmed. We observed a small number of long pili known as sex pili. This form of pili establishes direct contact between bacteria, providing a very typical figure of Mpf apparatus (FIG. 1C). These pili may be specialized in conjugation. The other form of pili forms small hair-like projections emerging out from the cell surfaces, probably involved in the bacteria's attachment to other cells. Without pili, many

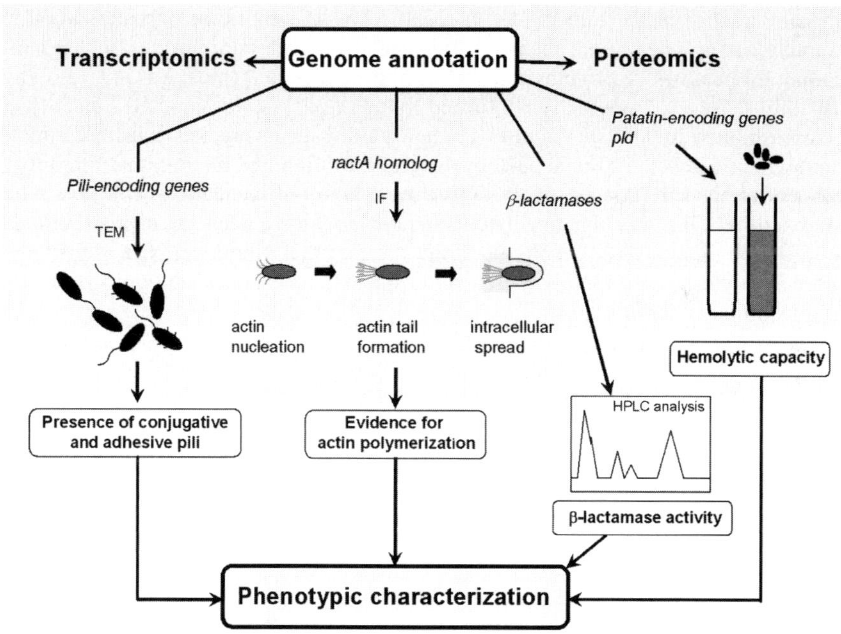

FIGURE 3. Schematic representation of phenotypic *R. felis* characters highlighted from genome sequence. Identification of genes known to confer specific features in other microorganisms prompted us to look for possible similar phenotype in *R. felis*. Pili and actin comet tails were thus visualized through transmission electronic microscopy (TEM) and immunofluorescence assay (IF), respectively. Following this strategy, we also evidenced hemolytic and γ-lactamase capacities of these bacteria. These results illustrate the fact that whole genome sequencing permit not only to develop classical transcriptomics and proteomics approaches but also to gain insights concerning poorly documented bacterial phenotypes.

disease-causing bacteria lose their invasion capability. The latter type appendages might be considered as virulence factors, as described for *Francisella tularensis.*

PHENOTYPIC POST-GENOMICS ANALYSIS

Some post-genomics studies were initiated by using transcriptomics and proteomics approaches. Transcription of some *R. felis* genes has been investigated. We also started to analyze the *R. felis* proteome through bidimensional electrophoresis coupled with mass spectrometry. Here, we envisaged post-genomics as a way to associate *in vivo* phenotypes of these bacteria to genomic features. Indeed, the obligate intracellular nature of *R. felis* hindered progress in the detailed characterization of its phenotypic diversity. This approach is schematically represented in FIGURE 3.

As previously mentioned, we also found a RickA homologue in *R. felis* genome.[26] Based on this finding, we performed immunofluorescence assays and evidenced that *R. felis* can use the actin cytoskeleton to disseminate through eukaryotic cells, as other SFG *rickettsiae*. Moreover, we identified *R. felis* multiplying in nucleus (FIG. 1). This phenomenon is strictly associated with the spotted fever group *rickettsiae* and linked to intracellular mobility provided by actin polymerization.[27] Another *R. felis* phenotypic character suggested from genomic analyses [3 ORFs encoding for patatin-like proteins and one for phospholipase D (pld)] was its hemolytic capability. We experimentally confirmed that *R. felis* lyse erythrocytes, this effect being inhibited by DTT.[18] Another genome-guided discovery was β-lactam inhibition, which reached 57% and 53% of the concentration and the minimal inhibitory concentration (MIC), respectively, following 2 hours of incubation of *R. felis* with amoxicillin. This was the first betalactamase activity evidenced in a *Rickettsia.* While preliminary, these results illustrate the fact that whole genome sequencing offers opportunities to rapidly gain a better understanding of phenotypic characters of a fastidious microorganism.

PERSPECTIVES AND CONCLUSIONS

The present work showed the usefulness of the genomic approach to rapidly identify specific features in such a bacterium. To date, 4 intracellular bacterial genomes were entirely sequenced in 7 years or less after their first identification or culture. *W. pipientis* was first cultured in 1997 and sequenced in 2004,[28] which allowed the identification of several genes involved in host-symbiont interactions. *Parachlamydia* was first identified in *amoeba* in 1997 and sequenced in 2004,[29] which allowed the unexpected identification of genes for conjugation.[30] *Tropheryma whipplei* was first cultured in eukaryotic cells in 2000. Its genome sequencing in 2003[31,32] allowed the identification of basic metabolic properties that successfully guided the establishment of a cell-free culture.[33] Moreover, the sequence of the *Wolbachia* genome of *Brugia malayi* was recently released and the bacteria has never been cultured.[34] The genome sequencing of *R. felis* provided evidences of the presence of conjugative plasmids. The genomic findings prompted us to identify two types of pili, a hemolytic activity, a β-lactamase activity, and intracellular motility. These results illustrate the fact that for such recently identified/cultured fastidious organisms, complete genome sequencing is a very potent and time-saving strategy facilitating identification of unrecognized phenotypic traits.

[*Competing interests statement:* The authors have no conflicting financial interests.]

REFERENCES

1. WOLBACH, S.B., J.L. TODD & F.W. PALFREY. 1922. The Etiology and Pathology of Typhus. Harvard University Press. Cambridge, MA.
2. RAOULT, D. & V. ROUX. 1997. Rickettsioses as paradigms of new or emerging infectious diseases. Clin. Microbiol. Rev. **10:** 694–719.
3. SIKORA, H. 1916. Beiträge zur Anatomie, Physiologie und Biologie der Kleiderlaus (Pediculus vestimenti Nitzsch). I. Anatomie des Verdauungstraktes. Arch. f. Schiffs-und Tropen-hyg **20:** 5–76.
4. ADAMS, J.R., E.T. SCHMIDTMANN & A.F. AZAD. 1990. Infection of colonized cat fleas, *Ctenocephalides felis* (Bouché), with a rickettsia-like microorganism. Am. J. Trop. Med. Hyg. **43:** 400–409.
5. AZAD, A.F., J.B. SACCI, W.M. NELSON, *et al.* 1992. Genetic characterization and transovarial transmission of a typhus-like rickettsia found in cat fleas. Proc. Natl. Acad. Sci. USA **89:** 43–46.
6. AZAD, A.F., S. RADULOVIC, J.A. HIGGINS, *et al.* 1997. Flea-borne rickettsioses: ecologic considerations. Emerg. Infect. Dis. **3:** 319–327.
7. RAOULT, D., B. LA SCOLA, M. ENEA, *et al.* 2001. A flea-associated rickettsia pathogenic for humans. Emerg. Infect. Dis. **7:** 73–81.
8. KELLY, P.J., N. MEADS, A. THEOBALD, *et al.* 2004. *Rickettsia felis*, *Bartonella henselae*, and *B. clarridgiae*, New Zealand. Emerg. Infect. Dis. **10:** 967–968.
9. PAROLA, P., J.P. CORNET, Y.O. SANOGO, *et al.* 2003. Detection of *Ehrlichia* spp., *Anaplasma* spp., *Rickettsia* spp., and other eubacteria in ticks from the Thai-Myanmar border and Vietnam. J. Clin. Microbiol. **41:** 1600–1608.
10. ROLAIN, J.M., M. FRANC, B. DAVOUST & D. RAOULT. 2003. Molecular detection of *Bartonella quintana*, *B. koehlerae*, *B. henselae*, *B. clarridgeiae*, *Rickettsia felis*, and *Wolbachia pipientis* in cat fleas, France. Emerg. Infect. Dis. **9:** 338–342.
11. SCHRIEFER, M.E., J.B. SACCI, JR., J.S. DUMLER, *et al.* 1994. Identification of a novel rickettsial infection in a patient diagnosed with murine typhus. J. Clin. Microbiol. **32:** 949–954.
12. ZAVALA-VELAZQUEZ, J.E., J.A. RUIZ-SOSA, R.A. SANCHEZ-ELIAS, *et al.* 2000. *Rickettsia felis* rickettsiosis in Yucatan. Lancet **356:** 1079–1080.
13. RICHTER, J., P.E. FOURNIER, J. PETRIDOU, *et al.* 2002. *Rickettsia felis* infection acquired in Europe and documented by polymerase chain reaction. Emerg. Infect. Dis. **8:** 207–208.
14. RADULOVIC, S., J.A. HIGGINS, D.C. JAWORSKI, *et al.* 1995. Isolation, cultivation, and partial characterization of the ELB agent associated with cat fleas. Infect. Immun **63:** 4826–4829.
15. RADULOVIC, S., J.A. HIGGINS, D.C. JAWORSKI & A.F. AZAD. 1995. In vitro and in vivo antibiotic susceptibilities of ELB rickettsiae. Antimicrob. Agents Chemother. **39:** 2564–2566.
16. RADULOVIC, S., J.A. HIGGINS, D.C. JAWORSKI & A.F. AZAD. 1996. In vitro and in vivo antibiotic susceptibilities of ELB rickettsiae. Antimicrob. Agents Chemother. **40:** 2912.
17. LA SCOLA, B., S. MECONI, F. FENOLLAR, *et al.* 2002. Emended description of *Rickettsia felis* (Bouyer *et al.* 2001), a temperature-dependent cultured bacterium. Int. J. Syst. Evol. Microbiol. **52:** 2035–2041.
18. OGATA, H., P. RENESTO, S. AUDIC, *et al.* 2005. The genome sequence of *R. felis* identifies the first case of conjugative plasmid in an obligate intracellular parasite. PLoS. Biol. In press.
19. GREUB, G., F. COLLYN, L. GUY & C.A. ROTEN. 2004. A genomic island present along the bacterial chromosome of the *Parachlamydiaceae* UWE25, an obligate amoebal

endosymbiont, encodes a potentially functional F-like conjugative DNA transfer system. BMC Microbiol. **4:** 48.

20. RUBTSOV, A.M. & O.D. LOPINA. 2000. Ankyrins. FEBS Lett. **482:** 1–5.
21. CAZALET, C., C. RUSNIOK, H. BRUGGEMANN, *et al.* 2004. Evidence in the *Legionella pneumophila* genome for exploitation of host cell functions and high genome plasticity. Nat. Genet. **36:** 1165–1173.
22. GERDES, K., S.K. CHRISTENSEN & A. LOBNER-OLESEN. 2005. Prokaryotic toxin-antitoxin stress response loci. Nature Rev. Microbiol. **3:** 371–382.
23. PANDEY, D.P. & K. GERDES. 2005. Toxin-antitoxin loci are highly abundant in free-living but lost from host-associated prokaryotes. Nucl. Acids Res. **33:** 966–976.
24. YEUNG, M.K. 2000. *Actinomyces*: surface macromolecules and bacteria-host interactions. *In* Gram-Positive Pathogens. V.A. Fischetti, R.P. Novick, J.J. Ferretti *et al.*, Eds.: 583–593. American Society for Microbiology. Washington, D.C.
25. WU, H. & P.M. FIVES-TAYLOR. 2001. Molecular strategies for fimbrial expression and assembly. Crit. Rev. Oral Biol. Med. **12:** 101–115.
26. CHUNG, S., P. MONDON, Y.C. CHANG & K.J. KWON-CHUNG. 2003. *Cryptococcus neoformans* with a mutation in the tetratricopeptide repeat-containing gene, CCN1, causes subcutaneous lesions but fails to cause systemic infection. Infect. Immun. **71:** 1988–1994.
27. TEYSSEIRE, N., C. CHICHE-PORTICHE & D. RAOULT. 1992. Intracellular movements of *Rickettsia conorii* and *R. typhi* based on actin polymerization. Res. Microbiol. **143:** 821–829.
28. ALT-MORBE, J., J.L. STRYKER, C. FUQUA, *et al.* 1996. The conjugal transfer system of *Agrobacterium tumefaciens* octopine-type Ti plasmids is closely related to the transfer system of an IncP plasmid and distantly related to Ti plasmid vir genes. J. Bacteriol. **178:** 4248–4257.
29. BERANEK, A., M. ZETTL, K. LORENZONI, *et al.* 2004. Thirty-eight C-terminal amino acids of the coupling protein TraD of the F-like conjugative resistance plasmid R1 are required and sufficient to confer binding to the substrate selector protein TraM. J. Bacteriol. **186:** 6999–7006.
30. KOONIN, E.V. & L. ARAVIND. 2000. The NACHT family—a new group of predicted NTPases implicated in apoptosis and MHC transcription activation. Trends Biochem. Sci. **25:** 223–224.
31. QIN, A., A.M. TUCKER, A. HINES & D.O. WOOD. 2004. Transposon mutagenesis of the obligate intracellular pathogen *Rickettsia prowazekii.* Appl. Environ. Microbiol. **70:** 2816–2822.
32. COLLINS, N.E., J. LIEBENBERG, E.P. DE VILLIERS, *et al.* 2005. The genome of the heartwater agent *Ehrlichia ruminantium* contains multiple tandem repeats of actively variable copy number Proc. Natl. Acad. Sci. USA **102:** 838–843.
33. BRAYTON, K.A., L.S. KAPPMEYER, D.R. HERNDON, *et al.* 2005. Complete genome sequencing of *Anaplasma marginale* reveals that the surface is skewed to two superfamilies of outer membrane proteins. Proc. Natl. Acad. Sci. USA **102:** 844–849.
34. FOSTER, J., M. GANATRA, I. KAMAL, *et al.* 2005. The *Wolbachia* genome of *Brugia malayi*: endosymbiont evolution within a human pathogenic nematode PLoS. Biol. **3:** e121.

Dissecting the *Rickettsia prowazekii* Genome

Genetic and Proteomic Approaches

AIMEE M. TUCKER,[a] LEWIS K. PANNELL,[b] AND DAVID O. WOOD[a]

[a]*Department of Microbiology and Immunology, Laboratory of Molecular Biology, and*
[b]*Proteomics and Mass Spectrometry, Cancer Research Institute,*
University of South Alabama College of Medicine, Mobile, Alabama 36688, USA

ABSTRACT: The obligate nature of *Rickettsia prowazekii* intracellular growth places severe restrictions on the analysis of rickettsial gene function and gene expression. Fortunately, this situation is improving as methods for the genetic manipulation and proteomic analysis of this fascinating human pathogen become available. In this paper, we review the current status of rickettsial genetics and the isolation of rickettsial mutants using a genetic approach. In addition, the examination of rickettsial gene expression through characterization of the rickettsial proteome will be described. This will include a description of a high-throughput, accurate mass approach that has identified 596 rickettsial proteins in a complex rickettsial protein sample.

KEYWORDS: *Rickettsia prowazekii*; genetics; proteomics

INTRODUCTION

Rickettsia prowazekii, the causative agent of epidemic typhus, has played a significant role in human history.[1] Outbreaks of this disease precipitated by wars, famines, and other human calamities proved devastating to louse-infested, starving populations unable to obtain basic hygienic amenities. Unlike other rickettsial species, which are vectored by ticks or fleas, *R. prowazekii* is not maintained in its louse vector. In fact, the infected human body louse also succumbs to *R. prowazekii* infection. Thus, maintenance of *R. prowazekii* in a human population was once thought to depend entirely on epidemic typhus survivors that harbor the bacterium in an uncharacterized state. Recrudescence of the disease (Brill-Zinsser disease), years or decades after the initial infection, provided a source of *R. prowazekii*, which in the presence of the louse vector, spread the disease to uninfected individuals. However, *R. prowazekii* has been found in at least one other mammalian host (the flying squirrel) and there is evidence of disease transmission to humans from this source.[2,3] Other, as yet unidentified, animal reservoirs may exist to maintain this pathogen between epidemics.

Address for correspondence: Dr. David Wood, Department of Microbiology and Immunology, Laboratory of Molecular Biology, University of South Alabama, Mobile, AL 36688. Voice: 251-460-6324; fax: 251-460-7269.
dowood@jaguar1.usouthal.edu

Ann. N.Y. Acad. Sci. 1063: 35–46 (2005). © 2005 New York Academy of Sciences.
doi: 10.1196/annals.1355.005

Unfortunately, a discussion of *R. prowazekii* and epidemic typhus is not just a historical exercise. More recent outbreaks of epidemic typhus have occurred, demonstrating that, in the presence of the age-old precipitating factors of overcrowding and lack of hygiene, this disease remains a threat for human populations of the new millennium.[4,5] In addition, *R. prowazekii* has been categorized as a select agent, a pathogen that has the potential to be used as a bioterrorist weapon.[6]

R. prowazekii is an obligate intracellular parasitic bacterium that grows only within the cytoplasm of its eukaryotic host cells. Thus, it differs from other obligate intracellular bacteria (*Chlamydia*, *Ehrlichia*, *Coxiella*) that reside within membrane-bound vesicles. *R. prowazekii* pathogenicity results from its ability to exploit the intracytoplasmic environment, replicate to high numbers within the host cell, lyse the host cell, and infect additional host cells. While antibiotics, such as doxycycline, are available for the treatment of rickettsial diseases, the limitations of tetracycline therapy, the prospect of antibiotic resistance, the small number of alternative antimicrobial agents, and the lack of an effective and safe vaccine all provide a strong stimulus for studying this novel human pathogen.

GENETIC ANALYSIS

Genetic manipulation of *R. prowazekii* has been hampered by the lack of robust genetic tools. This situation is rapidly changing as rickettsiologists take advantage of an increasing number of rickettsial genome sequence databases and the development of techniques, such as site-directed mutagenesis and transposon insertions, for generating and isolating rickettsial gene mutants.[7–12] However, the obligate intracellular nature of rickettsial growth continues to impose severe restrictions on the genetic manipulation and isolation of rickettsial mutants. For example, one of the most straightforward tasks in the genetic analysis of free-living bacteria such as *Escherichia coli*, the isolation of individual clones, is quite problematic for a bacterium that does not form colonies on the surface of a solid medium.

An additional challenge to *R. prowazekii* gene manipulation has been the lack of selectable markers for identifying and isolating the rickettsial transformants. While tetracycline and chloramphenicol would be obvious choices, based on the sensitivity of intracellular rickettsiae to these antibiotics, their use has been restricted due to their importance in the treatment of rickettsial disease. This led our lab to test antibiotic resistance genes obtained from *E. coli* for their effectiveness in the selection of rickettsial transformants. Two genes, *ereB* (erythromycin resistance) and *Rparr2* (rifampin resistance), have been used successfully.[8,9] Recently, chloramphenicol was used as a selectable marker in the transformation of a tick symbiont, *R. monacensis.*[7] As might be expected, this selection was very effective. Of special significance was the demonstration by the authors of this report of the expression of GFPuv in *R. monacensis*. The ability to detect individual fluorescent rickettsiae growing within their host cell shows great promise for studies examining the intracellular growth of these obligate parasitic bacteria.

In addition to new selectable markers, improvements in transposon technology have also advanced rickettsial gene manipulation. For example, insertional mutants of *R. prowazekii* have been obtained using the transposome system marketed by

TABLE 1. Transposon insertion sites

Gene Number and Annotation		
RP243	*emrA*	Multidrug resistance protein EmrA
RP263	ORF	Unknown
RP275	*lepA*	GTP-binding protein LepA
RP294	*gppA*	pppGpp phosphohydrolase
RP489	ORF	Unknown
RP689	ORF	Unknown
RP823	*ftsK*	Cell division protein FtsK
RP880	*mutL*	DNA mismatch repair protein MutL
Intergenic		Between RP229 and RP230
Intergenic		Between RP623 and RP624

Epicentre, Madison, Wisconsin.[8] This system, which electroporates the transposon DNA combined with the transposase directly into the rickettsiae, provides an effective means for generating insertional mutations of the rickettsial genome. Identification of insertion sites is straightforward since the transposon contains a replication origin that can be used to rescue the transposon and adjacent rickettsial DNA. The transposon also contains primer sites which allow sequencing of the adjacent rickettsial DNA and identification of the insertion site within the rickettsial genome. Currently, ten *R. prowazekii* genomic insertions have been identified, six of which were previously reported.[8] Insertions within coding regions are of special interest (TABLE 1). These mutants, once cloned, can be examined for phenotypic differences such as variable growth rates, stress responses, and/or the ability to grow in different host cells. Unfortunately, as mentioned above, we have found the most difficult step to be the isolation of pure clones. The selection of rickettsial transformants using either erythromycin or rifampin results in a high background of spontaneously resistant mutants. We have successfully used limiting dilution to clone two rickettsial mutants (*mutL* and RP689), which are currently being evaluated for phenotypic differences. To increase our chances of isolating clones, we are currently using a transposon containing both the *ereB* and *Rparr2* genes. This will permit double selection for clones exhibiting both erythromycin and rifampin resistance, reducing the background of spontaneous mutants.

Despite the success of direct rickettsial gene mutagenesis, the characterization of rickettsial gene function will continue to rely heavily on the expression of rickettsial gene products in surrogate hosts such as *E. coli*. For example, by screening a rickettsial *E. coli* clone bank, we identified the *R. prowazekii* gene (*sam*) coding for the first bacterial transporter of the essential metabolite *S*-adenosylmethionine.[13] With this gene function in hand, we were able to construct the first *E. coli metK* deletion strain, providing a suitable background for examining the function of rickettsial *metK* genes.[14] This permitted a test of the hypothesis that the *metK* genes of *R. prowazekii* Breinl and *R. typhi* Willmington coded for an enzyme with methionine adenosyltransferase activity. As investigators strive to correlate gene identification with actual function, the use of surrogate hosts will continue to be an important component of rickettsial investigations.

PROTEOMICS

The area of proteomics holds great promise for analyzing rickettsial gene expression. Two recent papers demonstrate the power of this approach. Chao *et al.* have published the first partial proteome of *R. prowazekii*, while Renesto *et al.*, using two-dimensional techniques, have provided a preliminary analysis of *R. conorii* proteins.[15,16] In our studies we have taken a similar path to that of Chao *et al.*, namely, the direct analysis of complex mixtures of proteins by mass spectrometry. We are developing protocols to provide comprehensive and reproducible analyses of rickettsial protein expression. To develop these protocols and permit direct comparisons between different protocols as well as with previously published proteomes, we employed a single sample prepared from the Madrid E strain of *R. prowazekii*.

The Madrid E strain was propagated in embryonated hen eggs and the rickettsiae isolated as described previously.[17] Rickettsiae were suspended in a sucrose-phosphate-glutamate-magnesium buffer (218 mM sucrose, 3.76 mM KH_2PO_4, 7 mM K_2HPO_4, 4.9 mM potassium glutamate, and 10 mM $MgCl_2$ [SPG-Mg]) and stored at −80°C until use. The rickettsiae were collected by centrifugation and suspended in 50 mM KPO_4, pH 7.0 containing the following: 1 mM PMSF, 10 µg/mL DNaseI, 10 µg/mL RNaseA, 2 µg/mL aprotinin, 1 µg/mL leupeptin, 1 µg/mL pepstatin A. Rickettsiae were disrupted using a French press at 20,000 PSI. Following lysis, additional protease inhibitors (1 mM AEBSF, 10 µM bestatin, 50 µM E-64, 1 µM pepstatin A) were added. The rickettsial lysate was centrifuged at 14,000 × *g* for 10 min at 4°C to remove unbroken rickettsiae and cellular debris. The supernatant was centrifuged at 80,000 × *g* for 90 min. The resulting supernatant was designated the soluble fraction and stored at −80°C. The insoluble pellet was subsequently treated with 8 M urea and the resulting extract designated the membrane fraction. Protein concentration of the soluble fraction (2.2 µg/µL) was determined using the BioRad DC protein assay kit. For proteomic analysis, saturated sodium bicarbonate was added to the sample to increase the pH to 8.0. Sequencing grade modified trypsin (Promega, Madison, WI) was added to final concentration of 1 pmol/L and incubated at 37°C overnight. Trypsin-treated samples were first separated on a Waters capillary liquid chromatograph using an acetonitrile/water (both containing 0.2% formic acid) gradient on a VC-10-C18-150 (soluble fraction) or VC-10-C4-150 (membrane fraction) column (Micro-Tech Scientific, Vista, CA) using a 1 µL/min flow rate. Data were acquired on a Waters QTOF Ultima high-resolution mass spectrometer using MassLynx software.

Tandem Mass Spectrometry (LC/MS/MS)

For MS/MS data, the ProteinLynx software (part of MassLynx) was used to convert the data to a PKL (peaklist) file format for input into our in-house Mascot search engine <http://www.matrixscience.com> using a custom *R. prowazekii* database established from the deduced proteome.[18] The Mascot-determined threshold was used to establish the significance of protein identification. All PKL files were also searched against the whole non-restricted NCBInr database to identify proteins which may have co-purified. In doing this, we identified porcine trypsin, which had been added to digest the proteins, two major vitellogenin egg proteins, and several keratins. All of the identified, non-rickettsial proteins were added to the rickettsial database and used to refine searching and identification.

TABLE 2. Comparison of MS/MS results

Laboratory:	Chao *et al.*[15]	Wood *et al.* (unpublished)
Extraction:	9 M urea	French press/8 M urea
Separation:	On-line 2D-LC, 13 elutions from strong ion exchange column followed by a C18-hydrophobicity column	1D-LC, C18 hydrophobicity column (soluble fraction) and C4 hydrophobicity column (membrane fraction)
Total proteins:	251	278
Unique to laboratory:	63	92

With use of the maximum injection volume of 6.4 µL, repeated 100-min MS/MS runs were performed and the resulting peaklist files were searched against the rickettsial database. There was some variability in the repeated injections, both in the proteins identified and the number of proteins identified per injection. A compilation of 7 injections yielded a total of 51 identifiable proteins from the rickettsial database. By decreasing the flow rates of the sample over the chromatography column, MS/MS sampling times were extended from 100 min to 180 min, slightly increasing the number of proteins identified above threshold from 51 to 65. However, 19 of these proteins were unique to the 180-min run. Considering that the samples injected for both run conditions were identical, the variation probably results from changes in the peptides chosen for sequencing in the second round of MS. Selection of peptides for sequencing is dependent on the peak intensity, and although the program is designed to limit repetitive sequencing of the same peptide peaks, the major limitation of tandem mass spectrometry is that only the most abundant peptides are chosen for sequencing.

To increase coverage of the proteome, we fractionated the original soluble fraction into five pI ranges by isoelectric focusing. In addition, elutions from six salt concentrations from strong cation exchange were analyzed. Finally, a more concentrated soluble fraction and an 8 M urea-extracted membrane fraction were analyzed. A compilation of the data from repeated injections of these numerous samples yielded results similar to those of Chao *et al.*[15] (TABLE 2). We identified 278 *R. prowazekii* proteins. While this number is similar to the 251 identified by Chao *et al.*, the two partial proteomes are not identical. Of our 278 proteins, 95 were unique to our proteome, while Chao *et al.* identified 65 proteins not found in our proteome. This probably reflects the different extraction and fractionation methods used to obtain the rickettsial protein samples. We used a French press to disrupt the rickettsiae and obtain a soluble fraction and an 8 M extraction of the membrane fraction to release proteins from the insoluble pellet. Chao *et al.* used 9 M urea and extensive fractionation to obtain analyzable samples. Despite extensive analysis by both labs, the MS/MS approach only yielded approximately 250 total proteins.

The MS/MS approach has several drawbacks. First, it identifies only the more abundant proteins in any sample. While this can be improved by protein fractionation, as discussed above, less abundant proteins may never be identified by this approach. Second, information on the relative intensities of peptide peaks within an analysis is lost, eliminating the possibility of comparing the relative abundance of proteins. This led us to analyze our samples using an accurate mass approach.

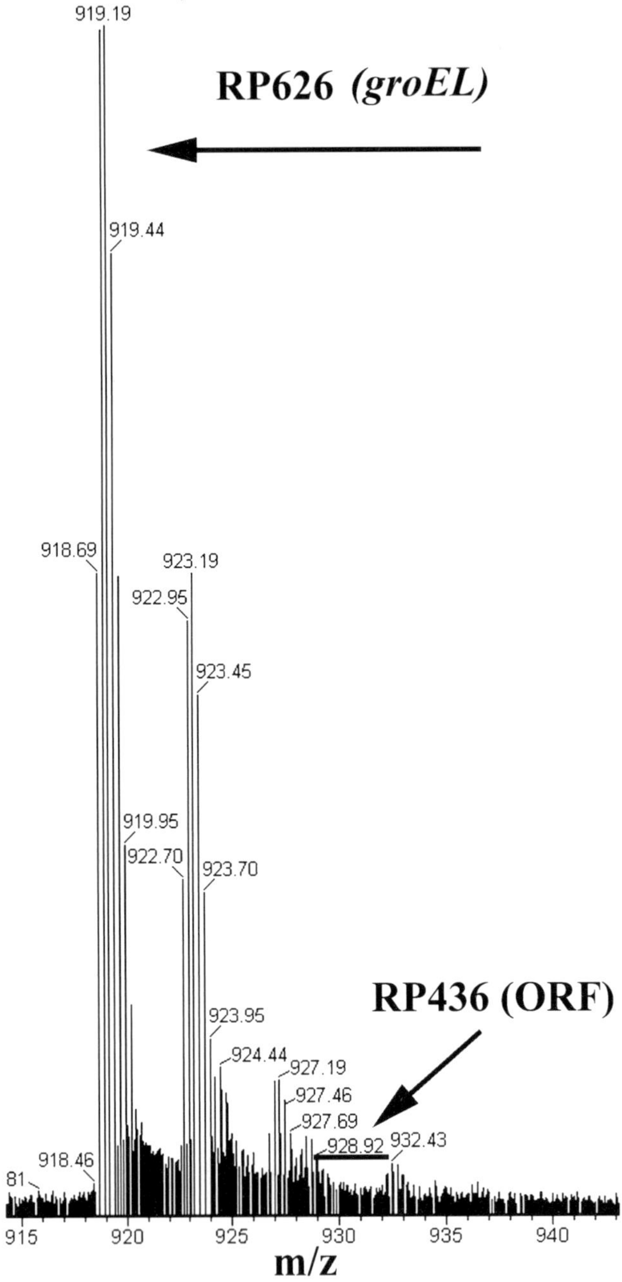

FIGURE 1. Mass spectrum demonstrating the dynamic range of accurate mass ion detection.

Accurate Mass (LC/MS)

The accurate mass approach provides several advantages in the analysis of complex peptide mixtures.[19, 20] First, analysis can be performed on the lowest intensity peak, providing identification of less abundant peptides as demonstrated in FIGURE 1. GroEL, one of the most abundant rickettsial proteins, is consistently identified by tandem mass spectrometry. However, a peptide corresponding to RP436, with 40-fold less intensity, is not identified by MS/MS, but is easily identified using the accurate mass approach, which has a much greater dynamic range. Second, maintenance of intensity data will allow relative abundance calculations and comparison of differential expression. To determine the feasibility of this approach, we once again analyzed a rickettsial protein preparation prepared from *R. prowazekii* grown in egg yolk sacs. Tryptic peptides were analyzed by LC/MS. During MS acquisition, a lock mass of fibrinopeptide B (Sigma, St. Louis, MO) was infused post-column into the LC effluent such that it gave approximately 150 counts per 5 seconds on the most abundant, doubly charged m/z 776.8368 ion (approximately one-tenth of the most intense peak in the spectrum). The application of a continuous lock mass allows for the correction of variations during long (180 min) runs due to room temperature changes which affect the mass determination using QTOF. After lock mass correction, the mass spectrometry data were optimized using the ReSpect™ algorithim marketed by Positive Probability, Ltd., Isleham, UK. This algorithim improves signal to noise, deconvolves the peaks, coverts electrospray mass spectra to zero-charge spectra, and corrects baselines. After this data conversion, in-house software analyzes the peak list generated at confidence levels of 95% or greater and determines those masses in the table that are unique within a 10 ppm error (this error represents twice the average error of the instrument). These masses are then searched against a rickettsial database generated by an *in silico* tryptic digest of the rickettsial proteome with carryover proteins included. By analyzing the MS/MS data, the majority of peptides detected were from either zero or one missed cut, indicating an efficient trypsin digest of the rickettsial proteins. Therefore, to generate the database for searching, we included peptide masses that would result from both zero and one missed cut. The protein number, name, and exact mass and sequence of each peptide were recorded into an internal rickettsial peptide database for our MS-only analyses. To ensure that all possible theoretical masses were represented in the rickettsial database, initial peptides with and without the first methionine were included. By increasing the number of peptides in the database in this way, and by incorporating known carry-over proteins (e.g., vitellogenins and keratins) as well, we actually reduce the probability of finding a peptide mass without overlapping masses within 10 ppm error. Therefore identification of a protein with a unique mass occurs under the most stringent conditions. Proteins are identified when unique masses from the peak list correspond to a peptide mass which has no overlapping masses in the database within 10 ppm. In this study multiple injections were performed on each sample, 10 for the soluble fraction and 5 for the membrane fraction. To increase the stringency of protein identification, one or more unique peptides from a protein must be detected in at least 8 out of the 10 or 4 out of the 5 injections.

Using this approach we identified 596 proteins (TABLE 3). which represent 71% of the *R. prowazekii* protein coding genes. Although this number is a significant improvement over the partial proteomes identified previously, it should be noted that

TABLE 3. ***Rickettsia prowazekii*** **proteins identified by accurate mass**

Gene Number					
RP001	RP070	RP145	RP216	RP287	RP356
RP002	RP071	RP146	RP219	RP289	RP358
RP003	RP072	RP148	RP221	RP290	RP359
RP005	RP073	RP150	RP222	RP291	RP361
RP006	RP074	RP151	RP223	RP292	RP362
RP007	RP075	RP152	RP225	RP293	RP363
RP008	RP077	RP153	RP226	RP294	RP364
RP009	RP081	RP154	RP227	RP295	RP365
RP011	RP082	RP155	RP228	RP296	RP366
RP012	RP083	RP157	RP229	RP297	RP371
RP013	RP085	RP158	RP233	RP298	RP372
RP014	RP086	RP160	RP234	RP300	RP373
RP015	RP087	RP161	RP236	RP301	RP374
RP017	RP089	RP163	RP237	RP302	RP375
RP018	RP090	RP165	RP238	RP304	RP376
RP022	RP091	RP170	RP239	RP305	RP379
RP025	RP092	RP171	RP240	RP307	RP384
RP026	RP093	RP172	RP241	RP308	RP386
RP029	RP094	RP173	RP243	RP310	RP387
RP030	RP097	RP174	RP245	RP313	RP389
RP031	RP100	RP175	RP246	RP314	RP390
RP032	RP102	RP176	RP247	RP315	RP393
RP033	RP103	RP177	RP248	RP316	RP394
RP034	RP104	RP178	RP249	RP317	RP395
RP035	RP105	RP179	RP251	RP318	RP397
RP036	RP106	RP180	RP252	RP319	RP400
RP037	RP107	RP182	RP253	RP320	RP401
RP038	RP108	RP183	RP254	RP321	RP402
RP041	RP109	RP184	RP256	RP322	RP403
RP042	RP110	RP185	RP258	RP323	RP404
RP043	RP115	RP186	RP259	RP325	RP405
RP044	RP116	RP190	RP260	RP326	RP406
RP045	RP117	RP191	RP261	RP327	RP407
RP047	RP118	RP193	RP262	RP328	RP409
RP048	RP119	RP194	RP263	RP329	RP410
RP051	RP121	RP196	RP264	RP332	RP411
RP052	RP122	RP197	RP265	RP333	RP412
RP053	RP123	RP198	RP269	RP334	RP413
RP054	RP124	RP200	RP271	RP335	RP415
RP055	RP128	RP201	RP273	RP338	RP416

TABLE 3. (*continued*) ***Rickettsia prowazekii*** **proteins identified by accurate mass**

Gene Number					
RP056	RP129	RP202	RP274	RP339	RP418
RP057	RP130	RP203	RP275	RP340	RP419
RP058	RP132	RP204	RP278	RP342	RP420
RP059	RP135	RP205	RP280	RP344	RP421
RP060	RP136	RP206	RP281	RP345	RP422
RP062	RP137	RP208	RP282	RP347	RP423
RP064	RP140	RP212	RP283	RP348	RP425
RP065	RP141	RP213	RP284	RP349	RP426
RP067	RP142	RP214	RP285	RP350	RP427
RP068	RP144	RP215	RP286	RP353	RP428
RP431	RP506	RP580	RP672	RP755	RP828
RP432	RP508	RP581	RP673	RP757	RP831
RP433	RP509	RP583	RP674	RP758	RP832
RP434	RP510	RP586	RP675	RP759	RP833
RP436	RP511	RP587	RP676	RP761	RP835
RP439	RP512	RP588	RP677	RP763	RP836
RP441	RP513	RP589	RP679	RP764	RP837
RP442	RP514	RP590	RP680	RP766	RP840
RP444	RP515	RP593	RP681	RP767	RP841
RP445	RP516	RP595	RP682	RP768	RP842
RP446	RP517	RP596	RP683	RP769	RP843
RP447	RP520	RP597	RP684	RP772	RP845
RP448	RP521	RP598	RP685	RP773	RP846
RP449	RP526	RP601	RP686	RP776	RP847
RP450	RP528	RP602	RP687	RP778	RP849
RP451	RP530	RP604	RP690	RP779	RP850
RP452	RP534	RP610	RP691	RP780	RP851
RP454	RP535	RP611	RP692	RP782	RP852
RP455	RP536	RP614	RP693	RP783	RP853
RP457	RP538	RP617	RP694	RP784	RP854
RP458	RP539	RP618	RP696	RP785	RP855
RP459	RP540	RP619	RP698	RP789	RP856
RP460	RP542	RP620	RP700	RP790	RP857
RP462	RP543	RP622	RP701	RP791	RP858
RP464	RP545	RP623	RP703	RP792	RP859
RP465	RP546	RP626	RP704	RP793	RP860
RP468	RP547	RP628	RP707	RP794	RP861
RP469	RP551	RP629	RP716	RP797	RP863
RP472	RP552	RP631	RP718	RP799	RP864
RP473	RP553	RP635	RP719	RP801	RP865

TABLE 3. **(*continued*) *Rickettsia prowazekii* proteins identified by accurate mass**

Gene Number					
RP474	RP555	RP637	RP720	RP802	RP866
RP475	RP556	RP638	RP721	RP803	RP867
RP476	RP558	RP639	RP722	RP804	RP868
RP478	RP559	RP643	RP723	RP805	RP869
RP479	RP560	RP645	RP726	RP806	RP870
RP482	RP561	RP646	RP730	RP807	RP871
RP486	RP562	RP647	RP733	RP808	RP872
RP488	RP563	RP648	RP734	RP809	RP874
RP489	RP564	RP652	RP735	RP810	RP875
RP490	RP565	RP653	RP737	RP811	RP876
RP492	RP566	RP656	RP738	RP815	RP878
RP494	RP567	RP658	RP739	RP818	RP880
RP495	RP568	RP659	RP740	RP819	RP882
RP496	RP569	RP661	RP741	RP820	RP883
RP497	RP571	RP665	RP742	RP821	RP884
RP498	RP572	RP666	RP743	RP822	RP885
RP499	RP573	RP667	RP747	RP823	

TABLE 4. ***Rickettsia prowazekii* proteins identified by MS/MS only**[a]

Gene Number					
RP040[b]	RP232[b]	RP463[b]	RP606[c]	RP650[b]	RP775[b]
RP099[c]	RP355	RP471	RP627[c]	RP654[c]	RP816[b]
RP112[c]	RP367	RP483[b]	RP634[b]	RP655[c]	RP844[b]
RP131[b]	RP370[b]	RP485[c]	RP636[b]	RP657	
RP138[c]	RP378[b]	RP487[b]	RP640[c]	RP660[c]	
RP139[c]	RP396^	RP503[c]	RP642[c]	RP762[b]	
RP231[b]	RP398[b]	RP527[b]	RP644[b]	RP771[c]	

[a]Data compiled from Chao *et al.*[15] and Wood *et al.* (unpublished).
[b]Proteins detected by accurate mass in <80% of repeat injections, and thus not reported in TABLE 3.
[c]Proteins without a theoretical unique mass at 10 ppm error.

there are a few drawbacks. As seen in TABLE 4, there are several proteins identified by LC/MS/MS that are absent from the accurate mass list. Of these, many are small proteins that do not contain a theoretical unique peptide. One example, RP627 (*groES*), is abundant in all samples analyzed by LC/MS/MS. When examined by LC/MS only, all of the peptide masses can be found in the peaklist, but none are unique under stringent conditions. Our conditions for protein identification require that at least one unique peptide be detected in no less than 80% of the repeat injections for each sample analyzed. Several proteins in TABLE 4 are detectable by accurate mass but are not included in TABLE 3 since they fall below this threshold. Also, there are four proteins detected by LC/MS/MS (TABLE 4) that should have been identified by LC/MS, given that they have theoretical unique masses. The absence of these proteins may be due to the differences in sample preparation and/or extraction methods. Two possible methods can be employed to overcome such obstacles. First, an alternative digestive enzyme that generates different, perhaps larger, peptides can be used in addition to trypsin. Alternatively, such proteins may be identified by sample fractionation prior to trypsin digestion. By analyzing less complex mixtures of peptides, the size of the peaklist is decreased, increasing the probability that a mass will be considered unique. This type of fractionation can be as intensive as the 13-step, 2-D on-line strong ion exchange used by Chao *et al.*,[15] or simpler methods can be employed. Off-line chromatography or pI fractionation of a sample using isoelectric focusing can effectively separate samples for analysis. Techniques such as these, combined with accurate mass, will enable researchers to identify a more complete proteome of *R. prowazekii*. As previously mentioned, accurate mass data also retain intensity values that will allow us to compare the relative abundance of proteins that are differentially expressed from species to species, during changing growth conditions, or during infection of different host cells.

All but one of our insertional mutants is represented in the list of expressed proteins. RP689 is difficult to identify by MS/MS or MS only owing to the high identity to its upstream homologue, RP688. Identification of the remaining proteins suggests that these proteins may be functional and that our mutants may have recognizable phenotypes. To learn more about the functionality of the gene products of this novel pathogen, we are currently examining our mutants for phenotypic and proteomic differences.

In conclusion, the characterization of rickettsial intracellular growth can now be approached by both genetic and proteomic techniques. Rickettsial genome sequences are available which provide gene identification, gene structure, and gene organization information as well as permit genome comparisons between rickettsial species.[18,21,22] Additional sequences are nearing completion. Comparisons of these sequences are leading to a new understanding of the diversity and evolution of this intriguing genus. Analysis of rickettsial protein expression by a variety of proteomic techniques is beginning to uncover rickettsial protein expression patterns and has the potential to identify critical differences during different stages of rickettsial growth, such as the transition from mammalian host to arthropod vector. Such differences could identify valuable targets for effective vaccines or new antimicrobial agents. In addition, it is now possible to generate both random and gene-specific mutations in *R. prowazekii*, opening the door to genetic analysis techniques that have been so successful in dissecting and deciphering gene function in free-living bacteria.

ACKNOWLEDGMENTS

We wish to thank Lonnie Driskell for excellent technical assistance and Brad Leyshon and Julio Ruiz for assistance in developing the accurate mass protocols. We also thank Robert Alecio, Tony Ferrige, and Stuart Ray of Positive Probability, Ltd., for providing critical expertise in the application of the ReSpect™ algorithim and data analysis.

The work was supported by Public Health Service Grants AI020384 and AI055913 from the National Institute of Allergy and Infectious Diseases.

[Competing interests statement: The authors declare that they have no competing interests.]

REFERENCES

1. WEISS, K. 1988. The role of rickettsioses in history. *In* Biology of Rickettsial Diseases, Vol. 1. D.H. Walker, Ed.: 1–14. CRC Press. Boca Raton, FL.
2. REYNOLDS, M.G. *et al.* 2003. Flying squirrel-associated typhus, United States. Emerg. Infect. Dis. **9:** 1341–1343.
3. BOZEMAN, F.M. *et al.* 1975. Epidemic typhus rickettsiae isolated from flying squirrels. Nature **255:** 545–547.
4. RAOULT, D. *et al.* 1998. Outbreak of epidemic typhus associated with trench fever in Burundi. Lancet **352:** 353–358.
5. TARASEVICH, I., E. RYDKINA & D. RAOULT. 1998. Outbreak of epidemic typhus in Russia. Lancet **352:** 1151.
6. Federal Register. 2005. **70**(52)**:** 13317.
7. BALDRIDGE, G.D. *et al.* 2005. Analysis of fluorescent protein expression in transformants of *Rickettsia monacensis*, an obligate intracellular tick symbiont. Appl. Environ. Microbiol. **71:** 2095–2105.
8. QIN, A. *et al.* 2004. Transposon mutagenesis of the obligate intracellular pathogen *Rickettsia prowazekii*. Appl. Environ. Microbiol. **70:** 2816–2822.
9. RACHEK, L.I. *et al.* 2000. Transformation of *Rickettsia prowazekii* to erythromycin resistance encoded by the *Escherichia coli ereB* gene. J. Bacteriol. **182:** 3289–3291.
10. RACHEK, L.I. *et al.* 1998. Transformation of *Rickettsia prowazekii* to rifampin resistance. J. Bacteriol. **180:** 2118–2124.
11. RENESTO, P., E. GOUIN & D. RAOULT. 2002. Expression of green fluorescent protein in *Rickettsia conorii*. Microb Pathog. **33:** 17–21.
12. TROYER, J.M., S. RADULOVIC & A.F. AZAD. 1999. Green fluorescent protein as a marker in *Rickettsia typhi* transformation. Infection and Immunity. **67:** 3308–3311.
13. TUCKER, A.M. *et al.* 2003. S-adenosylmethionine transport in *Rickettsia prowazekii*. J. Bacteriol. **185:** 3031–3035.
14. DRISKELL, L.O. *et al.* 2005. Rickettsial *metK*-encoded methionine adenosyltransferase expression in an *Escherichia coli metK* deletion strain. J. Bacteriol. **187:** 5719–5722.
15. CHAO, C.C. *et al.* 2004. Proteome analysis of Madrid E strain of *Rickettsia prowazekii*. Proteomics **4:** 1280–1292.
16. RENESTO, P. *et al.* 2005. Proteome analysis of *Rickettsia conorii* by two-dimensional gel electrophoresis coupled with mass spectrometry. FEMS Microbiol. Lett. **245:** 231–238.
17. WINKLER, H.H. 1976. Rickettsial permeability: an ADP-ATP transport system. J. Biol. Chem. **251:** 389–396.
18. ANDERSSON, S.G.E. *et al.* 1998. The genome sequence of *Rickettsia prowazekii* and the origin of mitochondria. Nature **396:** 133–143.
19. CARGILE, B.J. & J.L. STEPHENSON, JR. 2004. An alternative to tandem mass spectrometry: isoelectric point and accurate mass for the identification of peptides. Anal. Chem. **76:** 267–275.
20. SMITH, R.D. *et al.* 2002. The use of accurate mass tags for high-throughput microbial proteomics. OMICS J. Integrat. Biol. **6:** 61–90.
21. MCLEOD, M.P. *et al.* 2004. Complete genome sequence of *Rickettsia typhi* and comparison with sequences of other rickettsiae. J. Bacteriol. **186:** 5842–5855.
22. OGATA, H. *et al.* 2001. Mechanisms of evolution in *Rickettsia conorii* and *R. prowazekii*. Science **293:** 2093–2098.

New Perspectives on Rickettsial Evolution from New Genome Sequences of *Rickettsia*, particularly *R. canadensis*, and *Orientia tsutsugamushi*

MARINA E. EREMEEVA,[a] ANUP MADAN,[b] CHRIS D. SHAW,[c] KEVIN TANG,[d] AND GREGORY A. DASCH[a]

[a]*Viral and Rickettsial Zoonoses Branch, National Center for Infectious Diseases, Centers for Disease Control and Prevention, Atlanta, Georgia 30333, USA*

[b]*Laboratory of Neurobiology, University of Iowa, Iowa City, Iowa, USA*

[c]*School of Interactive Arts and Technology, Simon Fraser University Surrey, Surrey, British Columbia, Canada*

[d]*Scientific Resources Program, National Center for Infectious Diseases, Centers for Disease Control and Prevention, Atlanta, Georgia 30333, USA*

ABSTRACT: The complete genome sequences available for eight species of *Rickettsia* and information for other near relatives in the Rickettsiales including *Orientia* and species of Anaplasmataceae are a rich resource for comparative analyses of the evolution of these obligate intracellular bacteria. Differences in these organisms have permitted them to colonize varied intracellular compartments, arthropod vectors, and vertebrate reservoirs in both pathogenic and symbiotic relationships. We summarize some comparative aspects of the genomes of these organisms, paying particular attention to the recently completed sequence for *R. canadensis* McKiel strain and an estimated two-thirds of the genome sequence for a Thailand patient isolate of *Orientia tsutsugamushi*. The *Rickettsia* genomes exhibit a high degree of synteny punctuated by distinctive chromosome inversions and consistent phylogenetic relationships regardless of whether protein coding sequences or RNA genes, concatenated open reading frames or gene regions, or whole genomes are used to construct phylogenetic trees. The aggregate characteristics (number, length, composition, repeat identity) of tandem repeat sequences of *Rickettsia,* which often exhibit recent and rapid divergence between closely related strains and species of bacteria, are also very conserved in *Rickettsia* but differed significantly in *Orientia. O. tsutsugamushi* shared no significant synteny to species of *Rickettsia* or Anaplasmataceae, supporting its placement in a unique genus. Like *Rickettsia felis, Orientia* has many transposases and ankyrin and tetratricopeptide repeat

Address for correspondence: Marina Eremeeva, Viral and Rickettsial Zoonoses Branch, Mail Stop G-13, National Center for Infectious Diseases, Centers for Disease Control and Prevention, 1600 Clifton Road, NE, Atlanta GA 30333. Voice: 404-639-4612; fax: 404-639-4436.
MEremeeva@cdc.gov

NOTE: The findings and conclusions in this report are those of the authors and do not necessarily represent the views of the Centers for Disease Control & Prevention or Department of Health & Human Services.

Ann. N.Y. Acad. Sci. 1063: 47–63 (2005).
doi: 10.1196/annals.1355.006

domains. *Orientia* shares the important ATP/ADP translocase and proline-betaine transporter multigene families with *Rickettsia,* but has more gene families that may be involved in regulatory and transporter responses to environmental stimuli.

KEYWORDS: ***Rickettsia*; *Orientia*; genome; variable number of tandem repeats (VNTR); annotation**

INTRODUCTION

Since the first complete genome sequence of *Rickettsia prowazekii* Madrid E was obtained in 1998 and a close evolutionary relationship of rickettsiae to the ancestor of the mitochondria was proposed,[1] seven more genomes of *Rickettsia* have been sequenced. These include *Rickettsia conorii* strain Malish 7,[2,3] *Rickettsia typhi* Wilmington,[4] *Rickettsia felis* URRWCCal2,[5] *Rickettsia rickettsii* Sheila Smith CWPP (GenBank AADJ01000001), *Rickettsia sibirica* 246 (GenBank AABW000000001),[6] *Rickettsia akari* Hartford CWPP (GenBankAAFE01000001), and *Rickettsia canadensis* McKiel 2678 (present authors). The genomic sequences of *Rickettsia bellii* and *Orientia tsutsugamushi* are also being obtained by several groups, including ours, and it is likely that genome sequences of other species and strains in the Order Rickettsiales will be soon available because of the small genome sizes of these species, the interesting diversity of their microbial, cell-biological and ecological traits, the continued discovery of new rickettsial agents, and their importance for human and veterinary medicine. This additional genomic sequence information provides a vast amount of information for analyzing the evolution and functional organization of the genomes of intracellular organisms during their adaptation to different intracellular niches and hosts. In this paper, we summarize some comparative aspects of the genome sequences of the eight species of *Rickettsia* and first describe some attributes of the genomes of *R. canadensis* and *Orientia tsutsugamushi*.

PROPERTIES AND PHYLOGENY OF *RICKETTSIA CANADENSIS* AND *ORIENTIA TSUTSUGAMUSHI*

McKiel *et al.*[7] first described isolation of a novel rickettsia, *R. canada* [sic] strain 2678. The agent was isolated in embryonated chicken eggs from a pool of *Haemaphysalis leporispalustris* ticks collected from a domestic rabbit used as a sentinel animal in field studies of tick-transmitted diseases in snowshoe hares, *Lepus americanus,* and other small animals in the Richmond area near Ottawa, Ontario, Canada in 1962–63. A second isolate, strain H299, was recovered from a pool of 16 engorged ticks removed from a snowshoe hare shot in October 1964 about 20 miles south of the area where sentinel animals were stationed, but this strain was lost. Inoculation of strain 2678 into guinea pigs, mice, hamsters, and rabbits caused seroconversion of these animals and raised antibodies that cross-reacted with *R. typhi* and *R. prowazekii* in complement fixation tests, but toxin neutralization tests differentiated it from both *R. prowazekii* and *R. typhi.* Subsequent field work failed to detect this agent until another isolate CA410 of *R. canada* was obtained from

TABLE 1. Biological and molecular characteristics of *R. canadensis* shared with either typhus or spotted fever group rickettsiae

Characteristic	Typhus Group	Spotted Fever Group
Tick association		++
Abundant growth in yolk sac	++	
Small plaque formation	++	
Intranuclear growth		++
Hemolytic activity	++	
S-layer type		rOmpA + rOmpB
Lipopolysaccharide type	++	
Cross-protective activity	++	
Genome size		1.33 × TG[a]
G+C%	29.2	

[a]TG, typhus group; the values are obtained based upon DNA reassociation method.[15] The exact numbers are not shown since it appears that the original publication appears to have a systematic error in estimation of rickettsial genome size.

H. leporispalustris tick from a black-tailed jack rabbit, *Lepus californicus,* from Mendocino County in California.[8] Strains 2678 and CA410 differ somewhat in their protein profiles on SDS-polyacrylamide gel electrophoresis (PAGE) and in the reactivity and molecular weight of their rOmpA proteins with monoclonal antibodies as detected by Western blotting,[9] but only strain 2678 has been studied in much detail. Serologic evidence has been described that suggests *R. canadensis* may cause a febrile disease in man.[10]

The biological and phylogenetic placement of *R. canadensis* has been problematic. Some of its properties are summarized in TABLE 1. While *R. canadensis* is antigenically more closely related to typhus group rickettsiae, like pathogenic spotted fever group rickettsiae, it causes a generalized infection in ticks, can be transmitted by ticks, and is maintained trans-stadially and transovarially in them.[11,12] It also invades the nuclei of cells[11] and has both rOmpA and rOmpB proteins like spotted fever rickettsiae.[9,13] On the other hand, like typhus group rickettsiae, *R. canadensis* does not rapidly kill embryonated chicken eggs where it grows to high titers, it hemolyzes red blood cells, it is susceptible to erythromycin, and it forms small plaques more slowly than spotted fever group rickettsiae.[14] It also has a G+C% similar to that of typhus group rickettsiae.[15] By reassociation kinetics measurements, its genome size was estimated to be 35% bigger than those of *R. typhi* and *R. prowazekii* and 15% bigger than that of *R. rickettsii.*[9] *R. canadensis* is readily differentiated from *R. prowazekii* and *R. typhi* by specific activities of the enzymes glutamate dehydrogenase and glutamate oxaloacetate transaminase, its whole-cell protein profiles by SDS PAGE, and isoelectric focusing patterns of soluble proteins.[16] DNA-DNA hybridization[15] and sequence comparisons of specific rickettsial genes like those of 16S rRNA and *gro*EL (FIG. 1) place it at a similar distance from typhus and spotted fever group rickettsiae much like the mite- and flea-transmitted species, *R. akari and R. felis.*[17,18] Similar comparisons with partial sequences of the 17-kDa

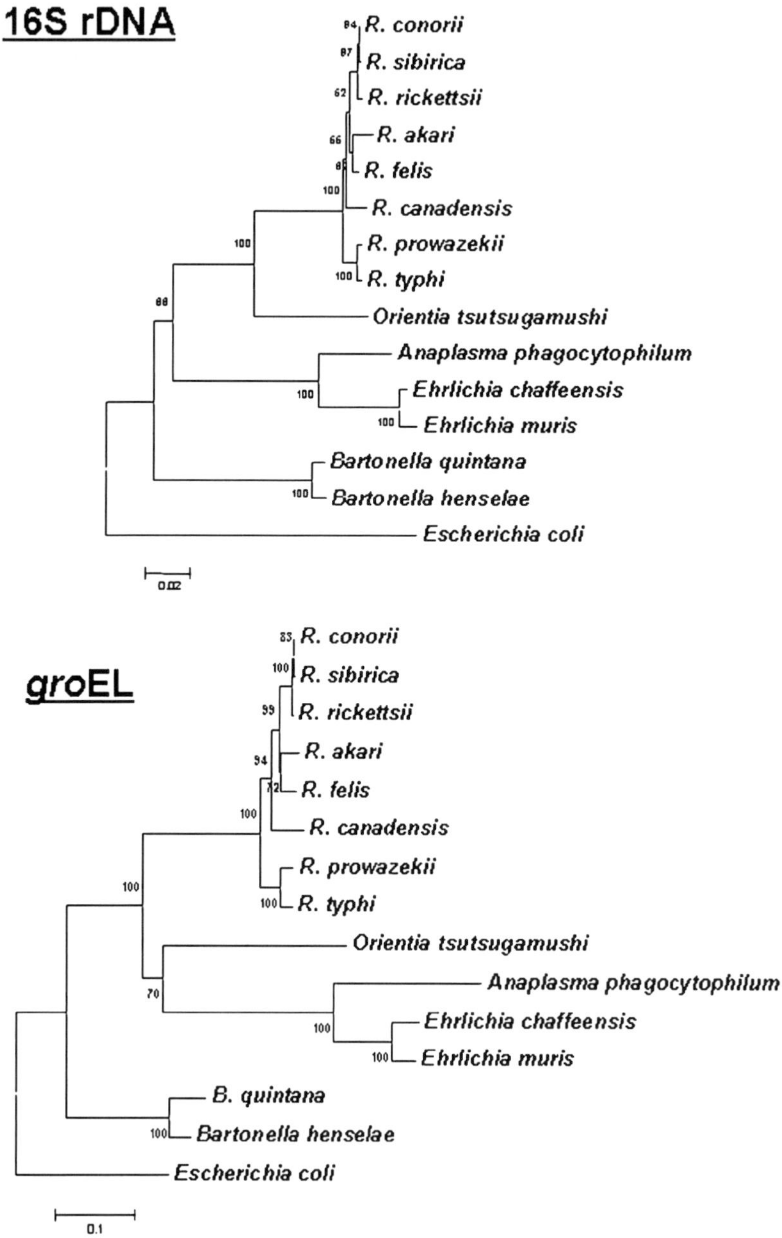

FIGURE 1. Phylogenetic relationships of selected Rickettsiales whose genomic sequences are available. Neighbor-joining phylogenetic trees based on 16S rRNA gene [*top*] and GroEL gene [*bottom*] alignments were drawn using the MEGA2 software.[42] Distance matrix was calculated using Kimura-2 parameters and based on 1,317 sites for 16S rRNA gene and 1,217 sites for GroEL. The scale bar represents % sequence divergence. Numbers at nodes are the percentage of 1,000 bootstrap resamplings that support the topology shown.

antigen, citrate synthase, and 23S rRNA genes have been made.[19–21] These data suggested that *R. canadensis* may be representative of a distinct lineage of rickettsiae which is poorly represented as yet among characterized isolates but which, like *R. bellii,* shares some ancestral characteristics with both classic typhus and spotted fever group rickettsiae; in that sense it may more closely resemble forms ancestral to this genus. Consequently, we obtained the complete genome sequence of the McKiel 2678 strain of *R. canadensis* and present here our initial observations on some of its genomic properties.

Orientia tsutsugamushi is the etiologic agent of scrub typhus, which is transmitted by larvae of numerous species of trombiculid mites. Although it has long been associated with the genus *Rickettsia* because of its similar obligate intracellular growth in the cytoplasm of infected host cells, in 1995 it was reclassified from *Rickettsia* to the genus *Orientia* due to its clear phenotypic and genotypic differences from *Rickettsia.*[22] These traits included its different cell wall structure and apparent lack of peptidoglycan and lipopolysaccharide, also characteristics of the phagosome-enclosed intracellular species in the genera *Anaplasma* and *Ehrlichia* but not *Rickettsia,* which has both molecules.[23] *Orientia* also has a unique profile of antigens and proteins which distinguish it from all the other Rickettsiales.[23,24] Despite its monospecific status and in contrast to species of *Rickettsia*, *O. tsutsugamushi* has long been recognized to exhibit substantial antigenic diversity.[25,26] The widespread application of restriction fragment length polymorphism (RFLP) analysis and DNA sequencing to PCR amplicons obtained from isolates and from infected patient, rodent and chigger samples[27–29] have confirmed that the significant genetic diversity found in this species[28,29] is not confined to the type-specific surface antigen gene, which is predominantly detected in serotyping.[22,26,29]

The 16S rDNA sequences of several prototype strains of *Orientia* formed a cluster with levels of similarity of greater than 98.5%,[30] suggesting that forming new species in this genus is as yet unwarranted. However, this cluster clearly separated *O. tsutsugamushi* from the genus *Rickettsia* (90.2–90.6% similarity) and from the Anaplasmataceae (FIG. 1). Interestingly, unlike the 16S rDNA tree, the phylogenetic tree with groEL gene[31] grouped *Orientia* more closely to *Anaplasma* and *Ehrlichia* than *Rickettsia,* but with a lower bootstrap value than that found with the 16S rDNA sequences (FIG. 1). The G+C% composition of *Orientia* is 28.1–30.5%,[22] a value slightly lower than that found for typhus rickettsiae. The genome size of *Orientia* by pulsed field gel electrophoresis analysis has been reported to be between 2.4 and 2.7 Mbp,[32] about twice that of *Rickettsia* (TABLE 2). Currently, efforts to sequence strains of *Orientia* from Japan (Gilliam-like), Korea (Boryong), Papua/New Guinea (Karp), and Thailand (Northeast border) are under way in other laboratories. In order to assure that some of the genetic diversity found in different isolates of *Orientia* can be analyzed, and because the isolates available from Thailand include many types not reported from other countries,[25,28] we chose to sequence the well-characterized human patient isolate AF PL-12 from Central Thailand.[33] Because this genome is larger than those of *Rickettsia* and it exhibits some of the complexity found in the slightly smaller *Bartonella henselae* genome, as it also contains many repeated regions that were not amenable to completion by direct shotgun sequencing analysis,[34] it may require some concerted effort to complete the *Orientia* genome sequences. Consequently, we report here some of our observations on the estimated 70% (1.57 Mb) of the full genome sequence that has been obtained.

TABLE 2. Putative numbers of open reading frames (ORFs) found in *Rickettsia* chromosomes using different recognition algorithms[a]

Species and Total bp	GenMark	Glimmer	Getorf ATG only (>50 aa)	Getorf with Alt. starts (>50 aa)	NCBI Annotation
R. canadensis *1,159,772*	1,032	1,177	1,505	2,267	MAI[b]
R. felis *1,485,148*	1,512	1,510	2,231	3,263	1,400
R. akari *1,231,204*	1,337	1,285	1,862	2,786	MAI
R. conorii *1,268,755*	1,404	1,532	1,962	2,862	1,374
R. rickettsii *1,257,710*	1,365	1,527	1,914	2,849	MAI
R. sibirica *1,250,021*	1,443	1,357	1,893	2,809	MAI
R. prowazekii *1,111,523*	903	982	1,328	1,889	835
R. typhi *1,111,496*	860	854	1,319	1,879	877

[a]Details on ORF recognition algorithms can be found at the following websites: <http://opal.biology.gatech.edu/GeneMark/>(GenMark), <http://www.genomics.jhu.edu/Glimmer/ (Glimmer), and < http://emboss.sourceforge.net/>(Getorf).

[b]Manual annotation incomplete.

GENERAL ATTRIBUTES OF THE GENOME SEQUENCES OF *R. CANADENSIS* AND SEVEN OTHER SPECIES OF *RICKETTSIA*

Surprisingly, the assembled genome size of 1,159,772 bp for *R. canadensis* was much smaller than that obtained by reassociation kinetics[15] and only about 48 Kb bigger than those of *R. typhi* and *R. prowazekii* (TABLE 2). Its estimated coding capacity based on Glimmer predicted open reading frames was approximately 75.2% and its G+C% content 29% as expected. Like the other species of *Rickettsia* whose genomes have been sequenced, the genome of *R. canadensis* encodes 33 tRNA genes, the three (5S, 16S, and 23S) ribosomal RNA genes, and three other RNA molecules, ssrA (tmRNA), rnpB (RNA component of ribonuclease P), and srp (signal recognition particle 4.5S RNA). Predicted open reading frames (ORF) based completely on automated GenMark and Glimmer analysis are generally close to the final results obtained by manual annotation for the four sequences that have complete annotations at NCBI (TABLE 2). Not surpisingly, assuming complete accuracy in sequencing, this is about ½ of the potential genes with greater than 50 aa size whether restricting the calls to ATG starts or including alternative start codons. This is because GenMark and Glimmer allow overlapping genes on the same strand, but rarely include open reading frames that overlap in opposite orientation, while Getorf is not restricted in this fashion and many small fragments overlap in the opposite orienta-

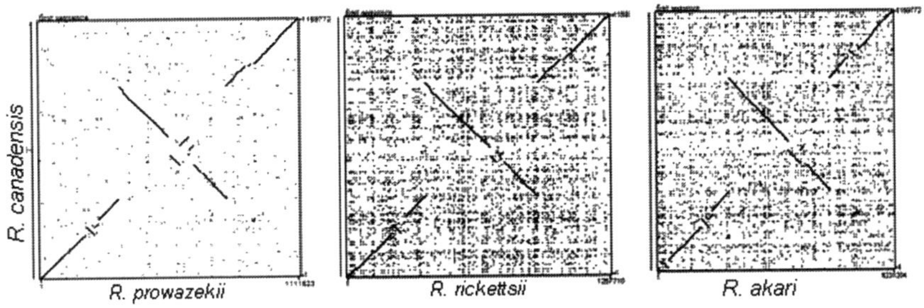

FIGURE 2. PipMaker plot <http://pipmaker.bx.psu.edu/cgi-bin/pipmaker?basic> comparison of genome sequences of *R. canadensis* with genome sequences of three other species of *Rickettsia*.

tion with larger ORFs. Although the number of ORFs predicted by Glimmer and GenMark might be expected to increase relative to *R. prowazekii* and *R. typhi* in direct proportion to their increased genome size, *R. canadensis* (4.3% larger genome, 9.5–37.3% increase in ORFs), the four spotted fever group rickettsiae (10.8–14.2% larger genomes, 13.6–67.5% increase in ORFs) and *R. felis* (33.7% larger genome, 61–76% increase in ORFs) have increasingly more predicted ORFs than expected for their respective % increases in genome sizes. Many of these predicted additional ORFs are small hypothetical "unique" proteins without homologues among these species or to other bacteria. This contrasts with the strong chromosome synteny and high gene homology of most well-identified functional proteins as described below; consequently, the reliability of ORF identification appears to decrease with increased genome size and many of these predicted ORFs may not be expressed or be essential.

PipMaker[35] was used to compare the genome sequence of *R. canadensis* to those of other species of *Rickettsia* (FIG. 2). As is evident from the full genome, strong diagonal lines found on these three plots and all the other pairwise comparisons (not shown) strong conservation of DNA sequences and specific gene orders is evident at both a local operon and genome-wide level among all eight of the genome sequences. This indicates that strong selective pressures have occurred in the genus to preserve the remarkable synteny observed among all of the species of *Rickettsia*. As is true for many other closely related bacteria, a cluster of relative inversions (upper left bottom right diagonals in the figure) has occurred in many of the species opposite the origin of replication (middle of PipPlots), but other parts of these genomes also have inversions less frequently. The presence of a unique large inversion encompassing the middle third of the chromosome was identified in *R. canadensis*. Inversion sites often occur close to tRNA genes. The presence of a significant level of off-diagonal signal is seen in all PipPlot pairwise comparisons including two of the four spotted fever group rickettsiae or three of these organisms (excluding *R. felis*) with *R. canadensis* (FIG. 2). However, the amount of the off-diagonal signal is greatly diminished when comparison is made to the genome sequences of *R. typhi* or *R. prowazekii* (FIG. 2) or between *R. canadensis* and *R. felis* (not shown). This signal appears to be due to conservation of numerous small repetitive DNA elements scattered throughout rickettsial genomes. *R. canadensis* apparently shares more of these elements with spotted fever group rickettsiae than with *R. prowazekii* or *R. typhi*.

TANDEM REPEAT SEQUENCES IN *RICKETTSIA* AND *ORIENTIA*

A wide variety of repetitive sequence elements are found in bacteria. These range from duplicated genes which exhibit varying degrees of homology like the ATP/ADP translocase genes, proline-betaine transporters, and *sca* gene families in *Rickettsia*, to the small palindromic repeat elements which are found in both coding and non-coding DNA, and direct large repetitive protein domains found in varying number in the rOmpA proteins. For the eight *Rickettsia* genomes and partial *Orientia* sequence we have examined in some detail the properties of repeated sequences (VNTR-variable number of tandem repeats) that vary in their copy number, composition, period length, and the amount and type of homology present between individual repeat copies (FIG. 3). The prevalence and complexity of VNTR vary widely among different species of bacteria. VNTR are thought to be fast-evolving loci because the number of repeats is commonly affected by slippage during replication. VNTR loci can be used to fingerprint differences between closely related strains and are therefore powerful tools for forensic science and molecular epidemiology.

A tandem repeat finder program was used to identify VNTR sites in all eight species of *Rickettsia* and in the partial sequence of *Orientia* available (FIG. 3).[36] The number of repeats was fairly similar among the species of *Rickettsia,* and differences did not correlate well with genome size or closest relative since *R. sibirica* (1.25 Mb) had the fewest repeats (347) while *R. typhi* (1.11 Mb) with 459 approached that of *R. felis* (1.49 Mb), which had 493 (FIG. 3A). However, the *Orientia* sequence (1.57 Mb), which was only slightly greater than that of *R. felis*, had more than 200 more repeats; it also differed markedly in the number of larger repeats than those found in *Rickettsia*. In species of both genera the vast majority of repeats had a very low copy number between 2 and 3 and the distribution of repeats with copy number was very similar. Not surprisingly, given the low G+C% composition of the total DNAs of these nine species, the VNTR also had a decided bias toward a low G+C% (FIG. 3B). However, the distributions of VNTRs for all species were greatly skewed toward values less than the average genome compositions. This is somewhat surprising as typically two-thirds of the VNTR are located within coding sequences which are somewhat higher in G+C% than intergenic regions. However, factors contributing to increases in the numbers of these low G+C% VNTRs may have also influenced the accumulation of A and T in these genomes that lowered their overall compositions. *Orientia*, and to a lesser extent *R. felis*, were atypical in having a greater number of VNTRs with high G+C% than the other species.

The presence of exact repeats of sequences provides a possible site for unequal homologous recombination, which may lead to loss or corresponding gain in the number of copies of a repeat between the two chromosomes exchanging the repeats. This may be responsible for alterations in the number of rOmpA 72 and 75 amino acid repeats in different strains of *R. conorii* and *R. rickettsii*.[37,38] On a smaller scale different strains of *R. rickettsii* have insertion/deletion (indel) events that may have occurred in this fashion,[39] and differences in homologous genes often occur in the number of copies of tandem repeats found in different species.[40] Alterations in the repeats that make them imperfect repeats may be less subject to these events. Consequently, we examined the extent to which imperfect repeats were included in the VNTR regions of the eight *Rickettsia* genome sequences and for *Orientia* and then the number of repeats with indel events. In different species 38–50% of VNTRs ex-

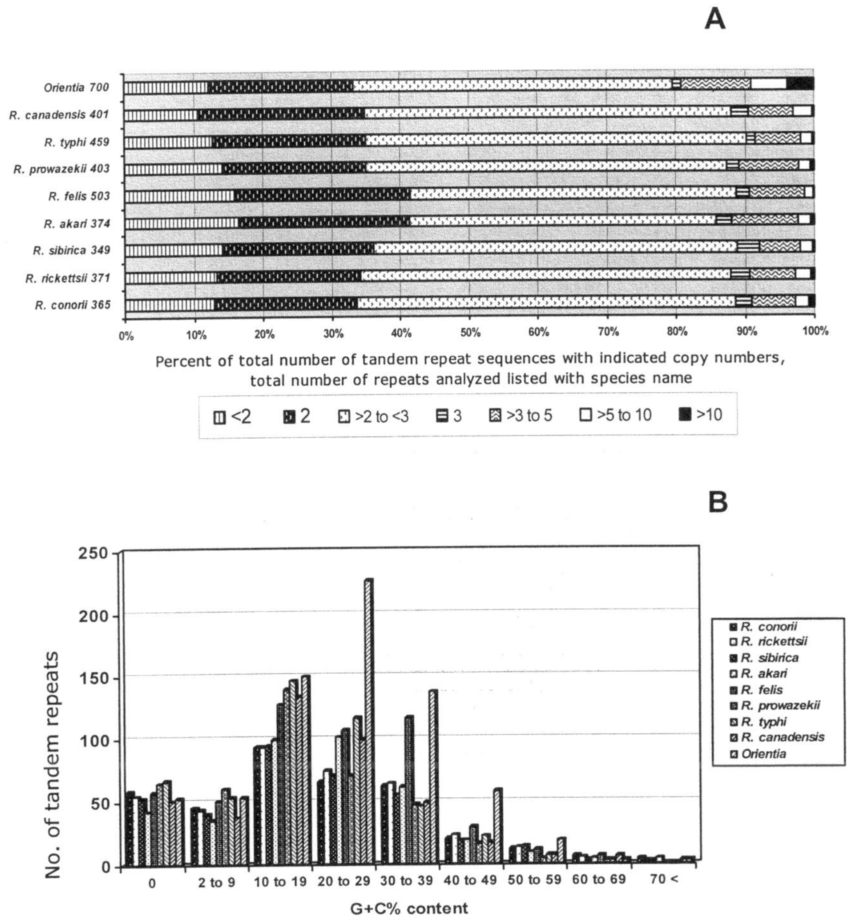

FIGURE 3. Comparative analysis of tandem repeat sequences found in genome sequences of eight *Rickettsia* and *Orientia*. (**A**) Percentage of repeats with different copy numbers (total number of repeats given beside each species name). (**B**) Distribution by G+C% composition of number of tandem repeat sequences.

hibited complete identity and another 30–42% exhibited 90–98% repeat sequence identity so these constituted the majority of VNTRs (FIG. 3C). Typically about 13–16% of the VNTR had 80–89% identity and only 2–4% had 70–79% identity. An even smaller number of indels were found in each of the species as 72–74% lacked indels and another 3–6% had only 1–5% of nucleotides as indels; 13–18% had 1–2 nucleotides as indels out of 20 in a VNTR (FIG. 3D). Consequently, one would expect that variation in VNTR copy numbers could be a significant source of inter and intraspecies variation in both *Rickettsia* and *Orientia*, and, other than the total number of sites available for evolutionary change by various genetic processes, these organisms are very similar in their VNTR characteristics.

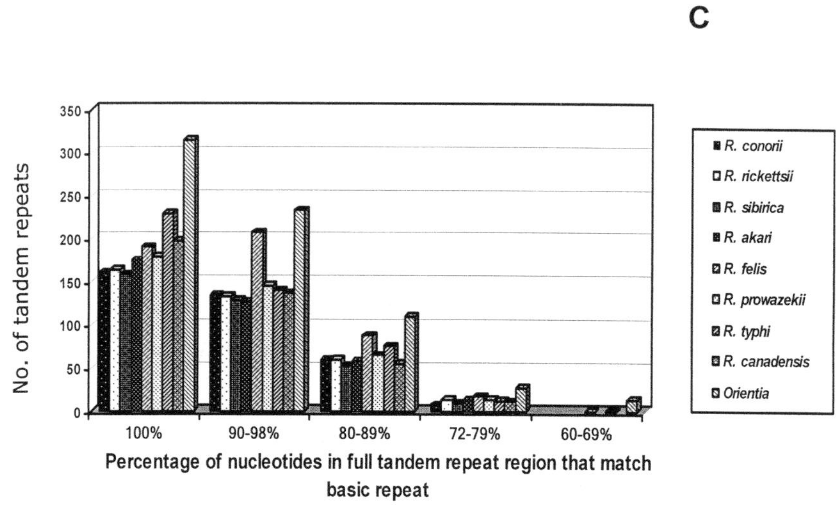

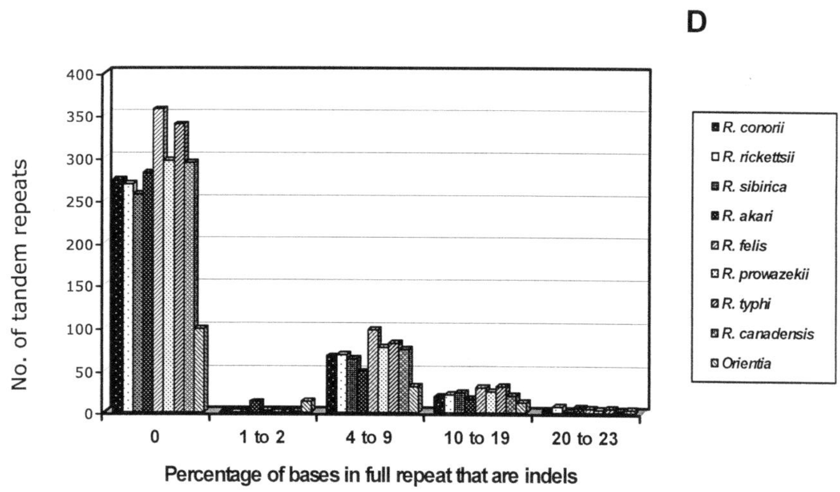

FIGURE 3—***continued.*** **(C)** Distribution of number of repeats by percentage of sequence homology to the individual repeat unit. **(D)** Prevalence of percentage of indel nucleotides in the tandem repeat sequences.

PHYLOGENETIC RELATIONSHIPS AMONG SPECIES OF *RICKETTSIA* AND *ORIENTIA*

As has been discussed above and shown in FIGURE 1, various genes have been used to examine phylogenetic relationships among different rickettsiae. Most commonly these have included 16S rRNA, *gro*EL, 17-kDa and 120-kDa cytoplasmic antigen genes, and rOmpA and rOmpB species-specific antigens, *rpo*B and *glt*A. Some

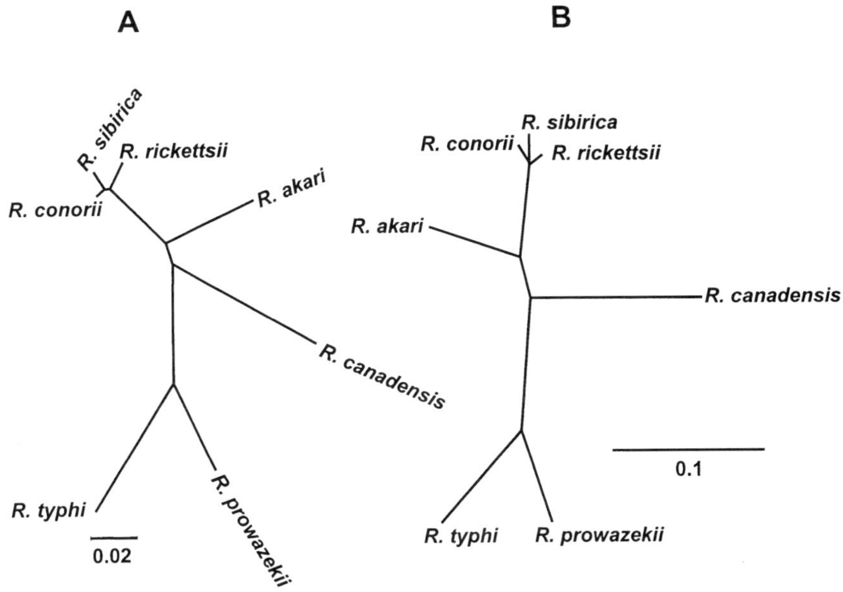

FIGURE 4. **(A)** Phylogenetic analysis of 14 concatenated T4SS complex protein sequences (8,032 amino acid sites of homologues of RT0034, RP103-RP108, RP286-RP291, RP294, and RP784) of *Rickettsia* constructed as in FIGURE 1. **(B)** *Rickettsia* phylogeny based on whole genome sequence comparisons using Mavid.[43]

of these genes exhibit relatively little variation (17-kDa and 16S rRNA), while others, like the 120-kDa, rOmpB and rpoB genes, have evolved more rapidly. In principle this type of analysis can be done for every gene that is present in all of the species of the genus (a limitation for rOmpA) or it is possible to concatenate a series of genes before tree construction to obtain an overall average for the species. In fact most of the individual gene trees have a very similar shape, with occasional exchanges of positions with poorly supported bootstrap values. Because many of the type 4 secretion system proteins (T4SS) are very large and are thought to be essential for intracellular life by all the species in the Rickettsiales, they appear to be an excellent choice for construction of phylogenetic trees (FIG. 4A). Indeed a tree constructed by examining the full genome sequences (FIG. 4B) greatly resembled that for the T4SS proteins, further supporting the validity of this approach. Because many T4SS proteins have now been identified in *Orientia* and in the Anaplasmataceae, we also constructed a phylogenetic tree for some of the VirB4 protein homologues (FIG. 5). This tree clearly places *Orientia* more closely to *Rickettsia* than to Anaplasmataceae, a result similar to that obtained for the 16S rDNA tree (FIG. 1). However, it also supports the taxonomic placement of *Orientia* as a unique genus.

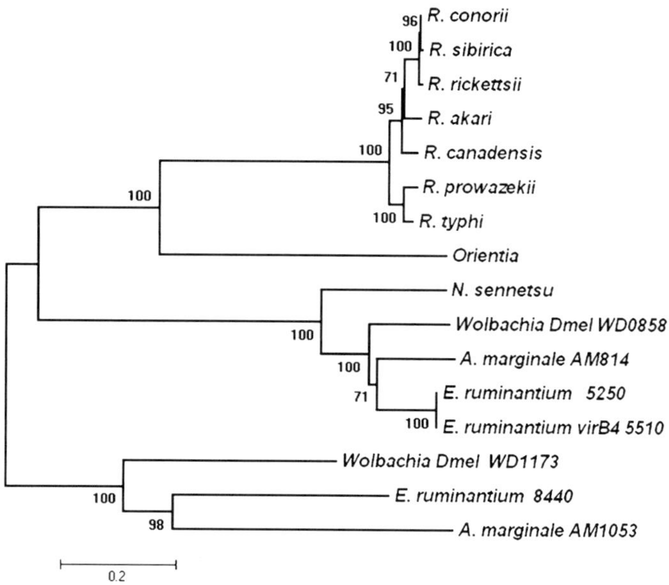

FIGURE 5. Phylogenetic relationship VirB4 amino acid sequences of species of Rickettsiales. Neighbor-joining phylogenetic tree based on VirB4 amino acid sequence similarities (738 sites) was drawn using the MEGA2 software as described in FIGURE 1. NCBI entrez genome identifiers are indicated for ORFs of species with paralogous sequences used in the tree.

SOME IMPORTANT ATTRIBUTES OF *ORIENTIA* FROM ITS PARTIAL ANNOTATION

Although the full sequence of the *Orientia* genome is not yet available, it contained 27 tRNA genes, the 5S, 16S, and 23S rRNA genes, DNA encoding signal recognition particle protein Ffh and its receptor FtsY, but not signal-recognition protein RNA, the RNA of ribonuclease P (*rnp*B) but not the protein gene (*rnp*A), and the tmRNA binding protein but not the tmRNA (*ssr*A). Only one of the 27 tRNA genes encoded a tRNA (Leu-CAA) that was not used by the species of *Rickettsia* but it is present in *Anaplasma marginale*, *Wolbachia* TRS and Dmel, and *Ehrlichia ruminantium*. Homologues were also found for other genes previously described for *Orientia* such as the 56-kDa and 47-kDa antigen genes, superoxide dismutase, and a 3,082-bp PCR target (GenBank L23765), but not the 22-kD antigen or groESL operon. The ADP/ATP translocase family of *Rickettsia* had three *Orientia* homologues (*tlc*1, 2, and 5) and the *Rickettsia* proline/betaine transporter family had four homologues in *Orientia*. The concatenated contigs obtained for the genome of *Orientia* were compared with the genome sequences of three species of Anaplasmataceae, *Anaplasma phagocytophilum*, *Neorickettsia sennetsu*, and *Wolbachia pipientis* from *Drosophila melanogaster* and to *R. canadensis* using PipMaker (FIG. 6). No strong diagonal lines were observed, in contrast to the results shown in FIGURE 2. Some off-diagonal signal was obtained with all four genomes, but particularly with *R. canadensis*. Unsuccessful attempts to identify genes with BLAST using nucleotide searches of nucleotide databases confirmed the strong evolutionary divergence of *Orientia* from the others, as shown in FIGS. 1 and 5. However, protein BLAST and SMART (Simple Modular Architecture Research Tool)[37] analyses of putative open reading frames identified using Glimmer and a new annotation tool called IMASS (developed by CS and GD) lead to the recognition of some significant attributes of the *Orientia* genome. First, a large number of repeated elements are present in the *Orientia* genome, most notably including 19 SMART domains found in more than one ORF, most frequently the 56 histidine kinase-like ATPases domains (HATPase-c) and the 37 domains found in ATPases associated with a variety of cellular activities (AAA) (TABLE 3). The number and type of SMART domains detected suggest that *Orientia* has a much larger range of regulatory proteins involved in responses to environmental stimuli than any known for *Rickettsia* including *R. felis*.[6] *R. felis* is also unusual among species of *Rickettsia* in having two plasmids, 82 transposase genes, 8 phage-related proteins, 22 ankyrin- and 11 tetratricopeptide (TPR)-containing ORFs.[6] In *Orientia* 82 transposase domains of six types have been detected (41 copies of transposase 11, 21 of transposase 14, 9 of transposase 31, 5 each of transposases 9 and 20, and 1 of transposase 8). The 42 ankyrin domain proteins found in *Orientia* varied in the numbers of repeats present (1–9), their lengths (28–56), sequences, and repeat patterns, and the sizes of their ORFs (57–938). TPR-containing ORFs were also common in *Orientia* and, although their repeat length was generally 34 amino acids, the number of repeats and sizes of

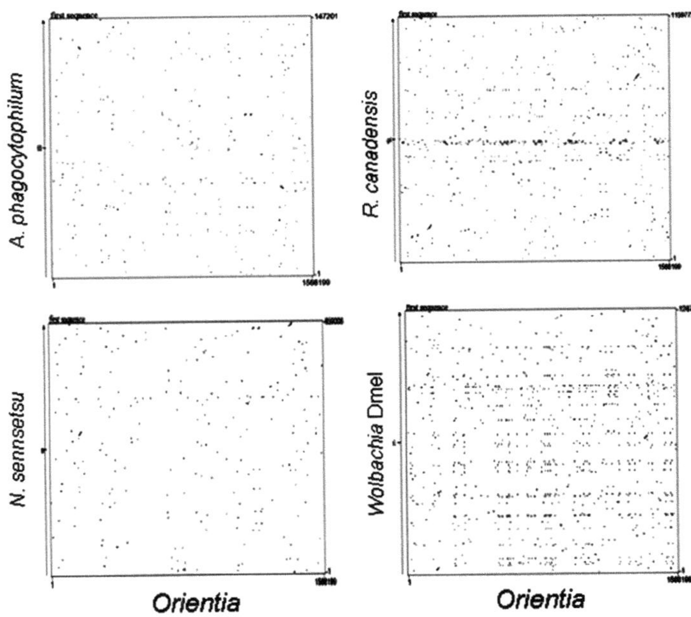

FIGURE 6. PipMaker Plot comparison of the genome sequences of *Orientia* with four other species of Rickettsiales.

TABLE 3. Type and prevalence of 223 SMART domains[a] found in the partial genome sequence of *Orientia*

SMART Domains Detected	No. Found
HATPase_c (histidine kinase-like ATPases)	56
AAA (ATPases associated with a variety of cellular activities)	37
HDc (metal-dependent phosphohydrolases with conserved "HD" motif)	23
HhH1 (helix-hairpin-helix DNA-binding motif class 1)	12
KH (K homology RNA-binding domain)	10
REC (cheY-homologous receiver domain)	7
S1 (ribosomal protein S1-like RNA-binding domain)	6
HisKA (his kinase A phosphoacceptor domain)	5
Elp3 (elongator protein 3, MiaB family, radical SAM)	4
CBS, HNHc, HTH_XRE, PHB, TOPRIM	3 each
DNAJ, KOW, PDZ, PlsC, S4	2 each
53EXOc, Ami_2, BHL, BRCT, CSP, DESDc, DSRM, DUF1, DUF2, ENDO3c, FES, GuKc, HELICc, HhH2, NHN_nucleases, LIGANc, LON, MUTSac, MUTSd, NGN, PAC, ParB, PBPb, PLDc, POLAc, rADc, RHOD, RIBOc, RL11, RPOLA_N, RPOLD, small_GTPase, STYKc, TOP1Ac, TOP1Bc, TOP2c, YqgFc, ZnF_C2HC, ZnF_CHCC	1 each

[a]<http://smart.embl.de>

TABLE 4. High-quality identification of some *Orientia* genes by BLAST

Conserved Genes	High-Interest Genes
endonuclease III (*nth*)	2-acylglycerophosphoethanolamine acyl-transferase-2 (*aas*)
ATP-dependent nuclease subunit A (*add*A)	3-octaprenyl-4-hydroxybenzoate carboxy-lyase (*ubi*X)
NAD-dependent DNA ligase (*lig*A)	ADP, ATP carrier protein (*tlc*2)
excinuclease A subunit (*uvr*A)	hemolysin C (*tly*C)
DNA mismatch repair protein MutS (*mut*S)	GTP-binding protein Era (*era*)
elongation factor P (*efp*)	heme exporter protein C (*ccm*C)
histidyl tRNA synthetase (*his*S)	nitrogen assimilation protein (*ntr*X)
isoleucyl-tRNA synthetase- (*ile*S)	nitrogen regulation protein (*ntr*Y)
lysyl-tRNA synthetase (*lys*S)	proton-sodium glutamate symport protein (*glt*P)
poly(A) polymerase (*pcn*B)	outer membrane assembly protein (*asm*A)
replicative DNA helicase (*dna*B)	signal peptidase I (*lep*B)
ribonuclease III (*rnc*)	dihydrodipicolinate synthetase (*dap*A)
succinyl CoA synthetase, alpha subunit (*suc*D)	integrase/recombinase (*xer*D)

the ORFs containing TPR varied considerably. Given the many elements *Orientia* shares with *R. felis*, which has two plasmids, including the numerous plasmid- and conjugation-related proteins, it would not be very surprising if some isolates of *Orientia* also have plasmids and may be capable of conjugation.

ACKNOWLEDGMENTS

The studies reported in this article were supported by NIAID Grants AI05326-01 and 50942. The authors thank our international fellows, Truong Thang and Jui-Shan Ma, and our student interns, Collins Rainey, Holly Lemon-Steiner, Shwante Rogers, Erin Humbles, Noe Galvan, Albert Garcia, Cheryl Chow, Sasha Yurgionas, Drew MacKellar, Nina Tioleco, Matt Erdman, and Sara Scherer, for their assistance in the annotations of the *Rickettsia* and *Orientia* genome sequences.

M. E. Eremeeva and A. Madan contributed equally to this work.

REFERENCES

1. ANDERSSON, S.G., A. ZOMORODIPOUR, J.O. ANDERSSON, *et al.* 1998. The genome sequence of *Rickettsia prowazekii* and the origin of mitochondria. Nature **396:** 133–140.
2. OGATA, H., S. AUDIC, V. BARBE, *et al.* 2000. Selfish DNA in protein-coding genes of *Rickettsia*. Science **290:** 347–350.
3. OGATA, H., S. AUDIC, P. RENESTO-AUDIFFREN, *et al.* 2001. Mechanisms of evolution in *Rickettsia conorii* and *R. prowazekii*. Science **293:** 2093–2098.
4. MCLEOD, M.P., X. QIN, S.E. KARPATHY, *et al.* 2004. Complete genome sequence of *Rickettsia typhi* and comparison with sequences of other rickettsiae. J. Bacteriol. **186:** 5842–5855.
5. OGATA, H., P. RENESTO, S. AUDIC, *et al.* 2005 The genome sequence of *Rickettsia felis* identifies the first putative conjugative plasmid in an obligate intracellular parasite. PLoS Biol **3:** e248.
6. MALEK, J.A., J.M. WIERZBOWSKI, W. TAO, *et al.* 2004. Protein interaction mapping on a functional shotgun sequence of *Rickettsia sibirica*. Nucleic Acids Res. **32:** 1059–1064.
7. MCKIEL, J.A., E.J. BELL, & D.B. LACKMAN. 1967. *Rickettsia canada*: a new member of the typhus group of rickettsiae isolated from *Haemaphysalis leporispalustris* ticks in Canada. Can. J. Microbiol. **13:** 503–510.
8. LANE, R.S., R.N. PHILIP & E.A. CASPER. 1981. Ecology of tick-borne agents in California. II. Further observations on rickettsiae. *In* Rickettsiae and Rickettsial Diseases. W. Burgdorfer & R. L. Anacker Eds.: 575–584. Academic Press. New York.
9. CHING, W.-M., G.A. DASCH, M. CARL & M.E. DOBSON. 1990. Structural analyses of the 120-kDa serotype protein antigens of typhus group rickettsiae: comparison with other S-layer proteins. Ann. N.Y. Acad. Sci. **590:** 334–351.
10. BOZEMAN, F.M., B L. ELISBERG, J.W. HUMPHRIES, *et al.* 1970. Serologic evidence of *Rickettsia canada* infection of man. J. Infect. Dis. **121:** 367–371.
11. BURGDORFER, W. 1968. Observations on *Rickettsia canada*, a recently described member of the typhus group rickettsiae. J. Hyg. Epid. Microbiol. Immunol. **12:** 26–31.
12. BRINTON, L.P. & W. BURGDORFER. 1971. Fine structure of *Rickettsia canada* in tissues of *Dermacentor andersoni* Stiles. J. Bacteriol. **105:** 1149–1159.
13. DASCH, G.A. & A.L. BOURGEOIS. 1981. Antigens of the typhus group of rickettsiae: importance of the species-specific surface protein antigens in eliciting immunity. *In* Rickettsiae and Rickettsial Diseases. W. Burgdorfer & R. L. Anacker Eds.: 61–70. Academic Press. New York.
14. WOODMAN, D.R., E. WEISS, G.A. DASCH & F.M. BOZEMAN. 1977. Biological properties of *Rickettsia prowazekii* strains isolated from flying squirrels. Infect. Immunol. **16:** 853–860.

15. MYERS, W.F. & C.L. WISSEMAN, JR. 1981. The taxonomic relationship of *Rickettsia canada* to the typhus and spotted fever groups of the genus *Rickettsia*. *In* Rickettsiae and Rickettsial Diseases. W. Burgdorfer & R. L. Anacker Eds.: 313–325. Academic Press. New York.
16. DASCH, G.A., J.R. SAMMS & E. WEISS. 1978. Biochemical characteristics of typhus group rickettsiae with special attention to the *Rickettsia prowazekii* strains isolated from flying squirrels. Infect. Immunol. **19:** 676–685.
17. STOTHARD, D.R., & P.A. FUERST. 1995. Evolutionary analysis of the spotted fever and typhus groups of *Rickettsia* using 16S rRNA gene sequences. Syst. Appl. Microbiol. **18:** 52–61.
18. ROUX, V., & D. RAOULT. 1995. Phylogenetic analysis of the genus *Rickettsia* by 16S rDNA sequencing. Res. Microbiol. **146**: 385–396.
19. AZAD, A.F., J.B. SACCI, JR., W.M. NELSON, *et al.* 1992. Genetic characterization and transovarial transmission of a typhus-like rickettsia found in cat fleas. Proc. Natl. Acad. Sci. USA **89:** 43–46.
20. ROUX, V., E. RYDKINA, M. EREMEEVA & D. RAOULT. 1997. Citrate synthase gene comparison, a new tool for phylogenetic analysis, and its application for the rickettsiae. Int. J. Syst. Bacteriol. **47:** 252–261.
21. ANDERSSON, S.G., D.R. STOTHARD, P. FUERST & C.G. KURLAND. 1999. Molecular phylogeny and rearrangement of rRNA genes in *Rickettsia* species. Mol. Biol. Evol. **16:** 987–995.
22. TAMURA, A., N. OHASHI, H. URAKAMI & S. MIYAMURA. 1995. Classification of *Rickettsia tsutsugamushi* in a new genus, *Orientia* gen. nov., as *Orientia tsutsugamushi* comb. nov. Int. J. Syst. Bacteriol. **45**: 589–591.
23. DASCH, G.A., E. WEISS & J.C. WILLIAMS. 1990. Antigenic properties of the Ehrlichiae and other Rickettsiaceae. *In* Ehrlichiosis: A Vector-borne Disease of Animals and Humans. J.C. Williams & I. Kakokma, Eds.: 32–58. Kluwer. Dordrecht, the Netherlands.
24. OAKS, E.V., R.M. Rice, D.J. KELLY & C.K. STOVER. 1999. Antigenic and genetic relatedness of eight *Rickettsia tsutsugamushi* antigens. Infect. Immunol. **57:** 249–253.
25. ELISBERG, B.L., J.M. CAMPBELL & F.M. BOZEMAN. 1968. Antigenic diversity of *Rickettsia tsutsugamushi*: epidemiologic and ecologic significance. J. Hyg. Epidemiol. Microbiol. Immunol.**12:** 18–25.
26. MURATA, M., Y. YOSHIDA, M. OSONO, *et al.* 1986. Production and characterization of monoclonal strain-specific antibodies against prototype strains of *Rickettsia tsutsugamushi*. Microbiol. Immunol. **30:** 599–610.
27. KELLY, D., G.A. DASCH, T.C. CHAN & T.M. HO. 1994. Detection and characterization of *Rickettsia tsutsugamushi* (Rickettsiales: Rickettsiaceae) in infected *Leptotrombidium (Leptotrombidium) fletcheri* chiggers (Acari: Trombiculidae) with the polymerase chain reaction. J. Med. Entomol. **31:** 691–699.
28. DASCH, G.A., D. STRICKMAN, G. WATT & C. EAMSILA. 1996. Measuring genetic varibililty in *Orientia tsutsugamushi* by PCR/RFLP analysis: a new approach to questions about its epidemiology, evolution, and ecology. *In* Rickettsiae and Rickettsial Diseases. J. Kazar & R. Toman, Eds.: 79–84. VEDA. Bratislava, Slovak Republic.
29. TAMURA, A. 1999. Genetic diversity in *Orientia tsutsugamushi*. *In* Rickettsiae and Rickettsial Diseases at the Turn of the Third Millenium. D. Raoult & P. Brouqui, Eds. : 67–73. Elsevier. Paris.
30. OHASHI, N., M. FUKUHARA, M. SHIMADA & A. TAMURA. 1995. Phylogenetic position of *Rickettsia tsutsugamushi* and relationship among its antigenic variants by analyses of 16S rRNA gene sequences. FEMS Microbiol. Lett. **125:** 299–304.
31. STOVER, C.K., D. MARANA, G. DASCH & E. OAKS. 1990. Molecular cloning and sequence analysis of the Sta58 major antigen gene of *Rickettsia tsutsugamushi*: sequence homology and antigenic comparison of Sta58 to the 60-kilodalton family of stress proteins. Infect. Immunol. **58:** 2076–2084.
32. TAMURA, A. 1996. Overview of *Orientia tsutsugamushi* based on recent findings. *In* Rickettsiae and Rickettsial Diseases. J. Kazar & R. Toman, Eds.: 62–71. VEDA. Bratislava, Slovak Republic.

33. Strickman, D., C.D. Smith, K.D. Corcoran, *et al.* 1994. Pathology of *Rickettsia tsutsugamushi* infection in *Bandicota savilei*, a natural host in Thailand. Am. J. Trop. Med. Hyg. **51:** 416–423.
34. Alsmark, C.M., A.C. Frank, E.O. Karlberg, *et al.* 2004. The louse-borne human pathogen *Bartonella quintana* is a genomic derivative of the zoonotic agent *Bartonella henselae*. Proc. Natl. Acad. Sci. USA **101:** 9716–9721.
35. Schwartz, S., Z. Zhang, K.A. Frazer, *et al.* 2000. PipMaker: a web server for aligning two genomic DNA sequences. Genome Res. **10:** 577–586.
36. Benson, G. 1999. Tandem repeats finder: a program to analyze DNA sequences. Nucleic Acids Res. **27:** 573–580.
37. Walker, D.H., H.M. Feng, J.I. Saada, *et al.* 1995. Comparative antigenic analysis of spotted fever group rickettsiae from Israel and other closely related organisms. Am. J. Trop. Med. Hyg. **52:** 569–576.
38. Matsumoto, M., Y. Tange, T. Okada, *et al.* 1996. Deletion in the 190 kDa antigen gene repeat region of *Rickettsia rickettsii*. Microb. Pathog. **20:** 57–62.
39. Eremeeva, M.E., R.M. Klemt, L.A. Santucci-Domotor, *et al.* 2003. Genetic analysis of isolates of *Rickettsia rickettsii* that differ in virulence. Ann. N.Y. Acad. Sci. **990:** 717–722.
40. Gilmore, R.D., Jr. 1993. Comparison of the rompA gene repeat regions of rickettsiae reveals species-specific arrangements of individual repeating units. Gene **125:** 97–102.
41. Letunic, I., R.R. Copley, S. Schmidt, *et al.* 2004. SMART 4.0: towards genomic data integration. Nucleic Acids Res. **32** [database issue]**:** D142–D144.
42. Kumar, S., K. Tamura, I.B. Jakobsen & M. Nei. 2001. MEGA2: Evolutionary genetics analysis software. Bioinformatics **17:** 1244–1245.
43. Bray, N. & L. Pachter. 2004. MAVID: constrained ancestral alignment of mutiple sequences. Genome Res. **14:** 693–699.
44. Shaw, C.D., M.E. Eremeeva, H.H. Shah & G.A. Dasch. 2005. Development of an Interactive Multigenome Analysis System (IMASS) for annotation of bacterial sequences. Abstract 52 (F). 2005 American Society for Microbiology Biodefense Research Meeting, Baltimore, MD.

Preliminary Assessment of Genome Differences between the Reference Nine Mile Isolate and Two Human Endocarditis Isolates of *Coxiella burnetii*

PAUL A. BEARE,[a] STEPHEN F. PORCELLA,[b] REKHA SESHADRI,[c]
JAMES E. SAMUEL,[d] AND ROBERT A. HEINZEN[a]

[a]*Coxiella Pathogenesis Section, Laboratory of Intracellular Parasites, and* [b]*Genomics Core Facility, Rocky Mountain Laboratories, NIAID, NIH, Hamilton, Montana 59840, USA*

[c]*Institute for Genomic Research, Rockville, Maryland 20850, USA*

[d]*Department of Medical Microbiology and Immunology, Texas A&M University, College Station, Texas 77843, USA*

ABSTRACT: **This study investigates the complete genome sequences of the Nine Mile, K, and G isolates to improve our understanding of the unique virulence properties of *C. burnetii* and to provide important insight into the genome architecture and genetic diversity of this pathogen.**

KEYWORDS: **endocarditis; genome; sequencing; Q fever; comparative genomics**

INTRODUCTION

Acute Q fever typically arises from inhalation of aerosolized bacteria and has protean influenzae-like manifestations such as periorbital headache, fever, and malaise. Workers in animal husbandry and other domestic livestock operations are at greatest risk of contracting disease. Rare chronic disease can occur, typically manifested as endocarditis or hepatitis, and there is recognition that these infections are increasing worldwide. *Coxiella* is a class III biohazard and a CDC select agent with potential for illegitimate use. A licensed vaccine for immunization against Q fever is not available in the United States (reviewed in Maurin and Raoult[1]).

C. burnetii is an obligate intracellular bacterium that replicates within an acidic vacuole with lysosomal characteristics.[1] Few virulence determinants are defined for the organism, but they likely include factors that allow survival and replication in its hostile intracellular niche and resistance to the host's innate and adaptive immune

Address for correspondence: Robert A. Heinzen, Rocky Mountain Laboratories, 903 S. 4th St., Hamilton, MT 59840. Voice: 406-375-9695; fax: 406-363-9380.
rheinzen@niaid.nih.gov

Ann. N.Y. Acad. Sci. 1063: 64–67 (2005).
doi: 10.1196/annals.1355.007

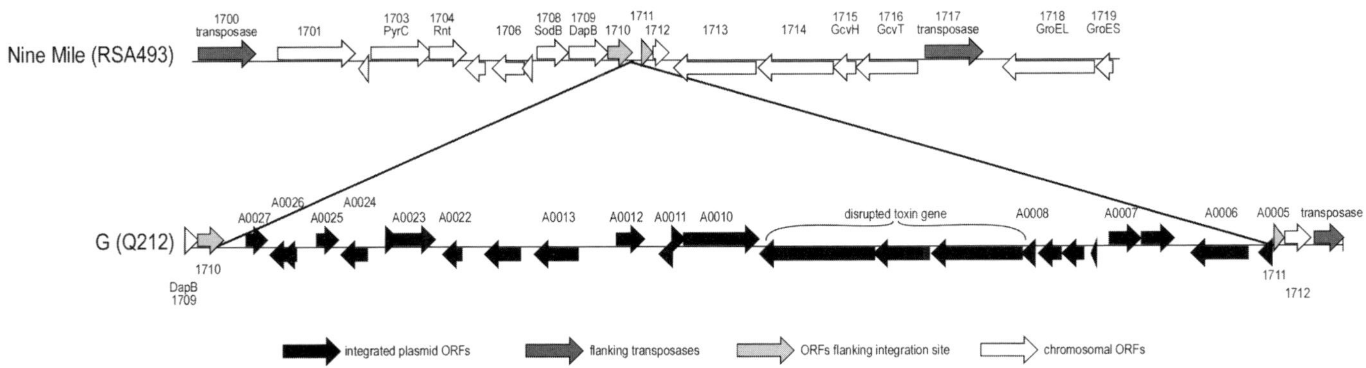

FIGURE 1. Insertion site in the G genome of a 16,624-bp DNA fragment containing QpRS plasmid-like sequences.

responses. Virulence genes would also include those that direct *Coxiella* biphasic development to produce a small cell variant that is resistant to environmental stress and remains infectious in contaminated soils for several years.[2]

Debate continues on whether a correlation exists between gene content and pathogenic potential of *C. burnetii* isolates. Early studies on a limited number of isolates showed isolates such as K and G from human chronic disease patients differ genetically from acute disease isolates.[3,4] This association became less firm with the analysis of more isolates.[1]

The genome sequence of the Nine Mile phase I (RSA493) isolate, biologically representative of human acute disease isolates, was recently deciphered.[5] It is roughly 2 megabases in size and encodes 2094 open reading frames (ORFs). To further evaluate the genetic diversity of *C. burnetii*, we are currently sequencing the genomes of the K (Q154) and G (Q212) isolates, human chronic endocarditis isolates that maintain an autonomously replicating plasmid and integrated plasmid sequences, respectively. A preliminary report is provided here.

MATERIALS AND METHODS

C. burnetii was propagated in embryonated hens' eggs and genomic DNA was purified as previously described.[3] Protein encoding ORFs were predicted by GLIMMER[6] using default parameters. ORFs were searched against a nonredundant amino acid database.

RESULTS AND DISCUSSION

Analysis was conducted on K and G genomes that are currently in the manual finishing stage and consisting of approximately 50 contigs each. Initial Blast searches and genome alignments indicate a high degree of synteny with the Nine Mile I genome. However, upon closer inspection, regions containing novel genes, rearrangements, or insertions/deletions are present in both genomes. For example, K and G are missing a number of genes between CBU0949 and CBU0954 (data not shown). Some of these deleted genes are predicted as nonfunctional in Nine Mile I,[5] and their loss therefore likely reflects ongoing reductive evolution. These plasticity-like zones are frequently flanked by transposon-like sequences. Genomic context and DNA Blast comparisons of predicted chromosomal ORFs indicate that the K and G genomes are more similar to each other than to the Nine Mile genome.

A 16,624-bp insertion containing QpRS plasmid-like sequences was detected in the G genome between CBU1710 (hypothetical) and CBU1711 (hypothetical) without ORF disruption. This is the same plasmid integration site previously described for the S isolate.[7] With the exception of a flanking transposase in G, flanking ORFs are syntenous with the Nine Mile I genome.

Comparison of the complete genome sequences of the Nine Mile, K, and G isolates will improve our understanding of the unique virulence properties of *C. burnetii* and provide important insight into the genome architecture and genetic diversity of this pathogen.

ACKNOWLEDGMENTS

This research was supported by the Intramural Research Program of the National Institutes of Health, National Institute of Allergy and Infectious Diseases, Bethesda, Maryland.

[*Competing interests statement:* The authors have no conflicting financial interests.]

REFERENCES

1. MAURIN, M. & D. RAOULT. 1999. Q fever. Clin. Microbiol. Rev. **12:** 518–553.
2. HEINZEN, R.A., T. HACKSTADT & J.E. SAMUEL. 1999. Developmental biology of *Coxiella burnetii*. Trends Microbiol. **7:** 149–154.
3. HENDRIX, L.R., J.E. SAMUEL & L.P. MALLAVIA. 1991. Differentiation of *Coxiella burnetii* isolates by analysis of restriction-endonuclease-digested DNA separated by SDS-PAGE. J. Gen. Microbiol. **137:** 269–276.
4. SAMUEL, J.E., M.E. FRAZIER & L.P. MALLAVIA. 1985. Correlation of plasmid type and disease caused by *Coxiella burnetii*. Infect. Immun. **49:** 775–779.
5. SESHADRI, R. *et al.* 2003. Complete genome sequence of the Q-fever pathogen *Coxiella burnetii*. Proc. Natl. Acad. Sci. USA **100:** 5455–5460.
6. DELCHER, A.L. *et al.* 1999. Improved microbial gene identification with GLIMMER. Nucleic Acids Res. **27:** 4636–4641.
7. WILLEMS, H. *et al.* 1997. Plasmid-homologous sequences in the chromosome of plasmidless *Coxiella burnetii* Scurry Q217. J. Bacteriol. **179**: 3293–3297.

Fur-Regulated Genes in *Coxiella burnetii*

HEATHER L. BRIGGS,[a] MARY J. WILSON,[a] REKHA SESHADRI,[b] AND JAMES E. SAMUEL[a]

[a]*TAMUS Health Science Center, Department of Medical Microbiology and Immunology, College Station, Texas, USA*

[b]*Institute of Genomic Research, Rockville, Maryland, USA*

ABSTRACT: In this paper, we describe the identification of an iron-acquisition gene homologue, ferrous iron transporter (feoB) in *C. burnetii.* The results of a genomic screen for putative Fur-regulated genes and Fur boxes and the development of a two-plasmid system to analyze these Fur boxes will also be illustrated.

KEYWORDS: ***Coxiella burnetii*; iron; *fur*; *feoB***

INTRODUCTION

Coxiella burnetii, the etiologic agent of Q fever, is an obligate, intracellular gram-negative bacterium. The bacterium is found in a variety of animal reservoirs such as arthropods, sheep, goats, and cattle.[1] Transmission of bacteria occurs primarily by the aerosol route. Therefore, Q fever is considered an occupational hazard for those in close contact with livestock.[2]

C. burnetii replicates within a vacuole with properties similar to the phagolysosome of host cells.[3] It is within this inhospitable environment that *C. burnetii* must acquire necessary nutrients such as iron. The ability to acquire iron is essential in the pathogenesis of the majority of bacteria.[4] Previous work by Dale Howe *et al.* has predicted an absolute requirement of iron by describing an inhibition of *C. burnetii* replication in J774A.1 murine macrophage-like cells incubated in the presence of deferoxamine, an iron chelator.[5] However, acquisition must be tightly regulated since excess iron results in the generation of oxygen radicals via the Fenton reaction. In gram-negative bacteria, iron acquisition proteins are commonly regulated by Fur, ferric uptake regulator. Homologues have been described in gram-positive and gram-negative bacteria including the phylogenetic relative of *Coxiella*, the intracellular pathogen *Legionella*.[4,6] The prototypic model for transcriptional regulation is that in an iron-replete environment, Fur binds Fe^{+2}. Fur and the co-repressor, iron, block the transcription of Fur-regulated genes by binding to a palindromic sequence known as a "Fur box," present in the promoter region.[7] This typically results in transcriptional

Address for correspondence: James E. Samuel, Ph.D., Department of Medical Microbiology and Immunology, Texas A&M University System Health Science Center, College Station, TX 77843-1114. Voice: 979-862-1684; fax: 979-845-3479.
jsamuel@tamu.edu

Ann. N.Y. Acad. Sci. 1063: 68–72 (2005).
doi: 10.1196/annals.1355.008

repression, although a few experimental models have noted activation of some promoters.[8,9]

We hypothesized that *C. burnetii* employs a functional Fur regulon to maintain necessary levels of iron. Previous work has included the identification of *C. burnetii fur* gene. Primers were designed based on similar regions in related *fur* genes, which were then used to amplify and clone the complete *C. burnetii fur* gene. The clone was shown to complement an *E. coli fur* deletion strain (unpublished data). To identify Fur-regulated genes, a FURTA screen, an approach developed in *E. coli*, was performed which resulted in the identification of one putative gene, *fur-regulated gene 1* (*frg1*, CBU0970) (unpublished data).[10]

MATERIALS AND METHODS

Media and Chemicals: Luria-Bertani media (Difco, Detroit, MI) were prepared according to a laboratory manual.[11] Antibiotics were incorporated into media at the following concentrations to maintain plasmids in *E. coli*: kanamycin 50 $\mu g\ mL^{-1}$, tetracycline at 12.5 $\mu g\ mL^{-1}$, and chloramphenicol at 30 $\mu g\ mL^{-1}$. *o*-Nitrophenyl-β-D-galactopyranoside (ONPG), deferoxamine, and ferric chloride were purchased from Sigma Chemical Co. (St. Louis, MO). All cultures were grown in LB media at 37°C on a shaker.

Isolation of Plasmid DNA: Plasmid minipreps were prepared by using the Fast-Plasmid Miniprep Kit (Eppendorf, Hamburg, Germany).

PCR Amplification: Primers were designed as indicated below and used at a final concentration of 1 μM per 50 μL reaction volume. The amplification procedure consisted of $94°\text{-}1[94°\text{-}1m|50°\text{-}1m|72°\text{-}7m]_{35}72°\text{-}6m|4°$-pause. Primers and *C. burnetii* RSA493, Nine Mile Phase I, DNA were mixed with PCR SuperMix (Invitrogen, Carlsbad, CA), and reactions were carried out using the DNA Engine PT-200 Peltier Thermal Cycler (MJ Research, Reno, NV). PCR products were subsequently cloned into PCR cloning vector pBlue-TOPO (Invitrogen, Carlsbad, CA). Primers used were: FeoB For (TTTTGGGAGTCTTGTCGGTC), FeoB Rev (TGGAGTGTGAGGTAAAGGTTCC), 769For (CAAACTAATGGGATAAGCACAGGC), and 769Rev (AATCATACGACTTCTGCGTGGC) (Integrated DNA Technologies, Inc., Coralville, IA).

DNA Sequence Analysis: DNA was sequenced at Gene Technologies Laboratories (Biology Department, Texas A&M University). Sequence homologies were compared using MacVector (Oxford Molecular Company, Madison, WI) and BLAST programs. The genome was searched using the Pustell DNA matrix search option in MacVector (Oxford Molecular Company, Madison, WI).

Genome Survey: The genomic data for the survey and promoter search were provided by TIGR. A search of the genome using the Pustell DNA matrix search in MacVector was performed to identify putative iron-acquisition homologues containing potential Fur boxes. Inclusion criteria included a maximum of 50% mismatch to each Fur box (Fur box consensus sequence, *frg1* (CBU0970), and *feoB* (CBU1766)), location in an intergenic region, presence of TATTA and Shine Delgarno regions, and located within 100 base pairs of the start site.[10]

Regulator/Promoter Two-Plasmid System: Putative Fur box sequences were cloned into a promoter trap vector, pBlue Topo (Invitrogen, Carlsbad, CA). The vector and the full *C. burnetii fur* clone were co-transformed into BN4020, an *E. coli fur* deletion strain.[12] pBlue TOPO was also co-transformed with pMH15, a plasmid containing the full *E. coli fur.*[13] β-galactosidase activity was assessed quantitatively for bacterial cultures as described.[14] The substrate for lacZ hydrolysis in this assay was o-nitrophenyl-β-D-galactopyranoside (ONPG). $FeCl_3$ was added for a final concentration of 50 μM. Deferoxamine, an iron chelator, was added for a final concentration of 200 μM.

RESULTS AND DISCUSSION

Genome Survey: The genome annotation resulted in the identification of *feoB* (CBU1766), a ferrous iron transporter. FeoB has been previously described as a Fur-regulated iron acquisition protein in *E. coli.*[15] Sequence analysis of the promoter region revealed a putative Fur box. Clustal analysis of the *feoB* Fur box and the *E. coli* Fur box consensus sequence showed approximately 68% similarity.[10] The identification of a ferrous iron uptake system is consistent with the lifestyle of the organism in which the environment would favor the formation of ferrous iron. However, it was unexpected that no other iron-acquisition homologues were identified. This suggests that the Fur regulon may consist of a limited set of iron uptake systems.

The matrix search of the genome resulted in eighteen potential Fur-regulated genes (TABLE 1). The closest match to the *feoB* and *frg1* fur boxes was CBU0769, a putative glutamine amidotransferase. Clustal analysis with the *feoB* Fur box showed 62% similarity and 79% similarity with the *frg1* Fur box. Due to the high percentage of similarity, CBU0769 was chosen as the first unknown to be tested in the regulator/promoter two-plasmid system. Also of note is the lack of identification of putative Fur-regulated genes directly involved with iron acquisition and the large number of hypotheticals. However, this is consistent with the role of Fur as a global regulator in gram-negative bacteria.[7]

Regulator/Promoter Two-Plasmid System: pBlue TOPO alone provided the background level of β-galactosidase activity. The *E. coli* plasmid (pMH15) containing the full *E. coli fur* gene was used as a control since it has been shown that it can interact with Fur boxes in other bacteria.[10,16] Since *feoB* is Fur-regulated in *E. coli*, it was used as a positive control to develop an assay to identify *C. burnetii* Fur-regulated Fur boxes.[15] When Miller units were compared between the bacteria containing pFeoB Fur grown in an iron-replete environment and an iron-depleted environment, there was a significant increase ($P \leq 0.001$) under iron-depleted conditions. These data were confirmed with *E. coli fur.* To confirm the assay as functional in identification, the putative CBU0769 Fur box was cloned and tested as with *feoB*. There was a significant increase ($P \leq 0.01$) under iron-depleted conditions. The difference in significance may be due to differential regulation by Fur.

C. burnetii is an acidophilic organism which has a Fur homologue and a ferrous iron transporter. At least 18 potential Fur-regulated genes have been identified and can be screened using the regulator/promoter two-plasmid system. At least one gene, CBU0769, shows Fur-regulation. Therefore, we predict that *C. burnetii* has a functional Fur regulon with a limited set of genes, suggesting a minimal number of iron uptake systems and a more global role of Fur.

TABLE 1. Putative Fur-regulated genes

ID	Gene	Putative identification
CBU0216		Hypothetical protein
CBU0280	dinP	DNA-damage-inducible protein P
CBU0432		Major Facilitator Family transporter
CBU0611		Putative surface antigen
CBU0769		Glutamine amdiotransferase
CBU0920		Fatty acid desaturase family protein
CBU0963	bcp	Bacterioferritin comigratory protein
CBU0968		Conserved hypothetical
CBU1106		Hypothetical protein
CBU1477		Antioxidant, AhpC/TSA family
CBU1493		Hypothetical protein
CBU1546		Hypothetical protein
CBU1556		Hypothetical protein
CBU1600		Conserved hypothetical
CBU1695	metG	Methionyl-tRNA synthetase
CBU1851		Hypothetical protein
CBU2012	hslU	Heat shock protein, HslVU

ACKNOWLEDGMENTS

This grant was supported by Grant RO1 AI037744 from the NIH.

[*Competing interest statement*: The authors declare that they have no conflict of interest.]

REFERENCES

1. HEINZEN, R.A., T. HACKSTADT & J.E. SAMUEL. 1999. Developmental biology of *Coxiella burnetii*. Trends Microbiol. **7:** 149–154.
2. MARRIE, T.J. 1990. Epidemiology of Q fever. *In* Q Fever, Vol. 1: The Disease. T.J. Marrie, Ed.: 49–70. CRC Press. Boca Raton, FL.
3. BERON, W. *et al.* 2002. *Coxiella burnetii* localizes in a Rab7-labeled compartment with autophagic characteristics. Infect. Immunol. **70:** 5816–5821.
4. ANDREWS, S.C., A.K. ROBINSON & F. RODRIGUEZ-QUINONES. 2003. Bacterial iron homeostasis. FEMS Microbiol. Rev. **27:** 215–237.
5. HOWE, D. & L.P. MALLAVIA. 1999. *Coxiella burnetii* infection increases transferrin receptors on J774A.1 cells. Infect. Immun. **67:** 3236–3241.
6. HICKEY, E.K. & N.P. CIANCIOTTO. 1994. Cloning and sequencing of the *Legionella pneumophila* fur gene. Gene **143:** 117–121.
7. ESCOLAR, L., J. PEREZ-MARTIN & V. DE LORENZO. 1999. Opening the iron box: transcriptional metalloregulation by the Fur protein. J. Bacteriol. **181:** 6223–6229.
8. DELANY, I., *et al.* 2001. The Fur repressor controls transcription of iron-activated and -repressed genes in *Helicobacter pylori*. Mol. Microbiol. **42:** 1297–309.

9. Foster, J.W. & H.K. Hall. 1992. Effect of *Salmonella typhimurium* ferric uptake regulator (fur) mutations on iron- and pH-regulated protein synthesis. J. Bacteriol. **174:** 4317–4323.
10. Stojiljkovic, I., A.J. Baumler & K. Hantke. 1994. Fur regulon in gram-negative bacteria. J. Mol. Biol. **236:** 531–545.
11. Maniatis, T.E., E.F. Fritsch & J. Sambrook. 1989. Molecular Cloning: A Laboratory Manual. Cold Spring Harbor Laboratory Press. Cold Spring Harbor, NY.
12. Bagg, A. & J.B. Neilands. 1985. Mapping of a mutation affecting regulation of iron uptake systems in *Escherichia coli* K-12. J. Bacteriol. **161:** 450–453.
13. Hantke, K. 1984. Cloning of the repressor protein gene of iron-regulated systems in *Escherichia coli* K12. Mol. Gen. Genet. **197:** 337–341.
14. Miller, J.H. 1972. Experiments in Molecular Genetics. Cold Spring Harbor Laboratory Press. Cold Spring Harbor, NY.
15. Kammler, M., C. Schon & K. Hantke. 1993. Characterization of the ferrous iron uptake system of *Escherichia coli*. J. Bacteriol. **175:** 6212–6219.
16. Desai, P.J., A. Angerer & C.A. Genco. 1996. Analysis of Fur binding to operator sequences within the *Neisseria gonorrhoeae* fbpA promoter. J. Bacteriol. **178:** 5020–5023.

A Minimal Set of DNA Repair Genes Is Sufficient for Survival of *Coxiella burnetii* under Oxidative Stress

K. MERTENS, L. LANTSHEER, AND J. E. SAMUEL

Department of Medical Microbiology and Immunology, Texas A&M University Health Science Center, College Station, Texas 77843-1114, USA

ABSTRACT: This paper studies the functional and regulatory role of RecA, but further investigations are necessary to clarify the control mechanism of the SOS response gene expression in C. burnetii.

KEYWORDS: ***Coxiella burnetii*; oxidative stress; SOS response; *recA*; *recFOR***

INTRODUCTION

The primary defense mechanism of the host cell against invading bacteria is oxidative stress, mediated by reactive oxygen (ROS) and nitrogen species (RNS). A variety of base modifications, single-strand breaks, and base adducts are generated during the reaction of ROS and RNS with DNA.[1] This leads to the induction of several DNA repair mechanisms, the SOS response, coordinated by RecA, and the repressor LexA.

Coxiella burnetii, the etiologic agent of acute and chronic Q fever in humans, replicates within a phagolysosome of eukaryotic cells.[2] In this environment, bacteria are constitutively exposed to oxidative stress, and maintenance of an effective DNA repair system for genomic stability would be a critical factor for survival. Analyses of the annotated sequence of Nine Mile phase I *C. burnetii* RSA493 (TIGR) provided insights into DNA repair mechanism. The functional and regulatory roles of *recA* in DNA repair and recombination was determined by complementation analysis in *Escherichia coli recA1*.

MATERIALS AND METHODS

Bacterial Strains and Plasmids: Nine Mile phase II strain *C. burnetii* RSA 439 was propagated and isolated as previous described.[3] *E. coli* TOP10 *recA1*, *E. coli* BL21, and the cloning vector pCR2.1 (Invitrogen Life Technologies) were cultivated

Address for correspondence: James E. Samuel, Department of Medical Microbiology and Immunology, Texas A&M University System Health Science Center, 407 Reynolds Bldg., College Station, TX 77843-1114. Voice: 979-862-1684; fax: 979-845-3479.
jsamuel@tamhsc.edu.

Ann. N.Y. Acad. Sci. 1063: 73–75 (2005). © 2005 New York Academy of Sciences.
doi: 10.1196/annals.1355.009

and isolated as described by the supplier. DNA isolation, manipulations, and bacterial transformations were carried out according to the methods of Sambrook *et al.*[4]

Cloning of* C. burnetii *and* E. coli *recA: Chromosomal DNA of *C. burnetii* RSA 439 phase II or *E. coli* BL21 was used as template for amplification of *recA*, including the upstream promoter region, with 5′CACGGTCTGGATTGGCATAGC′3 and 5′ACGCAAATCCGTCATTCTGCT′3 or 5′GTGAGTGAACCCGTCGTGGT′3 and 5′CGCAGATGCGACCCTTGTGT′3 as forward and reverse primer.

UV, MC, and MMS Sensitivity Assays: *E. coli* cultures in mid-log phase (OD_{600} of 0.6) were treated with 10 μL of either 0.01% MC or 15% MMS solution, loaded on sterile disks. Sensitivity for each treatment was determined by measuring the zone of growth inhibition. For UV treatment, bacterial cultures in mid-log phase were resuspended in 10 mM $MgSO_4$ and irradiated. Cells were serially diluted, plated on appropriate selection agar, and incubated in the dark. UV sensitivity was determined by cfu/mL calculation of treated and untreated cells.

RESULTS AND DISCUSSION

Genome comparison indicated that essential components of the SOS response (*lexA*, *umuCD*), the recombinational repair system (*recBCD*, *recE, recT*), and also MutM (GO glycosylase) and MutH (endonuclease), both part of the repair system under oxidative stress and mismach repair, are absent in *C. burnetii*. Despite the lack of MutM, which can be complemented by MutS, as shown for *E. coli*,[5] a fully functional nucleotide and base excision repair system is present in *C. burnetii*. For recombinational DNA repair, the *recFOR* pathway with all necessary downstream genes for homologous recombination is annotated and may compensate for the absence of *recBCD*.[6] RecA, but not the repressor protein LexA, is present in *C. burnetii*, suggesting a constituitive expression or the presence of an unknown regulation mechanism for the SOS response regulon. A similar situation was found for several species of the genus *Rickettsia* and may represent a common element lost in an evolutionary process of genome reduction in consideration of the intracellular lifestyle of these organisms.[7]

Complementation analyses demonstrated that the expression of the *C. burnetii recA* gene under control of its native promoter was able to induce SOS response and homologous recombination in the *E. coli recA1* strain, as shown in TABLE 1. Com-

TABLE 1. MC, MMS, and UV sensitivity of *E. coli* RecA complemented with wt *E. coli* or *C. burnetii* recA

	Zone of Inhibition (mm)		cfu × 10^6/mL after UV Treatment [mJ/cm^2]		
Plasmid	0.01% MC	15% MMS	Untreated	500	1000
pCR2.1	9.6 ± 0.6	18.6± 1.6	5.13 ± 4.4	0.013 ± 0.01	0
precAEc[a]	5.4 ± 0.7[b]	9.2 ± 0.6[b]	11.9 ± 5.3	8.27 ± 5.7	4.98 ± 3.1
precACb[a]	7.7 ± 0.8[b]	12.2 ± 1.0[b]	18.9 ± 5.2	14.7 ± 9.4	10.0 ± 5.7

[a]Wild-type *recA* gene of *E. coli* BL21 (Ec) or *C. burnetii* RSA 439 (Cb) cloned into pCR2.1
[b]Significance value <0.01

parable sensitivity was obtained for *E. coli recA1* in MC, UV, and MMS treatments either complemented with wild-type *E. coli* or *C. burnetii recA* gene. These data indicate that *C. burnetii* has an effective and functional DNA repair system to sustain genome stability under oxidative stress. Repair of base modifications by base and nucleotide excision repair and also of DNA strand-breaks via the *recFOR* pathway is sufficient for genome stability in the presence of a functional RecA. The functional and regulatory role of RecA was demonstrated, but still further investigations are necessary to clarify the control mechanism of the SOS response gene expression in *C. burnetii*.

ACKNOWLEDGMENTS

This study was supported by funding from NIH Grant AI037744.

[*Conflict of interest statement:* The authors of this research declare that they have no conflict of interest.]

REFERENCES

1. FANG, F.C. 2004. Antimicrobial reactive oxygen and nitrogen species: concepts and controversies. Nat. Rev. Microbiol. **2:** 820–832.
2. BACA, O.G. & D. PARETSKY. 1983. Q fever and *Coxiella burnetii*: a model for host-parasite interactions. Microbiol. Rev. **47:** 127–149.
3. SAMUEL, J.E., M.E. FRAZIER & L.P. MALLAVIA. 1985. Correlation of plasmid type and disease caused by *Coxiella burnetii*. Infect. Immun. **49:** 775–779.
4. SAMBROOK, J.R.D.W. 2001. Molecular Cloning. Cold Spring Harbor Laboratory Press. Cold Spring Harbor, NY.
5. WYRZYKOWSKI, J. & M.R. VOLKERT. 2003. The *Escherichia coli* methyl-directed mismatch repair system repairs base pairs containing oxidative lesions. J. Bacteriol. **185:** 1701–1704.
6. MORIMATSU, K. & S.C. KOWALCZYKOWSKI. 2003. RecFOR proteins load RecA protein onto gapped DNA to accelerate DNA strand exchange: a universal step of recombinational repair. Mol. Cell **11:** 1337–1347.
7. RENESTO, P., H. OGATA, S. AUDIC, J.M. CLAVERIE & D. RAOULT. 2005. Some lessons from *Rickettsia* genomics. FEMS Microbiol. Rev. **29:** 99–117.

Identification, Cloning, and Expression of Potential Diagnostic Markers for Q Fever

C. C. CHAO,[a] H. W. CHEN,[a] X. LI,[a] W. B. XU,[b] B. HANSON,[b]
AND W. M. CHING[a]

[a]*Rickettsial Diseases Department, Naval Medical Research Center, Silver Spring, Maryland, USA, and Department of Preventive Medicine and Biometrics, Uniformed Services University of Health Sciences, Bethesda, Maryland, USA*

[b]*PanBio, Incorporated, Columbia, Maryland, USA*

ABSTRACT: The clinical diagnosis of Q fever is difficult. Whole cell antigens are currently used in several serological methods, but antigens are limited due to the hazardous nature of *Coxiella burnetii* cultivation. In this report, we described the method of detecting immunodominant antigens of *C. burnetii* by using proteomic techniques with patient sera, and cloning and expressing the selected antigens using a novel vector known for its ease of expression, purification, and downstream application.

KEYWORDS: Q fever; 2D gel electrophoresis; LC-MS-MS; protein antigens; biotin

INTRODUCTION

Coxiella burnetii, the etiologic agent of Q fever, is an obligate intracellular bacterium. *C. burnetii* is widely distributed in nature and infects a variety of mammals, birds, reptiles, fishes, and ticks.[1] Two phase variants of *C. burnetii* have been described, the highly virulent phase I and the less virulent phase II. In humans, infection is usually the result of inhalation of contaminated aerosols associated with infected sheep, goats, and, to a lesser extent, cattle. The extreme infectivity of the bacterium makes it a potential bioweapon and it is classified as a group B agent by the US Centers for Disease Control.

The diagnosis of Q fever is difficult and relies mainly on serological examination, the most commonly used method being indirect immunofluorescence assay (IFA).[2] Acute and chronic infections are characterized by different serological profiles.[3] Whole cell antigens are currently used in several serological methods, but are limited due to the hazardous nature of cultivation of *C. burnetii*. In this report, we identified six protein antigens by western blot analysis of whole cell lysate separated on a two-dimensional (2D) gel using patient sera that showed positive IgG by IFA against both phase I and phase II cells. The protein antigens were identified using a ProteomeX

Address for correspondence: Chien-Chung Chao, Ph.D., RDD/IDD/NMRC, 503 Robert Grant Ave., RM 3N71, Silver Spring, MD 20910. Voice: 301-319-7313; fax: 301-319-7460.
chaoc@nmrc.navy.mil

Ann. N.Y. Acad. Sci. 1063: 76–78 (2005).
doi: 10.1196/annals.1355.010

workstation (LC-MS) consisting of a liquid chromatography and a downstream electrospray ion trap mass spectrometer (LCQ DecaXP plus, Thermo Electrons). The identified antigens were cloned into a novel vector (pETAB′C). The clone gene was expressed as a tripartite protein fused with biotinylated leader peptide and ubiquitin. Affinity purification was carried out as described by Wang and colleagues.[4]

MATERIALS AND METHODS

Two-Dimensional Gel Electrophoresis and Western Blot Analysis

Phase I and Phase II *C. burnetii* (Henszering strain) cells were purified as described. The pure organisms were washed with cold PBS once and resuspended in lysis buffer (9 M urea, 4% CHAPS, and 50 mM dithiothreitol). Equal volume of sample solution (100 μg of protein) was subjected to 2D gel electrophoresis using Bio-Rad system as described by the manufacturer. The gel was transferred onto a polyvinylidene difluoride (PVDF) membrane and blotted against patient sera to identify protein antigens.

LC-MS Analysis to Identify Protein Antigens

The proteins that showed reactivity with patient sera were located in the gel and excised from the gel for LC-MS analysis. The digested proteins were analyzed as described.[5]

Cloning and Construction of Vectors Carrying Genes of Interest

PCR reactions were carried out using genomic DNA purified from phase II organisms (*C. burnetii* grown in VERO cells) and primer pairs of each gene containing *Not*I site on both the 5′ and 3′ overhang. The correct amplicons were cloned into the pETAB′C vector provided by Dr. Yang and plated on agar plate with ampicillin. Correct orientation of inserts was verified by PCR reaction and the sequence of inserted gene was confirmed.

Expression and Purification of Biotinylated Proteins

Escherichia coli BL21(DE3) cells transformed with respective plasmids were grown at 37°C overnight in instant TB medium (Novagen) supplemented with 50 μg/mL ampicillin and 2 M biotin. The purification was carried out as described by Wang and colleagues.[4]

RESULTS AND DISCUSSIONS

The combination of 2D electrophoresis, Western blot, and LC-MS allowed us to identify six antigens. Two of them (hsp 60 and Com-1) have been reported before and four (RecA, elongation factor Tu, OmpA-like transmembrane domain, and FtsZ) were newly identified. These antigens were successfully cloned into a pETAB′C vector and the expressed recombinant antigens were biotinylated in *E. coli* culture

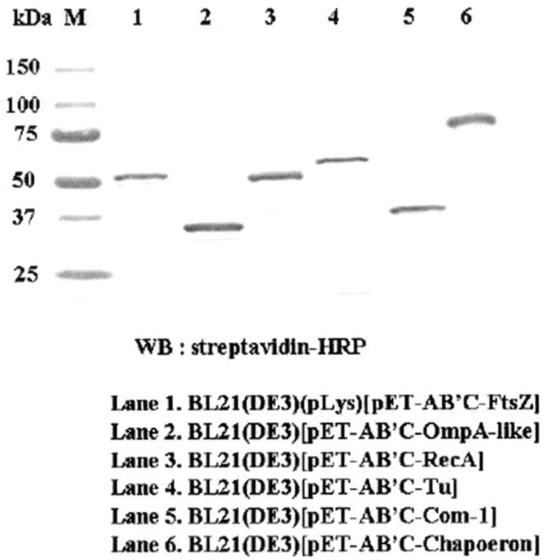

FIGURE 1. Western blot analysis of the expression of biotinylated protein antigens.

(FIG. 1). Highly pure expressed antigen was obtained using an avidin column with high efficiency. These biotinylated recombinant antigens can be used for the development of sensitive diagnostic assays.

ACKNOWLEDGMENTS

This work was supported by Work Unit No. 6000.RAD1.L.A0311.

Disclaimer: The opinions and assertions contained herein are the private ones of the authors and are not to be construed as official or reflecting the views of the Navy Department or the Department of Defense at large.

[*Conflict of interest statement:* The authors of this research declare that they have no conflict of interest.]

REFERENCES

1. SAWYER, L.A., D.B. FISHBEIN & J.E. MCDADE. 1987. Q fever: current concepts. Rev. Infect. Dis. **9:** 935–946.
2. TISSOT-DUPONT, H., X. THIRION & D. RAOULT. 1994. Q fever serology: cutoff determination for microimmunofluorescence. Clin. Diagn. Lab. Immunol. **1:** 189–196.
3. MAURIN, M. & D. RAOULT. 1999. Q fever. Clin. Microbiol. Rev. **12:** 518–553.
4. WANG, T., E. EVDOKIMOV, K. YIADOM, *et al.* 2003. Biotin-ubiquitin tagging of mammalian proteins in *Escherichia coli*. Protein Expr. Purif. **30:** 140–149.
5. CHAO, C.C., D. CHELIUS, T. ZHANG, *et al.* 2004. Proteome analysis of Madrid E strain of *Rickettsia prowazekii*. Proteomics **4:** 1280–1292.

Preliminary Transcriptional Analysis of *spoT* Gene Family and of Membrane Proteins in *Rickettsia conorii* and *Rickettsia felis*

C. ROVERY, M. V. LA, S. ROBINEAU, K. MATSUMOTO, P. RENESTO, AND D. RAOULT

Unité des Rickettsies, CNRS-UMR 6020, IFR48, Faculté de Médecine, 13 385 Marseille, France

ABSTRACT: *Rickettsiae* survival implicates adaptation to different environmental conditions. We hypothesized that multiple copies of genes in bacteria with reduced genomes might account for such a process. Transcription of *spoT* and *sca* paralogs was thus analyzed in *R. conorii* and *R. felis*.

KEYWORDS: *Rickettsia conorii*; *Rickettsia felis*; transcriptome; *spoT; sca*

INTRODUCTION

Rickettsia conorii and *R. felis* are obligate intracellular bacteria transmitted to humans by ticks and fleas, respectively.[1] Their survival implicates a great ability to adapt to different environments, including both the vector and the mammalian host. Molecular mechanisms involved in adaptation of *Rickettsia* to different host conditions are still unknown. As other intracellular parasites, rickettsiae possess small genomes. In this context of genomic reduction,[2] we hypothesized that genes found in multiple copies may play a role in such an adaptation process. Among these is *spoT* for which 7 and 15 copies were identified in *R. conorii*[3] and in *R. felis*,[4] respectively. In numerous bacterial species, this gene was described as an effector of stress adaptation system (stringent response) allowing regulation of the nucleotide guanosine-3,5-(bis)pyrophosphate (ppGpp) concentration.[5] Persistence of vector-borne pathogens in immunocompetent hosts can also be achieved by varying the immunodominant surface protein(s).[6] Accordingly, transcriptional variation of Sca family membrane proteins was also investigated. Finally, the transcription and the expression of the major immunodominant rickettsial outer membrane protein (rOmpA) was also examined.

Address for correspondence: Prof. Didier Raoult, Unité des Rickettsies, CNRS-UMR 6020, IFR48, Faculté de Médecine, 27, Bd Jean Moulin, 13 385 Marseille, France. Voice.: +(33) 491 32 43 75; fax: +(33) 491 38 77 72.
didier.raoult@medecine.univ-mrs.fr

**Ann. N.Y. Acad. Sci. 1063: 79–82 (2005). © 2005 New York Academy of Sciences.
doi: 10.1196/annals.1355.011**

MATERIALS AND METHODS

Bacterial Strains and Growth Conditions

R. conorii strain seven (ATCC, VR613) were propagated in various cell lines (Vero cell, C6/36) or within ticks (*Rhipicephalus sanguineus*) as previously described.[7] *R. felis felis* strain Marseille were grown at 28°C in *Xenopus laevis*–derived XTC-2 cell line.[8] To determine the transcriptional pattern following starvation, infected cells were incubated in phosphate buffered saline (PBS) for 6 hours.

RNA Extraction and RT-PCR

The extraction procedure (Rneasy Mini Kit, Qiagen) including Rnase-Free Dnase treatment (Qiagen) and RNA analysis (Agilent 2100 bioanalyzer, Agilent Technologies, Englewood, NJ) was performed as described.[7]

Immunofluorescence

All samples were fixed for 10 min with methanol and washed three times with PBS–0.05% Tween 20 before incubation with primary antibodies (Abs) (rabbit anti–*R. conorii* polyclonal Abs 1:5,000 dilution and a monoclonal mouse anti rOmpA 1:10,000 dilution). After washings, the slides were incubated with fluorescein isothiocyanate (FITC)-conjugated anti-rabbit immunoglobulin G (IgG) Abs (1:1,000 dilution; Beckman-Coulter, Roissy, France) and anti-mouse Cy3 conjugate (1:1,000 dilution, Molecular Probes, Eugene, OR). Images were obtained with a laser scanning confocal fluorescence microscope (Leica, Lyon, France) paired to a Scanware software. The percentage of *R. conorii* expressing rOmpA was determined by counting 100 bacteria for each condition. For each optical field, the number of red and/or green marked cells was counted.

RESULTS AND DISCUSSION

By using highly specific primers, we examined transcription of the 15 *spoT* paralogs identified within *R. felis* genome. Different conditions were tested, namely 28°C (control), 4°C/37°C (thermal stress), and PBS (nutrient stress). In previous experiments, we demonstrated that *R. conorii spoT* paralogs presented a variable transcription according to the experimental treatment.[7] In contrast, concerning *R. felis*, data obtained showed that transcription of the 15 *spoT* paralogs was unchanged. Thus, transcription of *spoT* genes in *R. felis* is modified neither by nutrient starvation nor by temperature shifts. Therefore, modulation of these genes under other conditions of bacterial stress cannot be excluded.

More sets of data illustrate that genomic changes in bacterial surface proteins occur in the course of infection.[9] Modifications have been evidenced according to the host, as during *B. burgdorferi* passage from ticks to mammals.[10,11] The temperature-linked variation of rickettsial antigens was also reported.[12] RT-PCR targeting the 12 members of the large *R. felis* Sca family performed on the same samples as above were all positive and unchanged whatever the culture conditions. We then investigated possible changes in *R. conorii* rOmpA expression depending on the host environ-

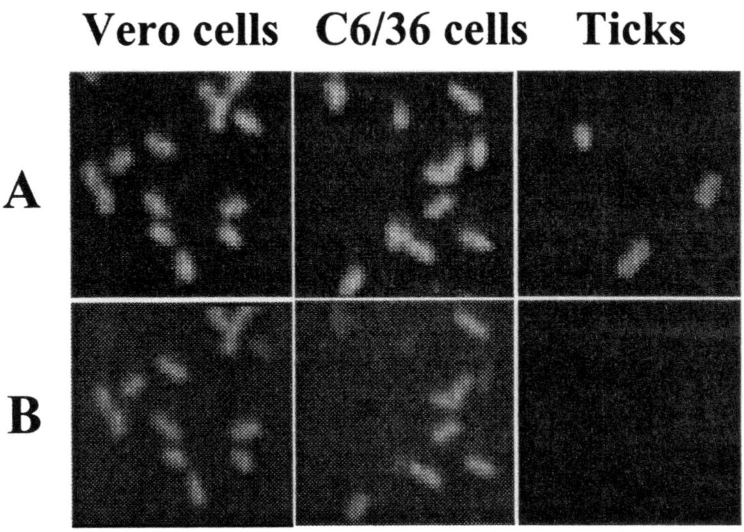

FIGURE 1. Visualization of rOmpA in *R. conorii* maintained within various host cells. (**A**) Staining with polyclonal *anti-R.conorii* Abs. (**B**) Staining with anti-rOmpA Abs.

ment. When eukaryotic cell monolayers were used as host cells (infected Vero or C6/36 cells), a strong correlation was always observed between *rpsL* and *rompA* transcription. In contrast, concerning tick samples, a lack of rOmpA transcription was observed while *rpsL* was positive. This led us to look for the expression of this protein by immunofluorescence assays to confirm this result. As illustrated in FIGURE 1, *R. conorii* rOmpA was observed on more than 95% of rickettsiae propagated within Vero cells, this value being 54.9% for C6/36 infected cells. In contrast, the majority of rickettsiae in the tick hemolymph (85.7%) did not stain with the Abs.

Data obtained using specific Abs raised against *R. conorii* and rOmpA, support the idea that rOmpA might be differentially expressed and that its expression might correspond to a certain cell adaptation. It can also be hypothesized that like other arthropod-associated pathogens, such as *Ehrlichia canis* or *B. burgdorferi*,[11] changes in the outer surface proteins occur during alternating infections in ticks and mammals. Undoubtedly, this point merits further investigation since antigenic variation represents a challenge in the development of vaccines against vector-borne pathogens.

[*Conflict of interest statement:* The authors of this research declare that they have no conflict of interest.]

REFERENCES

1. RAOULT, D. & V. ROUX. 1997. Rickettsioses as paradigms of new emerging infectious diseases. Clin. Microbiol. Rev. **10:** 694–719.
2. ANDERSSON, J.O. & S.G.E. ANDERSSON. 1999. Genome degradation is an ongoing process in *Rickettsia*. Mol. Biol. Evol. **16:** 1178–1191.

3. Ogata, H., S. Audic, P. Renesto-audiffren, *et al.* 2001. Mechanisms of evolution in *Rickettsia conorii* and *R. prowazekii.* Science **293:** 2093–2098.
4. Ogata, H., P. Renesto, S. Audic, *et al.* 2005. The genome sequence of *Rickettsia felis* identifies the first putative conjugative plasmid in an obligate intracellular parasite. PLoS Biol. **3**(8)**:** e248.
5. Chatterji, D. & A.K. Ohja. 2001. Revisiting the stringent response; ppGpp and starvation signaling. Curr. Opin. Microbiol. **4:** 160–165.
6. Deitsch, K.W., E.R. Moxon & T.E. Wellems. 1997. Shared themes of antigenic variation and virulence in bacterial, protozoal, and fungal infections. Microbiol. Mol. Biol. Rev. **61:** 281–293.
7. Rovery, C., P. Renesto, N. Crapoulet, *et al.* 2005. Transcriptional response of *Rickettsia conorii* exposed to temperature variation and stress starvation. Res. Microbiol. **156:** 211–218.
8. Raoult, D., B. La Scola, M. Enea, *et al.* 2001. A flea-associated rickettsia pathogenic for humans. Emerg. Infect. Dis. **7:** 73–81.
9. Solnick, J.V., L.M. Hansen, N.R. Salama, *et al.* 2004. Modification of *Helicobacter pylori* outer membrane protein expression during experimental infection of rhesus macaques. Proc. Natl. Acad. Sci. USA **101:** 2106–2111.
10. Brooks, C.S., P.S. Hefty, S.E. Jolliff & D.R. Akins. 2003. Global analysis of *Borrelia burgdoferi* genes regulated by mammalian host-specific signals. Infect. Immun. **71:** 3371–3383.
11. Schwan, T.G., W.T. Piesman, W.T. Golde, *et al.* 1995. Induction of an outer surface protein on *Borrelia burgdoferi* during tick feeding. Proc. Natl. Acad. Sci. USA **92:** 2909–2913.
12. Policastro, P.F., U.G. Munderloch, E.R. Fischer & T. Hackstadt. 1997. *Rickettsia rickettsii* growth and temperature-inducible protein expression in embryonic tick cell lines. J. Med. Microbiol. **46:** 839–845.

Phylogenic Analysis of Rickettsial Patatin-like Protein with Conserved Phospholipase A_2 Active Sites

GUILLAUME BLANC,[a] PATRICIA RENESTO,[b] AND DIDIER RAOULT[b]

[a]*IGS-CNRS UPR 2589,* [b]*Unité des Rickettsies, CNRS UMR 6020, 13385 Marseille, France*

ABSTRACT: Genome analysis of *Rickettsia felis* highlighted the presence of three patatin-like protein (PLP) genes (*pat1*, *pat2A*, and *pat2B*), whereas only one PLP gene (*pat1*) is found in the other sequenced rickettsial genomes. Here, we aligned the rickettsial PLPs with characterized patatins from plants and found that they possess all the conserved amino acid residues identified as important for phospholipase A_2 activity. We also carried out a phylogenic analysis of the rickettsial PLPs together with bacterial and eukaryotic homologs. The phylogeny of the rickettsial Pat1 proteins is in conflict with the currently recognized *Rickettsia* phylogeny. Possible scenarios that might explain this incongruence are discussed and involve either gene conversion or gene duplication events.

KEYWORDS: patatin-like protein; patatins; phospholipase A_2

INTRODUCTION

Rickettsia felis is a flea-borne bacterium responsible for human spotted fever.[1] Sequencing of its 1.6 Mb genome[2] revealed specific features. We have most particularly focused our interest on putative virulence factors and identified three *R. felis* ORFs able to encode for proteins with a patatin-like domain. One of these ORFs is located on the chromosome (*pat1*), while the two other are located on the two *R. felis* plasmids (*pat2A* and *pat2B*) and exhibit 100% sequence identity. Patatin is the major storage glycoprotein found in potatoes and is endowed for phospholipase A_2 (PLA_2) activity.[3] A rickettsial patatin-like protein (PLP) has been previously described in *R. typhi*.[4] The *R. felis* chromosomal *pat1* locus is conserved in all the rickettsial genomes sequenced to date.[2] In this work, we analyzed the sequence conservation between the rickettsial PLPs and characterized patatins, and constructed a phylogenetic tree to shed new light on their evolution.

Address for correspondence: Prof. Didier Raoult, Unité des Rickettsies, CNRS UMR 6020, 13385 Marseille, France. Voice: +(33) 491 32 43 75; fax: +(33) 491 38 77 72.
didier.raoult@medecine.univ-mrs.fr

**Ann. N.Y. Acad. Sci. 1063: 83–86 (2005). © 2005 New York Academy of Sciences.
doi: 10.1196/annals.1355.012**

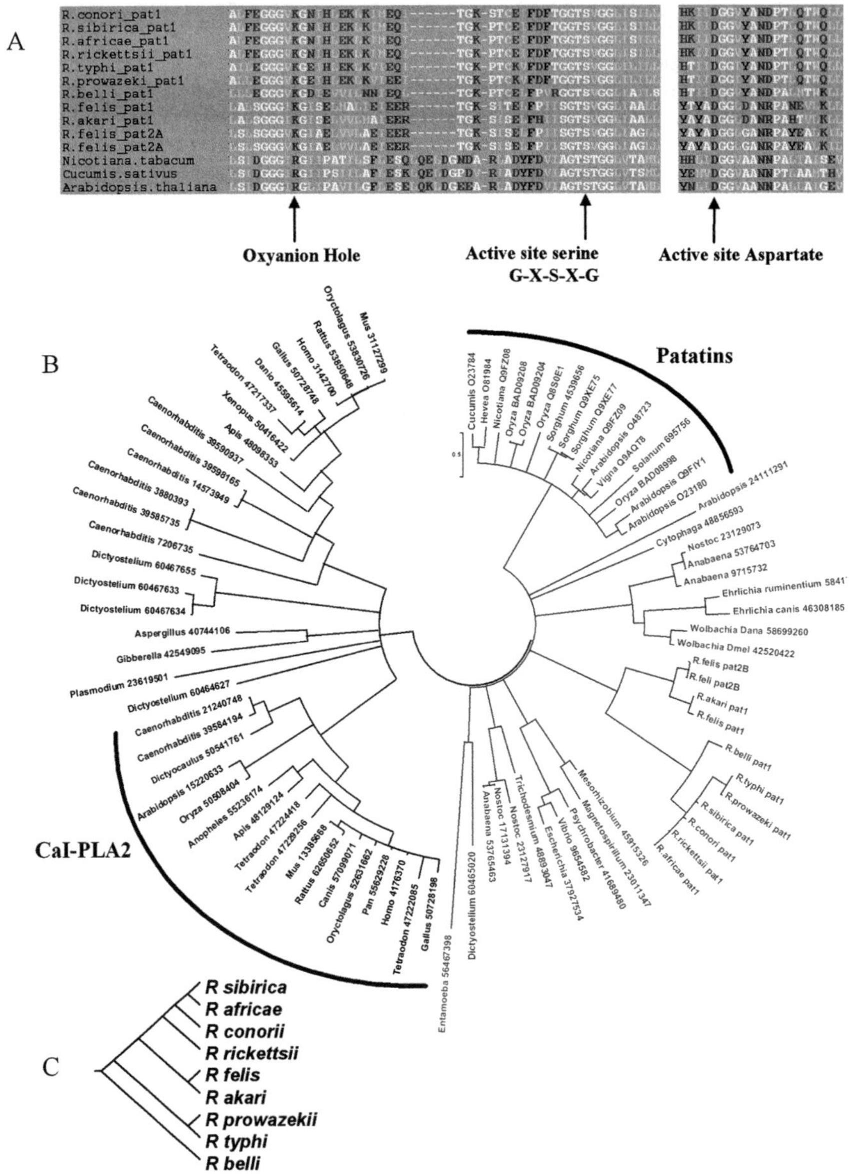

FIGURE 1. Multiple alignment and phylogenetic analyses of the Rickettsia PLPs. (**A**) Multiple alignment including the rickettsial PLPs and three plant patatins around three residues identified as important for PLA_2 activity in plants (oxyanion hole, active site serine, and aspartate). (**B**) Phylogenetic tree of the PLPs. Branches with bootstrap support <50 were collapsed in multifurcation. Sequences are named by their genus name and their Genbank identifier. Plant patatins and CaI-PLA_2 proteins are indicated. Black and gray colors delineate group 1 and 2 proteins, respectively. (**C**) Currently recognized phylogeny of *Rickettsia* spp. (Modified from Roux and colleagues.[6])

MATERIALS AND METHODS

Patatin-like proteins were searched in the Genpep database and the *Rickettsia* proteomes using the BLASTP program and the *R. felis* Pat1 protein as query. Proteins matching with E-value < 1e-5 were kept for further analyses. We used the CLUSTALW program to align protein sequences. Localization of the amino acid residues important for PLA_2 activity was done according to Hirschberg and colleagues.[3] We constructed the phylogenetic tree from protein alignment with the MEGA3 software using the JTT+Gamma ($\alpha = 1.129$) model. The α parameter for the Gamma distribution was estimated using ProtTest.

RESULTS AND DISCUSSION

Alignment of the rickettsial PLP sequences with characterized plant patatin highlighted conserved regions (FIG. 1A), including three conserved residues identified as important for PLA_2 activity:[3] (1) a conserved glycine-rich region with a conserved arginine or lysine residue, which probably served as an oxyanion hole, (2) a serine hydrolase motif, G-X-S-X-G, and (3) an active site aspartate residue within the D-X-G/A motif. These sites were also found conserved in other bacterial PLPs.[5] The serine-aspartate catalytic dyad is required for the activity of $cPLA_2$ and its conservation in *R. felis* suggests that these proteins could display enzymatic activity (not shown). It has long been thought that the membranolytic activity of PLA_2 was involved in both hemolytic activity and the escape of *Rickettsia* from early phagosomal compartments. We suggest that the rickettsial PLPs might play a role in such process.

A cross-kingdom phylogenic tree was constructed from the alignment of Pat1 homologs identified in Genbank. The phylogenetic tree is not entirely resolved with several branches having low bootstrap support (>50), but clearly delineates two main protein groups (FIG. 1B). The first group includes the calcium-independent PLA_2 proteins ($CaI\text{-}PLA_2$) and the likes, whereas the second group contains the plant patatins. All rickettsial PLPs, including the *R. felis* plasmid Pat2 proteins, cluster in a single clade that falls in group 2 (FIG. 1B). *Wolbachia* and *Erhlichia* species (*Rickettsiaceae* order) harbor a single PLP gene that is also mostly related to the plant patatins (FIG. 1B). They may inherit the *pat* gene through vertical transmission from a common ancestor with *Rickettsia*. However, the *Nostoc* and *Anabeana* (cyanobacteria) cluster branches as an outgroup relative to the *Wolbachia* and *Erhlichia* clade. This suggests that a lateral gene transfer occurred between the *Nostoc-Anabeana* and the *Wolbachia-Erhlichia* ancestors, for which the direction remains to be determined. Although the *pat1* locus is conserved and exhibits a nearly perfect colinearity among the eight sequenced *Rickettsia* genomes,[2] the phylogenetic relationships between the *Rickettsia* Pat1 proteins are markedly different from the known *Rickettsia* phylogeny (FIG. 1B and 1C). The *R. felis* and *R. akari* Pat1 proteins branch before the separation of *R. bellii* and the spotted fever–typhus *Rickettsia* spp. Furthermore, the *R. felis* and *R. akari* Pat1 proteins cluster with the two Pat2 proteins, which are encoded on the *R. felis* plasmids. Two possible scenarios may account for this phylogenetic incongruence: (1) An ancestral *pat* gene underwent a tandem duplication event before the radiation of the *Rickettsia* spp., resulting in *pat1* and *pat2*, further followed by differential gene losses among the different *Rickettsia* lineages and duplication of *pat2* on the ancestral *R. felis* plasmid. (2) A gene conversion event occurred between an ancestral *pat2* (donor) and the *pat1* (acceptor) loci in the *R. felis–R. akari* ancestor. These two scenarios imply that the *pat2* gene was present in the *R. felis–R. akari* ancestor. In addition, our results suggest that the *R. felis* plasmid was present in the *R. felis–R. akari* ancestor and later lost in the *R. akari* lineage.

[*Conflict of interest statement:* The authors of this research declare that they have no conflict of interest.]

REFERENCES

1. RAOULT, D., B. LA SCOLA, M. ENEA, *et al.* 2001. A flea-associated Rickettsia pathogenic for humans. Emerg. Infect. Dis. **7:** 73–81.
2. OGATA, H., P. RENESTO, S. AUDIC, *et al.* 2005. The genome sequence of *Rickettsia felis* identifies the first putative conjugative plasmid in an obligate intracellular parasite. PLoS Biol. **3**(8)**:** e248.
3. HIRSCHBERG, H.J., J.W. SIMONS, N. DEKKER & M.R. EGMOND. 2001. Cloning, expression, purification, and characterization of patatin, a novel phospholipase A. Eur. J. Biochem. **268:** 5037–5044.
4. MCLEOD, M.P., X. QIN, S.E. KARPATHY, *et al.* 2004. Complete genome sequence of *Rickettsia typhi* and comparison with sequences of other rickettsiae. J. Bacteriol. **186:** 5842–5855.
5. BANERJI, S. & A. FLIEGER. 2004. Patatin-like proteins: a new family of lipolytic enzymes present in bacteria? Microbiology **150:** 522–525.
6. ROUX, V., E. RYDKINA, M. EREMEEVA & D. RAOULT. 1997. Citrate synthase gene comparison, a new tool for phylogenetic analysis, and its application for the *Rickettsiae*. J. Syst. Bacteriol. **47:** 252–261.

Proteomic Analysis of *Rickettsia prowazekii*

C. C. CHAO,[a] D. CHELIUS,[b] T. ZHANG,[b] E. MUTUMANJE,[a] AND W. M. CHING[a]

[a]*Rickettsial Diseases Department, Naval Medical Research Center, Silver Spring, Maryland, and Department of Preventive Medicine and Biometrics, Uniformed Services University of Health Sciences, Bethesda, Maryland, USA*

[b]*Thermo Electrons, San Jose, California, USA*

ABSTRACT: *Rickettsia prowazekii* is an obligate intracellular gram-negative bacterium. Comparative proteomics study of a virulent strain (Breinl) versus an avirulent strain (Madrid E) was performed using an integrated liquid chromatography and mass spectrometer. About 30% of predicted proteins were detected and identified. Among the detected proteins, more than 30 proteins were of unknown function in both strains. Although several proteins were detected in only one strain, the overall distribution of detected proteins in different COGs (clusters of orthologs groups) was very similar between the two strains. Functional analysis of differentially expressed proteins, either qualitatively or quantitatively, may lead to the discovery of pathogenesis-related factors.

KEYWORDS: ***Rickettsia prowazekii*; proteomics; LC-MS-MS**

INTRODUCTION

R. prowazekii is the causative agent of epidemic typhus. The natural infection is normally caused by rubbing of infected louse or its feces into a bite or skin abrasion and has caused significant health problems for military personnel during times of war and civil disturbance.[1,2] Infection can also occur by inhalation, permitting aerosolized *R. prowazekii* to be deployed as a biological weapon.[1] Consequently, *R. prowazekii* is listed as a select agent by the United States.[1,2]

The genomic DNA sequence of the avirulent strain of *R. prowazekii* (Madrid E) has been completed.[3] Differences in the genome of avirulent and virulent strains are evident as shown by Ge and colleagues[4] in that 24 genes in the avirulent Madrid E strain have significantly lower hybridization signals than in the virulent Breinl strain. These results suggest that some of these genes may be important for strain virulence. In this report, we analyzed the protein expression profiles of these two strains.

Address for correspondence: Chien-Chung Chao, Ph.D., RDD/IDD/NMRC, 503 Robert Grant Ave., RM 3N71, Silver Spring, MD 20910. Voice: 301-319-7313; fax: 301-319-7460.
chaoc@nmrc.navy.mil

**Ann. N.Y. Acad. Sci. 1063: 87–89 (2005). © 2005 New York Academy of Sciences.
doi: 10.1196/annals.1355.013**

TABLE 1. Comparison of proteins detected in Madrid E and Breinl strains of *R. prowazekii*

Description	Madrid E	Breinl
Total detected proteins	251	250
Single peptide in all three runs	14	13
Multiple peptides in only one run	8	9
Multiple peptides in two or three runs	229	228
Hypothetical proteins detected	68	66

MATERIALS AND METHODS

Preparation of Rickettsia prowazekii

The preparation of *Rickettsia prowazekii* was carried out as described previously.[5]

Reduction, Alkylation, Digestion of Proteins, 2D-LC/MS/MS, and Data Analysis

The lysed rickettsia cells were reduced, alkylated, and digested with trypsin, and the digested sample (15 μg of total protein) was analyzed as described by Chao and colleagues.[5]

RESULTS AND DISCUSSIONS

The total number of proteins detected in Madrid E and Breinl strains were 251 and 250 (TABLE 1), respectively. This is equivalent to 30% of the total number of proteins based on ORFs. This limited efficacy may be due to the broad dynamic range of the expressed proteins. Among these detected proteins, 37 from Madrid E and 33 from Breinl were of unknown function. Most of the proteins were identified by multiple peptides or by one single peptide in all three runs. The distribution of detected proteins in different COGs was very similar between the two strains. Among the 24 genes considered as potential DNA vaccine candidates,[6] 12 of them were confirmed expressed (RP333, 344, 043, 775, 326, 833, 451, 586, 290, 291, 292, 293). Three of these 12 proteins (RP333, RP775, and RP586) were identified only in Madrid E and not in Breinl strain. Understanding the role of these three proteins is important to better comprehend the differences between the virulent and avirulent strains.

ACKNOWLEDGMENTS

This work was supported by Work Unit Number 6000.RAD1.L.A0242.

Disclaimer: The opinions and assertions contained herein are the private ones of the authors and are not to be construed as official or reflecting the views of the Navy Department or the Department of Defense at large.

[*Conflict of interest statement:* The authors of this research declare that they have no conflict of interest.]

REFERENCES

1. KELLY, D.J., D. STRICKMAN, G.A. DASCH, *et al.* 2002. The past and present threat of Rickettsial diseases to military medicine and international public health. Clin. Infect. Dis. **34:** 145–169.
2. MORE, J.B. & C.E. PEDERSEN. 1980. The impact of Rickettsial diseases on military operations. Mil. Med. **145:** 780–785.
3. ANDERSSON, S.G., A. ZOMORODIPOUR, J.O. ANDERSSON, *et al.* 1998. The genome sequence of *Rickettsia prowazekii* and the origin of mitochondria. Nature **396:** 133–140.
4. GE, H., E.Y.-Y. CHUANG, S. ZHAO, *et al.* 2004. Comparative genomics of *Rickettsia prowazekii* Madrid E and Breinl strains. J. Bacteriol. **186:** 556–565.
5. CHAO, C.C., D. CHELIUS, T. ZHANG, *et al.* 2004. Proteome analysis of Madrid E strain of *Rickettsia prowazekii*. Proteomics **4:** 1280–1292.
6. COKER, C., M. MAJID & S. RADULOVIC. 2003. Development of *Rickettsia prowazekii* DNA vaccine: cloning strategies. Ann. N.Y. Acad. Sci. **990:** 957–964.

Rickettsia conorii and *R. prowazekii* Proteome Analysis by 2DE-MS

A Step toward Functional Analysis of Rickettsial Genomes

PATRICIA RENESTO,[a] SAÏD AZZA,[a] ALAIN DOLLA,[b] PATRICK FOURQUET,[c] GUY VESTRIS,[a] JEAN-PIERRE GORVEL,[c] AND DIDIER RAOULT[a]

[a]*Unité des Rickettsies, CNRS UMR 6020,* [b]*Bioénergétique et Ingénierie des Protéines–Institut de Biologie Structurale et Microbiologie,*
[c]*Centre d'Immunologie de Marseille-Luminy, 13385 Marseille, France*

ABSTRACT: In this work, we present a comparative two-dimensional (2D) PAGE analysis of *Rickettsia conorii* and *Rickettsia prowazekii*. This analysis reveals protein spots that were either unique to or common to both strains, some of them being identified by matrix-assisted laser desorption ionization–time of flight mass spectrometry.

KEYWORDS: ***Rickettsia conorii*; *Rickettsia prowazekii*; 2D-electrophoresis**

INTRODUCTION

Rickettsia species are small gram-negative bacilli, divided in two antigenically defined groups: the spotted fever group and the typhus group.[1] During the last few years, two rickettsial genomes have been sequenced, that is, those of *R. prowazekii*[2] and *R. conorii,*[3] which are responsible for typhus and Mediterranean spotted fever, respectively. These genomic sequences provided significant insights into the molecular physiology and evolution of these bacteria, which possess small reduced genomes.[3] A comprehensive comparative analysis of both genomes highlighted protein candidates susceptible to the new generation of rickettsial vaccines or to be targeted by new antimicrobial drugs.[4] The aim of this work was to further expand our knowledge about which proteins are actually expressed by these microorganisms and encoded by virtual annotated genes.

Address for correspondence: Patricia Renesto, Unité des Rickettsies, CNRS UMR 6020. Voice: +(33) 491 32 43 75; fax: +(33) 491 38 77 72.
patricia.renesto@medecine.univ-mrs.fr

**Ann. N.Y. Acad. Sci. 1063: 90–93 (2005). © 2005 New York Academy of Sciences.
doi: 10.1196/annals.1355.014**

MATERIALS AND METHODS

To identify rickettsial proteins that are expressed, we have developed two-dimensional gel electrophoresis (2D-PAGE) coupled with matrix-assisted laser desorption ionization–time of flight mass spectrometry (MALDI-TOF MS) protocol. The major drawback, when considering such strictly intracellular bacteria was to remove eukaryotic contaminants. Indeed, identification of proteins by MALDI-TOF MS provides peptide mass fingerprints and not sequence information, and contaminating eukaryotic proteins may hamper an efficient detection. In this work, *R. conorii* (strain seven, ATCC, VR613) and *R. prowazekii* (strain Brein L) grown in Vero cells were extensively purified and disrupted with a high pressure of nitrogen gas. Subcellular rickettsial fraction enriched in membrane proteins was resolved by 2D-PAGE as previously described.[5]

RESULTS AND DISCUSSION

We report here a preliminary comparison of membrane-enriched fractions of *R. conorii* and *R. prowazekii* separated by 2D-PAGE and detected by silver-staining. Comparison of both patterns revealed that, whereas several main spots are found at the same position, many positional shifts and differentially present or absent spots are also observed (FIG. 1). Peptide mass fingerprinting using MALDI-MS allowed us to identify eight distinct proteins that were assigned easily between the two strains (TABLES 1 and 2) and that are located at the same position within the 2D-PAGE patterns. In all cases, observed pI and molecular mass values were in agreement with those expected deduced from *in silico* analysis. Heat shock proteins were particularly

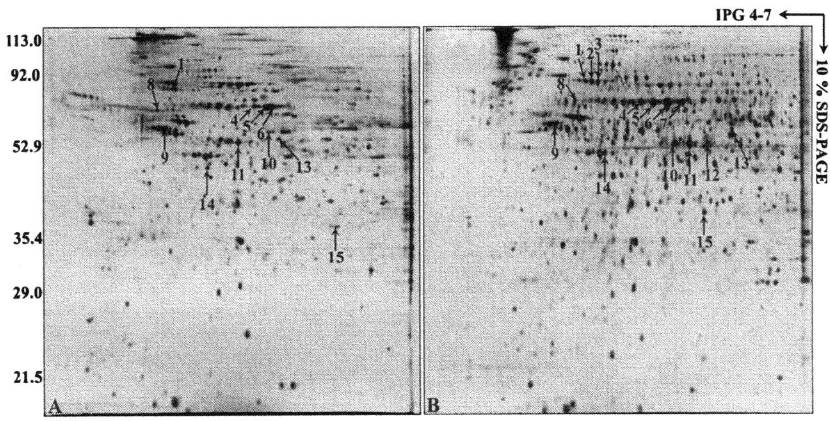

FIGURE 1. *R. conorii* (**A**) and *R. prowazekii* (**B**) membrane-enriched fractions resolved by 2D-PAGE: 100 μg proteins were loaded on IPG strips pH 4–7, 18 cm (Amersham Biosciences). The gel strips were focused on a Multiphor electrophoresis unit and the second dimension was run on vertical 10% acrylamide SDS-PAGE gels (Protean II; Bio-Rad). The gels were silver-stained and spots excised for MALDI-TOF MS identification. Proteins successfully identified in *Table 1* and *Table 2* are numbered. Relative molecular masses (kDa) are indicated on the left.

TABLE 1. ***R. conorii*** **proteins identified from 2D-PAGE**

					In Silico Data	2D-PAGE Data	Spot Number	ORFs
Spot Number	ORFs	Gene	Protein Description	Score	MW (kDa)	pI	MW (kDa)	pI
1	RC0233	*dnaK*	DnaK-Hsp-70 protein	195	67.98	5.0 2	70.92	5.14
4	RC0968	*groEL*	groEL; 60 kD chaperonin	82	58.67	5.62	59.06	5.80
5	RC0968	*groEL*	groEL; 60 kD chaperonin	113	58.67	5.62	58.73	5.91
6	RC0968	*groEL*	groEL; 60 kD chaperonin	75	58.67	5.62	58.74	5.97
8	RC1015	*ftsZ*	Cell division protein ftsZ	56	48.48	4.86	57.84	4.93
9	RC1235	*atpD*	ATP synthase beta chain	73	54.49	4.93	55.02	4.58
10	RC1008	*tuf*	Elongation factor EF-tu	121	42.95	5.42	46.70	5.67
11	RC1008	*tuf*	Elongation factor EF-tu	116	42.95	5.42	50.31	5.57
13	RC1216	*serS*	Serine-tRNA ligase	49	48.66	5.62	47.10	6.00
14	RC1198	*mreB*	Rod shape-determining prot mreB	81	37.5	5.29	41.74	5.42
15	RC0113	*tsf*	Elongation factor EF-Ts	118	33.78	5.21	38.47	5.38

TABLE 2. ***R. prowazekii*** **proteins identified from 2D-PAGE**

					In Silico Data	2D-PAGE Data	Spot Number	ORFs
Spot Number	ORFs	Gene	Protein Description	Score	MW (kDa)	pI	MW (kDa)	pI
1	RP185	*dnaK*	DnaK-Hsp-70 protein	69	68.45	5.2	75.45	5.28
2	RP185	*dnaK*	DnaK-Hsp-70 protein	140	68.45	5.2	74.80	5.33
3	RP185	*dnaK*	DnaK-Hsp-70 protein	149	68.45	5.2	74.48	5.38
4	RP626	*groEL*	groEL; 60 kD chaperonin	91	58.95	5.62	68.35	5.82
5	RP626	*groEL*	groEL; 60 kD chaperonin	101	58.95	5.62	68.62	5.72
6	RP626	*groEL*	groEL; 60 kD chaperonin	74	58.95	5.62	66.83	5.93
7	RP626	*groEL*	groEL; 60 kD chaperonin	78	58.95	5.62	66.44	6.05
8	RP666	*ftsZ*	Cell division protein ftsZ	78	48.89	5.05	68.81	5.19
9	RP801	*atpD*	ATP synthase beta chain	193	51.35	4.85	68.13	5.04
10	RP661	*tuf*	Elongation factor EF-tu	145	43.01	5.77	60.07	5.98
11	RP661	*tuf*	Elongation factor EF-tu	88	43.01	5.77	59.93	6.11
12	RP661	*tuf*	Elongation factor EF-tu	80	43.01	5.77	60.35	6.25
13	RP783	*serS*	Serine-tRNA ligase	92	48.84	5.95	65.43	6.45
14	RP768	*mreB*	Rod shape-determining prot mreB	90	37.5	5.39	56.50	5.44
15	RP087	*tsf*	Elongation factor EF-Ts	83	34.17	5.83	41.08	6.23

abundant. As previously described,[5] several spots resulted in the same protein identification, suggesting the presence of numerous isoforms. Such post-translational modifications are likely to be more abundant concerning *R. prowazekii*. This could explain the fact that, within the range of pI 4–7, 674 and 918 spots were numerated for *R. conorii* and *R. prowazekii*, respectively, while 1,374 and 834 ORFs were annotated in both genomes.[3]

In summary, this work opens the way to characterization of the proteome of rickettsia species, to compare protein profile of either different isolates or of bacteria maintained under different experimental conditions, and to identify immunogenic proteins as potential vaccine targets. The ability to rapidly identify such proteins can provide numerous advantages and capabilities in a diversity of fields, from microbiology to medical diagnosis of rickettsial diseases.

ACKNOWLEDGMENTS

This work was supported by the French CNRS Grant "Protéomique et Génie des Protéines" No. PGP03-009.

[*Conflict of interest statement:* The authors of this research declare that they have no conflict of interest.]

REFERENCES

1. Raoult, D. & V. Roux. 1997. Rickettsioses as paradigms of new or emerging infectious diseases. Clin. Microbiol. Rev. **10:** 694–719.
2. Andersson, S.G., A. Zomorodipour, J.O. Andersson, *et al.* 1998. The genome sequence of *Rickettsia prowazekii* and the origin of mitochondria. Nature **396:** 133–140.
3. Ogata, H., S. Audic, P. Renesto-Audiffren, *et al.* 2001. Mechanisms of evolution in *Rickettsia conorii* and *R. prowazekii*. Science **293:** 2093–2098.
4. Renesto, P., H. Ogata, S. Audic, *et al.* 2005. Some lessons from *Rickettsia* genomics. FEMS Microbiol. Rev. **29:** 99–117.
5. Renesto, P., S. Azza, A. Dolla, *et al.* 2005. Proteome analysis of *Rickettsia conorii* by two-dimensional gel electrophoresis coupled with mass spectrometry. FEMS Microbiol. Lett. **245:** 231–238.

Phylogenetic Study of *Rickettsia* Species Using Sequences of the Autotransporter Protein-Encoding Gene *sca2*

MAXIME NGWAMIDIBA,[a] GUILLAUME BLANC,[b] HIROYUKI OGATA,[b] DIDIER RAOULT,[a] AND PIERRE-EDOUARD FOURNIER[a]

[a]*Unité des Rickettsies, IFR 48, CNRS UMR 6020, Faculté de Médecine, Université de la Méditerranée, 13385 Marseille Cedex 05, France*

[b]*Information Génomique et Structurale, UPR 2589 31, 13402 Marseille Cedex 20, France*

ABSTRACT: The analyses of genome sequences from *Rickettsia conorii* and *R. prowazekii* have allowed the identification of five genes encoding autotransporter proteins, including *ompA* and four genes annotated in the *R. prowazekii* genome as "surface cell antigen" (*sca*) genes. Of these, *ompA* and *sca5* (*ompB*) are known to encode membrane-exposed antigenic proteins playing a major role in the host's immune response, and *sca4* encodes a truncated autotransporter protein. In order to study further the phylogeny of the genus *Rickettsia*, we attempted amplification and sequencing of the *sca2* genes from the 20 currently validated *Rickettsia* species. Sixteen species exhibited a complete *sca2* gene, ranging from 2,727 bp in *R. bellii* to 5,580 bp in *R. rhipicephali*. *R. helvetica* and *R. canadensis* had a split gene, and *R. prowazekii* and *R. typhi* had remnant fragments of *sca2*. We also identified in *R. akari*, *R. prowazekii*, and *R. typhi* a duplication of the *sca2* gene. The phylogenetic trees inferred from both the nucleotide and protein sequences of *sca2* showed four clusters of rickettsiae, that is, the *R. rickettsii*, *R. massiliae*, *R. akari*, and typhus groups, which were supported by significant bootstrap values.

KEYWORDS: *Rickettsia*; phylogeny; *sca* genes; DNA sequences

INTRODUCTION

Members of the genus *Rickettsia* are obligate intracellular, gram-negative bacteria, responsible for human spotted fevers and typhus. These bacteria are surrounded by a crystalline proteic layer,[1] also referred to as S-layer, that represents 10–15% of their total proteic mass[2] and is made from immunodominant surface proteic antigens.[3] Prior to 2001, two surface-exposed proteins, that is, rOmpA and rOmpB, had been identified as major antigenic determinants eliciting an early and dominant immune response in patients infected with rickettsiae.[4–6] The two proteins are encoded by the surface cell antigen (*sca*) genes *ompA* and *ompB*, respectively.[7,8] They exhibit

Address for correspondence: Pierre-Edouard Fournier, Unité des Rickettsies, IFR 48, CNRS UMR 6020, Faculté de Médecine, Université de la Méditerranée, 27 Boulevard Jean Moulin, 13385 Marseille Cedex 05, France. Voice: +(33) 04.91.38.55.17; fax: +(33) 04.91.83.03.90. pierre-edouard.fournier@medecine.univ-mrs.fr

Ann. N.Y. Acad. Sci. 1063: 94–99 (2005). © 2005 New York Academy of Sciences. doi: 10.1196/annals.1355.015

an autotransporter protein structure.[9] In addition to these two genes, the *sca4* gene encodes a truncated autotransporter protein that has lost its autotransporter domain.[10] All three genes were demonstrated to be good tools to study phylogenetic relation ships among *Rickettsia* species, but were not amplified from all species.[7,8,10] The comparison of genome sequences from *R. prowazekii*[11] and *R. conorii*[12] allowed the identification of another two paralogous autotransporter genes annotated as *sca1* and *sca2*. Here, we investigated whether the *sca2* gene could be a good phylogenic tool for *Rickettsia* sp.

MATERIALS AND METHODS

We first searched "*in silico*" the seven rickettsial genome sequences available in GenBank for the presence of the *sca2* gene. We also searched the genomic sequence of *R. bellii* (unpublished data). Then, we amplified and sequenced the gene in the remaining 12 validated *Rickettsia* species. When primers failed to amplify a gene fragment, the GenomeWalker DNA walking method was performed using the Universal Genome Walker Kit (CLONTECH, Palo Alto, CA). Sequencing was performed using an ABI Prism 3100 automated sequencer (PE-Applied Biosystems). We used ClustalW to carry out multiple alignments of nucleotide and derived amino acid sequences.[13] Alignments were manually corrected to remove gapped and ambiguous positions before analysis. Neighbor-Joining (NJ) and Maximum Parsimony (MP) phylogenetic reconstructions were carried out using the MEGA2 software (version 2.1).[14] Maximum Likelihood (ML) trees were performed with the programs PROTML (MOLPHY software package) and PAUP[15] for the protein and nucleotide alignments, respectively. Statistical support for internal branches was assessed by bootstrap resampling for MP and NJ analyses and Resampling of Estimated Log-Likelihood (RELL) for ML analysis.[16]

RESULTS

Sca2 fragments were amplified from all tested *Rickettsia* species, except *R. bellii*. However, at the homologous location of the *sca2* gene in the *R. conorii* and *R. prowazekii* genomes, we found in the *R. akari* genome two consecutive genes, that is, *sca2* and a second autotransporter protein-encoding gene that we named *sca6* (FIG. 1). At this same location in the *R. bellii* genome, we found a gene that had characteristics of both *sca2* and *sca6* genes. Thus, it is likely that the *sca2/6* gene present in *R. bellii* is the preduplication ancestral gene of *sca2* and *sca6*.[17] The size of *sca2* genes ranged from 2,727 bp for *R. bellii* to 5,580 bp for *R. rhipicephali*. The gene was split in *R. canadensis* and *R. helvetica*, and present as a remnant in *R. prowazekii* and *R. typhi*. The overall pairwise nucleotide sequence identities of *sca*2 varied from 62.8% between *R. felis* and *R. helvetica* to 98.4% between *R. massiliae* and *R. rhipicephali*, as compared to a range of 95.2–99.8% for sequences of the *ompA* gene,[7] 70–99.6% for the *ompB* gene,[8] and 76.3–99.7% for the *sca4* gene.[10]

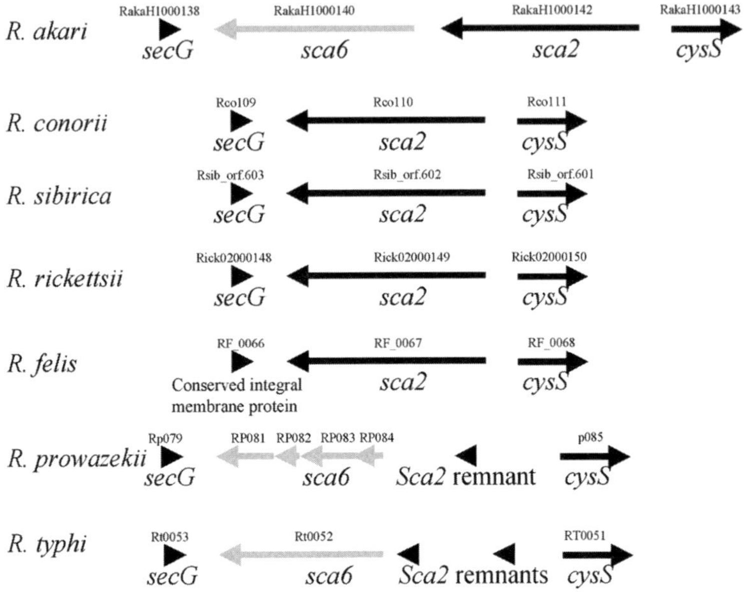

FIGURE 1. Aligned portions of the genomes of *R. conorii*, *R. rickettsii*, *R. sibirica*, *R. akari*, *R. prowazekii*, and *R. typhi*, containing the *sec*G (*white arrows*), *sca2* (*gray arrows*), and *cys*S (*black arrows*) genes, and, when present, the *sca6* gene (*cross-hatched arrows*). *Sca2* remnants in *R. prowazekii* and *R. typhi* are indicated. ORF numbering according to each genome is indicated. Positions within the genomes are indicated with respect to their origins of replication.

The phylogenetic relationships among *Rickettsia* species inferred from the comparison of *sca2* sequences provided similar phylogenetic organizations with the various methods. A first cluster, previously named *R. rickettsii* group,[18] included *R. parkeri*, *R. conorii*, *R. africae*, *R. sibirica*, *R. slovaca*, *R. rickettsii*, *R. honei*, and *R. japonica*. This cluster was supported by bootstrap values of 78–100% (Fig. 2). A second cluster, the *R. massiliae* group, was made of *R. montanensis*, *R. aeschlimannii*, *R. massiliae*, and *R. rhipicephali*. This cluster was supported by bootstrap values of 57–100%. A third cluster, previously named *R. akari* group, was made of *R. felis*, *R. australis*, and *R. akari*. All bootstrap values for this cluster were 100% in all phylogenetic reconstructions. Finally, members of the typhus group were grouped together with a 100% bootstrap value. *R. bellii* was the most outer species. When compared to phylogenic classifications obtained from the study of other *sca* genes, the *sca2*-based phylogeny was the most reliable, with 14/17 nodes supported by bootstrap values ≥80%, and was similarly reliable than *ompB*-based phylogeny (14/16), as compared to 4/11 for *ompA*, and 12/16 for *sca4*.

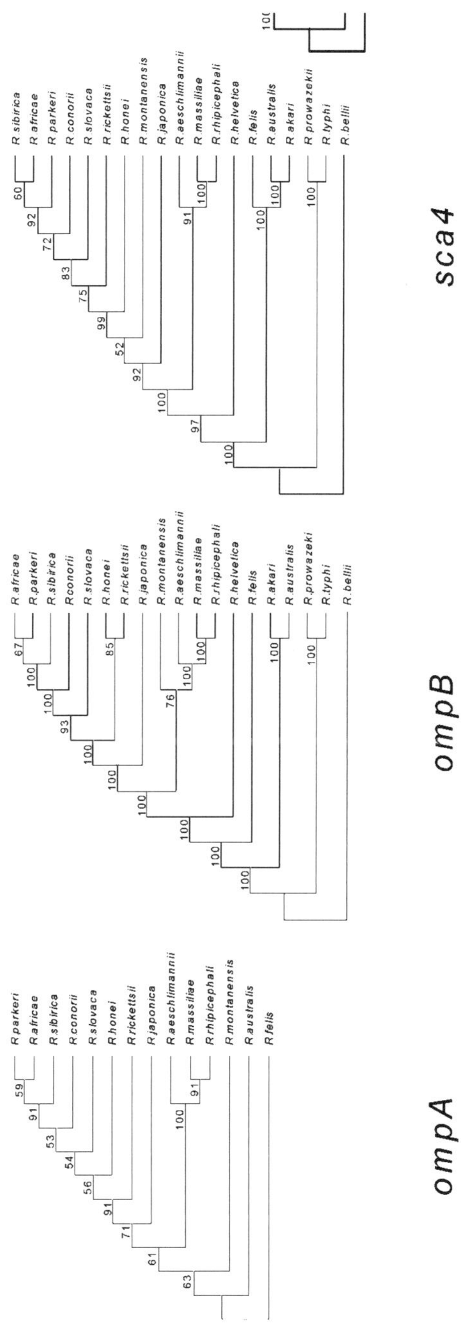

FIGURE 2. Unrooted trees showing the phylogenetic relationships among rickettsiae, as inferred from sequence analysis of each of the three genes by the maximum parsimony method. The numbers at the nodes are the proportion of 100 bootstrap resamplings that support the topology shown.

DISCUSSION

We have observed that the gene annotated as *sca2* in the *R. prowazekii* and *R. typhi* genomes is in fact another *sca* family gene, which we named *sca6* (FIG. 1). This organization of the *sca2* locus, with *sca2* adjacent to *sca6*, is probably ancestral to the split between typhus and spotted fever groups, as remnants of the *sca2* gene are found beside the *sca6* gene in *R. prowazekii* and *R. typhi*.

We obtained unique sequences for the 20 studied species. *Sca*2 was the less conserved *sca* gene among *Rickettsia* species, thus making this gene a potential identification tool for spotted fever group rickettsiae. The *sca2*-based phylogenetic analysis of *Rickettsia* species was highly reliable, with 82% of nodes supported by bootstrap values equal to or higher than 80% (FIG. 2). By comparison with those obtained from other *sca* genes, the phylogenic organization inferred from *sca2* sequences was as reliable as that based on *ompB* and more reliable than those based on *ompA* and *sca4*. Four clusters supported by significant bootstrap values were identified. A first cluster included *Rickettsia* species previously classified within the *R. rickettsii* group.[18] A second cluster was made of members of the *R. massiliae* group. The third cluster incorporated members of the *R. akari* group, and the fourth cluster included members of the typhus group. *Sca2* was the first *sca* gene detected in *R. canadensis*. As observed for other *sca* genes, *R. bellii* appeared to have diverged early from other species.

The *sca2*-based phylogenic organization was similar to those obtained using *ompA*, *ompB*, and *sca4* sequences.[7,8,10] This suggests that, in the different *Rickettsia* species, *sca* genes have undergone similar evolutionary forces. However, the presence of split *sca2* genes in two species also suggests that *sca2* may be undergoing a degradation process.

We have demonstrated that the *sca2* gene may be used as a valuable tool for the identification and phylogenic classification of *Rickettsia* species. Whether this gene is functional is currently unknown. However, further studies should aim at determining whether it plays a role in the immune response observed in patients with rickettsioses.

[*Conflict of interest statement:* The authors of this research declare that they have no conflict of interest.]

REFERENCES

1. PALMER, E.L., M.L. MARTIN & L. MALLAVIA. 1974. Ultrastucture of the surface of *Rickettsia prowazekii* and *Rickettsia akari*. Appl. Microbiol. **28:** 713–716.
2. CHING, W.M., H. WANG, B. JAN & G.A. DASCH. 1996. Identification and characterization of epitopes on the 120-kilodalton surface protein antigen of *Rickettsia prowazekii* with synthetic peptides. Infect. Immun. **64:** 1413–1419.
3. CHING, W.M., M. CARL & G.A. DASCH. 1992. Mapping of monoclonal antibody binding sites on CNBr fragments of the S-layer protein antigens of *Rickettsia typhi* and *Rickettsia prowazekii*. Mol. Immunol. **29:** 95–105.
4. ANACKER, R.L., G.A. MCDONALD, R.H. LIST & R.E. MANN. 1987. Neutralizing activity of monoclonal antibodies to heat-sensitive and heat-resistant epitopes of *Rickettsia rickettsii* surface proteins. Infect. Immun. **55:** 825–827.

5. GILMORE, R.D., JR., N. JOSTE & G.A. MCDONALD. 1989. Cloning, expression, and sequence analysis of the gene encoding the 120 kD surface-exposed protein of *Rickettsia rickettsii*. Mol. Microbiol. **3:** 1579–1586.
6. TEYSSEIRE, N. & D. RAOULT. 1992. Comparison of Western immunoblotting and micro-immunofluoresence for diagnosis of Mediterranean spotted fever. J. Clin. Microbiol. **30:** 455–460.
7. FOURNIER, P.E., V. ROUX & D. RAOULT. 1998. Phylogenetic analysis of spotted fever group rickettsiae by study of the outer surface protein rOmpA. Int. J. Syst. Bacteriol. **48:** 839–849.
8. ROUX, V. & D. RAOULT. 2000. Phylogenetic analysis of members of the genus *Rickettsia* using the gene encoding the outer-membrane protein rOmpB (ompB). Int. J. Syst. Evol. Microbiol. **50:** 1449–1455.
9. HENDERSON, I.R., F. NAVARRO-GARCIA & J.P. NATARO. 1998. The great escape: structure and function of the autotransporter proteins. Trends Microbiol. **6:** 370–378.
10. SEKEYOVA, Z., V. ROUX & D. RAOULT. 2001. Phylogeny of *Rickettsia* spp. inferred by comparing sequences of "gene D," which encodes an intracytoplasmic protein. Int. J. Syst. Evol. Microbiol. **51:** 1353–1360.
11. ANDERSSON, S.G., A. ZOMORODIPOUR, J.O. ANDERSSON, *et al.* 1998. The genome sequence of *Rickettsia prowazekii* and the origin of mitochondria. Nature **396:** 133–140.
12. OGATA, H., S. AUDIC, P. RENESTO-AUDIFFREN, *et al.* 2001. Mechanisms of evolution in *Rickettsia conorii* and *R. prowazekii*. Science **293:** 2093–2098.
13. CHENNA, R., H. SUGAWARA, T. KOIKE, *et al.* 2003. Multiple sequence alignment with the Clustal series of programs. Nucleic Acids Res. **31:** 3497–3500.
14. KUMAR, S., K. TAMURA, I.B. JAKOBSEN & M. NEI. 2001. MEGA2: molecular evolutionary genetics analysis software. Tempe, AZ.
15. PAUP. 1998. Phylogenetic analysis using parsimony. Computer Program. Sinauer. Sunderland, MA.
16. HASEGAWA, M. & H. KISHINO. 1994. Accuracies of the simple methods for estimating the bootstrap probability of a maximum-likelihood tree Mol. Biol. Evol. **11:** 142–145.
17. BLANC, G., M. NGWAMIDIBA, H. OGATA, *et al.* 2005. Molecular evolution of *Rickettsia* surface antigens: evidence of positive selection. Mol. Biol. Evol. In press.
18. ROUX, V. 1999. Phylogenetic analysis and taxonomic relationships among the genus *Rickettsia*. *In* Rickettsiae and Rickettsial Diseases at the Turn of the Third Millennium. D. Raoult & P. Brouqui, Eds.: 52–66. Elsevier. Marseille.

Molecular Characterization of a Group of Proteins Containing Ankyrin Repeats in *Orientia tsutsugamushi*

NAM-HYUK CHO, JO-MIN KIM, EUN-KYUNG KWON, SE-YOON KIM, SEUNG-HOON HAN, HYUK CHU, JUNG-HEE LEE, MYUNG-SIK CHOI, AND IK-SANG KIM

Department of Microbiology and Immunology, Seoul National University College of Medicine, Seoul 110-799, Republic of Korea

ABSTRACT: *Orientia tsutsugamushi*, an obligate intracellular bacterium, is the causative agent of scrub typhus. The sequencing and analysis of full genomic DNA of *O. tsutsugamushi* has revealed at least 19 genes thus far encoding proteins with different numbers of ankyrin repeat domains. We have cloned several genes containing ankyrin repeats from the genome and produced fusion proteins to characterize their functions in host cells. It is likely that the proteins with ankyrin repeat domains expressed in *O. tsutsugamushi*–infected cells may control the synthesis or stability of host proteins to modulate the various cellular functions after infection. The exploitation of host factors by ankyrin repeat proteins of *O. tsutsugamushi* may also play a critical role in its pathogenesis.

KEYWORDS: *Orientia tsutsugamushi*; ankyrin repeat; intracellular bacterium; EF-1α

Orientia tsutsugamushi, an obligate intracellular bacterium, is the causative agent of scrub typhus.[1] The disease is characterized by fever, rash, eschar, pneumonitis, meningitis, and disseminated intravascular coagulation, which leads to severe multiorgan failure. While we are performing the sequencing and analysis of full genomic DNA of *O. tsutsugamushi*, it has revealed an abundance of genes, at least 19 genes thus far, encoding proteins with different numbers of ankyrin repeat domains. These domains are commonly found in diverse eukaryotic and prokaryotic proteins that regulate various cellular functions such as cell cycle, signal transduction, transcription, and structures.[2,3] Interestingly, it was also reported that *Wolbachia pipientis*, another obligate intracellular bacterium that infects arthropods and nematodes, contains 23 genes containing ankyrin repeats.[4] *Rickettsia felis* also contains numerous ankyrin repeats[5] as well as *C. burnetii*,[6] in contrast to other rickettsial relatives such as Ehrlichia, Rickettsia, and Anaplasma where just a few genes containing ankyrin repeats were found in their genome. Moreover, an ankyrin domain protein described

Address for correspondence: Nam-Hyuk Cho, Department of Microbiology and Immunology, Seoul National University College of Medicine, Seoul 110-799, Republic of Korea. Voice: +82-2-740-8392; fax: +82-2-743-0881.
chonh@snu.ac.kr

Ann. N.Y. Acad. Sci. 1063: 100–101 (2005).
doi: 10.1196/annals.1355.016

from *Ehrlichia phagocytophila* appears to be transported into the host cell where it has been reported to bind host chromatin during apoptosis.[7] We have cloned several genes containing ankyrin repeats from the genome of *O. tsutsugamushi* and produced fusion proteins to characterize their functions in the host cells. The expression of ankyrin repeat proteins was examined by immunoblot using polyclonal antibodies produced from immunized mice. We have also searched their binding partners from host cell lysates by GST-pull down assay for the functional study of ankyrin repeat proteins. We have found that two ankyrin-repeats proteins could interact with elongation factor-1α[8] and inhibit the cell division when they were expressed in ECV304 cell lines. It is likely that the proteins with ankyrin repeat domains expressed in *O. tsutsugamushi*–infected cells may control the synthesis or stability of host proteins to modulate the various cellular functions after infection. The exploitation of host factors by ankyrin repeat proteins of *O. tsutsugamushi* may also play a critical role in its pathogenesis.

[*Conflict of interest statement:* The authors of this research declare that they have no conflict of interest.]

REFERENCES

1. SEONG, S.Y., M.S. CHOI & I.S. KIM. 2001. *Orientia tsutsugamushi* infection: overview and immune responses. Microbes Infect. **3:** 11–21.
2. MOSAVI, L.K. *et al.* 2004. The ankyrin repeat as molecular architecture for protein recognition. Protein Sci. **13:** 1435–1448.
3. SEDGWICK, S.G. & S.J. SMERDON. 1999. The ankyrin repeat: a diversity of interactions on a common structural framework. Trends Biochem. Sci. **24:** 311–316.
4. MCGRAW, E.A. & S.L. O'NEILL. 2004. *Wolbachia pipientis*: intracellular infection and pathogenesis in *Drosophila*. Curr. Opin. Microbiol. **7:** 67–70.
5. OGATA, H. *et al.* 2005. The genome sequence of *Rickettsia felis* identifies the first putative conjugative plasmid in an obligate intracellular parasite. PLoS Biol. **3:** 248.
6. SESHADRI, R. *et al.* 2003. Complete genome sequence of the Q-fever pathogen *Coxiella burnetii*. Proc. Natl. Acad. Sci. USA **100:** 5455–5460.
7. CATUREGLI, P. *et al.* 2000. ankA: an *Ehrlichia phagocytophila* group gene encoding a cytoplasmic protein antigen with ankyrin repeats. Infect. Immun. **68:** 5277–5283.
8. LAMBERTI, A. *et al.* 2004. The translation elongation factor 1A in tumorigenesis, signal transduction, and apoptosis: review article. Amino Acids **26:** 443–448.

Ehrlichia ruminantium

A Promiscuous Genome

MARIA ALLSOPP,[a] HELENA STEYN,[a] ERICH ZWEYGARTH,[a] AND BASIL ALLSOPP[b]

[a]*Onderstepoort Veterinary Institute, P. Bag X5, Onderstepoort 0110, South Africa*

[b]*Department of Veterinary Tropical Diseases, Faculty of Veterinary Science, University of Pretoria, P. Bag X04, Onderstepoort 0110, South Africa*

ABSTRACT: **The intracellular bacterium, *Ehrlichia ruminantium*, is the causative agent of heartwater, a tick-borne disease of livestock. Because vaccines need to incorporate components from several virulent isolates, it is essential to have information on the extent of genetic variation among isolates. We therefore amplified and sequenced a panel of seven core function genes.**

KEYWORDS: ***Ehrlichia ruminantium*; phylogenetic analysis; recombination**

INTRODUCTION

The intracellular bacterium, *Ehrlichia ruminantium*, is the causative agent of heartwater throughout sub-Saharan Africa, Madagascar, and some islands of the Caribbean. The disease is tick-borne and it causes substantial livestock losses, threatening food security and productivity in both the commercial and small-scale farming sectors. Immunization by infection and treatment is currently practised in South Africa, and it is known that a variety of immunotypes of the organism occur in the field, and that cross-protection between them varies widely from total to minimal.[1] Because future vaccines may therefore need to incorporate components from several virulent isolates, it is essential to have information on the extent of genetic variation among isolates. We therefore amplified and sequenced a panel of seven core function genes (TABLE 1), some of which have been extensively used for the characterization of other Rickettsiales, from 12 different cultured stocks (TABLE 1) originally isolated in different areas of Africa and the Caribbean.

MATERIALS AND METHODS

DNA extracted from *E. ruminantium* culture supernatants was subjected to PCR amplification of the appropriate genes. Single, well-defined amplicons were directly

Address for correspondence: Basil Allsopp, Department of Veterinary Tropical Diseases, Faculty of Veterinary Science, University of Pretoria, P. Bag X04, Onderstepoort 0110, South Africa. Voice: +27 12 5298426; fax: +27 12 5298312.
Basil.Allsopp@up.ac.za

**Ann. N.Y. Acad. Sci. 1063: 102–104 (2005). © 2005 New York Academy of Sciences.
doi: 10.1196/annals.1355.017**

TABLE 1. Identities of the sequences of 7 core function genes from 12 different *E ruminantium* stocks

			Sequence Identity of Gene or Genetic Region						
Stock	Code	Origin	16S	pCS20	gltA	groESL	ftsZ	sodB	nuoB
Welgevonden	Welg	RSA	Welg	Welg	Welg	Welg	Welg	Welg	Welg
Mara87/7	M87	RSA	M87	M87	M87	M87	M87	M87	M87
Ball3	B3	RSA	B3	Welg	B3	B3	B3	Welg	M87
Blaauwkrans	Blk	RSA	Welg	Blk	Blk	Welg	Blk	Blk	Blk
UmBanein	UmB	Sudan	M87	UmB	UmB	B3	Welg	Welg	Welg
Kiswani	Kis	Kenya	Kis	Kis	Kis	Kis	Kis	Kis	Welg
Gardel	Gar	Caribbean	Gar	Gar	Gar	Gar	Gar	Gar	Gar
Kümm1	Km1	RSA	Km1	Km1	Km1	Km1	Km1	Km1	Km1
Kümm2	Km2	RSA	Km2	Km2	na	Km2	Km2	M87	Km2
Senegal	Sen	Senegal	Km1	Km1	Sen	Km1	Sen	Sen	Sen
Sankat	Sank	Ghana	Km1	Km1	Sank	Km1	Sank	Sank	Sank
Pokoase	Pok	Ghana	Km1	Km1	Km1	Pok	Sen	Km1	Km1

Abbreviation: na, not amplified.

sequenced using appropriately diluted amplification primers. Where multiple bands were obtained, the band corresponding to the correct sized amplicon was gel-purified using the protocol recommended for the Qiagen MinElute system (Qiagen, Hilden, Germany). Gel-purified amplicons were cloned into pGEM-T vector (Promega, Madison, USA) and recombinant plasmids were purified using the High Pure Plasmid Isolation kit (Roche Diagnostics, Mannheim, Germany) according to the manufacturers' protocols. To obtain a consensus and to reduce the possibility of polymorphisms due to PCR errors, at least four recombinants containing inserts of a given gene were sequenced. Sequences for each gene were aligned and subjected to phylogenetic analysis using PHYML.[2]

RESULTS AND DISCUSSION

TABLE 1 shows the sequence identities of each gene for the 12 *E. ruminantium* stocks examined. All the Gardel sequences were unique to that stock, reflecting its isolation to the island of Guadeloupe. All the Kümm 2 sequences, with the exception of sodB, were unique to that stock, and were also the most distant from all the others, reflecting the unusual phenotype of that stock.[3] The situation for all the other stocks is more complex. The southern African stocks Welgevonden, Mara87/7, and Kümm1 were the first to be sequenced and they initially also appeared to have unique sequences for each gene. When more southern and eastern African stocks were sequenced, however, some sequences were unique to the new stocks, but others were identical to either Welgevonden or Mara 87/7. There was less overall variability among the western African stocks, confirming the results seen previously in a smaller study, and confirming the suggestion that *E. ruminantium* originated in southern

Africa.[4] With respect of the western African sequences, these were either unique to the stock or identical to those of the southern African Kümm1 stock, with the sole exception that Senegal and Pokoase share the same ftsZ sequence. These findings led to the topologies of the gene trees (not shown) varying from gene to gene, but there were consistent features shared by all the trees. Firstly, the southern (except Kümm1) and eastern African isolates clustered together; secondly, the western African isolates clustered together, and Kümm1 was found in this cluster; thirdly, the position of Gardel was unstable, although most frequently it clustered with weak bootstrap support with the southern African isolates. This latter observation suggests that the Caribbean *E. ruminantium* Gardel genotype came, not from western Africa as had long been assumed, nor from southern Africa, but possibly from somewhere more central, such as Angola.[4] We suggest that the reason for the different phylogenies of the different genes is that extensive recombination takes place between different genotypes in the field. We have frequently detected more than one *E. ruminantium* genotype in DNA from single ticks, so it is possible that recombination occurs during the period when the organisms are extracellular within the tick, immediately after feeding and before intracellular infection is established.

[*Competing interests statement:* The authors have no conflicting financial interests.]

REFERENCES

1. COLLINS, N.E., A. PRETORIUS, M. VAN KLEEF, *et al.* 2003. Development of improved attenuated and nucleic acid vaccines for heartwater. Dev. Biol. (Basel) **114:** 95–110.
2. GUINDON, S. & O. GASCUEL. 2003. A simple, fast, and accurate algorithm to estimate large phylogenies by maximum likelihood. Syst. Biol. **52:** 696–704.
3. ZWEYGARTH, E., A.I. JOSEMANS, M.F. VAN STRIJP, *et al.* 2002. The Kümm isolate of *Ehrlichia ruminantium: in vitro* isolation, propagation and characterization. Onderstepoort J. Vet. Res. **69:** 147–153.
4. ALLSOPP, M.T.E.P., H. VAN HEERDEN, H.C. STEYN & B.A. ALLSOPP. 2003. Phylogenetic relationships among *Ehrlichia ruminantium* isolates. Ann. N.Y. Acad. Sci. **990:** 685–691.

Coxiella burnetii Infection

JAN KAZAR

Research Base of the Slovak Medical University, Bratislava, Slovak Republic

ABSTRACT: *Coxiella burnetii* is an obligate intracellular bacterium that causes a worldwide zoonosis, Q fever, and can be misused as a biological warfare agent. Infection in animals (coxiellosis) is mostly persistent. Infection in humans is often asymptomatic, but it can manifest as an acute disease (usually a self-limited flu-like illness, pneumonia, or hepatitis) or as a chronic form (mainly endocarditis, but also hepatitis and chronic fatigue syndrome). *C. burnetii* infection in pregnant women may result in abortions, premature deliveries, and stillbirths. Infection in nature is maintained and transmitted by ticks as the principal vector and reservoir. Cattle, sheep, and goats are the most important source of human infections. Humans contract *C. burnetii* infection mostly by aerosol in contact with contaminated environs, wind playing an important factor in spreading the infection. The wide distribution of *C. burnetii* contributes to a high resistance of its extracellular small cell variant to environmental conditions. Its intracellular large cell variant, adapted to survive under harsh conditions of phagolysosomes, enables long-term survival and persistence of *C. burnetii*, namely in monocytes/macrophages. Host factors such as underlying disease and cell-mediated immunity play a decisive role in the clinical expression of *C. burnetii* infection. Complete genome analysis of *C. burnetii* will certainly contribute to better understanding of the pathogenesis of *C. burnetii* infection and will improve Q fever diagnosis and immunoprophylaxis.

KEYWORDS: *Coxiella burnetii*; ticks; hosts; Q fever; epidemiology; pathogenesis; diagnosis; therapy; prevention; biological weapon

INTRODUCTION

In general, the outcome of infection in vertebrates results from an interaction of the microbial agent with its host. It is especially true with intracellular parasites, including *Coxiella burnetii*. This paper will try to summarize the peculiarities of *C. burnetii*; its interactions with the host cells, vectors, animals, and humans; and diagnosis, therapy, and prevention of *C. burnetii* infection.

BACTERIOLOGY

C. burnetii is an obligate intracellular microorganism that cannot be grown in axenic medium. It is a small pleomorphic rod (0.2–0.4 μm wide, 0.4–1.0 μm long)

Address for correspondence: Jan Kazar, Research Base of the Slovak Medical University, Bratislava, Slovak Republic. Voice: +421259369100; fax: +421254771094.
jan.kazar@szu.sk

**Ann. N.Y. Acad. Sci. 1063: 105–114 (2005). © 2005 New York Academy of Sciences.
doi: 10.1196/annals.1355.018**

with a membrane similar to that of gram-negative bacterium.[1,2] Based on 16S rRNA sequence analysis, this bacterium belongs to a separate genus *Coxiella* of the gamma subdivision of *Proteobacteria*[3] with the genera *Legionella*, *Franciscella*, and *Rickettsiella* as its closest relatives.[1]

DNA-DNA hybridization showed a low degree of genetic heterogeneity among *C. burnetii* strains,[4] but a considerable heterogeneity among *C. burnetii* isolates of different origin was demonstrated by restriction fragment length polymorphism (RFLP) analysis[5] and pulsed field gel electrophoresis.[6] The genome size among different *C. burnetii* strains was found to be highly variable as well.[7] Plasmids were described for *C. burnetii*, but the assumption that the plasmid type and size are related to the acute versus chronic form of Q fever[8] has not been confirmed.[9]

C. burnetii displays antigenic variations analogous to the smooth-rough variation in the family *Enterobacteriaceae*[10] When propagated in nonimmunocompetent substrates (cell cultures or embryonated eggs), *C. burnetii* converts from a very infectious naturally occurring (in infected animals, humans or arthropods) phase I to a laboratory acquired phase II that is accompanied by a change of physicochemical and biological properties of the agent and dramatic changes in lipopolysaccharide (LPS) structure.[2] It remains unclear whether chromosomal deletions in the LPS biosynthetic regions can explain all cases of *C. burnetii* phase variation.[11]

C. burnetii is very resistant to heat, pressure, and chemical stress[12] so that it can survive for months in environs. This fact together with its high infectivity and easy spreading to humans placed *C. burnetii* in the "Category B" of warfare agents.[13] As an obligate intracellular parasite, it can multiply only within living cells, namely in phagolysosomes, under harsh conditions of acidic pH.[14] *C. burnetii* undergoes a complex intracellular cycle,[15] leading to the formation of spore-like forms. Intracellular developmental stages of *C. burnetii* include metabolically inactive "small-cell variant" (SCV), corresponding to the extracellular form of *C. burnetii*, and "large-cell variant" (LCV), corresponding to the metabolically active intracellular form of the agent.[1] According to Samuel and colleagues,[16] a pressure-insensitive small dense cell (SDC) rather than pressure-sensitive SCV represents the form most likely to survive extracellularly. Recently it has been demonstrated that the LCV is the replicative form of *C. burnetii*.[17] Factors inducing the sporulation-like process are unknown, but the role of life cycle–specific major outer protein, P1, that functions as a porin, is considered.[16]

PATHOGENESIS OF *C. BURNETII* INFECTION

In *C. burnetii* pathogenesis, one must take into account phase variants of the agent. *C. burnetii* enters monocytes/macrophages, the only known target cells,[1] by phagocytosis that differs in phase I and phase II cells. Whereas the CR3 receptor is engaged in the entry of phase II *C. burnetii* and this is readily internalized via the phagolysosomal pathway, the natural phase I bind to human monocytes via the complex of leukocyte response integrin and integrin-associated protein and it is only poorly internalized by monocytes/macrophages and can survive within these cells.[18] Therefore, the results obtained with phase II *C. burnetii* should be interpreted carefully.

As to the virulence determinants of *C. burnetii*, apart from the LPS, other factors such as acid phosphatase, superoxide dismutase, catalase, *com1* protein, and other surface proteins, and macrophage infectivity potentiator, were suggested.[19] Recent findings indicate that *C. burnetii* LPS is involved not only in phagocytosis, but also in filamentous actin reorganization and inflammatory response through Toll-like receptor 4.[20] It has been found that *C. burnetii* survival in the phagolysosomal-like parasitophorous vacuole requires specific iron systems, secretion of enzymes to detoxify the compartment (catalase and SOD), and downregulation of an oxidative burst (acid phosphatase).[16] *C. burnetii* encodes functional components of a type IV secretion system that could play an important role in creating the specialized vacuole that supports its multiplication.[21] *C. burnetii* and *Legionella pneumophila* are the only two bacteria known today to utilize a type-IVB secretion system for pathogenesis[22] as revealed by sequencing their genomes and can be explained by a significant homology of these agents.[23]

C. burnetii has the ability to induce persistent infections both in humans and animals.[11,24] The host factors, namely certain conditions such as immunosuppression and underlying disease,[1,25] and the level of the cell-mediated immunity[18] play a decisive role in the outcome of *C. burnetii* infection. Host control of *C. burnetii* is mediated primarily by activated monocytes/macrophages that leads to the production of reactive oxygen and nitrogen intermediates with potent antimicrobial activities.[26] The downregulation of macrophage responses to lymphokines and induction of suppressor factors may also allow *C. burnetii* to survive within these cells,[18] e.g., defective phagosome maturation and impaired *C. burnetii* killing was observed in patients with chronic Q fever.[27] *C. burnetii* multiplication and parasitophorous vacuole maturation was inhibited by nitric oxide.[28] Whereas acute Q fever is associated with cytokine overproduction, persistent amounts of tumor necrosis factor were associated with the occurrence of endocarditis in patients with valvulopathy.[29] The roles of this factor, interferon-gamma, and other cytokines are discussed at length by Mege.[30]

C. BURNETII INFECTION IN TICKS

Infected ticks are probably most important in keeping the natural cycle of *C. burnetii* infection going. Every tick species, parasitizing a susceptible host in a known area of endemicity, can be expected to harbor and spread *C. burnetii*, thus representing the principal vector and reservoir of the agent.[9] *C. burnetii* can be carried out by more than 40 naturally infected tick species that transmit the agent both vertically (transtadially or transovarially to their progeny and horizontally (via bite or in feces) to wild vertebrates and wild birds, thus creating wildlife coxiellosis.[31] The tick species that are the most frequent vectors of *C. burnetii* belong to the genera Ixodes, Rhipicephalus, Amblyomma, and Dermacentor.[32]

C. BURNETII INFECTION IN HOST ANIMALS (COXIELLOSIS)

Ticks do not transmit *C. burnetii* by bite to humans, but can do so to domestic animals. This results in creation of livestock coxiellosis that can be maintained later by a direct contact of animals in question or with their fomites.[31] Cattle, sheep, and goats shedding *C. burnetii* in their urine, feces, milk, and mainly birth products represent the most important source of human infection,[33] though it can be contracted also from pets, namely cats[34] and dogs,[35] and sometimes even from domestic poultry[33] or pigeons.[36] *C. burnetii* infection in farm animals is usually dormant and may result in abortion in goats and sheep.[31] High prevalence of *C. burnetii* was found in samples of bulk tank milk from U.S. dairy herds.[37] In other countries the role of cows in spreading *C. burnetii* infection is being replaced by sheep[38] and goats.[39]

Wild animals do not represent a direct source of human *C. burnetii* infection, but they contribute to the maintaining of the agent in nature. Apart from the most important small wild rodents, *C. burnetii* infection was demonstrated also in insectivores, lagomorphs, carnivores, ungulates, marsupials, monkeys, bats, and birds, and even in reptiles and fish.[33] In the United Kingdom, wild rats were suggested as important reservoir of *C. burnetii*[40] and, because they can serve as prey for domestic cats, they could maintain *C. burnetii* between sporadic human epidemics. Migratory birds are able to spread *C. burnetii* over long distances via their feces and ectoparasites.[33] Recently, a wildlife reservoir as a potential source of Q fever has been suggested.[41]

C. BURNETII INFECTION IN HUMANS (Q FEVER)

Q fever is a worldwide zoonosis that occurs in all geographic and climatic zones, where the source and natural conditions of *C. burnetii* infection and circulation exist and where it is sought.[9] New Zealand, due probably to a relative geographic remoteness and strict control measures, is the only larger country without Q fever.[42]

Human Q fever is an airborne infection usually through the inhalation of contaminated aerosols.[1] Due to a long-term survival of the agent in contaminated environs, under certain conditions Q fever can be considered a windborne infection spread from farmlands to the urban areas and to many unexpected places.[43] Of other ways of transmission, alimentary route remains controversial because of a discrepancy between some outbreaks connected with ingestion of contaminated raw milk or milk products[44] and inability to induce Q fever when contaminated milk was fed to volunteers.[9] The route of infection can probably determine the clinical manifestation of Q fever.[45] Increased surveillance has revealed an importance of vertical or transplacental transmission of *C. burnetii*.[46] Sexual, person-to-person, and percutaneous (including tick-borne) transmission are rare,[9] and nosocomial infection is also possible.[47]

Q fever is a highly variable disease ranging from acute to fatal chronic infection, but subclinical and asymptomatic infections are also common.[1] Proposed reasons for regional variations of clinical manifestations include differences in *C. burnetii* virulence, routes of infection, or average infectious dose, but they lack convincing evidence. Though some *C. burnetii* strains of lower virulence for laboratory animals were described,[48,49] they can hardly explain varying severity of the disease during the same Q fever outbreak. However, different RFLP patterns revealed evolutionary relationships among groups that corresponded to the geographical origin of the *C. burnetii* isolates[50] and a difference in virulence potential of isolates associated with acute (the presence of an immunodominant 28-kDa protein) and chronic diseases has been suggested.[51]

Acute Q fever, after incubation period of 1–3 weeks, manifests mostly as flu-like disease or atypical pneumonia, less often as hepatitis, isolated and/or prolonged fever, bone, exanthematous, neurological or ocular disease. Pericarditis and myocarditis are infrequent, the latter being life-threatening.[1] Other manifestations are very rare[9] and new ones can appear. Q fever during pregnancy corresponds mainly to placentitis and can cause death in utero, abortion, or premature birth.[52] High incidence of Q fever pneumonia and flu-like disease in children was reported from Japan.[53] Though children are frequently exposed to *C. burnetii*, they are less frequently symptomatic than adults and may have milder disease.[54]

Chronic Q fever, on the other hand, is serious and often fatal illness. It evolves slowly years after primary infection in about 5% of patients infected with *C. burnetii*, mostly in men over 40 with underlying heart disease and/or impaired immunity.[1] The major clinical presentation is endocarditis, much less often are infections of vascular grafts or aneurysms, chronic hepatitis, osteoarticular and chronic pulmonary infections.[1] Since 1997, due to a reduction in the delay of the disease diagnosis and the use of novel effective antibiotic regimes, clinical presentation of Q fever endocarditis has dramatically changed with significant decrease of heart failure, hepatomegaly, inflammatory syndrome, anemia, leukopenia, and abnormal liver function.[55] Clinical symptomatology of acute and chronic Q fever is summarized by others.[56,57]

C. burnetii infection can become chronic fatigue syndrome.[58] In its development, ongoing *C. burnetii* persistence, cytokine dysregulation,[59] and variation in immune response genes leading to cell-mediated hypersensitivity[60] have been hypothesized.

Though Q fever can be considered primarily an occupational disease of workers in close contact with farm animals or processing their products, it may occur also in visitors to areas at risk, workers in the cotton-processing plants, researchers and laboratory personnel, students of veterinary medicine, travellers to areas with Q fever occurrence, and even innocent bystanders.[9] Most cases recruit from grown-up people, in men more frequently than in women.[9] Higher occurrence and severity in men can be partly explained by professional character of Q fever and by sex hormonal factors.[61] Ethnic or race factors are of no importance. As to the seasonal appearance, acute Q fever in Europe is more frequently reported in spring and early summer.[1]

DIAGNOSIS OF *C. BURNETII* INFECTION

Clinical diagnosis of acute Q fever is difficult because its acute form can resemble that of nearly any infectious disease.[1] As to chronic Q fever, *C. burnetii* is an underestimated cause of endocarditis, i.e., early diagnosis is the key to good prognosis that emphasizes the need for systematic serologic examination in case of valvular dysfunction.

Though *C. burnetii* can be isolated in laboratory animals, embryonated eggs, and preferably in cell cultures (shell-vial method with centrifugation of the clinical specimen), it requires careful collection and handling of specimens, experienced personnel, and biosafety level 3 laboratories.[62] Different direct immunodetection methods using mostly monoclonal antibodies have been used with varying results.[9] Polymerase chain reaction (PCR) is an important and simple tool to detect and differentiate *C. burnetii* strains.[63] It allows not only detection of the agent in clinical specimens, cell cultures, and milk, but also retrospective diagnosis with frozen or paraffin-embedded samples.[64] Real-time PCR was used to evaluate *C. burnetii* antibiotic susceptibilities.[65] An adapted nested-PCR was helpful in establishing an early diagnosis of chronic Q fever.[66] However, in acute Q fever, PCR was not so sensitive and should be performed together with serology.[67]

Q fever is diagnosed in most cases by serology. It is easy to perform and not so expensive, but diagnosis does require detection of phase II (acute Q fever) and phase I (chronic Q fever) antibodies.[9] Microimmunofluorescence test is a method of choice with the cut-off values of 50 (IgM) and 200 (IgG) of phase II antibodies in acute Q fever and of 800 of phase I antibodies in chronic Q fever, respectively, when testing a single serum sample only.[62] Other tests include complement fixation, microagglutination, ELISA, Western blotting, dot blotting, slide agglutination, indirect hemolysis, radioimmunoassay, and cross-adsorption.[62]

TREATMENT OF *C. BURNETII* INFECTION

Rapid and proper Q fever diagnosis is indispensable for early and efficient treatment of the disease. When diagnosis is not available, in seriously ill patients at least the empiric treatment must be started within the first 3 days of illness.[68] In specific treatment tetracycline is being replaced by other antibiotics, e.g., in acute Q fever, doxycycline, ofloxacin, and pefloxacin for 14 to 21 days were successfully used.[1] The combination of pefloxacin and rifampin was used to treat patients with prolonged Q fever.[68] Fluoroquinolones penetrating into the cerebrospinal fluid have been used in patients with Q fever meningoencephalitis, but they are contraindicated in children and pregnant women.[1] In this population, macrolides may represent a potential alternative. However, the possibility of *C. burnetii* resistance to antibiotics should also be kept in mind.[69]

In chronic Q fever, relapses occur on withdrawal of antibiotic monotherapy so that combined regimes, e.g., doxycycline with chloroquine (for at least 18 months) or with ofloxacin (for at least 3 years), that reduced the death rate to less than 5% have been proposed.[70] In such combinations, chloroquine increasing the acidic pH of lysosomes can enhance the antibacterial action of doxycycline.[71]

CONTROL OF *C. BURNETII* INFECTION

Controlling *C. burnetii* infection includes nonspecific and specific preventive measures. The former were summarized elsewhere.[72] Specific measures include vaccination of at-risk individuals. At-risk individuals should include persons exposed professionally to *C. burnetii* infection, but patients at risk for chronic Q fever development should also be considered.

So far, three types of human vaccines have been developed and tested effectively: (1) the only registered phase I corpuscular vaccine in Australia,[73] (2) phase I corpuscular chloroform-methanol–treated vaccine in the USA,[74] and (3) soluble chemovaccine—an LPS-protein complex extracted from phase I cells by trichloroacetic acid—in Slovakia.[75] According to our previous recommendation,[76] an efficient Q fever vaccine should consist of phase I *C. burnetii* cells, e.g., phase I corpuscular vaccine, or be prepared from phase I cells, e.g., soluble chemovaccine. It was confirmed also by failure of phase II corpuscular vaccine to protect goats against *C. burnetii* infection with its consequent spread to humans.[44] A need for one or more Q fever vaccines, e.g., the suitability of particular *C. burnetii* strain as a vaccine candidate, was partly answered by demonstration of cross-protection among four

C. burnetii strains of different origin[77] and by a complete protection of our laboratory personnel exposed for about 30 years to infection with tens of *C. burnetii* strains by the soluble vaccine prepared from one *C. burnetii* strain.

Genome sequencing and analysis of *C. burnetii*[78] will certainly help to develop an efficient subunit Q fever vaccine. As a matter of fact, in a recent study analyzing the immunodominant antigens, as many as 54 clones expressing immunoreactive proteins have been found in phase I *C. burnetii*.[79]

[*Conflict of interest statement:* The author of this research declares that there is no conflict of interest.]

REFERENCES

1. MAURIN, M. & D. RAOULT. 1999. Q fever. Clin. Microbiol. Rev. **12:** 518–553.
2. KOVACOVA, E. & J. KAZAR. 2002. Q fever: still a query and underestimated infectious disease. Acta Virol. **46:** 193–210.
3. STEIN, A., N.A. SAUNDERS, A.G. TAYLOR & D. RAOULT. 1993. Phylogenetic homogeneity of *Coxiella burnetii* strains as determined by 16S ribosomal RNA sequencing. FEMS Microbiol. Lett. **113:** 339–344.
4. VODKIN, M.H., J.C. WILLIAMS & E.H. STEPHENS. 1986. Genetic heterogeneity among isolates of *Coxiella burnetii*. J. Gen. Microbiol. **132:** 455–463.
5. HENDRIX, L.R., J.E. SAMUEL & L.P. MALLAVIA. 1991. Differentiation of *Coxiella burnetii* isolates by analysis of restriction-endonuclease-digested DNA separated by SDS–PAGE. J. Gen. Microbiol. **137:** 269–276.
6. THIELE, D., H. WILLEMS, G. KOPF & H. KRAUSS. 1993. Polymorphism in DNA restriction patterns of *Coxiella burnetii* isolates investigated by pulsed field gel electrophoresis and image analysis. Eur. J. Epidemiol. **9:** 419–425.
7. WILLEMS, H., C. JAGER & G. BALJER. 1998. Physical and genetic map of the obligate intracellular bacterium *Coxiella burnetii*. J. Bacteriol. **180:** 3816–3822.
8. SAMUEL, J.E., M.E. FRAZIER & L.P. MALLAVIA. 1985. Correlation of plasmid type and diseases caused by *Coxiella burnetii*. Infect. Immun. **49:** 775–779.
9. KAZAR, J. 1999. Q fever: current concept. *In* Rickettsiae and Rickettsial Diseases at the Turn of the Third Millennium. D. Raoult & P. Brouqui, Eds.: 304–319. Elsevier. New York.
10. BACA, O.O. & L.P. MALLAVIA. 1983. Q fever and *Coxiella burnetii*: a model for host-parasite interactions. Microbiol. Rev. **47:** 127–149.
11. THOMPSON, H.A., T.A. HOOVER, M.H. VODKIN & E.I. SHAW. 2003. Do chromosomal deletions in the lipopolysaccharide biosynthetic regions explain all cases of phase variation in *Coxiella burnetii* strains? Ann. N.Y. Acad. Sci. **990:** 664–670.
12. HEINZEN, R.A., T. HACKSTADT & J.E. SAMUEL. 1999. Developmental biology of *Coxiella burnetii*. Trends Microbiol. **7:** 149–154.
13. ROTZ, L.D., A.S. KHAN, S.R. LILLIBRIDGE, *et al.* 2002. Public health assessment of potential terrorism agents. Emerg. Infect. Dis. **8:** 225–230.
14. HACKSTADT, T. & J.C. WILLIAMS. 1981. Biochemical stratagem for obligate parasitism of eukaryotic cells by *Coxiella burnetii*. Proc. Natl. Acad. Sci. USA **78:** 3240–3244.
15. MCCAUL, T.F. & J.C. WILLIAMS. 1981. Developmental cycle of *Coxiella burnetii*: structure and morphogenesis of vegetative and sporogenic differentiations. J. Bacteriol. **147:** 1063–1078.
16. SAMUEL, J.E., K. KISS & S. VARGHEES. 2003. Molecular pathogenesis of *Coxiella burnetii* in a genomic era. Ann. N.Y. Acad. Sci. **990:** 653–663.
17. COLEMAN, S.A., E.R. FISCHER, D. HOWE, *et al.* 2004. Temporal analysis of *Coxiella burnetii* morphological differentiation. J. Bacteriol. **186:** 7344–7352.
18. MEGE, J.L., M. MAURIN, C. CAPO & D. RAOULT. 1997. *Coxiella burnetii*: the "query" fever bacterium. A model of immune subversion by a strictly intracellular microorganism. FEMS Microbiol. Rev. **19:** 209–217.

19. BACA, O.G. & L.P. MALLAVIA. 1997. The identification of virulence factors of *C. burnetii*. *In* Rickettsial Infection and Immunity. B. Anderson, H. Friedman & M. Bendinelli, Eds.: 131–147. Plenum Press. New York.
20. HONSTETTRE, A., E. GHIGO, A. MOYNAULT, *et al.* 2004. Lipopolysaccharide from *Coxiella burnetii* is involved in bacterial phagocytosis, filamentous actin reorganization, and inflammatory response through Toll-like receptor 4. J. Immunol. **172:** 3695–3703.
21. ZAMBONI, D.S., S. MCGRATH, M. RABINOVITCH & C.R. ROY. 2003. *Coxiella burnetii* express type IV secretion system proteins that function similarly to components of the *Legionella pneumophila* Dot/Icm system. Mol. Microbiol. **49:** 965–976.
22. SEGAL, G., M. FELDMAN & T. ZUSMAN. 2005. The Icm/Dot type-IV secretion systems of *Legionella pneumophila* and *Coxiella burnetii*. FEMS Microbiol. Rev. **29:** 65–81.
23. VOGEL, J.-P. 2004. Turning a tiger into a house cat: using *Legionella pneumophila* to study *Coxiella burnetii*. Trends Microbiol. **12:** 103–105.
24. HARRIS, R.J., P.A. STORM, A. LLOYD, *et al.* 2000. Long-term persistence of *Coxiella burnetii* in the host after primary Q fever. Epidemiol. Infect. **14:** 543–549.
25. RAOULT, D. 1990. Host factors in the severity in Q fever. Ann. N.Y. Acad. Sci. **590:** 33–38.
26. BRENNAN, R.E., K. RUSSEL, G. ZHANG & J.E. SAMUEL. 2004. Both inducible nitric oxide synthase and NADPH oxidase contribute to the control of virulent phase I *Coxiella burnetii* infections. Infect. Immun. **72:** 6666–6675.
27. GHIGO, E., A. HONSTETTRE, C. CAPO, *et al.* 2004. Link between impaired maturation of phagosomes and defective *Coxiella burnetii* killing in patients with chronic Q fever. J. Infect. Dis. **190:** 1767–1772.
28. HOWE, D., L.F. BARROWS, N.M. LINDSTROM & R.A. HEINZEN. 2002. Nitric oxide inhibits *Coxiella burnetii* replication and parasitophorous vacuole maturation. Infect. Immun. **70:** 5140–5147.
29. HONSTETTRE, A., G. IMBERT, E. GHIGO, *et al.* 2003. Dysregulation of cytokines in acute Q fever: role of interleukin-10 and tumor necrosis factor in chronic evolution of Q fever. J. Infect. Dis. **187:** 956–962.
30. MEGE, J.L. 2005. Immunopathology of Q fever. Ann. N.Y. Acad. Sci. In press.
31. LANG, G.H. 1990. Coxiellosis (Q fever) in animals. *In* Q Fever: The Disease. T. J. Marrie, Ed.: 23–48. CRC Press. Boca Raton, FL.
32. PAROLA, P. & D. RAOULT. 2001. Ticks and tick-borne diseases in humans: an emerging infections threat. Clin. Infect. Dis. **32:** 897–928.
33. REHACEK, J. & I.V. TARASEVICH. 1988. Q fever. *In* Acari-borne Rickettsiae and Rickettsioses in Eurasia. M. Gresikova, Ed.: 204–343. VEDA. Bratislava.
34. LANGLEY, J.M., T.J. MARRIE, A. COVERT *et al.* 1988. Poker players' pneumonia: an outbreak of Q fever following exposure to a parturient cat. N. Engl. J. Med. **319:** 354–356.
35. KOMIYA, T., K. SADAMASU, H. TORINIWA, *et al.* 2003. Epidemiological survey on the route of *Coxiella burnetii* infection in an animal hospital. J. Infect. Chemother. **9:** 151–155.
36. STEIN, A. & D. RAOULT. 1999. Pigeon pneumonia in Provence: a bird-borne Q fever outbreak. Clin. Infect. Dis. **29:** 617–620.
37. KIM, S.G., E.H. KIM, C.J. LAFFERTY & E. DUBOVI. 2005. *Coxiella burnetii* in bulk tank milk samples in the United States. Emerg. Infect. Dis. **11:** 619–621.
38. HELLEBRAND, W., T. BREUER & L. PETERSEN. 2001. Changing epidemiology of Q fever in Germany. Emerg. Infect. Dis. **7:** 789–796.
39. SERBEZOV, V., J. KAZAR, V. NOVKIRISHKI, *et al.* 1999. Q fever in Bulgaria and Slovakia. Emerg. Infect. Dis. **5:** 388–394.
40. WEBSTER, J.P., G. LLOYD & D.W. MACDONALDS. 1995. Q fever (*Coxiella burnetii*) reservoir in wild brown rat (*Rattus norvegicus*) populations in the UK. Parasitology **110:** 31–35.
41. MADARIAGA, M.G. 2005. Q fever wildlife reservoir. Emerg. Infect. Dis. **11:** 776–777.
42. HILBINK, F., M. PENROSE, E. KOVACOVA & J. KAZAR. 1993. Q fever is absent from New Zealand. Int. J. Epdemiol. **22:** 645–949.
43. TISSOT-DUPONT, H., M.-A. AMADEI, M. NEZRI & D. RAOULT. 2004. Wind in November; Q fever in December. Emerg. Infect. Dis. **10:** 1264–1269.
44. FISHBEIN, D.B. & D. RAOULT. 1992. A cluster of *Coxiella burnetii* infections associated with exposure to vaccinated goats and their unpasteurized dairy products. Am. J. Trop. Med. Hyg. **47:** 35–40.

45. Marrie, T.J., A. Stein, D. Janigan & D. Raoult. 1996. Route of infection determines the clinical manifestations of acute Q fever. J. Infect. Dis. **173:** 484–487.
46. Langley, J.M., T.J. Marrie, J.C. Leblanc, *et al.* 2003. *Coxiella burnetii* seropositivity in parturient women is associated with adverse pregnancy outcome. Am. J. Obstet. Gynecol. **189:** 228–232.
47. Osorio, S., C. Sarria, P. Gonzales-Ruano, *et al.* 2003. Nosocomial transmission of Q fever. J. Hosp. Infect. **54:** 162–163.
48. Moos, A. & T. Hackstadt. 1987. Comparative virulence of intra- and interstrain lipopolysaccharide variants of *C. burnetii* in the guinea pig model. Infect. Immun. **55:** 1144–1150.
49. Oda, H. & K. Yoshiie. 1989. Isolation of a *Coxiella burnetii* strain that has low virulence for mice from a patient with acute Q fever. Microbiol. Immunol. **33:** 969–973.
50. Jager, C., H. Willems, D. Thiele & G. Bajler. 1998. Molecular characterization of *Coxiella burnetii* isolates. Epidemiol. Infect. **120:** 157–164.
51. Zhang, G., H. To, K.E. Russell, *et al.* 2005. Identification and characterization of an immunodominant 28-kilodalton *Coxiella burnetii* outer membrane protein specific to isolates associated with acute diseases. Infect. Immun. **73:** 1561–1567.
52. Stein, A. & D. Raoult. 1998. Q fever during pregnancy: a public health problem in southern France. Clin. Infect. Dis. **34:** 28–31.
53. To, H., N. Kako, G.Q. Zhang, *et al.* 1996. Q fever pneumonia in children in Japan. J. Clin. Microbiol. **34:** 647–651.
54. Maltezou, H.C. & D. Raoult. 2002. Q fever in children. Lancet Infect. Dis. **2:** 686–691.
55. Houpikian, P.G., T. Habib, T. Mesana & D. Raoult. 2002. Changing clinical presentation of Q fever endocarditis. Clin. Infect. Dis. **34:** 28–31.
56. Marrie, M. & D. Raoult. 1997. Q fever: a review and issues to the next century. Int. J. Antimicrob. Agents **8:** 145–161.
57. Raoult, D., H. Tissot-dupont, C. Foucalt, *et al.* 2002. Q fever 1985–1998: clinical and epidemiologic features of 1,383 infections. Medicine **79:** 109–123.
58. Marmion, B.P., M. Shannon, I. Maddocks, *et al.* 1996. Protracted debility and fatigue after acute Q fever. Lancet **347:** 977–978.
59. Pentilla, I.A., R.J. Harris, P.A. Storm, *et al.* 1998. Cytokine dysregulation in the post-Q fever syndrome. Quart. J. Med. **91:** 549–560.
60. Helbig, K.J., S.L. Heatley, R.J. Harris, *et al.* 2003. Variation in immune response genes and chronic Q fever. Concepts: preliminary test with post-Q fever fatigue syndrome.Genes Immun. **4:** 82–85.
61. Leone, M., A. Honstettre, H. Lepidi, *et al.* 2004. Effect of sex on *Coxiella burnetii* infection: protective role of 17beta-estradiol. J. Infect. Dis. **189:** 339–345.
62. Fournier, P.E., T.J. Marrie & D. Raoult. 1998. Diagnosis of Q fever. J. Clin. Microbiol. **36:** 1823–1834.
63. Mallavia, L.P., L.L. Whitting, M.F. Minnick, *et al.* 1998. Strategy for detection and differentiation of *Coxiella burnetii* strains using the polymerase chain reaction. Ann. N.Y. Acad. Sci. **590:** 572–581.
64. Yuasa, Y., K. Yoshiie, T. Takasaki & H. Oda. 1996. Retrospective survey of chronic Q fever in Japan by using PCR to detect *Coxiella burnetii* in paraffin-embedded clinical samples. J. Clin. Microbiol. **34:** 824–827.
65. Brennan, R.E. & J.E. Samuel. 2003. Evaluation of *Coxiella burnetii* susceptibilities by real-time PCR assay. J. Clin. Microbiol. **41:** 1869–1874.
66. Fenollar, F., P.E. Fournier & D. Raoult. 2004. Molecular detection of *Coxiella burnetii* in the sera of patients with Q fever endocarditis or vascular infection. J. Clin. Microbiol. **42:** 4919–4924.
67. Fournier, P.E. & D. Raoult. 2003. Comparison of PCR and serology assays for early diagnosis of acute Q fever. J. Clin. Microbiol. **41:** 5094–5098.
68. Raoult, D. 1993. Treatment of Q fever. Antimicrob. Agents Chemother. **37:** 1733– 1736.
69. Spyridaki, I., A. Psaroulaki, E. Kokkinakis, *et al.* 2002. Mechanisms of resistance to fluoroquinolones in *Coxiella burnetii*. J. Antimicrob. Chemother. **49:** 379–382.
70. Raoult, D., P. Houpikian, H. Tissot-dupont, *et al.* 1999. Treatment of Q fever endocarditis: comparison of 2 regimens containing doxycyclin and ofloxacin or hydrochloroquine. Arch. Intern. Med. **15:** 167–173.

71. RAOULT, D., M. DRANCOURT & G. VESTRIS. 1990. Bactericidal effect of doxycycline associated with lysosomotropic agents on *Coxiella burnetii* in P388D1 cells. Antimicrob. Agents Chemother. **34:** 1512–1514.
72. WOLDEHIVET, Z. 2004. Q fever (coxiellosis): epidemiology and pathogenesis. Res. Vet. Sci. **77:** 93–100.
73. ACKLAND, J.R., D.A. WORSWICK & B.P. MARMION. 1994. Vaccine prophylaxis of Q fever: a follow-up study of the efficacy of Q-Vax (SL). Med. J. Aust. **160:** 704–708.
74. FRIES, L.F., D.M. WAAG & J.C. WILLIAMS. 1993. Safety and immunogenicity in human volunteers of a chloroform-methanol residue vaccine for Q fever. Infect. Immun. **61:** 1251–1258.
75. KAZAR, J., R. BREZINA, A. PALANOVA, *et al.* 1982. Immunogenicity and reactogenicity of a Q fever chemovaccine in persons professionally exposed to Q fever in Czechoslovakia. Bull. WHO **60:** 389–394.
76. KAZAR, J. & J. REHACEK. 1987. Q fever vaccines: present status and application in man. Zbl. Bacteriol. Microbiol. Hyg. **267:** 74–78.
77. LESNY, M., J. KAZAR, P. PROPPER & M. LUKACOVA. 1991. Virulence and cross-immunity study on guinea pigs infected with different *Coxiella burnetii* strains. *In* Rickettsiae and Rickettsial Diseases. J. Kazar & D. Raoult, Eds.: 666–673. VEDA. Bratislava.
78. SESHADRI, R., I.T. PAULSEN, J.A. EISEN, *et al.* 2003. Complete genome sequence of the Q-fever pathogen *Coxiella burnetii*. Proc. Natl. Acad. Sci. USA **100:** 775–779.
79. ZHANG, G.Q. & J.E. SAMUEL. 2003. Identification and cloning of potentially protective antigens of *Coxiella burnetii* using sera from mice experimentally infected with Nine Mile phase I. Ann. N.Y. Acad. Sci. **990:** 510–520.

Coxiella burnetii Whole Cell Lysate Protein Identification by Mass Spectrometry and Tandem Mass Spectrometry

LUDOVIT SKULTETY,[a] LENKA HERNYCHOVA,[b] RUDOLF TOMAN,[a] MARTIN HUBALEK,[b] KATARINA SLABA,[a] JANA ZECHOVSKA,[b] VERONIKA STOFANIKOVA,[a] JURAJ LENCO,[b] JIRI STULIK,[b] AND ALES MACELA[b]

[a]*Laboratory for Diagnosis and Prevention of Rickettsial and Chlamydial Infections, Institute of Virology, Slovak Academy of Sciences, 845 05 Bratislava, Slovak Republic*

[b]*Institute of Molecular Pathology and Proteome Center for the Study of Intracellular Parasitism of Bacteria, Purkyne Military Medical Academy, 500 01 Hradec Kralove, Czech Republic*

ABSTRACT: The whole cell lysate of *Coxiella burnetii* strain RSA 493 was separated by two-dimensional electrophoresis and more than 500 protein spots were found on silver-stained reference map. Spots from the gels were subjected to identification based on peptide mass fingerprinting (PMF). In order to identify additional proteins, tandem mass spectrometry (MS/MS) using electrospray and matrix-assisted laser desorption/ionization techniques was applied. The three independent approaches resulted in the identification of 197 open reading frames (ORFs). Fifty-two proteins were identified by PMF and at least with one of the MS/MS methods, 37 proteins with both MS/MS instruments, and 19 proteins with all three techniques applied. All predicted *C. burnetii* ORFs were compared with the Clusters of Orthologous Groups database. The data related to identified proteins were stored and indexed in a file that can be read and searched using Microsoft Access.

KEYWORDS: *Coxiella burnetii*; proteins; mass spectrometry; tandem mass spectrometry

INTRODUCTION

Coxiella burnetii is the causative agent of Q fever, a zoonosis that is ubiquitous throughout the world and causes several outbreaks each year.[1] Diagnosis of the disease is complicated by the observation that symptoms of infection are often either

Address for correspondence: Ludovit Skultety, Laboratory for Diagnosis and Prevention of Rickettsial and Chlamydial Infections, Institute of Virology, Slovak Academy of Sciences, 845 05 Bratislava, Slovak Republic. Fax: +421-2-54774284.
viruludo@savba.sk

Ann. N.Y. Acad. Sci. 1063: 115–122 (2005).
doi: 10.1196/annals.1355.019

subclinical or extremely mild. *C. burnetii* proteins represent the major immunoreactive antigens in the serological diagnosis of Q fever.[2,3] In spite of the fact that the *C. burnetii* genome has recently been completely sequenced and annotated,[4] there is a lack of information on protein composition and structure. Proteomic methods are promising tools for obtaining new data in this respect and can be utilized for both diagnosis and prophylactic purposes. Our investigations have focused on the mass spectrometry (MS) and tandem mass spectrometry (MS/MS) identifications of most abundant proteins of *C. burnetii* in the virulent phase I as resolved by two-dimensional electrophoresis (2-D electrophoresis) or liquid chromatography (LC).

MATERIALS AND METHODS

Cultivation and purification of the *C. burnetii* strain RSA 493 (Nine Mile) in virulent phase I was accomplished as described.[5,6] Purified cells (50 mg) were suspended in 10 mL of lysis buffer consisting of 28 mM Tris-HCl, 22 mM Tris-Base, 200 mM dithiothreitol 0.3% sodium dodecylsulfate, and one tablet of Complete Mini-Protease Inhibitors. Incubation (3 min) in boiling water has been used for disruption of *C. burnetii* cells. An RNase and DNase treatment was used to digest DNA and RNA and the proteins were precipitated by a mixture of chloroform, methanol, and water.[7]

Bacterial proteins were solubilized and separated by two-dimensional (2-D) electrophoresis as described previously.[8] An improved silver staining compatible with protein digestion and mass spectrometric (MS) analysis[9] were applied. The spots selected from the preparative gels were excised and gel pieces were digested by a sequence grade trypsin (Promega). Peptide mass fingerprint (PMF) spectra were recorded by a matrix assisted laser desorption/ionization (MALDI) MS instrument Voyager DE STR (Applied Biosystems, Framingham, MA, USA) as described earlier.[8] Each mass spectrum was obtained by averaging 100 nitrogen laser shots and was evaluated by a DataExplorer Software (Applied Biosystems). A Protein-Prospector program (University of California, San Francisco Mass Spectrometry Facility, CA, USA, version 3.4.1.) was used for all searching against the *C. burnetii* [Species Codes: COXBU, Database: NCBInr.05.10.2004 (National Center for Biotechnology Information; 2004.10.19)] and all species nonredundant databases [NCBInr.05.10.2004 or Swiss-Prot and TrEMBL (Swiss Institute of Bioinformatics; 2004.12.07)].

In another set of experiments, a reduced and alkylated tryptic digest of *C. burnetii* whole cell lysate was separated on a C18 column using an increasing gradient of acetonitrile and then the spectra were recorded on an electrospray (ESI) MS/MS instrument Micromass Q-Tof Ultima API (Waters). The data were acquired by means of a Data Dependent Analysis (DDA) according to the procedure described earlier.[10] A ProteinLynx Global*SERVER* (Waters) was used for all searching against the databases mentioned above. Unimolecular dissociation spectra of the C18-separated tryptic digest were recorded also by a MALDI MS/MS instrument 4700 Proteomics Analyzer (Applied Biosystems). Each mass spectrum was obtained by averaging 300 Nd:YAG laser shots per spot. The data were analyzed by GPS Explorer™ Software (Applied Biosystems), which invoked a Mascot® database search to produce the protein identification.

RESULTS AND DISCUSSION

The silver-stained 2-D electrophoresis reference map of the whole cell lysate of *C. burnetii* is shown in FIGURE 1. Though the complete genome is predicted to encode 2,134 coding sequences,[4] only more than 500 distinct protein spots were counted in the gel by processing scanned image using the Melanie III software package. This result is in a good agreement with findings reported by Zhang and colleagues.[11] We have also observed many strong, low molecular weight (<20 kDa) spots in the high pI range of 7–10. On the other hand, most distinct spots of high intensity were of higher (>45 kDa) weight in the low pI range of 4–6. In the intermediate (20–45 kDa) mass range, the protein species were fairly evenly distributed.

All abundant spots were subjected to identification by PMF. The proteins were identified according to their probability score (>100), number of peptide masses matched to the identified proteins (>4), and percentage of sequence coverage (>20%). Multiple proteins resulting from potential posttranslational modifications were observed and thus 71 different proteins were identified as the products of known open reading frames (ORFs). However, in a case when more than one protein is isolated from a single spot and/or a low mass accuracy or posttranslational modifications are evident, there is a need for further verification. Thus, the ESI MS/MS technique was applied for both confirmation of the PMF data and identification of those proteins that were initially missed. In this way, an additional 16 proteins were described.

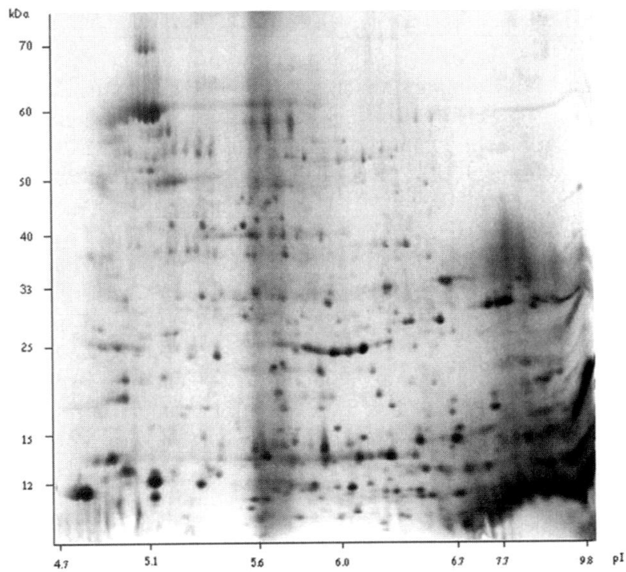

FIGURE 1. Silver-stained 2-D electrophoresis reference map of *C. burnetii* strain RSA 493.

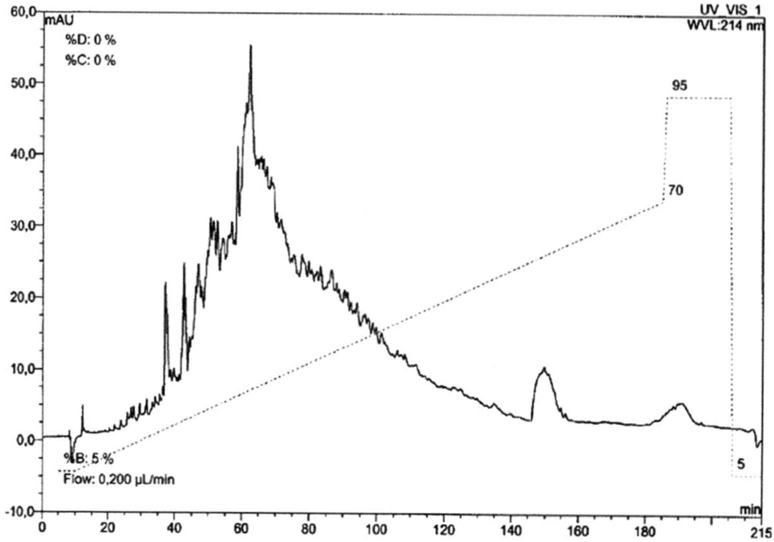

FIGURE 2. UV trace of the tryptic peptides of *C. burnetii* whole cell lysate separated on an LC Packings PepMap100 C18 column (150 mm × 75 µm) at a flow rate 200 nL/min.

In order to find more proteins and to confirm simultaneously the presence of those already identified, two LC–MS/MS approaches were used. The purified *C. burnetii* whole cell lysate was digested with trypsin and peptides were separated on a C18 column. An example of such a separation is given in FIGURE 2. A huge surface under the peaks clearly illustrates complexity of the sample and limitations of LC for the separation of complex peptide mixture. MS and MS/MS data were acquired by either hybrid ESI MS/MS or MALDI MS/MS instruments. Eight different DDA experiments were conducted by a Q-Tof Ultima instrument using various mass ranges of the survey window. The total number of proteins found was 92 (FIG. 3), 71 of which were separated by LC and the remainder by 2-D electrophoresis. Only validated peptide search results based on the three or more consecutive ions of the Y series are reported. Both the total number of the MS/MS-interpreted peptides (>2) belonging to the protein as well as the probability score (>4) have been required for all reported proteins to assure an unambiguous identification. The data generated by MALDI MS/MS instrument yielded to the identification of 147 proteins of known ORFs (FIG. 3). Likewise, only validated peptide search results based on the Mascot MOWSE score >60 and more then two peptides were required to report the protein. The only exemptions to these rules were those proteins that have also been identified by another technique.

The three independent approaches resulted in the identification of 197 ORFs (FIG. 3). As many as 52 proteins were identified by PMF and at least with one of the MS/MS methods, 37 ORFs were identified with both MS/MS methods, 30 by both MALDI instruments, and 19 proteins with all three techniques applied. All the

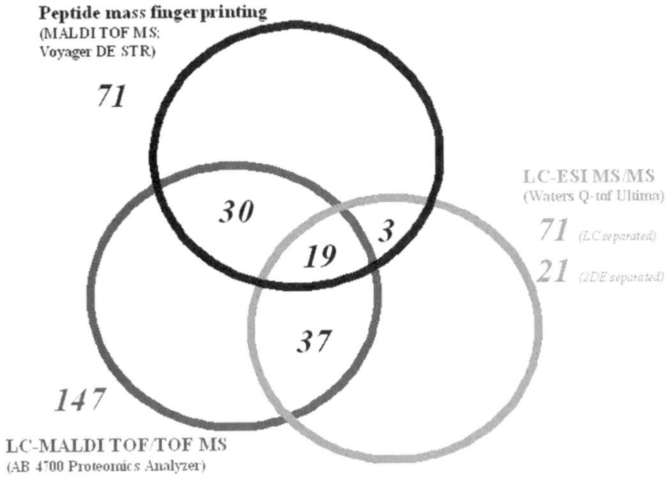

FIGURE 3. Distribution of the *C. burnetii* ORF identifications among the mass spectrometry techniques applied.

obtained data were then stored and indexed in the *C. burnetii* protein database that can be read and searched using Microsoft Access (see supplementary material).

Since *C. burnetii* lives and grows within an acidic phagosome in the host cell, it is likely that basic proteins serve to titrate excessive protons, which enter the cytoplasm of the bacterium.[12] It was suggested with the *in silico* analysis of the *C. burnetii* genome that about two-thirds of the proteins in this organism have a basic pI,[4] making it an ideal candidate for MALDI analysis. Using this ionization method, 169 ORFs were identified and only one third of the proteins was characterized by ESI (FIG. 3). It is evident from FIGURE 4 that many small (<20 kDa) ORFs had pI greater than 8 and the larger (>45 kDa) proteins were rather acidic. However, most proteins were fairly evenly distributed in the given pI range. Thus, our studies have not confirmed that basic proteins are preferentially ionized by MALDI and it appears that LC decoupled from the MS detection system is more suitable for analyzing highly complex protein mixtures as more running time is left for acquiring MS spectra of the separated peptides.

All predicted *C. burnetii* ORFs were compared with the Clusters of Orthologous Groups (COGs) database.[13] This indicated that more than 27% of proteins could be involved in metabolism and almost as many in cellular processes as well as in information, storage, and processing. The remaining proteins were rather poorly characterized (COG category R and S) or had no related COGs as there were no hits found (FIG. 5). Thirty-seven ORFs exhibited significant matches with COG category J (translation or essential components of ribosomal structures), 24 COGs might be involved in energy production and conversion (COG category C), and 21 in posttranslational modification and protein turnover–chaperones (COG category O). Other COG categories have only less than 16 representatives. Nevertheless, two candidates CBU0691 and CBU0683[4] for synthesizing two unusual sugars (virenose and dihy-

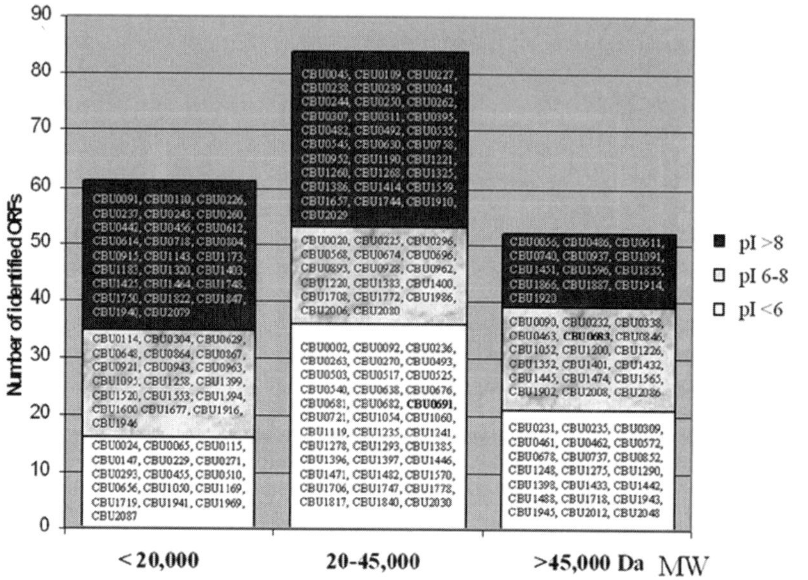

FIGURE 4. Distribution of the identified *C. burnetii* ORFs as a function of MW and pI.

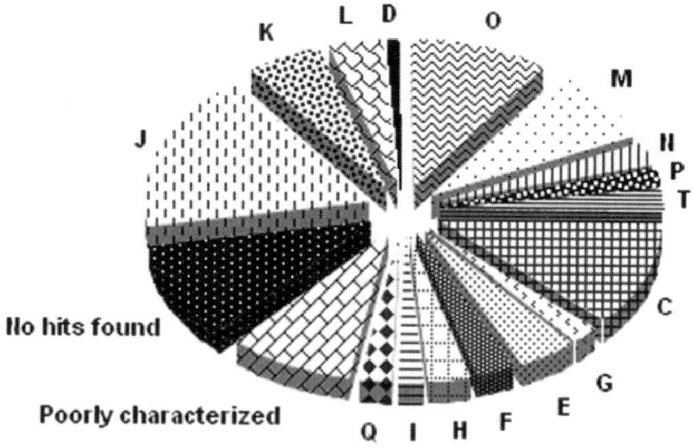

FIGURE 5. COG class distribution among the *C. burnetii* ORFs.

drohydroxystreptose) were found among them. Both sugars have not been found in other enterobacterial lipopolysaccharides (LPS) and can be considered as important chemotaxonomic markers of *C. burnetii*.[5,14] Basic alignment and homology studies indicated that the large group of LPS genes encoding the synthesis of O-polysaccharide chain was deleted in the *C. burnetii* Nine Mile phase II cells.[15] In accordance with this, an LPS isolated from these cells was found to be of rough (R) type.[6]

Immunogenicity and uniqueness are the key factors in determining suitability of candidate molecules towards exclusive recognition of strains/isolates. In addition, knowledge about factors that determine virulence of strains is indispensable for new leads in antimicrobial therapy and vaccine development. Until now, we have confirmed several immunoreactive proteins (CBU0091, CBU0109, CBU0395, CBU0867, CBU1221, CBU1268, CBU1718, CBU1910) that were previously cloned by Zhang and colleagues.[11] In the near future, we will focus on the identification of additional immunogenic, species and/or strain specific, virulence-related proteins that could help us to elucidate mechanisms involved in the pathobiology of *C. burnetii*.

ACKNOWLEDGMENTS

This study was supported by the following grants: the grant LN00A033 from the Ministry of Education, Youth and Sports, Czech Republic; the grants MO 9079201303 and MO 9079201301 from the Ministry of Defense, Czech Republic; the NATO Collaborative Linkage grant LST.CLG.978998; the grant APVT-51-032804 from the Science and Technology Assistance Agency; and the grants No. 3021/25, 5030/25 from the Scientific Grant Agency of the Ministry of Education of the Slovak Republic and the Slovak Academy of Sciences.

The authors acknowledge excellent technical assistance of Dr. D. Uria (Waters), Dr. M. Glueckmann (Applied Biosystems), Mrs. M. Benkovicova, A. Firychova, and J. Michalickova.

[*Conflict of interest statement:* The authors of this research declare that they have no conflict of interest.]

REFERENCES

1. Marrie, T.J. 1990. Acute Q fever. *In* Q Fever, Vol. I. The Disease. T.J. Marrie, Ed.: 125–160. CRC Press. Boca Raton, FL.
2. Marrie, T.J. & D. Raoult. 1997. Q fever: a review and issues for the next century. Int. J. Antimicrob. Agents. **8:** 145–161.
3. Williams, J.C. & D.M. Waag. 1991. Antigens, virulence factors, and biological response modifiers of *Coxiella burnetii*: strategies for vaccine development. *In* Q Fever: The Biology of *Coxiella burnetii*. J.C. Williams & H.A. Thompson, Eds.: 175–222. CRC Press. Boca Raton, FL.
4. Seshadri R., I.T. Paulsen, J.A. Eisen, *et al.* 2003. Complete genome sequence of the Q-fever pathogen *Coxiella burnetii*. Proc. Natl. Acad. Sci. USA **100:** 5455–5460.
5. Skultety, L., R. Toman & V. Patoprsty. 1998. A comparative study of lipopolysaccharides from two *Coxiella burnetii* strains considered to be associated with acute and chronic Q fever. Carbohydr. Polymers **35:** 189–194.
6. Toman, R. & L. Skultety. 1996. Structural study on a lipopolysaccharide from *Coxiella burnetii* strain Nine Mile in avirulent phase II. Carbohydr. Res. **283:** 175–185.

7. WESSEL, D. & U.I. FLUGGE. 1984. A method for the quantitative recovery of protein in dilute solution in the presence of detergents and lipids. Ann. Biochem. **138:** 141–143.
8. SKULTETY, L., L. HERNYCHOVA, R. TOMAN, *et al.* 2004. Initial peptide mass fingerprinting analysis of proteins obtained by lysis of *Coxiella burnetii* cells. Acta Virol. **48:** 29–34.
9. MORTZ, E., T.N. KROGH, H. VORUM, *et al.* 2001. Improved silver staining protocols for high sensitivity protein identification using matrix-assisted laser desorption/ionization–time of flight analysis. Proteomics **1:** 1359–1363.
10. PAVKOVA, I., M. HUBALEK, J. ZECHOVSKA, *et al.* 2005. *Francisella tularensis* live vaccine strain: proteomic analysis of membrane proteins enriched fraction. Proteomics **5:** 2460–2467.
11. ZHANG, G.Q., K. KISS, R. SESHADRI, *et al.* 2004. Identification and cloning of immunodominant antigens of *Coxiella burnetii.* Infect. Immun. **72:** 844–852.
12. SESHADRI, R. & J.E. SAMUEL. 2001. Characterization of a stress-induced alternate sigma factor, RpoS, of *Coxiella burnetii* and its expression during the development cycle. Infect. Immun. **69:** 4874–4883.
13. TATUSOV, R.L., N.D. FEDOROVA, J.D. JACKSON, *et al.* 2003. The COG database: an updated version includes eukaryotes. BMC Bioinformatics **11:** Art. No. 41 [online: http://www.biomedcentral.com/1471-2105/4/41].
14. TOMAN, R., L. SKULTETY, P. FTACEK, *et al.* 1998. NMR study of virenose and dihydrohydroxystreptose isolated from *Coxiella burnetii* phase I lipopolysaccharide. Carbohydr. Res. **306:** 291–296.
15. HOOVER, T.A., D.W. CULP, M.H. VODKIN, *et al.* 2002. Chromosomal DNA deletions explain phenotypic characteristics of two antigenic variants, phase II and RSA 514 (Crazy), of the *Coxiella burnetii* Nine Mile strain. Infect. Immun. **70:** 6726–6733.

Replication of *Coxiella burnetii* Is Inhibited in CHO K-1 Cells Treated with Inhibitors of Cholesterol Metabolism

DALE HOWE AND ROBERT A. HEINZEN

Coxiella Pathogenesis Section, Laboratory of Intracellular Parasites, Rocky Mountain Laboratories, National Institute of Allergy and Infectious Diseases, National Institutes of Health, Hamilton, Montana 59840, USA

ABSTRACT: *Coxiella burnetii* directs the synthesis of a large parasitophorous vacuole (PV) that is required for its replication. While some lysosomal characteristics of the PV have been described, the origin and composition of the PV membrane remain largely undefined. Cholesterol is an essential component of mammalian membranes where it lends mechanical stability and serves as a platform for signaling proteins. Using infected Chinese hamster ovary cells as a model, we examined whether cholesterol is trafficked to the *C. burnetii* PV membrane and the effects of inhibitors of cholesterol metabolism on *C. burnetii* replication. When infected cells were stained with filipin, a fluorescent polyene antifungal agent that binds cholesterol, obvious staining of PV was observed indicating the PV membrane is cholesterol-rich. Furthermore, replication of *C. burnetii* was significantly inhibited in cells treated with the cholesterol metabolism inhibitors lovastatin, ketoconazole, imipramine, progesterone, and U18666A. These data suggest that cholesterol is an important component of the *C. burnetii* PV membrane and that normal cellular cholesterol metabolism is required for optimal *C. burnetii* replication.

KEYWORDS: parasitophorous vacuole; membrane; lipid; filipin; cholesterol; *Coxiella*

INTRODUCTION

Coxiella burnetii, an obligate intracellular pathogen, requires an acidic parasitophorous vacuole (PV) for replication. Although the PV has characteristics of a phagolysosome,[1] recent studies indicate PV maturation diverges from typical endosomal maturation. For example, fusion of lysosomes with phagosomes containing viable *C. burnetii* is delayed[2] and mature *C. burnetii* PV freely fuse with other endolysosomal vacuoles.[3] *C. burnetii* PV also appear to interact with the autophagic pathway to acquire characteristics of autophagolysosomes.[4] Maturation of the *C. burnetii* PV is directed by the pathogen as protein synthesis is required for biogenesis of the large and spacious PV.[3]

Address for correspondence: Robert A. Heinzen, Laboratory of Intracellular Parasites, Rocky Mountain Laboratories, National Institute of Allergy and Infectious Diseases, 903 S. 4th St., Hamilton, Montana, 59840. Voice: 406-375-9695; fax: 307-363-9380.
rheinzen@niaid.nih.gov

**Ann. N.Y. Acad. Sci. 1063: 123–129 (2005). © 2005 New York Academy of Sciences.
doi: 10.1196/annals.1355.020**

During the course of *C. burnetii* infection, PV expand to occupy nearly all of the host cell cytoplasm. These large vacuoles are resistant to mechanical disruption[5] and appear to have a low buoyant density (unpublished observation). Because membranes with a high cholesterol content have similar properties,[6] we hypothesized that the *C. burnetii* PV membrane may be cholesterol-rich. In this study, we identify cholesterol as a structural component of the *C. burnetii* PV and show that *C. burnetii* replication is reduced following treatment with inhibitors of cholesterol metabolism.

MATERIALS AND METHODS

Coxiella burnetii *and Cell Culture*

C. burnetii (Nine Mile strain in phase II) was propagated and harvested as previously described.[7] Chinese hamster ovary (CHO K-1) epithelial cells (CRL-9618, American Type Culture Collection) were maintained in DMEM/F-12 supplemented with 5% fetal bovine serum (FBS) (Invitrogen, Carlsbad, CA) and incubated at 37°C in 5% CO_2. Semi-confluent CHO K-1 monolayers were infected with *C. burnetii* at a multiplicity of infection of 10 for 2 h at room temperature. The inoculum was removed and fresh media with or without inhibitors was added. Inhibitors of cholesterol metabolism were used at the following final concentrations: lovastatin (1 μM), ketoconazole (10 μM), imipramine (100 μM), progesterone (100 μM), and U18666A (5 μM) (Sigma-Aldrich, St. Louis, MO).

Microscopy

For fluoresent microscopy, infected CHO K-1 cells on 12-mm coverslips were fixed with 4% paraformaldehyde in phosphate-buffered saline (PBS; 150 mM NaCl, 10 mM $NaPO_4$, pH 7.2) for 10 min, followed by permeabilization for 10 min with 0.1% saponin in PBS containing 10% goat serum. *C. burnetii* were stained with antiserum from a convalescent guinea pig followed by Alexa Fluor 594 goat anti–guinea pig IgG (H&L) (Invitrogen). Cellular cholesterol was then stained with filipin (50 μg/mL) (Sigma-Aldrich) as previously described.[8] Samples were viewed with a Nikon TE-2000 E inverted microscope equipped with a CoolSNAP HQ digital camera (Roper Scientific, Tuscon, AZ). Images were acquired using Metamorph software (Universal Imaging, Dowingtown, PA) and processed using Image J (written by Wayne Rasband at the U.S. National Institutes of Health and available by anonymous FTP from zippy.nimh.nih.gov) and Adobe Photoshop (Adobe Systems, San Jose, CA).

FIGURE 1. The *C. burnetii* PV membrane contains cholesterol and inhibitors of cholesterol metabolism disrupt PV biogenesis. Infected CHO K-1 cells were treated with inhibitors and fixed at 4 days postinfection. *C. burnetii* was stained by indirect immunofluoresence, then cholesterol was counterstained with filipin. Parallel images are depicted. Filipin labeled the *C. burnetii* PV membrane (*arrowheads*) in untreated and treated cells. Bars: 5 μm.

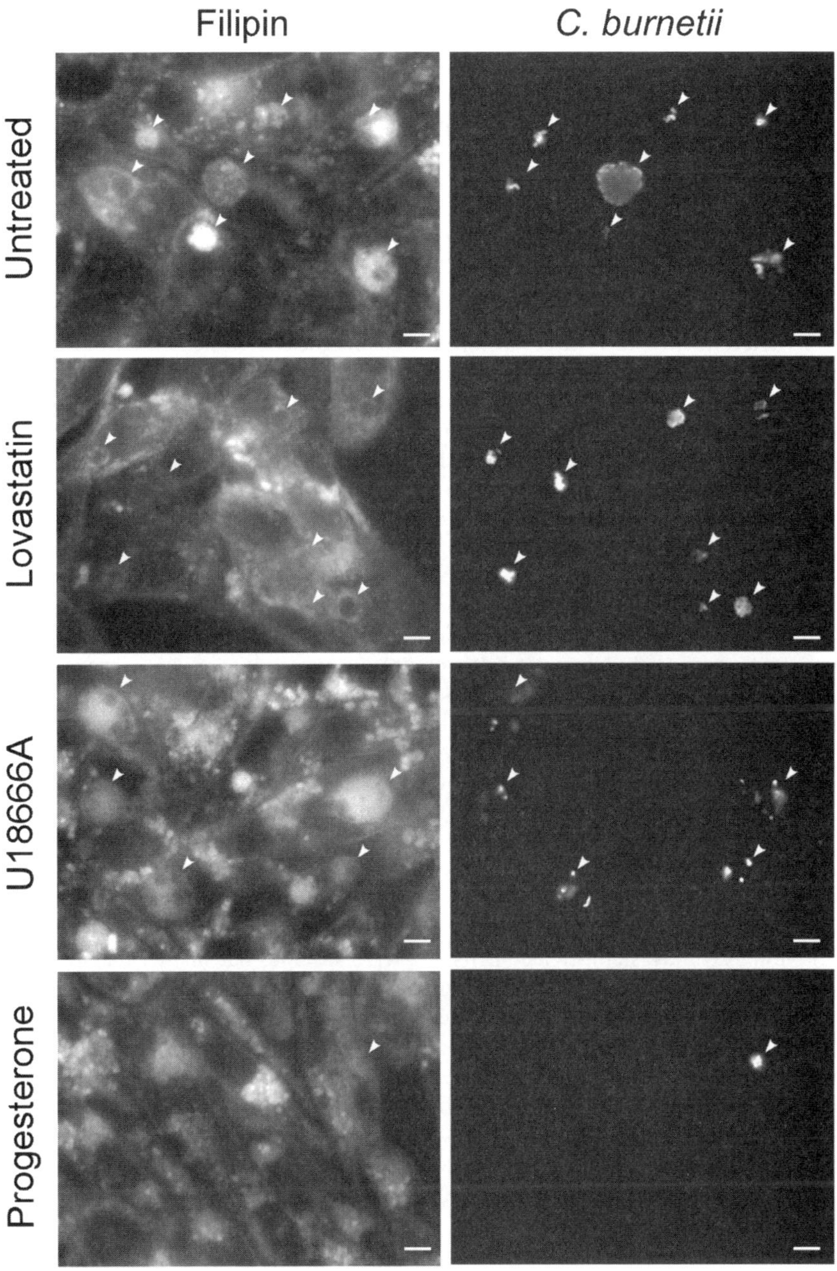

FIGURE 1. *See previous page for legend.*

Quantitative PCR of C. burnetii *and CHO K-1 Genome Equivalents*

C. burnetii and CHO K-1 genome equivalents were quantified using TaqMan qPCR. Infected cells were harvested at 6 days postinfection and total DNA was extracted using an UltraClean microbial DNA Isolation Kit (MoBio Laboratories Inc., Carlsbad, CA). Primers and probe specific for *C. burnetii dotA* and CHO K-1 *gapdh* were designed with PrimerExpress software (Applied Biosystems, Foster City, CA). DNA was amplified using a Prism 7000 sequence detection system (Applied Biosystems).

RESULTS

To determine whether the *C. burnetii* PV membrane contains cholesterol, infected cells were stained with filipin, a fluorescent polyene antifungal that binds cholesterol.[8] CHO K-1 cells were employed as a host cell in this study as they are an established model system for *in vitro* cholesterol studies.[9,10] *C. burnetii* PV membranes stained at an intensity similar to that of the plasma membrane where 75–90% of cholesterol normally resides,[11] confirming the presence of cholesterol in the PV membrane (FIG. 1). Filipin also decorated cholesterol-rich particles in the cell cytoplasm, typical of CHO K-1 cells.[10]

Because cholesterol appeared to be a prominent lipid in the PV membrane, we examined the effect of restricting access to cholesterol on PV development. Infected cells were treated with inhibitors of cholesterol metabolism. Lovastatin, an inhibitor of 3-hydroxy-3-methylglutaryl coenzyme A reductase,[12] and ketoconazole, an inhibitor of lanosterol 14α-desmethylase,[13] were used to block steps in cholesterol biosynthesis. Imipramine,[14] 3-β-[2-(diethylamino) ethoxy]androst-5-en-17-one (U18666A), [9] and progesterone[15] were used to inhibit transport of LDL-derived cholesterol from lysosomes. PV membranes in cells treated with lovastatin or U18666A labeled with filipin at an intensity similar to that of PV in untreated cells (FIG. 1). Conversely, in cells treated with progesterone, imipramine (data not shown), or ketoconazole (data not shown), few PV developed that stained diffusely with filipin, suggesting a reduced level of cholesterol in these PV membranes.

Treatment with inhibitors of cholesterol metabolism generally affected PV morphology. In lovastatin-treated cells, PV were spacious but smaller than those of untreated cells. In cells treated with progesterone, imipramine, or ketoconazole, small, tightly fitting PV were observed that usually contained a single organism. Treatment with U18666A had no obvious effect on PV morphology. In summary, inhibition of host cell cholesterol metabolism in most cases disrupts PV morphology and reduces, but does not eliminate, cholesterol trafficking to the PV membrane.

Disruption of PV morphology following treatment with cholesterol metabolism inhibitors appeared to coincide with reduced *C. burnetii* replication as immunofluorescent staining revealed fewer organisms in treated cells than in untreated cells. To investigate this possibility, *C. burnetii* genome equivalents were quantified by qPCR following inhibitor treatments. In untreated cells, *C. burnetii* genome equivalents increased approximately 6-fold during a 6-day time course (FIG. 2). In cells treated with lovastatin or U18666A, *C. burnetii* genome equivalents increased approximately 3.5-fold and 2.5-fold, respectively. *C. burnetii* genome equivalents

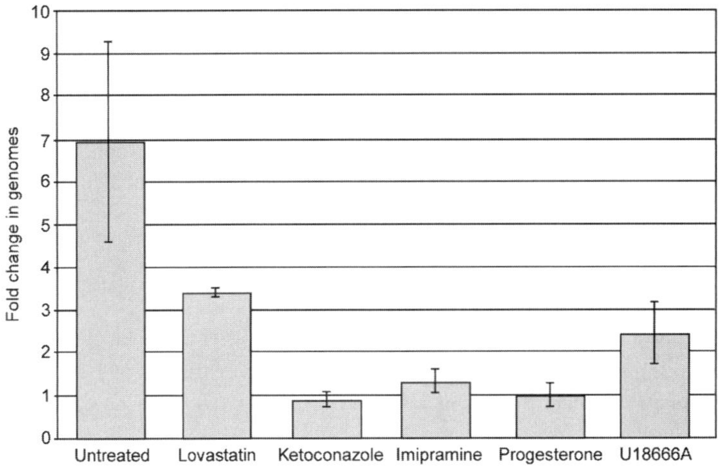

FIGURE 2. *C. burnetii* replication is reduced by inhibitors of cholesterol metabolism. CHO K-1 cells were infected with *C. burnetii* and incubated in the presence of inhibitors for 6 days. Immediately after infection and at 6 days postinfection, total DNA was extracted and *C. burnetii* genome equivalents were quantified by qPCR. Results are expressed as fold change in genomes at 6 days postinfection normalized to genome equivalents extracted immediately after infection. The mean of three independent experiments is shown with error bars representing the standard deviations. All drugs significantly inhibited *C. burnetii* replication ($P < 0.01$) as calculated using one-way analysis of variance followed by a Dunnett's post-hoc test.

did not significantly increase in cells treated with progesterone, imipramine, or ketoconazole. To confirm that infection by *C. burnetii* and inhibitor treatments did not affect CHO K-1 cell division, CHO K-1 genome equivalents were quantified by qPCR. CHO K-1 genomes increased approximately 5-fold in both infected and uninfected cultures and this increase was not significantly changed by inhibitor treatments (data not shown).

DISCUSSION

PV are critical to the pathogenesis of *C. burnetii*, yet little is known about the structure of the PV membrane and the source of its constituent lipids. In this study, filipin staining indicated that PV membranes contain roughly the same amount of cholesterol as the plasma membrane. Cholesterol, whether from exogenous or endogenous sources, appears to be important for robust *C. burnetii* replication as agents that block specific steps in either pathway inhibit growth. Although the general appearance of PV is unaltered in lovastatin-treated cells, PV are smaller than normal and *C. burnetii* replication is inhibited by approximately 55%. Interestingly, PV in cells treated with U18666A are normal in size; however, *C. burnetii* replication is inhibited by approximately 73%. *C. burnetii* do not replicate in cells treated with progesterone, imipramine, or ketoconazole and PV in these cells are undeveloped and have reduced cholesterol in their membranes.

The results of this study show that exogenously acquired or endogenously synthesized cholesterol is required for normal PV biogenesis and optimal *C. burnetii* replication. The specific roles of cholesterol in the *C. burnetii* PV membrane are unknown. However, similar to the functions of cellular cholesterol, PV cholesterol might target transmembrane proteins that function in signal transduction, nutrient transport, or membrane fusion. In addition, cholesterol may provide structural support for this large organelle that can occupy more of the host cell volume than the nucleus.[16]

ACKNOWLEDGMENTS

We thank Anita Mora for assistance with graphics. This research was supported by the Intramural Research program of the National Institutes of Health, National Institute of Allergy and Infectious Diseases.

[*Competing interest statement*: The authors declare that they have no conflicts of interest.]

REFERENCES

1. HEINZEN, R.A. *et al.* 1996. Differential interaction with endocytic and exocytic pathways distinguish parasitophorous vacuoles of *Coxiella burnetii* and *Chlamydia trachomatis*. Infect. Immun. **64:** 796–809.
2. HOWE, D. & L.P. MALLAVIA. 2000. *Coxiella burnetii* exhibits morphological change and delays phagolysosomal fusion after internalization by J774A.1 cells. Infect. Immun. **68:** 3815–3821.
3. HOWE, D. *et al.* 2003. Maturation of the *Coxiella burnetii* parasitophorous vacuole requires bacterial protein synthesis but not replication. Cell Microbiol. **5:** 469–480.
4. GUTIERREZ, M.G. *et al.* 2005. Autophagy induction favours the generation and maturation of the *Coxiella*-replicative vacuoles. Cell Microbiol. **7:** 981–993.
5. HEINZEN, R.A. & T. HACKSTADT. 1997. The *Chlamydia trachomatis* parasitophorous vacuolar membrane is not passively permeable to low-molecular-weight compounds. Infect. Immun. **65:** 1088–1094.
6. NEEDHAM, D., T.J. MCINTOSH & E. EVANS. 1988. Thermomechanical and transition properties of dimyristoylphosphatidylcholine/cholesterol bilayers. Biochemistry **27:** 4668–4673.
7. HACKSTADT, T. *et al.* 1992. Evidence for proteolytic cleavage of the 120-kilodalton outer membrane protein of rickettsiae: identification of an avirulent mutant deficient in processing. Infect. Immun. **60:** 159–165.
8. KRUTH, H.S. *et al.* 1986. Type C Niemann-Pick disease: abnormal metabolism of low density lipoprotein in homozygous and heterozygous fibroblasts. J. Biol. Chem. **261:** 16769–16774.
9. LISCUM, L. & J.R. FAUST. 1989. The intracellular transport of low density lipoprotein-derived cholesterol is inhibited in Chinese hamster ovary cells cultured with 3-beta-[2-(diethylamino)ethoxy]androst-5-en-17-one. J. Biol. Chem. **264:** 11796–11806.
10. UNDERWOOD, K.W. *et al.* 1998. Evidence for a cholesterol transport pathway from lysosomes to endoplasmic reticulum that is independent of the plasma membrane. J. Biol. Chem. **273:** 4266–4274.
11. PRINZ, W. 2002. Cholesterol trafficking in the secretory and endocytic systems. Semin. Cell Dev. Biol. **13:** 197–203.
12. CATRON, D.M. *et al.* 2004. *Salmonella enterica* serovar Typhimurium requires nonsterol precursors of the cholesterol biosynthetic pathway for intracellular proliferation. Infect. Immun. **72:** 1036–1042.

13. IGLESIAS, J. & G.F. GIBBONS. 1989. Regulation of hepatic cholesterol biosynthesis: effects of a cytochrome P-450 inhibitor on the formation and metabolism of oxygenated sterol products of lanosterol. Biochem. J. **264:** 495–502.
14. LANGE, Y., J. YE & J. CHIN. 1997. The fate of cholesterol exiting lysosomes. J. Biol. Chem. **272:** 17018–17022.
15. BUTLER, J.D. *et al.* 1992. Progesterone blocks cholesterol translocation from lysosomes. J. Biol. Chem. **267:** 23797–23805.
16. HECHEMY, K.E. *et al.* 1993. Three-dimensional reconstruction of *Coxiella burnetii*–infected L929 cells by high-voltage electron microscopy. Infect. Immun. **61:** 4485–4488.

Protective Immunity against Q Fever Induced with a Recombinant P1 Antigen Fused with HspB of *Coxiella burnetii*

QINGFENG LI,[a] DONGSHENG NIU,[a] BOHAI WEN, MEILING CHEN, LING QIU, AND JINGBO ZHANG

Beijing Institute of Microbiology and Epidemiology, and State Key Laboratory of Pathogen and Biosecurity, Beijing 100071, China

ABSTRACT: The gene fragments encoding outer membrane protein 1 (P1) and heat-shock protein B (HspB) amplified from genomic DNA of *Coxiella burnetii* Xinqiao by PCR were inserted into prokaryotic expression vector pQE30 to construct recombinant expression plasmids pQE30/*p1* and pQE30/*hspB*, respectively. The *p1* fragment from pQE30/*p1* was ligated with *hspB* of pQE30/*hspB* to construct pQE30/*p1-hspB*. Recombinant proteins, P1, HspB, and P1-HspB, were expressed in *Escherichia coli* cells transformed with pQE30/*p1*, pQE30/*hspB*, and pQE30/*p1-hspB*, respectively. The purified recombinant proteins and whole-cell antigen (WCA) of *C. burnetii* were used to immunize BALB/c mice. The antibody detection, T-cell proliferation assay, and cytokine detection demonstrated that the animals immunized with P1-HspB or WCA exhibited stronger humoral and cellular immune responses compared with animals immunized with P1 or HspB individually. Seven days after challenge of 10-fold 50% infection dose of *C. burnetii*, mice were euthanized and their spleens were collected. The splenic weights of mice immunized with P1-HspB or WCA were significantly lighter than that of mice immunized with P1 or HspB. By real-time PCR assay, the coxiella loads of spleens of mice immunized with P1-HspB or WCA were also significantly lower than that of mice immunized with P1 or HspB. The data from this study indicate that fusion antigen P1-HspB is a good immunogen for eliciting immunoresponses against *C. burnetii*, and it may be a more suitable candidate for preparing subunit vaccine against Q fever.

KEYWORDS: *Coxiella burnetii*; fusion protein; protective immunity; subunit vaccine

INTRODUCTION

Q fever is a zoonotic disease with a worldwide distribution and it is caused by *Coxiella burnetii*, an obligate intracellular gram-negative bacterium. Many species

[a]Contributed equally to this work.

Address for correspondence: Bohai Wen, Beijing Institute of Microbiology and Epidemiology and State Key Laboratory of Pathogen and Biosecurity, 20 Dong-Da-Jie Street, Fengtai, Beijing 100071, China. Phone: +86-10-63820718; fax: +86-10-63815259.
wenbohai@yahoo.com

**Ann. N.Y. Acad. Sci. 1063: 130–142 (2005). © 2005 New York Academy of Sciences.
doi: 10.1196/annals.1355.021**

of mammals, birds, and ticks are reservoirs of *C. burnetii* in nature,[1] and it can cause Q fever via aerosol, arthropod-borne carriage, and possibly milk ingestion.[2] Human Q fever can be either acute or chronic. Acute Q fever is a flu-like illness that is effectively treated by antibiotics. Chronic Q fever is a severe, sometimes fatal disease including endocarditis, chronic hepatitis, chronic pulmonitis, and so on.[1]

Although the current methods of treating acute Q fever are efficacious, patients with chronic Q fever have responded poorly to various antibiotic therapies.[3] For this reason, an effective vaccine against *C. burnetii* is more desirable for the control of Q fever and biological attack of this pathogen.

The present vaccines to Q fever available were composed of either formalin-killed whole *C. burnetii* cells (WCbs) or chloroform-methanol residue of *C. burnetii* cells (CMRs).[4,5] WCbs' protective ability is well documented, but the adverse reactions induced by WCb vaccine, including fever, anorexia, malaise and tenderness, erythema, and edema at the inoculation site, are also well documented.[4,6] Although CMR vaccines are shown to be better tolerated in animals than WCb vaccine,[7] large-scale culture and purification of *C. burnetii* and preparation of CMR vaccine are time-consuming, labored, and even hazardous. Therefore, it is desired to develop novel vaccine against Q fever, such as recombinant protein or DNA vaccines, based on the protective antigens of *C. burnetii*.[2,8] Vodkin and Williams demonstrated that a 62-kDa heat-shock protein B (HspB) of *C. burnetii* was immunogenic in mice, indicating that the antigen may mediate protection against *C. burnetii*.[9] Later, Williams *et al.* found that a partially purified 29-kDa protein (P1) from *C. burnetii* could confer protection from a lethal challenge in mice.[8] These studies suggest that the two antigens may elicit immune responses against *C. burnetii* infection.

In the present study, the gene encoding P1 was ligated with the gene encoding HspB inserted into a prokaryotic expression vector. A fusion protein containing the antigenic determinants of P1 and HspB was expressed in *E. coli* cells transformed with the expression vector inserted with a fusion gene encoding P1 and HspB antigen. The protective efficacies against Q fever induced with the fusion protein was evaluated in mice, and the results obtained in the present study demonstrate that the fusion protein is capable of inducing much stronger immune protection against Q fever compared with the recombinant P1 or HspB antigen individually.

MATERIALS AND METHODS

Preparation of DNA and PCR Amplification

C. burnetii Xinqiao strain isolated from ticks in Chongqing, China was propagated in the yolk sac of chicken embryos. Genomic DNA of *C. burnetii* was extracted from the Xinqiao strain-infected yolk sac membrane with phenol-chloroform method described previously.[10] A primer pair, p1F (5′-ACAGGATCCGGCGGTCCTGATATCCCCATG-3′) and p1R (5′-GCGGAGCTCCAGGTAATTAACGGTTGCGG-3′), was designed based on the published *p1* gene sequences (GenBank accession number: AY249911); the other primer pair, hspBF (5′-GCCGAGCTCGTGACGTTGGGACCAAAAGG-3′) and hspBR (5′-ATACTGCAGCCGCCCATTCCTCCCATGCC-3′), was designed according to *hspB* gene sequence (GenBank accession number: AY251297) of *C. burnetii*. The restriction sites in the primer sequences were underlined. The primers were synthesized by Shanghai Sangon Company (Shanghai, China).

The target DNA fragments were amplified by PCR from genomic DNA extracted from *C. burnetii* Xinqiao. The two genes were amplified in a mixture of 200 M (each) deoxynucleoside triphosphate, 0.3 M (each) primer, and 0.6 U of *Taq* polymerase in 10 mM Tris-HCl buffer (pH 8.3) supplemented with 2.0 mM $MgCl_2$ and 50 mM KCl. For amplification of *p1* fragment, the PCR reaction was performed at 94°C for 5 min and then for 30 cycles of 94°C for 25 s and 65°C for 50 s, followed by a final incubation at 72°C for 7 min. The amplification of *hspB* fragment was performed at the same conditions as that of *p1* fragment except for 30 cycles of 94°C for 1 min and 72°C for 1 min.

Construction of Recombinant Expression Plasmids

The amplified *p1 and hspB* gene fragments were purified from agarose gel with a kit for DNA purification after electrophoresis of PCR productions. The purified truncated *p1* and *hspB* genes were digested with DNA endonuclease pairs (*Bam*HI/ *Sac*I for *p1*, and *Sac*I/ *Pst*I for *hspB*), respectively. The prokaryotic expression plasmid pQE30 was digested with the homologous enzyme pair. The digested truncated *p1* and *hspB* genes were ligated with the digested pQE30 with T4 ligase to construct

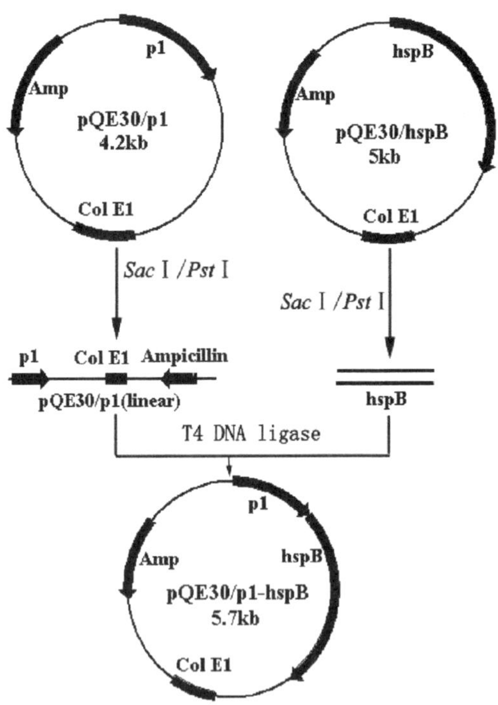

FIGURE 1. Strategy for construction of pQE30/*p1-hspB* that expresses the P1HspB fusion protein antigen of the *C. burnetii*.

the recombinant plasmids pQE30/*p1* and pQE30/*hspB*, respectively, according to the standard methods.[11] The *hspB* gene fragment was obtained from pQE30/*hspB* by endonuclease digestion and it ligated with *p1* gene fragment of pQE30/*p1* to construct pQE30/*p1-hspB* (FIG 1). *E. coli* M15 cells were transformed with the resulting ligation mixtures, respectively, and the transformed colonies were screened on medium containing ampicillin and kanamycin according to the standard protocols.[12]

Expression and Identification of Recombinant Proteins

E. coli cells harboring the recombinant plasmids were propagated in Luria-Bertani medium (LB, pH 7.0) and induced to express the target genes by IPTG according to methods described previously.[13] The proteins of *E. coli* cells were assessed in SDS-PAGE (5% stacking gel and 10% separation gel) and the expressed recombinant protein were identified by immunoblot assays according to the standard methods described by Towbin *et al.*[14]

Purification of Recombinant Proteins and Whole Cell Antigen

According to the manufacture's protocols, the recombinant protein tagged with six consecutive histidine residues was purified from the cellular debris by affinity chromatography with nickel-nitrilotriacetic resin (Ni-NTA, Qiagen GmbH) under native conditions.[13]

C. burnetii Xinqiao propagated in the yolk sac of chicken embryos was separated from host cell components by isopycnic centrifugation in Renografin density gradients, and the purified *C. burnetii* cells were inactivated as whole-cell antigen (WCA) with 1% formaldehyde as described previously.[15] The concentration of WCA was determined using BCA protein assay reagent (Bio Basic, Inc., Toronto, Canada) with bovine serum albumin as the standard.[16]

Immunization of Mice with Antigens

The specific pathogen-free BALB/c mice purchased from the Laboratory Animal Center of Beijing were male and 6 to 8 weeks of age. Each mouse was immunized subcutaneously with 30 μg of purified antigen mixed with Freund's complete adjuvant. After four weeks, the mouse was intraperitoneally given booster injections twice at 2-week intervals with 15 μg of homologous antigen emulsified in Freund's incomplete adjuvant. Phosphate-buffered saline (PBS) emulsified in Freund's adjuvant was used to inject mice as a mock immunization.

Antibody Responses

The indirect immunofluorescence assay (IFA) was performed to detect antibodies (IgGs) in mouse sera. Briefly, the WCAs of *C. burnetii* Xinqiao (phase I) and *C. burnetii* Grita (phase II) were placed onto 12-well Teflon-coated slides, respectively, and the WCAs in the wells were air-dried and fixed with cold acetone. The WCAs were incubated with serially diluted mouse sera in a moist chamber at 37°C for 60 min. After three rinses in phosphate-buffered saline, the WCAs were incubated with fluorescein isothiocyanate-conjugated goat anti-mouse IgG at 37°C for 60 min. The IgG titers of sera were determined under a fluorescence microscope.

Proliferation Assay of Splenic Cells

Ten days after the second booster, three mice in each group were killed and spleens were ground into single-cell suspensions in RPMI 1640 medium supplemented with 10% fetal bovine serum. The splenic cell suspension was applied in cell proliferation assay with the MTT (3-[4,5-dimethylthiazol-2-yl]-2,5-diphenyltetrazolium bromide) test described previously.[13]

IL-2 Levels in Murine Sera

IL-2 production was determined by using a murine IL-2 double-sandwich ELISA kit (Biosouce, Wuhan, China) according to the manufacturer's instructions. Briefly, 100 μL of murine sera were added to each well of a 96-well plate coated with monoclonal antibodies to murine IL-2 for at 37°C for 120 min. After five washes with washing buffer, 50 μL of biotin-conjugated antibodies to murine IL-2 were added to each well and the plate incubated at 37°C for 60 min. The plate was washed five times with washing buffer, and then 50 μL of peroxidase-conjugated streptavidin was added and it was incubated at 37°C for 60 min. Plate was washed five times with washing buffer prior to the addition of TMB substrate. Plates were read at 492 nm on microplate reader.

Evaluation of Immunoprotectivity

A total of 50 mice were randomly divided into five groups of 10 each and each group was immunized once and boosters given twice with an antigen (P1, HspB, P1-hspB, or WCA) or PBS according to the above immunization protocols. Ten days after the second booster immunization, each group was challenged with 10-fold 50% infection dose of *C. burnetii* stock suspensions calculated by the method of Reed and Muench.[17] Seven days later, mice were sacrificed, and the spleens were removed. Each spleen was weighed in scales and total DNA was extracted from its homogenate with phenol-chloroform method.[10] The extracted total DNA of each spleen was suspended in 30 μL of double-distilled water and the DNA solution was stored at –70°C. The levels of protection afforded by each antigen were assessed by using a real-time quantitative PCR assay specific for *C. burnetii.*[18] Two μL of DNA solution was applied in each real-time PCR reaction as templates to assess coxiella load of each spleen. The real-time PCR reactions were performed in DNA sequence detection system (ABI Prism TM, 7900 HT).

Statistical Analysis

Multiple comparisons by analysis of variance were performed using the SAS version 8 for windows 98. A P value < 0.05 was considered statistically significant.

RESULTS

Expression and Purification of the Recombinant P1, HspB, and P1-HspB Protein

In SDS-PAGE analysis, proteins with apparent sizes of approximately 29 kDa, 54 kDa, and 83 kDa were observed in *E. coli* cells transformed with pQE30/*p1*,

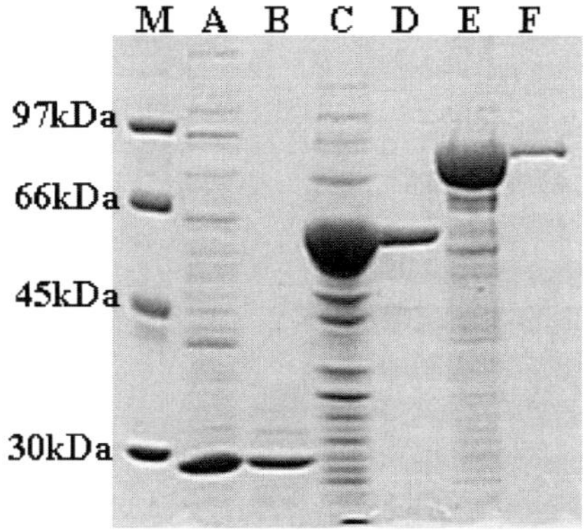

FIGURE 2. SDS-PAGE analysis of recombinant proteins P1, HspB, and P1-HspB. *Lane* M, protein molecular mass markers; *lanes* A, C, E, inclusion bodies extracted from *E. coli* cells harboring pQE30/*p1*, pQE30/*hspB*, and pQE30/*p1-hspB*, respectively; *lanes* B, D, F, purified P1, HspB, and P1-HspB proteins.

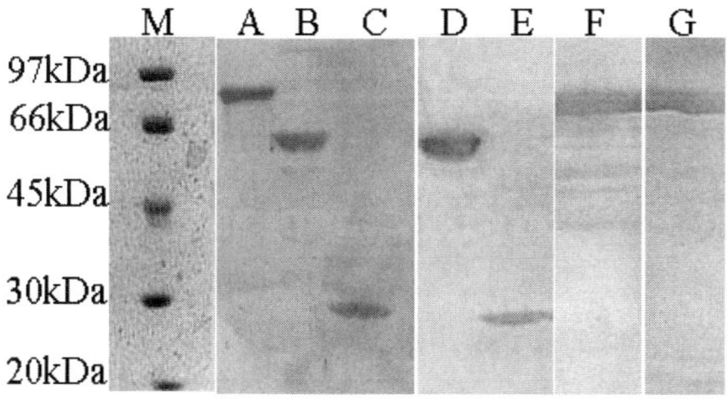

FIGURE 3. Specificity and cross-reactivity analysis of recombinant proteins with immunosera in immunoblot assays. *Lane* M, protein molecular mass markers; *lanes* A, B, C, antiserum to whole cell antigen of *C. burnetii* reacted with P1-HspB, HspB, P1, respectively; *lanes* D and E, antiserum to P1-HspB reacted with HspB, P1, respectively; *lane* F, antiserum to HspB reacted with P1-HspB; *lane* G, antiserum to P1 reacted with P1-HspB.

pQE30/*hspB*, and pQE30/*p1-hspB*, respectively. The recombinant proteins purified from *E. coli* cell debris by Ni-NTA affinity chromatography are shown in FIGURE 2. Immunoblot assays showed that recombinants P1, HspB, and P1-HspB were recognized by *C. burnetii*-immunized mouse serum; P1 and HspB were both recognized by mouse sera to P1-HspB. which was also recognized by mouse sera to P1 or HspB (FIG. 3).

Humoral Responses

Serum samples were obtained on weeks 1 to 9 after the primary immunization. The titers of phase I and II antibodies (IgGs) in sera from mice immunized with P1 or HspB were lower than those of mice immunized with P1-HspB or WCA. The titers of phase I and II IgGs in sera from P1-immunized mice were both at low levels, with their maximum levels being detectable on week 1 after first booster immunization and a rapid decrease seen two weeks later. The high titers of phase I and II IgGs were determined in mice immunized with WCA or P1-HspB on weeks 1 and 2 after the first booster injection and they persisted for over 5 weeks (FIG. 4).

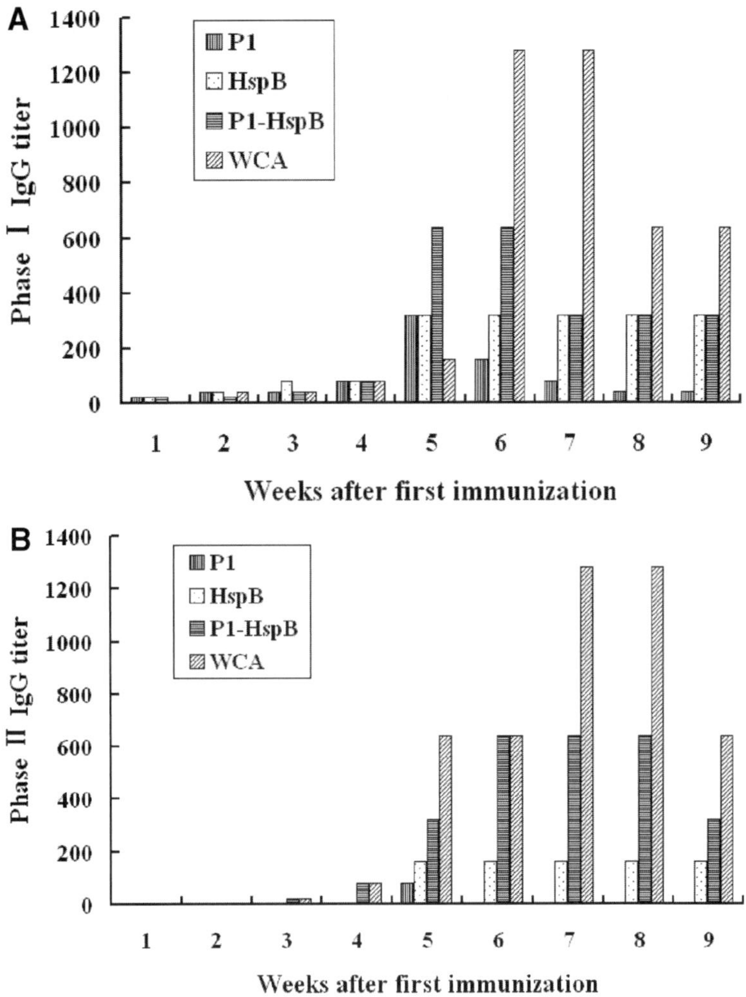

FIGURE 4. Titers of phase I (**A**) and II (**B**) IgG antibodies in sera from mice immunized with the different antigens were determined by immunofluorescence assay (IFA) with *C. burnetii* Xinqiao antigen. The pooled sera of 10 mice were two-fold diluted (1:20 to 1:2560) in PBS. The mice were given booster injections with homologous antigens on days 30 and 40 after the primary immunization.

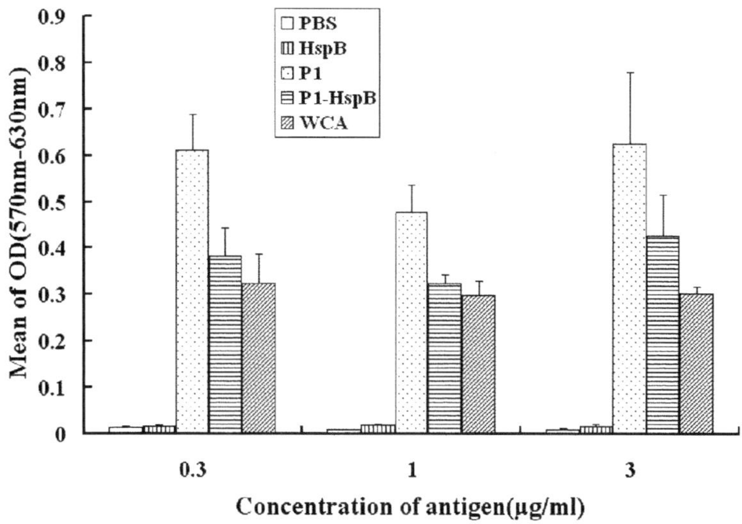

FIGURE 5. Splenic cell proliferative responses to recombinant antigens analyzed by 3-[4,5-dimethylthiazol-2-yl]-2,5-diphenyltetrazolium bromide on day 10 after the second booster injection. The recombinant proteins in various concentrations of (0.3, 1, and 3g/mL) were used as stimulating antigens. *Error bars* show the average with standard deviation for three mice per group.

Cell-Mediated Immune Responses

The proliferative responses of splenic cells from mice immunized with P1, P1-HspB, or WCA were significantly greater than those from HspB-immunized mice after stimulation with homologous antigens ($P < 0.05$) (FIG. 5). The IL-2 levels in the sera from mice immunized with P1 or P1-HspB were much higher than those of HspB-immunized mice ($P < 0.05$), but not significantly different from that of WCA-immunized mice ($P > 0.05$) (FIG. 6). Significant differences in IL-2 levels were observed between P1-, HspB-, or P1-HspB-immunized mice and the negative controls ($P < 0.05$) (FIG. 6).

Splenic Weights

Seven days post challenge, the mice were sacrificed and their spleens were collected. For the weights of spleens, there was no significant difference between P1-HspB- and WCA-immunized mice ($P > 0.05$). However, the splenic weights of P1-HspB- or WCA-vaccinated mice were significantly lighter than that of P1- or HspB-immunized mice ($P < 0.05$) (FIG. 7).

Loads of C. burnetii *in Spleens*

The loads of *C. burnetii* in murine spleens were determined by using the real-time quantitative PCR specific for this pathogen. The burden of *C. burnetii* in spleens of mice immunized with P1-HspB was higher than that of WCA-immunized mice, but

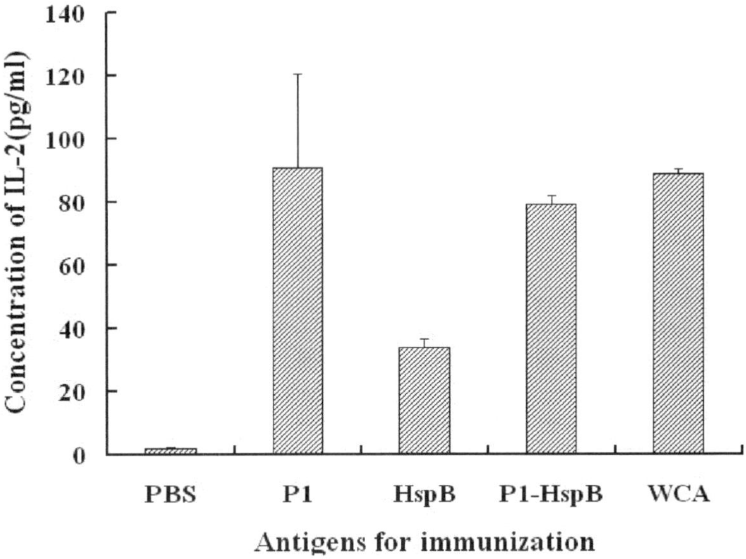

FIGURE 6. Interleukin-2 (IL-2) level in sera from antigen-immunized mice. The serum samples were obtained on day 7 after the second booster injection. The concentration of IL-2 in each mixed serum was analyzed by a double sandwich enzyme-linked immunosorbent assay. *Error bars* show the average with standard deviation for triplicate tests of each mixed serum from ten mice per group.

there was no significant difference between them ($P > 0.05$). The coxiella burden in spleens of P1-HspB-vaccinated mice was significantly lower than that of P1- or HspB-immunized mice ($P < 0.05$). There was no significant difference between P1- or HspB-immunized mice and mice injected with PBS in analysis of splenic weight (FIG. 8).

DISCUSSION

In this study, the choice of P1 is motivated by the fact that the protein is a cell surface component, characterized by susceptibility to iodination reaction, resistance to detergent solubilization at low temperatures, reactivity with immune serum to *C. burnetii*, and natural abundance.[19] The HspB of *C. burnetii* was demonstrated to belong to Hsp60 family and it was recognized as an immunogen.[9] P1 protein was also immnogenic and the immunity induced by it was more efficacious in clearance of *C. burnetii* from spleens of mice compared with immunity induced by another protein or lipopolysaccharide of *C. burnetii*.[8] Therefore, we cloned and expressed genes *p1* and *hspB* to prepare recombinant proteins P1, HspB, and P1-HspB.

Although the truncated P1 protein does not contain the N-terminal 23 residues and truncated HspB protein does not contain the N-terminal 28 residues as deduced from the open reading frames of their encoding genes, they may present epitopes

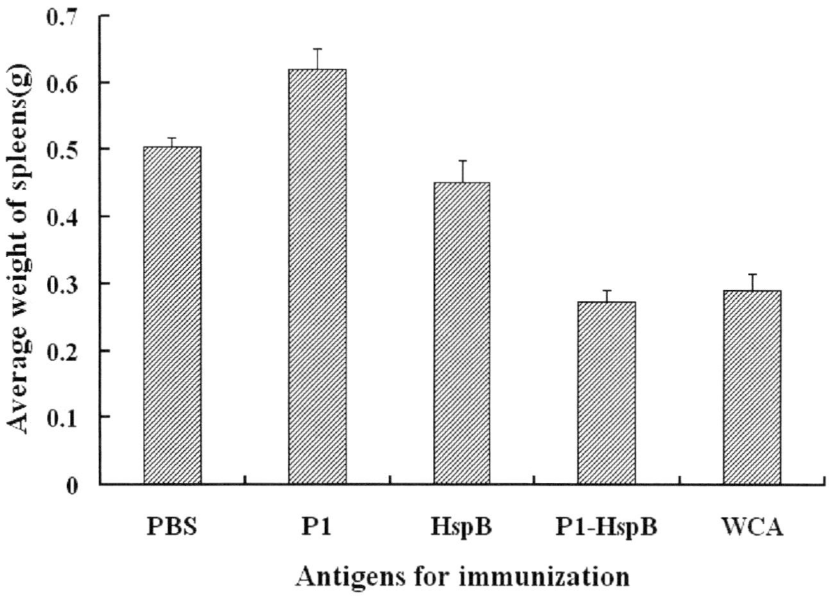

FIGURE 7. Comparison of spleen weights of mice immunized with different antigens. The spleen weight of each group is the average with standard deviation for ten mice.

similar to those found in the full-length native proteins. In immunoblot assay, P1-HspB reacted with immunoserum to P1, HspB, or WCA of *C. burnetii*, and the immunoserum to P1-HspB also reacted with P1 and HspB. These strongly demonstrate that the fusion antigen P1-HspB contains the epitopes of both P1 and HspB.

The humoral immunoresponses of mice immunized with these antigens of *C. burnetii* were monitored by IFA. Phase I and II IgGs in mice immunized with P1-HspB appeared as early as and decreased as slowly as those in mice immunized with WCA, suggesting that P1-HspB could induce strong humoral immunoresponses similar to WCA of *C. burnetii*. Otherwise, the antibody titer of HspB-immunized mice was much higher and lasted much longer than that of P1-immunized mice. These suggest that the high level of long-lived phase I and II antibodies were well induced by HspB. Although it was not as efficient as HspB in eliciting the humoral immunoresponses, P1 was recognized as an efficient antigen in eliciting cell-mediated immunoresponses (CMI). The proliferative level of splenic cells from mice immunized with P1, P1-HspB, or WCA was much higher than that in HspB-immunized mice in response to homologous antigens. This finding demonstrates that the P1-HspB fusion antigen has a much stronger capability of eliciting the CMI than HspB. In addition, the levels of IL-2 of mice immunized with P1 or P1-HspB was also similar to those of WCA-immunized mice and markedly higher than those of HspB-immunized mice. These results indicate that P1 subunit played an important role in eliciting the CMI.

The BALB/c mouse was used as a sublethal-infection model of *C. burnetii* with splenomegaly as a reporter for vaccinogenic activity in evaluating the protective efficacies of vaccine candidates against Q fever.[20] In the present study, comparison

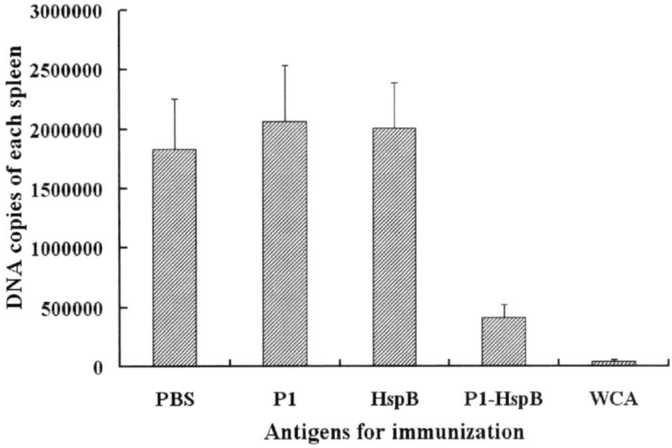

FIGURE 8. Comparison of burdens of *C. burnetii* in spleens of mice immunized with different antigen. The burden of each group is the average with standard deviation for ten mice.

of spleen weights of mice immunized with different antigens showed that the splenic weights of mice immunized with P1-HspB or WCA of *C. burnetii* were significantly lighter than that of P1- or HspB-immunized mice. The developed real-time PCR specific for *C. burnetii*[18] is a much more sensitive method to evaluate the protective efficacies of vaccine candidates against Q fever in animal models. In real-time PCR assay, the coxiella burdens of spleens of mice immunized with P1-HspB were significantly lower than those of mice immunized with P1 or HspB. These results strongly suggest that the protection against coxiella infection conferred by P1-HspB is much more efficient than that offered by P1 or HspB.

Many reports demonstrated that CMI was crucial for the development of resistance to the intracellular replication of *C. burnetii*.[21,22] However, a role for antibody was also shown to alter the course of *C. burnetii* infections in mice that received specific antiserum before infection.[22,23] In the present study, although both P1 and HspB could induce CMI and humoral immunoresponses, the immunoresponses elicited by P1 or HspB could not efficiently protect mice from coxiella infection. However, the efficient protection against *C. burnetii* was offered by immunization of fusion protein P1-HspB, suggesting that both CMI induced by P1 and humoral immunoresponses elicited by HspB play important roles in resisting *C. burnetii.*

It has been reported that many pathogens, including *C. burnetii*, may undergo a heat shock response during phagocytosis, resulting in the increased production of heat-shock proteins (Hsps).[24] Among the Hsps, immune responses (both antibody and T cell responses) to Hsp60 are most frequently observed.[24] These Hsps can be processed and presented as foreign determinants in the context of MHC class I or II. The MHC-peptide complex is subsequently recognized by T cells.[24] In addition, the potential of Hsps as adjuvants to enhance the immunogenicity of peptides or polysaccharide-based vaccines has been recognized.[24] A high and long-lasting antibody titer of anti-malaria synthetic peptide (NANP) was detected in mice immunized with NANP conjugated with mycobacterial Hsp60 or Hsp70 in the absence of adjuvants.[25] Based on the reports,[26,27] it may be postulated that the efficient protection elicited by P1-HspB may partially contribute to HspB that activates helper T cells and cytotoic T cells to assist in the production of antibodies to coxiella by B cells and to kill coxiella-infected cells, respectivly.

In conclusion, the data presented in this paper suggest that the P1-HspB fusion protein containing the antigenic properties of both P1 and HspB antigen of *C. burnetii* is a more efficient protein in eliciting humoral and cellular immunity against Q fever and may be a more suitable candidate for preparing subunit vaccines against Q fever.

ACKNOWLEDGMENTS

This research was supported by a Grant No. 30271214 from the National Natural Science Foundation of China.

[*Competing interest statement*: The authors declare that they have no conflicts of interest.]

REFERENCES

1. MAURIN, M. & D. RAOULT. 1999. Q fever. Clin. Microbiol. Rev. **12:** 518–553.
2. MADARIAGA, M.G., K. REZAI, G.M. TRENHOLME, *et al.* 2003. Q fever: a biological weapon in your backyard. Lancet Infect. Dis. **3:**709–721.
3. RAOULT, D. 1993. Treatment of Q fever. Antimicrob. Agents Chemother. **37:** 1733–36.
4. MARMION, B.P., R.A. ORMSBEE, M. KYRKOU, *et al.* 1990. Vaccine prophylaxis of abattoir-associated Q fever: eight years' experience in Australian abattoirs. Epidemiol. Infect. **104:** 275–287.
5. FRIES, L.F., D.M. WAAG, J.C. WILLIAMS, *et al.* 1993. Safety and immunogenicity in human volunteers of a chloroform-methanol residue vaccine for Q fever. Infect. Immun. **61:** 1251–1258.
6. WILHELMSEN, C.L. & D.M. WAAG. 2000. Guinea pig abscess/hypersensitivity model for study of adverse vaccination reactions induced by Q fever vaccines. Comp. Med. **50:**374–378.
7. ELLIOTT, J.J., D.L. RUBLE, G.M. ZAUCHA, *et al.* 1998. Comparison of Q fever cellular and chloroform-methanol residue vaccines as skin test antigens in the sensitized guinea pig. Acta Virol. **42:** 147–155.
8. WILLIAMS, J.C., T.A. HOOVER, D.M. WAAG, *et al.* 1990. Antigenic structure of *Coxiella burnetii*: a comparison of lipopolysaccharide and protein antigens as vaccines against Q fever. Ann. N. . Acad. Sci. **590:** 370–380.
9. VODKIN, M.H. & J.C. WILLIAMS. 1988. A heat shock operon in *Coxiella burnetti* produces a major antigen homologous to a protein in both *mycobacteria* and *Escherichia coli*. J. Bacteriol. **170:** 1227–1234.
10. WEN, B.H., R. JIAN, Y. ZHANG, *et al.* 2002. Simultaneous detection of *Anaplasma marginale* and a new *Ehrlichia* species closely related to *Ehrlichia chaffeensis* by sequence analyses of 16S ribosomal DNA in *Boophilus microplus* ticks from Tibet. J. Clin. Microbiol. **40:** 3286–3290.
11. JIN, D. & M. LI. 1992. Molecular Cloning: A Laboratory Manual, 2nd ed.: 48–56 [in Chinese]. Press of Science. Beijing, China.
12. JIN, D. & M. LI. 1992. Molecular cloning: a laboratory manual, 2nd ed.: 854–855 [in Chinese]. Press of Science. Beijing, China.

13. YU, Y., B.H. WEN, B.G. WEN, *et al.* 2005. Induction of protective immunity against scrub typhus with a 56-kilodalton recombinant antigen fused with 47-kilodalton antigen of *Orientia tsutsugamushi* Karp. Am. J. Trop. Med. Hyg. **72:** 458–464.
14. TOWBIN, H., T. STAEHELIN & J. GORDON. 1979. Electrophoretic transfer of proteins from polyacrylamide gels to nitrocellulose sheets: procedure and some applications. Proc. Natl. Acad. Sci. USA **76:** 4350–4354.
15. WILLIAMS, J.C., M.G. PEACOCK & T.F. MCCAUL. 1981. Immunological and biological characterization of *Coxiella burnetii*, phases I and II, separated from host components. Infect. Immun. **32:** 840–851.
16. SMITH, P.K., R.I. KROHN, G.T. HERMANSON, *et al.* 1985. Measurement of protein using bicinchoninic acid. Anal. Biochem. **150:** 76–85. [Erratum: Anal. Biochem. **163:** 279.]
17. REED, L.J. & H. MUENCH. 1938. A simple method of estimating fifty percent end-points. Am. J. Hyg. **27:** 493–497.
18. ZHANG, J.B, B.H. WEN, M.L. CHEN, *et al.* 2005. Detection of *Coxiella burnetii* by real-time quantitative PCR. Chinese J. Zoonoses **21:** 652–655.
19. VARGHEES, S, K. KISS, G. FRANS, *et al.* 2002. Cloning and porin activity of the major outer membrane protein P1 from *Coxiella burnetii.* Infect. Immun. **70**: 6741–6750.
20. ZHANG, G., K. KISS, R. SESHADRI, *et al.* 2004. Identification and cloning of immuno-dominant antigens of *Coxiella burnetii.* Infect. Immun. **72:** 844–852.
21. JERRELIS, T.R., L.P. MALLAVIA & D.J. HINRICHS. 1975. Detection of long-term cellular immunity to *Coxiella burnetii* as assayed by lymphocyte transformation. Infect. Immun. **11:** 280–286.
22. KAZAR, J., E. EL-NAJDAWI, R. BREZINA, *et al.* 1977. Search for correlates of resistance to virulent challenge in mice immunized with *Coxiella burnetii.* Acta Virol. **21:** 422–430.
23. HUMPHRES, R.C. & D.J. HINRICHS. 1981. Role of antibody in *Coxiella burnetii* infection. Infect. Immun. **31:** 641–645.
24. JINDAL, S. 1996. Heat shock proteins: applications in health and disease. Trends Biotechnol. **14:** 17–20
25. PERRAUT, R, A.R. LUSSOW, S. GAVOILLE, *et al.* 1993. Successful primate immunization with peptides conjugated to purified protein derivative or mycobacterial heat shock proteins in the absence of adjuvants. Clin. Exp. Immunol. **93:** 382–386.
26. KAUFMANN, S.H., U. VATH, J.E. THOLE. 1987. Enumeration of T cells reactive with Mycobacterium tuberculosis organisms and specific for the recombinant mycobacterial 64-kDa protein. Eur. J. Immunol. **17**:351–357.
27. BUCHMEIER, N.A. & F. HEFFRON. 1990. Induction of *Salmonella* stress proteins upon infection of macrophages. Science **248:**730–732.

Immunization Experiments with Recombinant *Coxiella burnetii* Proteins in a Murine Infection Model

JUDITH TYCZKA, SANDRA EBERLING, AND GEORG BALJER

Institute for Infectious Diseases of Animals, Justus Liebig University of Giessen, D-35392 Giessen, Germany

ABSTRACT: Previous attempts to develop Q fever vaccines were less successful in that the vaccines caused unacceptable side effects or failed to be protective. In this study, we tested the efficacy of a mixture of eight recombinant *Coxiella burnetii* (*C. b.*) proteins in sublethal challenge infections with mice. Eight potential *C. b.* virulence genes (Omp, Pmm, HspB, Fbp, Orf410, Crc, CbMip, and MucZ) were overexpressed in *E. coli* as *his*-tagged fusion proteins and partially purified. All recombinant proteins but rPmm proved to be antigenic in BALB/c mice when administered as protein mixtures. For efficacy testing, mice were immunized with an adjuvanted mixture of the eight recombinant proteins and subsequently challenged intraperitoneally with the *C. b.* isolate Nine Mile RSA493 (1.8 × 10^8 *C. b.*). Only animals vaccinated with the licensed Q fever vaccine Q-Vax™ (vaccination control) exhibited milder symptoms and minor gain of spleen and liver weights. In summary, clinical examinations and dissection of mice immunized with the eight recombinant *C. b.* proteins did not indicate a protective immune response after test infection.

KEYWORDS: Q fever; *Coxiella burnetii*; mice; vaccination; recombinant proteins; challenge; protection

INTRODUCTION

Q fever is caused by infections with the obligate intracellular bacterium *Coxiella burnetii* (*C. b.*). The zoonosis occurs worldwide, but mostly is diagnosed when large numbers of individuals are affected. The sources of infection in these outbreaks typically are domestic ruminants, which shed *C. b.* in large numbers with birth products or other excretions during parturition or abortion.[1] Q fever is considered an occupational hazard among livestock workers, veterinarians, research laboratory workers, and personnel of research animal facilities. Shortly after identification of the infectious agent, researchers strived for the development of vaccines,[2] but to date, to the best of our knowledge, a licensed vaccine [Q-Vax™] is only available in Australia. This vaccine consists of formalin-killed whole cells of *C. b.* Phase I (WCV I). Un-

Address for correspondence: Judith Tyczka, Institute for Hygiene and Infectious Diseases of Animals, Justus Liebig University of Giessen, Frankfurter Str. 85-89, D-35392 Giessen, Germany. Voice: +49 641 9938308; fax: +49 641 9938309

judith.tyczka@vetmed.uni-giessen.de

Ann. N.Y. Acad. Sci. 1063: 143–148 (2005). © 2005 New York Academy of Sciences.
doi: 10.1196/annals.1355.022

fortunately, like in other WCV I vaccines, the use of Q-Vax™ is hampered by the risk of severe side effects, especially in sensitized persons.[3] Attempts to develop a potent and safe vaccine utilizing inactivated Phase II, attenuated live Phase II, or chemically extracted Phase II organisms were unsuccessful.[4–6] Chloroform-methanol residues of Phase I organisms were demonstrated to be immunogenic and protective in different species, including nonhuman primates.[7,8] However, when used in higher doses, adverse reactions occurred similar to those seen with Q-Vax™,[9] and mass production of highly infectious Phase I *C. b.* poses a significant biohazard. Therefore, efforts to develop recombinant subunit protein vaccines have been undertaken since the 1990s. As immunization of laboratory animals with single recombinant proteins did not evoke protective immune responses,[10] we tested the efficacy of a mixture of eight recombinant *C. b.* proteins in sublethal challenge infections with mice.

MATERIALS AND METHODS

Microorganisms and Growth Conditions: *C. b.* Nine Mile RSA493 was propagated and harvested as previously described.[11] Bacteria were counted by Gimenez stain and stored at –70°C.

Expression, Purification, and Characterization of Recombinant C. b. Proteins: Eight open reading frames (ORFs) from the genome of *C. b.* were chosen on the basis of their similarities with virulence-associated genes of other bacterial species. ORFs encoding Omp (GenBank Acc. No. Z11828), HspB (M20482), Fbp (X75356), and Pmm (X79075) were cloned into expression vector pET-15b, whereas ORFs of CbMip (U14170), Crc (AF064961), MucZ (L42518), and Orf410 (X75356) were cloned in pET-24b(+). The clones were used for transformation of *E. coli* BL21(DE3). Production of N- (pET-15b) or C-terminal [pET-24b(+)] *his*-tagged fusion proteins was induced by 1 mM IPTG. Host cells were lysed in a French®Pressure Cell (Sopra, Büttelborn, Germany), and the recombinant proteins were partially purified using Ni^{2+}-NTA agarose (Qiagen, Hilden, Germany) under denaturing conditions (6 M GuHCl). Subsequent to gradual dialysis against distilled water, fusion proteins were concentrated (Centricon YM 10, Millipore, Eschborn, Germany) and stored in Tris-Buffer (pH 8.5) with protease inhibitors (complete-mini, Roche Diagnostics, Mannheim, Germany) at –70°C. *E. coli* BL21(DE3) transformed with either pET-15b or pET-24b(+) were processed correspondingly to obtain appropriate control preparations (*E. coli* protein). Protein concentrations were estimated using BCA*Protein Assay Reagent (Pierce, IL, USA). Purified proteins were characterized by SDS-PAGE and Western blotting utilizing standard techniques.[12] Antigenicity was proven by immunizing BALB/c mice two times at a 14-day interval with either single recombinant proteins or protein mixtures both adjuvanted with BAY R1005[13] (Bayer, Leverkusen, Germany). Sera were collected and tested by immunoblotting[12] against recombinant proteins. All recombinant proteins but rPmm proved to be antigenic when administered as protein mixtures.

Vaccination with Subsequent Challenge Infection: In two independent experiments, 8-week-old female BALB/c mice (6/group, randomly arranged; Charles River, Sulzfeld, Germany) were immunized subcutaneously twice at a 14-day interval with a mixture of the eight recombinant proteins (rOmp, rHspB, rFbp, rPmm, rCbMip, rCrc, rMucZ, and rOrf410; 20 μg each) adjuvanted with BAY R1005. For controls, mice were injected with Q-Vax™ (vaccination control; 1 μg/mouse;[4,14] CSL Limited, Victoria, Australia); *E. coli* protein, BAY R1005, or PBS (negative controls). Five weeks after the booster immunization, animals were challenged intraperitoneally with 1.8×10^8 *C. b.* Nine MileRSA493 and housed in a BSL3 containment. The courses of disease were monitored by daily reports of clinical signs (ruffled fur, bent backs, reduced movement) and classification of findings (severe, moderate, minor, or healthy) was based on clinical presentation of ≥2/3 per group. At day 7 and day 14 *p.i.* three mice per group were sacrificed and spleen and liver weights were measured. Untreated and noninfected animals served as controls.

RESULTS

Clinical Findings in Challenged Mice: Mice mock-vaccinated with PBS or adjuvant initially showed symptoms of moderate illness for 48 h followed by severe illness from day 3 till day 10 (FIG. 1). At day 11 a first improvement could be noticed and at day 14 all animals presented healthy again. Mice immunized with the adjuvanted recombinant proteins or with adjuvanted *E. coli* protein presented virtually identically, albeit signs of severe illness occurred slightly earlier (day 2). In contrast, animals vaccinated with Q-Vax™ presented better. Only this group kept well during the first 24 hours and the period of severe illness was shorter (day 3 till day 9). Moderate or minor symptoms occurred till day 12 and all mice were clinically healthy at day 13.

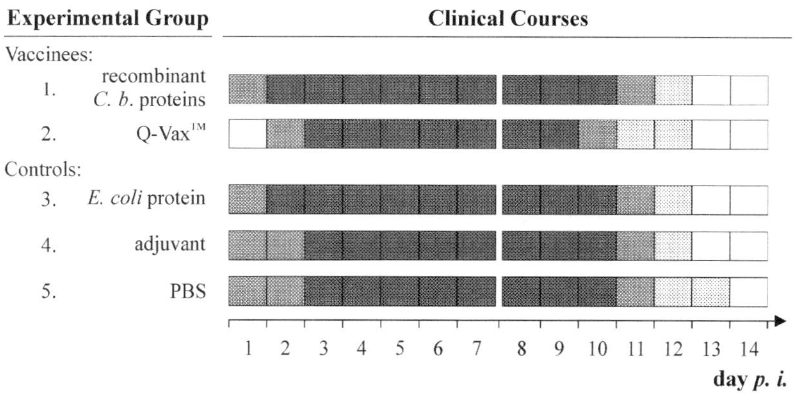

FIGURE 1. Clinical courses of vaccinated and control mice after challenge with *C. b.* Mice were immunized with the eight recombinant *C. b.* proteins (1), Q-Vax™ (2) or animals were mock-vaccinated with different control preparations [*E. coli* protein (3), adjuvant (4), PBS (5)]. Evaluation of disease courses was based on daily reports of clinical pictures (see MATERIALS AND METHODS section for details). ▇ = severe illness; ▇ = moderate illness; ░ = minor illness; ☐ = healthy

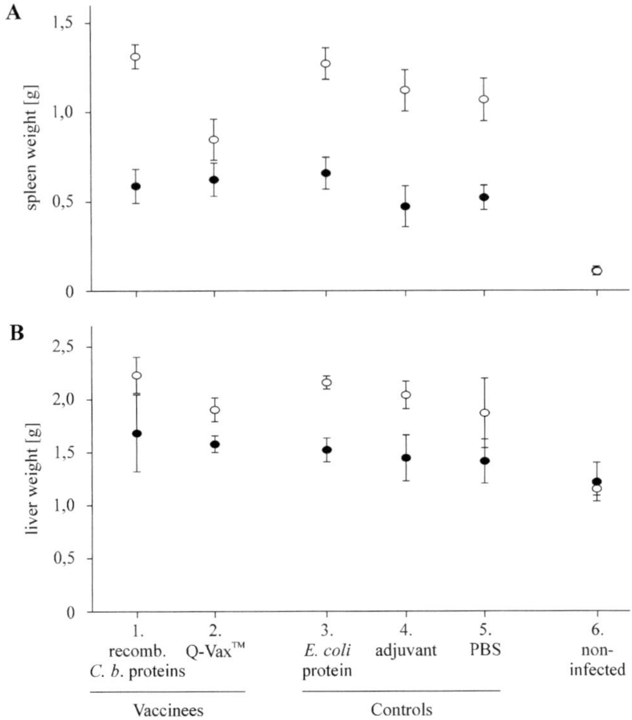

FIGURE 2. Comparison of spleen and liver weights from vaccinated and control mice at day 7 and day 14 after infection: (**A**) spleen weights; (**B**) liver weights. Mice were immunized with the eight recombinant *C. b.* proteins (1), Q-Vax™ (2) or animals were mock-vaccinated with different control preparations [*E. coli* protein (3), adjuvant (4), PBS (5)]. For comparison, organ weights of untreated and noninfected mice (6) are displayed. The organ weight of each group is the average with standard deviation among two times six mice. *Solid circles* = organ weights at day 7 *p.i.*; *open circles* = organ weights at day 14 *p.i.*

Evaluation of Spleen and Liver Weights during Dissection: All mice infected with *C. b.* exhibited profound spleno- and hepatomegaly at the time of dissection. However, challenged groups differed in average organ weights only moderately at day 7 (FIG. 2). Spleens were enlarged by four- (0.47 g; adjuvant) to six-fold (0.66 g; *E. coli* protein) when compared to noninfected controls (0.11 g). Average liver enlargements per group were less obvious, ranging between 1.42 g (PBS) and 1.68 g (recombinant *C. b.* proteins) compared to 1.22 g in noninfected controls. In contrast, differences between vaccination groups became evident at day 14. Compared to day 7 average spleen weights doubled for most challenged groups [range: +93% (*E. coli* protein) to +138% (adjuvant)]. Only mice vaccinated with Q-Vax™ gained less splenic weight (+36%). Compared to splenic enlargements, in most vaccination groups liver weights increased less evidently and rose by an average of 37% [range: +32% (PBS) to +42% (*E. coli* protein)]. Again, only vaccination with Q-Vax™ appeared to be partially protective as the average liver enlargement was +21% only.

DISCUSSION

The cell-mediated immune response is thought to be essential in the elimination of infections with intracellular pathogens like *C. b.*[15] Studies on Q fever and its prevention revealed that both cellular and humoral immune responses are involved in host resistance.[8,10,16] In our investigations, antigenicity for the recombinant *C. b.* proteins was proven by demonstrating seroconversions in immunized mice for all proteins but rPmm (data not shown). To determine whether the cellular immune response is adequately co-stimulated and results in protection, we challenged immunized mice with high doses of *C. b.* Nine Mile RSA493 known to induce severe illness and profound spleno- and hepatomegaly in naive animals.[10] In our model, only mice vaccinated with Q-Vax™ were partially protected, whereas animals immunized with the recombinant *C. b.* proteins presented similar to mock-vaccinated controls. Currently, experiments are under way to enumerate *C. b.* in spleens and livers of challenged mice to elucidate effects the immunization might have had on the elimination of the pathogen.

A lack of protection was reported earlier for vaccination trials utilizing single recombinant proteins. Immunization with rCom, rP1, rCbMip, or rP28 did not protect mice against severe illness and profound splenomegaly after *i. p.* infection with 1×10^8 *C. b.* Nine Mile RSA493.[10] In contrast, a partially purified 67-kDa antigen from *C. b.* QiYi was able to protect mice against an *i.p.* challenge with 10^3 ID_{50}.[17] Similarly, P1 protein purified from *C. b.* conferred protection from a lethal challenge and reduced the number of infectious *C. b.* in the spleens of challenged mice.[18] Although no LPS was detectable in the P1 preparations used for the trial, mice immunized with this preparation developed antibodies against Phase I LPS.[18] It is therefore reasonable to speculate that protective antigen(s) or unspecific immunostimulators copurified with the proteins of *C. b.* whole cells may have accounted for the protective efficacy of the vaccines. Either substances may be missing from preparations of recombinant proteins purified from *E. coli*. Previous attempts to overcome this problem by using adjuvants were not successful.[10] However, combining different recombinant proteins seems to improve their immunogenicity. In our preceding study, some of the recombinant *C. b.* proteins (rCrc, rMucZ) did not elicit antibody formation when administered separately, but were immunogenic in combination with other recombinant proteins (data not shown). Although protection could not yet be demonstrated, our approach to immunize mice with mixtures of recombinant *C. b.* proteins is a significant step forward to enhance the efficacy of the vaccine. We assume that the supplementation of mixtures of recombinant *C. b.* proteins with co-stimulatory antigens and/or appropriate adjuvants eventually will result in the development of protective recombinant subunit Q fever vaccines.

ACKNOWLEDGMENTS

We thank Christian Menge for critical reading of the manuscript. In part, this study was funded as a contract-research-project for the Bundeswehr Medical Service.

[*Conflict of interest statement:* The authors of this research declare that they have no conflict of interest.]

REFERENCES

1. MAURIN, M. & D. RAOULT. 1999. Q fever. Clin. Microbiol. Rev. **12:** 518–553.
2. SMADEL, J.E., M.J. SNYDER & F.C. ROBBINS. 1948. Vaccination against Q fever. Am. J. Hyg. **47:** 71.
3. MARMION, B.P., R.A. ORMSBEE, *et al.* 1984. Vaccine prophylaxis of abattoir-associated Q fever. Lancet **2:** 1411–1414.
4. ORMSBEE, R.A., E.J. BELL, *et al.* 1964. The influence of phase on the protective potency of Q fever vaccine. J. Immunol. **92:** 404–412.
5. JOHNSON, J.W., G.A. EDDY & C.E. PEDERSEN, JR. 1976. Biological properties of the M-44 strain of *Coxiella burnetii*. J. Infect. Dis. **133:** 334–338.
6. KAZAR, J., R. BREZINA, *et al.* 1982. Immunogenicity and reactogenicity of a Q fever chemovaccine in persons professionally exposed to Q fever in Czechoslovakia. Bull. WHO **60:** 389–394.
7. WILLIAMS, J.C., T.A. DAMROW, *et al.* 1986. Characterization of a Phase I *Coxiella burnetii* chloroform-methanol residue vaccine that induces active immunity against Q fever in C57BL/10 ScN mice. Infect. Immun. **51:** 851–858.
8. WAAG, D.M., M.J. ENGLAND, *et al.* 2002. Comparative efficacy and immunogenicity of Q fever chloroform:methanol residue (CMR) and Phase I cellular (Q-Vax) vaccines in cynomolgus monkeys challenged by aerosol. Vaccine **20:** 2623–2634.
9. FRIES, L.F., D.M. WAAG & J.C. WILLIAMS. 1993. Safety and immunogenicity in human volunteers of a chloroform-methanol residue vaccine for Q fever. Infect. Immun. **61:** 1251–1258.
10. ZHANG, G.Q. & J.E. SAMUEL. 2003. Identification and cloning of potentially protective antigens of *Coxiella burnetii* using sera from mice experimentally infected with Nine Mile Phase I. Ann. N.Y. Acad. Sci. **990:** 510–520.
11. LORENZ, H., C. JAGER, *et al.* 1998. PCR detection of *Coxiella burnetii* from different clinical specimens, especially bovine milk, on the basis of DNA preparation with a silica matrix. Appl. Environ. Microbiol. **64:** 4234–4237.
12. SAMBROCK, J., E.F. FRITSCH & T. MANIATIS. 1989. Molecular Cloning: A Laboratory Manual. Cold Spring Harbor Laboratory Press. Cold Spring Harbor, NY.
13. LOCKHOFF, O. 1991. Glycolipids as immunomodulators: synthesis and properties. Angew. Chem. Int. Ed. Engl. **30:** 1611–1620.
14. WAAG, D.M., M.J. ENGLAND & M.L. PITT. 1997. Comparative efficacy of a *Coxiella burnetii* chloroform:methanol residue (CMR) vaccine and a licensed cellular vaccine (Q-Vax) in rodents challenged by aerosol. Vaccine **15:** 1779–1783.
15. KAUFMANN, S.H. 1995. Immunity to intracellular microbial pathogens. Immunol. Today **16:** 338–342.
16. GAJDOSOVA, E. & R. BREZINA. 1989. Cell-mediated immune response to *Coxiella burnetii* antigens in Q fever convalescents and vaccinees. Acta Virol. **32:** 358–368.
17. ZHANG, X.N., N. ZHI, *et al.* 1994. Protective immunity induced by 67 K outer membrane protein of Phase I *Coxiella burnetii* in mice and guinea pigs. Acta Virol. **38:** 327–332.
18. WILLIAMS, J.C., T.A. HOOVER, *et al.* 1990. Antigenic structure of *Coxiella burnetii*: a comparison of lipopolysaccharide and protein antigens as vaccines against Q fever. Ann. N.Y. Acad. Sci. **590:** 370–380.

Structural and Functional Characterization of the Glycan Antigens Involved in Immunobiology of Q Fever

PAVOL VADOVIC, KATARINA SLABA, MARCELA FODOROVA, LUDOVIT SKULTETY, AND RUDOLF TOMAN

Laboratory for Diagnosis and Prevention of Rickettsial and Chlamydial Infections, Institute of Virology, SAS, 845 05 Bratislava, Slovakia

ABSTRACT: *Coxiella burnetii* is the causative agent of Q fever. The bacterium is extremely infectious and is classified as a category biological weapon. A lipopolysaccharide I (LPS I) belongs to the main components of the *C. burnetii* outer membrane and its structure-function relationship studies are of potential interest. Size-exclusion chromatography revealed noticeable differences in distribution and chemical composition of the O-polysaccharide chains in LPS I. It is likely that *C. burnetii* is capable of synthesizing chemically distinct subclasses of O-specific polysaccharide molecules differing in their antigenic reactivities. Methylation-linkage analysis indicated the presence of terminal virenose (Vir), dihydrohydroxystreptose (Strep), and mannose (Man), 4-substituted Vir, and 4-substituted Man in the O-specific chain. Serological data indicate that Vir and Strep might be involved in the immunobiology of Q fever.

KEYWORDS: *Coxiella burnetii*; lipopolysaccharide; composition; structure; immunobiology; Q fever

INTRODUCTION

Coxiella burnetii is the etiological agent of Q fever, a zoonosis that is endemic throughout the world. The disease can occur as an acute disabling illness or develop towards a chronic form. A lipopolysaccharide I (LPS I) belongs to the main components of the *C. burnetii* outer membrane and has important biological properties.[1,2] Two branched sugars, virenose (Vir) and dihydrohydroxystreptose (Strep), have been detected[3,4] in the O-polysaccharide chain of the LPS I but their location in the O-specific chain has not been clarified with certainty thus far. Further, there have been ongoing discussions of their possible role in the immunobiology of *C. burnetii*. In order to throw more light on these problems, we have started detailed structural

Address for correspondence: Rudolf Toman, Laboratory for Diagnosis and Prevention of Rickettsial and Chlamydial Infections, Institute of Virology, Slovak Academy of Sciences, Dubravska cesta 9, 845 05 Bratislava, Slovakia. Voice: 421-2-59302418; fax: 421-2-54774284.
virutoma@savba.sk

Ann. N.Y. Acad. Sci. 1063: 149–153 (2005). © 2005 New York Academy of Sciences.
doi: 10.1196/annals.1355.023

studies of LPS I and investigations related to the influence of Vir and Strep on the serological activity of the O-polysaccharide chain of LPS I.

MATERIALS AND METHODS

Cultivation and purification of the *C. burnetii* phase I and II cells from the *C. burnetii* strain Nine Mile (NM I and NM II, respectively) were accomplished as described.[3,5] Crude LPS I and II were isolated and purified as reported.[3,5] Lipid A was removed from LPS I by centrifugation after hydrolysis with 1% acetic acid at 100°C for 1 h and keeping the solution in a freezer overnight. Compositional analyses of LPS I, PS, and fractions A and B were performed as given[3] elsewhere. Immune rabbit sera were prepared by inoculation[6] of animals with the corpuscular antigens NM I and NM II. With NM I, the corresponding phase I and II serum is obtained. With NM II, only the phase II serum is obtained. The phase I serum was obtained by saturation of the phase I and II serum with NM II. SDS-PAGE and ELISA were carried out as published[3,7] earlier.

RESULTS AND DISCUSSION

LPS I was isolated from the purified *C. burnetii* phase I cells by a conventional hot phenol-water method. It was found in the aqueous layer and contained 8–10% of protein and the presence of appreciable amount of nucleic acids could also be detected. When the *C. burnetii* cells were treated with RNAse, DNAse, trypsin, and proteinase K prior to the hot phenol-water extraction the amount of these substances could be reduced to less than 3%. The final purification of LPS I was then accomplished again by a consecutive treatments with RNAse, DNAse, and proteinase K. On SDS-PAGE, LPS I gave two strong bands in the region of about 14–16 kDa and a group of unevenly distributed bands in the region of about 17–23 kDa. The slower-migrating LPS species extending above the 24 kDa region were stained poorly or not at all with the silver staining procedure. Thus, the banding pattern of LPS I revealed an unusual microheterogeneity of the O-polysaccharide chains that is quite rarely encountered with the enterobacterial LPSs.

Compositional sugar analysis of LPS I was accomplished by combination of both colorimetric assays and techniques used in gas chromatography or gas chromatography–mass spectrometry. Analyses showed the presence of 28.4 mol% D-mannose (Man), 18.1 mol% D-*glycero*-D-*manno*-heptose (Hep), 25.5 mol% Vir, 5.0 mol% Strep, 1.6% D-glucose (Glc), 6.2 mol% 3-deoxy-D-*manno*-oct-2-ulosonic acid (Kdo), and 15.2 mol% D-glucosamine (GlcN). After mild acid hydrolysis of LPS I and lipid A removal the remaining PS was fractionated on a column of Sephadex G-50. Nine fractions differing one from another in the composition of constituent sugars were obtained, thus confirming considerable microheterogeneity of the O-polysaccharide chains. At present, two fractions A and B (TABLE 1) are of interest in our ongoing structure-function relationship studies. Particularly, a role of an unusually high content of Vir in fraction A will be investigated in the immunobiology of Q fever.

TABLE 1. Sugar composition of fractions A and B obtained from polysaccharide after separation on Sephadex G-50

	Composition (mol%)						
Fraction	Vir	Man	Gal	Glc	Hep	Strep	GlcN
Polysaccharide	32.3	32.6	tr	1.8	14.4	6.7	12.2
A	48.9	17.2	tr	3.6	8.5	8.6	13.2
B	17.8	41.8	tr	2.0	21.9	3.5	13.0

Abbreviations: Vir, virenose (6-deoxy-3-C-methyl-D-gulose); Man, D-mannose; Gal, D-galactose; Glc, D-glucose; Hep, D-*glycero*-D-*manno*-heptose; Strep, dihydrohydroxystreptose [3-C-(hydroxymethyl)-L-lyxose]; GlcN, D-glucosamine; tr, trace.

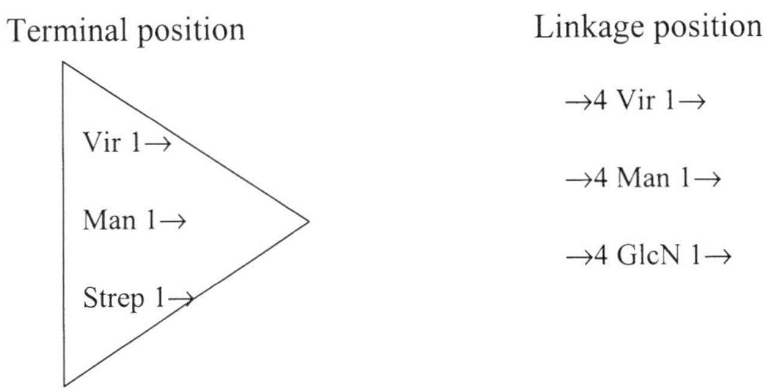

FIGURE 1. Two terminal Man, 2,3- and 3,4-disubstituted Hep are from the core region of LPS I and thus, other terminal and substituted sugars should be located in the O-polysaccharide chain with linkages.

Methylation-linkage analysis provides valuable information on the linkage positions in the investigated LPSs or polysaccharides. However, with *C. burnetii* PS and fractions A and B, the widely applied methylation procedures according to Hakomori[8] and Ciucanu and Kerek[9] led to a complete degradation of Vir and Strep in the O-polysaccharide chain. We found that a gradual addition of sodium hydride to a solution of PS or fractions A and B in dimethyl sulfoxide during the alkoxidation step resulted in the survival of both sugars that were then methylated with methyl iodide. Thus, the methylation analyses of PS and fractions A and B revealed the presence of terminal Vir, Strep, and Man, 4-substituted Vir, 4-substituted Man, and 2,3- and 3,4-disubstituted Hep. From amino sugars, 4-substituted GlcN was detected. The methylation data demonstrated the pyranose form of Vir, Man, Hep, and GlcN, and the furanose form of Strep. From our previous studies[5] it can be anticipated that two terminal Man, 2,3- and 3,4-disubstituted Hep are from the core region of LPS I and thus, other terminal and substituted sugars should be located in the O-polysaccharide chain with linkages (FIG. 1). In previous works[3,4] it has been suggested that Vir and Strep are located in terminal positions. In this work, we show that this is probably true only for Strep as Vir is also (1–4)-linked. Similarly, Man is present in terminal position but about 23% of it is also involved in 1–4 linkages.

TABLE 2. Assay of antibodies in two anti–*Coxiella burnetii* hyperimmune rabbit sera by ELISA with polysaccharide antigens derived from the bacterium

	Serum/Antibody Titers ($\times 10^{-2}$)		
Antigen	Anti-NM I Phase I	Anti-NM II Phase II	Normal
LPS I	256	4	<1
LPS II	4	16	<1
PS	128	2	<1
HPS	4	<1	<1

Abbreviations: LPS I, lipopolysaccharide from *C. burnetii* strain Nine Mile phase I cells; LPS II, lipopolysaccharide from *C. burnetii* strain Nine Mile phase II cells; PS, polysaccharide from LPS I; HPS, a product of mild hydrolysis of PS; NM I, phase I cells of *C. burnetii* strain Nine Mile; NM II, phase II cells of *C. burnetii* strain Nine Mile.

A portion of PS was hydrolyzed under mild conditions to obtain HPS in which the Vir and Strep residues were selectively removed from the O-specific chain. Other sugars were not cleaved under these conditions of hydrolysis. Serological activity of LPS I, PS, and HPS was examined with two different rabbit sera in ELISA (TABLE 2). LPS II[5] was used for comparison. The phase I serum against NM I bound strongly to the corresponding LPS I followed by PS. The weakest binding was observed with HPS and LPS II. The phase II serum against NM II gave a noticeable reaction only with LPS II. A remarkable decrease in the serological activity of HPS as compared to PS may indicate that most phase I antibodies are directed against the epitopes containing Vir and Strep. At present, however, it is not known with certainty whether the immunoreaction proceeds only with both sugars in terminal positions or also with those Vir residues located in the O-polysaccharide backbone.

In order to elucidate more deeply this and other problems related to the role of LPS I in immunobiology of Q fever, a more detailed knowledge of its structural features is necessary. Thus, a further logical step should include detailed linkage and sequential analyses of the constituent sugars in the O-specific chain of LPS I. Besides conventional structural methods, application of novel mass spectrometry and nuclear magnetic resonance techniques will be crucial, especially in analyzing and sequencing larger oligo- and polysaccharide fragments. For this reason, elaboration/application of effective stepwise or functionally specific degradation methods yielding the desired oligosaccharides will be of great importance.

ACKNOWLEDGMENTS

We thank Ludmila Hasikova and Margita Benkovicova for technical help. This work was supported in part by grant No. 2/3021/25 of the Scientific Grant Agency of Ministry of Education of the Slovak Republic and the Slovak Academy of Sciences.

[*Conflict of interest statement:* The authors of this research declare that they have no conflicts of interest.]

REFERENCES

1. DELLACASAGRANDE, J., E. GHIGO, S. MACHERGUI-EL HAMMAMI, *et al.* 2000. $\alpha_V\beta_3$ Integrin and bacterial lipopolysaccharides are involved in *Coxiella burnetii*–stimulated production of tumor necrosis factor by human monocytes. Infect. Immun. **68:** 5673–5678.
2. HONSTETTRE, A., E. GHIGO, A. MOYNNAULT, *et al.* 2004. Lipopolysaccharide from *Coxiella burnetii* is involved in bacterial phagocytosis, filamentous actin reorganization, and inflammatory responses through toll-like receptor 4. J. Immunol. **172:** 3695–3703.
3. SKULTETY L., R. TOMAN & V. PATOPRSTY. 1998. A comparative study of lipopolysaccharides from two *Coxiella burnetii* strains considered to be associated with acute and chronic Q fever. Carbohyd. Polymers. **35:** 189–194.
4. TOMAN, R., L. SKULTETY, P. FTACEK, *et al.* 1998. NMR study of virenose and dihydrohydroxystreptose isolated from *Coxiella burnetii* phase I lipopolysaccharide. Carbohyd. Res. **306:** 291–296.
5. TOMAN, R. & L. SKULTETY. 1996. Structural study on a lipopolysaccharide from *Coxiella burnetii* strain Nine Mile in avirulent phase II. Carbohyd. Res. **283:** 175–185.
6. GAJDOSOVA, E., E. KOVACOVA, R. TOMAN, *et al.* 1994. Immunogenicity of *Coxiella burnetii* whole cells and their outer membrane components. Acta Virol. **38:** 339–344.
7. SLABA, K., L. SKULTETY & R. TOMAN. 2005. Efficiency of various serological techniques for diagnosing *Coxiella burnetii* infection. Acta Virol. **49:** 123–127.
8. HAKOMORI, S.I. 1964. A rapid permethylation of glycolipid, and polysaccharide catalyzed by methylsulfinyl carbanion in dimethyl sulfoxide. J. Biochem. **55:** 205–208.
9. CIUCANU, I. & F. KEREK. 1984. A simple and rapid method for the permethylation of carbohydrates. Carbohyd. Res. **131:** 209–217.

Lack of Dendritic Cell Maturation Following Infection by *Coxiella burnetii* Synthesizing Different Lipopolysaccharide Chemotypes

JEFFREY G. SHANNON, DALE HOWE, AND ROBERT A. HEINZEN

Coxiella Pathogenesis Section, Laboratory of Intracellular Parasites, Rocky Mountain Laboratories, National Institute of Allergy and Infectious Diseases, National Institutes of Health, Hamilton, Montana 59840, USA

ABSTRACT: *Coxiella burnetii* is an obligate intracellular bacterium and the etiologic agent of the zoonotic disease Q fever. Symptomatic infection is normally characterized by flu-like symptoms; however, in some cases, a persistent infection can ensue that may reactivate months or years after initial exposure to cause chronic disease. The mechanisms by which this obligate parasite evades clearance by the host immune response during persistent infection are unknown. We have previously demonstrated that lipopolysaccharide (LPS) length is critical in determining the response of human dendritic cells (DC) to *C. burnetii*. Here, we investigated whether LPS chemotype affects DC maturation or activation. Immature human DC were infected with three virulent strains of *C. burnetii* (Nine Mile phase I, S, or Priscilla) that produce chemically distinct LPS molecules. None of these strains stimulated significant upregulation of cell surface markers of DC maturation. Moreover, these strains were equally deficient in inducing DC IL-12p70 production or p38 mitogen-activated protein kinase phosphorylation. Infection of DC by virulent *C. burnetii* without stimulating significant maturation or inflammatory cytokine production may be a mechanism of immune evasion that results in persistent infection of an otherwise immunocompetent host. Our data indicate that LPS chemotype is not a determinant of DC maturation or cytokine production in response to *C. burnetii.*

KEYWORDS: *Coxiella*; dendritic cell; immune evasion; lipopolysaccharide

INTRODUCTION

Coxiella burnetii is an obligate intracellular, gram-negative bacterial pathogen that can infect a wide range of vertebrate hosts and causes a flu-like disease in humans termed Q fever. *C. burnetii* can also establish a persistent infection that may later reactivate and result in chronic endocarditis or hepatitis.[1] Factors that determine if *C. burnetii* infection results in acute or chronic disease include the immunological status of the host and possibly strain-specific virulence factors.[2,3]

Address for correspondence: Robert A. Heinzen, Rocky Mountain Laboratories, NIAID, NIH, 903 South 4th Street, Hamilton, MT 59840. Voice: 406-375-9695; fax 406-363-9380. rheinzen@niaid.nih.gov

Ann. N.Y. Acad. Sci. 1063: 154–160 (2005). © 2005 New York Academy of Sciences. doi: 10.1196/annals.1355.024

Dendritic cells reside in the peripheral epithelial tissues in an immature state (iDC) where they serve as sentinels against invading microorganisms. Contact with a pathogen typically results in the conversion of iDC to mature DC (mDC). High levels of MHC class II and T cell costimulatory molecules are expressed on mDC, giving them the unique ability to stimulate the proliferation of naïve T cells. Furthermore, depending on the nature of the invading microbe, DC can skew the immune system towards T_h1, T_h2 or regulatory T cell response.[4,5]

We previously compared the virulent *C. burnetii* Nine Mile phase I (NMI) strain, producing full-length LPS, to the isogenic avirulent Nine Mile phase II (NMII) strain, producing severely truncated LPS, and found that full-length LPS of NMI was required to prevent DC maturation and inflammatory cytokine production.[6] Virulent *C. burnetii* strains are known to produce chemically distinct LPS molecules, and LPS chemotype has been speculated to play a role in disease outcome (i.e., acute or chronic disease).[2,7] In this study, we examined whether the chemical composition of full-length LPS of *C. burnetii* influences DC responses to the pathogen.

MATERIALS AND METHODS

Bacterial Strains

The Nine Mile phase I (NMI; RSA493), Nine Mile phase II (NMII; RSA439), S (Q217), and Priscilla (Q177) strains of *C. burnetii* were propagated in African green monkey kidney (Vero) fibroblasts. Organisms were purified from infected cells by Renografin density gradient centrifugation.[8] Purified bacteria were suspended in K-36 buffer (0.1 M KCl, 0.015 M NaCl, 0.05 M K_2HPO_4, 0.05 M KH_2PO_4, pH 7.0). LPS from *E. coli* serotype O111:B4 was purchased from Sigma (St. Louis, MO) and used at 500 ng/mL.

Monocyte-Derived Dendritic Cells

Human monocyte-derived dendritic cells were prepared as previously described.[6] For *Coxiella* infection experiments, cells were replated in 6 well plates at a concentration of 2×10^6 cells per mL in DC medium. Purified bacteria were added directly to the culture medium at an MOI of 20. The inoculum was not removed.

Flow Cytometry

DCs were harvested by incubation for 5 min in cold 0.1M EDTA in PBS, followed by gentle scraping and centrifugation ($500 \times g$, 5 min, 4°C). The following monoclonal antibodies were used to characterize DC phenotypes: antiCD83-APC, antiCD86-PE, antiCD209-PerCP-Cy5.5, antiCD80-FITC, antiCD40-APC, anti-CD11c-PE, and antiHLA-DR-PECy7 (BD PharMingen, San Diego, CA). AnnexinV-FITC (Caltag, Burlingame, CA) was used to determine cell viability. Approximately 5×10^5 DCs were stained with antibodies in FACS wash (PBS, 2% fetal bovine serum, 2.5 mM $CaCl_2$) for 15 min on ice, then washed twice with FACS wash and fixed with 4% paraformaldehyde. Samples were run on a FACS-Calibur flow cytometer (Becton Dickinson, San Jose, CA) and analyzed using FlowJo software (TreeStar, San Carlos, CA).

Immunoblot

Approximately 2×10^6 DC for each experimental condition were harvested by centrifugation ($500 \times g$, 5 min) and resuspended in 100 µL of cell lysis buffer (1× PBS, 1% Triton X-100, and a Complete Protease Inhibitor tablet [Roche Molecular Biochemicals, Indianapolis, IN]). Lysates were centrifuged ($10{,}000 \times g$, 10 min) and supernatants were added to 5× SDS PAGE sample buffer. Samples were electrophoresed on an 12% SDS polyacrylamide gel. Proteins were transferred to a PVDF membrane that was incubated with rabbit polyclonal anti-phosphoP38 antibody (Cell Signalling Technology, Beverly, MA) and anti-rabbit IgG-HRP antibody. HRP was detected using Supersignal West Pico Chemiluminescent Substrate (Pierce, Rockford, IL). The membrane was then incubated for 15 min at 37°C in Restore Western Blot Stripping Buffer (Pierce, Rockford, IL) and reprobed with rabbit polyclonal anti-totalp38 antibody (Cell Signaling Technology, Beverly, MA), followed by anti-rabbit IgG-HRP antibody to verify equal loading of samples.

Cytokine Measurement

The IL-12p70 concentration in culture supernatants was determined using an OptEIA ELISA kit (BD Pharmingen, San Diego, CA). The sensitivity of this assay is 4 pg/mL.

RESULTS

C. burnetii strains can be grouped according to a variety of factors including virulence (phase I or phase II), association with acute or chronic disease, LPS chemotype, and restriction fragment length polymorphisms.[1] For this study, we chose three strains of virulent *C. burnetii* that produce LPS molecules representative of the three chemotypes (or "chemogroups") defined by Hackstadt.[7] Nine Mile phase I (NMI) is a tick isolate and is representative of acute disease isolates producing LPS in chemogroup 1. The Priscilla strain is a goat abortion isolate and the S strain is a human liver biopsy isolate. They are representative of chronic disease isolates producing LPS in chemogroups 2 and 3, respectively.

To measure DC maturation after infection, immature human monocyte-derived DC were infected for 48 h, then analyzed by flow cytometry for surface expression of the maturation markers CD80, CD83, CD86, CD40, and HLA-DR. Treatment with *E. coli* LPS served as a positive control for DC maturation. DC did not mature after infection with the NMI, S, or Priscilla strains (FIG. 1). Additionally, none of these strains affected DC viability as determined by annexinV staining (data not shown). These data indicate that differences in LPS chemotype do not determine the effect of *C. burnetii* on DC maturation.

To determine if the three *C. burnetii* strains could productively infect human DC, cells were incubated with each strain for 48 h, then observed by immunofluorescence microscopy. All three strains infected and replicated within DC as evidenced by their ability to form large, spacious parasitophorous vacuoles (data not shown).

IL-12p70 production by DC in response to intracellular pathogens is essential in driving a Th1 immune response important in clearance of these organisms. We there-

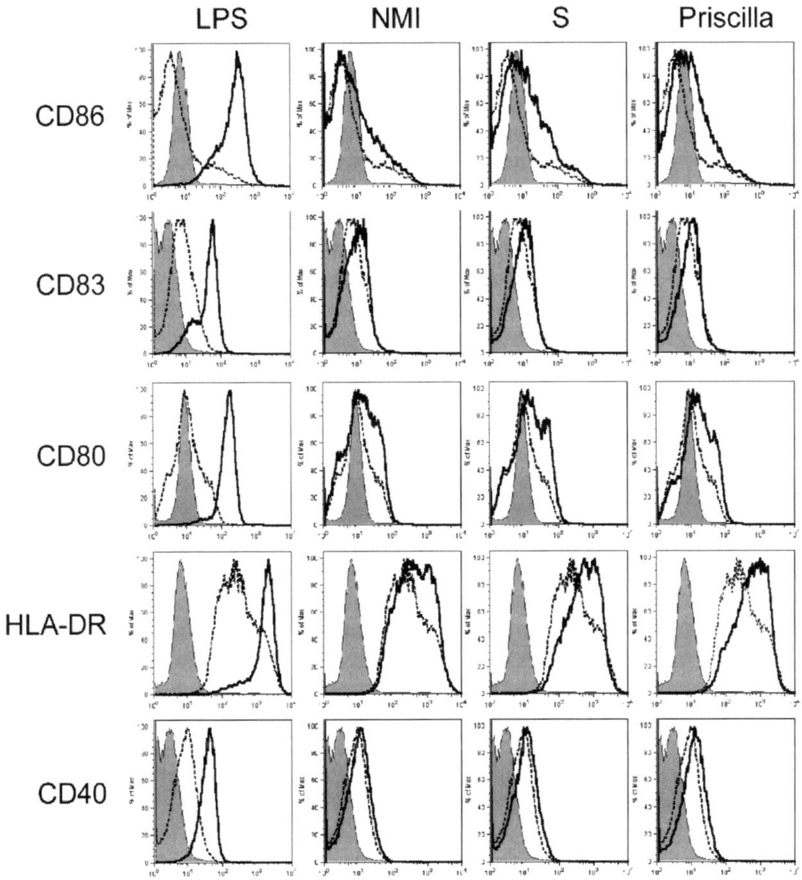

FIGURE 1. FACS analysis of DC maturation in response to 3 strains of virulent *C. burnetii*. Human monocyte-derived DC were either mock infected, LPS treated, or infected with *C. burnetii* Nine Mile phase I (NMI), S, or Priscilla for 48 h. Infected cells were then fixed and stained for the maturation markers CD86(B7.2), CD83, CD80(B7.1), HLA-DR(MHC classII), and CD40. Cell staining was measured by flow cytometry. Treatment with *E. coli* LPS served as a positive control for DC maturation. The dashed histogram depicts staining of mock infected cells. The solid histogram depicts staining of treated/infected cells. The shaded histogram depicts isotype control staining. The results shown are from 1 experiment and are representative of 5 independent experiments.

fore determined if any of the *C. burnetii* strains could induce IL-12 production by DC *in vitro*. Infection by all three virulent strains induced similar low levels of IL-12. In contrast, high levels of IL-12 were produced in response to the avirulent NMII strain (FIG. 2).

Many bacterial pathogens induce DC maturation via toll-like receptor ligation. Bacterial LPS generally signals through TLR4, or in some cases TLR2. Peptidoglycan and bacterial lipoproteins are ligands for TLR2 and unmethylated CpG DNA

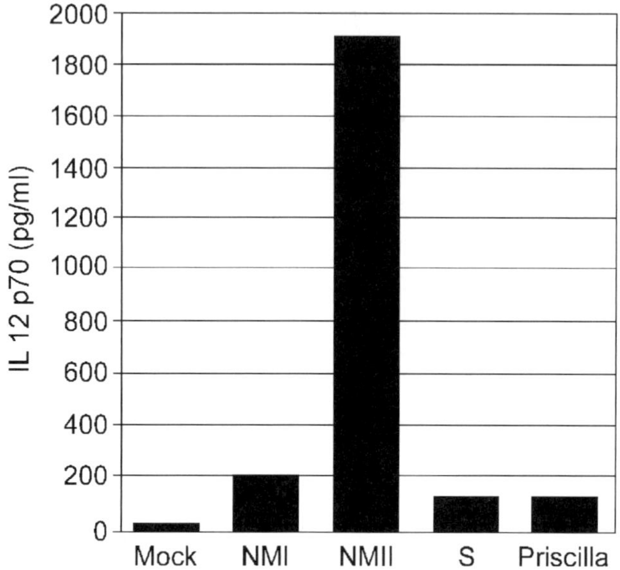

FIGURE 2. Lack of DC IL-12 production in response to 3 strains of virulent *C. burnetii*. Human DC were either mock infected or infected for 48 h with *C. burnetii* Nine Mile phase I (NMI), Nine Mile phase II (NMII), S, or Priscilla. Cell culture supernatants were collected and their IL-12p70 concentrations were determined by ELISA. The results shown are from one experiment and are representative of 3 independent experiments.

motifs stimulate through TLR9. Ligation of these receptors results in a cascade of signaling events including, in part, the phosphorylation of cellular p38 MAP kinase (MAPK). Therefore, to further examine TLR signaling during *C. burnetii* infection, we examined extracts of infected DC by Western blot to determine the amount of phosphorylated p38 MAPK present. Infection by the three virulent strains did not affect the level of p38 phosphorylation (FIG. 3). In contrast, infection by the avirulent NMII strain dramatically increased the amount of phosphorylated p38 MAPK.

DISCUSSION

The ability of dendritic cells to respond to invading pathogens is generally important in generating an effective immune response. We show here that three strains of virulent *C. burnetii*, each producing a chemically distinct LPS, can infect DC while stimulating virtually no maturation or activation of these cells, indicating that LPS chemotype does not affect these phenomena.

Mature DC express high levels of T cell costimulatory molecules necessary for induction of T cell proliferation. They also upregulate expression of lysosomal proteases required for antigen presentation. In contrast, immature DC are essentially unable to stimulate T cell proliferation or present antigen via MHC class II. We pro-

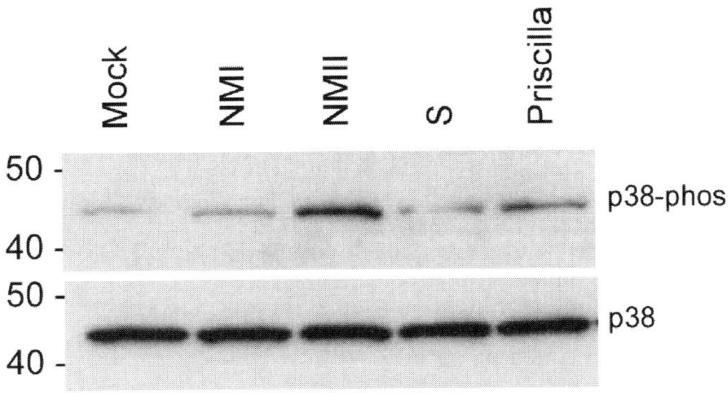

FIGURE 3. LPS chemotype is not a determinant of DC p38 MAPK phosphorylation in response to infection by *C. burnetii*. Human DC were either mock infected or infected with *C. burnetii* Nine Mile phase I (NMI), Nine Mile phase II (NMII), S, or Priscilla for 48 h. Cell extracts were run on an SDS-PAGE gel, blotted, and probed with anti-phospho-p38 MAPK antibody (*upper panel*). The blot was then then stripped and reprobed with anti-total-p38 MAPK antibody as a loading control (*lower panel*). The results shown are representative of 3 independent experiments.

pose that the lack of DC maturation after infection by virulent *C. burnetii* results in an immune response that lacks the potency required for complete clearance of the organism, thereby allowing for persistence. Indeed, the small amount of IL-12 elicited by infection by virulent *C. burnetii* is unlikely to drive the strong Th1 response that is typically required for clearance of intracellular pathogens.

The three *C. burnetii* strains examined in this study synthesize distinct LPS chemotypes as determined by serology and/or gel mobility.[7] Strains within LPS chemogroup 1, such as NMI, are from acute disease patients, arthropods, or milk. Strains within chemogroups 2 and 3, such as Priscilla and S, are almost exclusively from chronic Q fever patients. We observed no difference in the DC stimulatory capacity of these strains, suggesting LPS chemotype-specific DC responses are not involved in Q fever disease manifestations.

ACKNOWLEDGMENTS

We thank Ron Messer for assistance with flow cytometry and Anita Mora for graphics. This research was supported by the Intramural Research Program of the National Institutes of Health, National Institute of Allergy and Infectious Diseases.

REFERENCES

1. Maurin, M. & D. Raoult. 1999. Q fever. Clin. Microbiol. Rev. **12:** 518–553.
2. Moos, A. & T. Hackstadt. 1987. Comparative virulence of intra- and interstrain lipopolysaccharide variants of *Coxiella burnetii* in the guinea pig model. Infect. Immun. **55:** 1144–1150.

3. RAOULT, D., T. MARRIE & J. MEGE. 2005. Natural history and pathophysiology of Q fever. Lancet Infect. Dis. **5:** 219–226.
4. MOSER, M. & K.M. MURPHY. 2000. Dendritic cell regulation of TH1-TH2 development. Nat. Immunol. **1:** 199–205.
5. JONULEIT, H., *et al.* 2000. Induction of interleukin 10–producing, nonproliferating CD4(+) T cells with regulatory properties by repetitive stimulation with allogeneic immature human dendritic cells. J. Exp. Med. **192:** 1213–1222.
6. SHANNON, J.G., D. HOWE & R.A. HEINZEN. 2005. Virulent *Coxiella burnetii* does not activate human dendritic cells: role of lipopolysaccharide as a shielding molecule. Proc. Natl. Acad. Sci. USA **102:** 8722–8727.
7. HACKSTADT, T. 1986. Antigenic variation in the phase I lipopolysaccharide of *Coxiella burnetii* isolates. Infect. Immun. **52:** 337–340.
8. HACKSTADT, T., *et al.* 1992. Evidence for proteolytic cleavage of the 120-kilodalton outer membrane protein of rickettsiae: identification of an avirulent mutant deficient in processing. Infect. Immun. **60:** 159–165.

TLR2 Is Necessary to Inflammatory Response in *Coxiella burnetii* Infection

SORAYA MEGHARI,[a] AMÉLIE HONSTETTRE,[a] HUBERT LEPIDI,[a] BERNARDT RYFFEL,[b] DIDIER RAOULT,[a] AND JEAN-LOUIS MEGE[a]

[a]*Unité des Rickettsies, CNRS UMR 6020, Université de la Méditerranée, 13005 Marseille, France*

[b]*CNRS, 3B rue de la Ferollerie, 45071 Orléans, France*

ABSTRACT: The resolution of Q fever, a zoonosis caused by *Coxiella burnetii*, depends on efficient innate and adaptive immune responses. Such responses are influenced by Toll-like receptors (TLRs). TLR4 is involved only in part in immune responses against *C. burnetii*, suggesting a role for TLR2. We investigated *C. burnetii* infection in wild-type and TLR2$^{-/-}$ mice. *C. burnetii* organisms were similarly eliminated by wild-type and TLR2$^{-/-}$ mice. In contrast, the formation of granulomas, a marker for efficient cell-mediated immunity, was markedly impaired. These results show that TLR2 is required for inflammatory and immune response to *C. burnetii*, but is dispensable for bacterial clearance.

KEYWORDS: ***Coxiella burnetii*; TLR2; granuloma**

INTRODUCTION

Q fever is a zoonosis caused by *Coxiella burnetii*, an obligate intracellular microorganism that replicates in myeloid cells. In the primary infection, a minority of patients present acute symptoms such as isolated fever, hepatitis, or pneumonia. Q fever may become chronic in patients with valve lesions, arterial aneurysm, or arterial prosthesis. The most frequent clinical manifestation of chronic Q fever is endocarditis.[1] The control of Q fever depends on host immune response as manifested by granuloma formation and systemic immune response. However, immune response does not lead to *C. burnetii* eradication, and relapses may occur when cell-mediated immunity is depressed.[2] In chronic Q fever, defective immune response is associated with lack of granulomas, impaired antigen-mediated lymphoproliferation and microbial killing, and cytokine dysfunction.[1–3]

The development of protective immune response against *C. burnetii* requires coordination of innate and adaptive immune responses. Toll-like receptors (TLRs) are a family of receptors that recognizes microbial molecules.[4] In particular, TLR4 and TLR2 recognize Gram-negative, and Gram-positive bacteria and mycobacteria,

Address for correspondence: Jean-Louis Mege, Unité des Rickerrsies, Faculté fr Médecine, 26 Bld Jean Moulin, 13385 Marseille Cedex 5, France. Voice: 33 4 91 32 43 75; fax: 33 4 91 38 77 72. Jean-Louis. Mege@medecine.univ-mrs.fr

Ann. N.Y. Acad. Sci. 1063: 161–166 (2005). © 2005 New York Academy of Sciences. doi: 10.1196/annals.1355.025

respectively.[5] We have recently shown that TLR4 is involved in the recognition of *C. burnetii* lipopolysaccharide, initial activation of macrophages, and inflammatory response associated with *C. burnetii* infection since granuloma formation is decreased in TLR4$^{-/-}$ mice. However, the clearance of *C. burnetii* is not impaired in these mice.[6] It is likely that TLR2 is also involved in the recognition of *C. burnetii* and the control of its replication. Indeed, macrophages from TLR2$^{-/-}$ mice were defective in cytokine production upon *C. burnetii* infection but permissive for *C. burnetii* growth.[7]

In this report, we investigated the role of TLR2 in a murine model of *C. burnetii* infection. Bacterial clearance was not affected in TLR2$^{-/-}$ mice compared to wild-type (wt) mice. In contrast, the absence of TLR2 prevented the formation of granulomas. These results demonstrated that TLR2, as well as TLR4,[6] is not essential for bacterial clearance but is essential for granuloma formation.

MATERIALS AND METHODS

C. burnetii *Preparation*

C. burnetii organisms (Nine Mile strain in phase I) were cultured as previously described.[6] BALB/c mice were infected with 10^8 organisms for 10 days. Spleen homogenates were added to L929 cells for two passages. Infected cells were sonicated, and bacteria were purified on Renografin gradient and stored at –80°C. Bacterial viability was assessed using the LIVE/DEAD *Bac*Light bacterial viability kit (Molecular Probes, Eugene, OR). Only *C. burnetii* preparations containing more than 90% of viable organisms were used.

Bacterial Infection of Mice

The generation of TLR2$^{-/-}$ mice (C57BL/6 background) was described elsewhere.[8] Female C57BL/6 (wt) and TLR2$^{-/-}$ mice were infected by intraperitoneal route with 5×10^5 *C. burnetii* organisms. The clinical status of mice was recorded daily. They were serially killed before infection and after different infection times. Spleen and liver were aseptically excised. Tissue samples were fixed or not with 10% formalin, and then embedded in paraffin.

Histologic Analysis and Immunohistologic Detection of C. burnetii

The 5-μm sections of paraffin-embedded tissues were stained with hematoxylin-eosin-saffron. Granulomas were detected by optical examination, and quantified as previously described.[6] The results are expressed as the number of granuloma found per surface unit (mm^2). Immunohistologic detection of *C. burnetii* was performed as follows.[6] Tissue sections were deparaffinized in xylene and rehydrated in graded alcohol. Each tissue section was incubated with rabbit antibodies to *C. burnetii* (diluted at 1:200) for 60 min, then with biotin-conjugated antibodies directed against rabbit immunoglobulins followed by peroxidase-labeled streptavidin with amino-ethylcarbazole as substrate. Slides were counterstained with Mayer hematoxylin for 10 min. Negative controls were performed using normal rabbit serum. The bacteria were numbered by optical examination, and the tissue area was determined by image analysis. The results are expressed as the number of bacteria found per mm^2 of tissue.

RESULTS

Role of TLR2 in C. burnetii *Infection* in Vivo

Mortality or morbidity was not observed in wt and TLR2$^{-/-}$ mice up to 21 days, suggesting that mice remained resistant to *C. burnetii* despite the lack of TLR2. Tissue infection was assessed by immunodetection of *C. burnetii*. In wt and TLR2$^{-/-}$ mice, *C. burnetii* organisms were detected in liver and spleen, whereas lungs, heart, and mesenteric lymph nodes remained devoid of organisms. The organisms were found in intracellular location as coarse or fine grains, and immunopositive cells corresponded to macrophages inside granulomas. The time course of spleen and liver infection was similar in wt mice and TLR2$^{-/-}$ mice. Organisms were detectable at day 4 (data not shown); bacterial load reached a peak at day 7 and decreased thereafter (FIG. 1, A and C). The number of bacteria was moderately increased at day 7

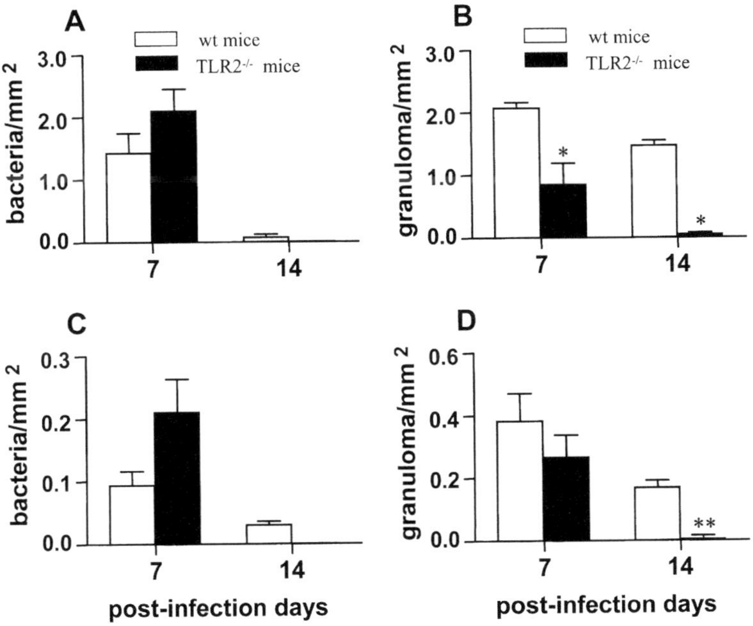

FIGURE 1. *C. burnetii* load and tissue granulomas. (**A–D**). Wild-type and TLR2$^{-/-}$ mice were infected and killed at days 7 and 14. Bacteria present in the spleen (**A**) and the liver (**C**) were quantified by image analysis. The results, expressed as the number of bacteria per square millimeter, are the mean ± SD of 5 mice/time point. The number of granulomas in the spleen (**B**) and the liver (**D**) was determined microscopically. The results, expressed as the number of granulomas per square millimeter of tissue, are the mean ± SD of 5 mice/time point. Results were compared with Student's *t* test: *P<0.002; **P<0.001.

in $TLR2^{-/-}$ mice compared to wt mice. Hence, TLR2 is dispensable for *C. burnetii* clearance *in vivo*.

Role of TLR2 in Granuloma Formation

As bacteria were detected within liver and splenic granulomas, we investigated granuloma expression in both tissues. In wt and $TLR2^{-/-}$ mice, lesions appeared as aggregates mainly composed of macrophages and lymphocytes and few polymorphonuclear leukocytes without suppuration. The granulomatous reactions were focal, and scattered throughout liver lobules, portobiliary spaces, and splenic red pulp. Granulomas were detected after 4 days of infection (data not shown); their number became maximum at day 7 and decreased thereafter (FIG. 1, B and D). In $TLR2^{-/-}$ mice, the number of splenic granulomas was markedly lower than that of wt mice at days 7 and 14 ($P<0.002$, FIG. 1B). In the liver of $TLR2^{-/-}$ mice, the number of granulomas was similar to that of wt mice at day 7, but was significantly decreased at day 14 ($P<0.001$, FIG. 1D). These results clearly show that TLR2 is critical for the formation of granulomas in *C. burnetii*–infected mice.

DISCUSSION

In this report, we provide evidence that TLR2 is involved in host response to *C. burnetii* but appears as dispensable for the clearance of *C. burnetii in vivo*. This finding is consistent with our previous report that shows the lack of TLR2 effect on *C. burnetii* replication in macrophages.[6] It has been recently demonstrated that TLR2-deficient macrophages are highly susceptible to *C. burnetii* infection.[7] The clonal versus non-clonal character of Nine Mile strain of *C. burnetii* may account for these differences.[7] Using highly virulent phase I organisms (this study and Honstettre and colleagues[6]) instead avirulent phase II organisms[7] likely explains the different intracellular fates of *C. burnetii*. Our previous report shows that the clearance of *C. burnetii* is similar in $TLR4^{-/-}$ and wt mice.[6] Since TLR2 is also dispensable for *C. burnetii* clearance, it is likely that TLR2 and TLR4 recognize a common microbial component such as peptidoglycan, but this recognition mechanism is not sufficient to elicit microbicidal program *in vivo*.

TLR2 is essential for granuloma formation since its absence is associated with decreased number of granulomas. In contrast, their organization is not altered since they contain essentially macrophages and T cells. Granulomas represent a form of delayed-type hypersensitivity or Th1 immune response, contributing to protection against intracellular organisms.[9] TLR2 has been reported to provide beneficial signals in staphylococcal sepsis[10] or pneumococcal meningitis.[11] In addition, TLR2 is overexpressed in lesions from tuberculous form of leprosy in which Th1 immune response was prominent compared to lesions from disseminated lepromatous form of the disease in which Th1 immune response is prevented.[12] However, TLR2 may also favor the persistence of pathogens. Indeed, $TLR2^{-/-}$ mice are more resistant to disseminated *Candida* infection, which results from increased candidacidal capacity of macrophages and decreased interleukin-10 production.[13] Similarly, immunosuppression mediated by *Yersinia enterocolitica* results from TLR2-mediated interleukin-10 release.[14] The effect of TLR2 absence on granuloma formation we observed is consistent with that of TLR4 deficiency.[6] Nevertheless, the lack of TLR4 affects the number and the organization of granulomas whereas the lack of TLR2 mainly affects the number of granuloma. As TLR4 and TLR2 use the adaptor MyD88 to signal into the cells, it is likely that MyD88 controls granuloma formation in *C. burnetii* infection. It has been shown that mice deficient for MyD88 have a profound defect in antigen-specific Th1 immune response including antigen-specific lymphoproliferation and interferon-γ production.[4] The mechanism by which TLR2 controls inflammatory response to *C. burnetii* is still speculative. It may include mediator production and leukocyte transendothelial migration since TLR are known to be involved in chemokine production and may affect leukocyte migration.[15]

Both TLR2 and TLR4 are required for granuloma formation in *C. burnetii* infection. Whereas TLR4 is probably involved in initial responses, TLR2 is rather implicated in sustained responses. Nevertheless, decreased granuloma formation does not affect the resistance of mice to *C. burnetii*. It is likely that TLR2 and TLR4 counterbalance the lacking TLR since both TLRs stimulate the same transductional pathways.

[*Competing interests statement:* The authors state that they have no conflicting financial interests.]

REFERENCES

1. RAOULT, D., T. MARRIE & J.L. MEGE. 2005. Natural history and pathophysiology of Q fever. Lancet Infect. Dis. **5:** 219–226.
2. MAURIN, M. & D. RAOULT. 1999. Q fever. Clin. Microbiol. Rev. **12:** 518–553.
3. HONSTETTRE, A., G. IMBERT, E. GHIGO, *et al.* 2003. Dysregulation of cytokines in acute Q fever: role of interleukin-10 and tumor necrosis factor in chronic evolution of Q fever. J. Infect. Dis. **187:** 956–962.
4. SCHNARE, M., G.M. BARTON, A.C. HOLT, *et al.* 2001. Toll-like receptors control activation of adaptive immune responses. Nat. Immunol.**2:** 947–950.
5. TAKEDA, K. & S. AKIRA. 2003. Toll receptors and pathogen resistance. Cell Microbiol. **5:** 143–153.
6. HONSTETTRE, A., E. GHIGO, A. MOYNAULT, *et al.* 2004. Lipopolysaccharide from *Coxiella burnetii* is involved in bacterial phagocytosis, filamentous actin reorganization, and inflammatory responses through Toll-like receptor 4. J. Immunol. **172:** 3695–3703.
7. ZAMBONI, D.S., M.A. CAMPOS, A.C. TORRECILHAS, *et al.* 2004. Stimulation of Toll-like receptor 2 by *Coxiella burnetii* is required for macrophage production of pro-inflammatory cytokines and resistance to infection. J. Biol. Chem. **279:** 54405–54415.
8. TORRES, D., M. BARRIER, F. BIHL, *et al.* 2004. Toll-like receptor 2 is required for optimal control of *Listeria monocytogenes* infection. Infect. Immun. **72:** 2131–2139.
9. SANDOR, M., J.V. WEINSTOCK & T.A WYNN. 2003. Granulomas in schistosome and mycobacterial infections: a model of local immune responses. Trends Immunol. **24:** 44–52.
10. TAKEUCHI, O., K. HOSHINO & S. AKIRA. 2000. TLR2-deficient and MyD88-deficient mice are highly susceptible to *Staphylococcus aureus* infection. J. Immunol. **165:** 5392–5396.
11. KOEDEL, U., B. ANGELE, T. RUPPRECHT, *et al.* 2003. Toll-like receptor 2 participates in mediation of immune response in experimental pneumococcal meningitis. J. Immunol. **170:** 438–444.
12. KRUTZIK, S.R., M.T. OCHOA, P.A. SIELING, *et al.* 2003. Activation and regulation of Toll-like receptors 2 and 1 in human leprosy. Nat. Med. **9:** 525–532.
13. NETEA, M.G., R. SUTMULLER, C. HERMANN, *et al.* 2004. Toll-like receptor 2 suppresses immunity against *Candida albicans* through induction of IL-10 and regulatory T cells. J. Immunol. **172:** 3712–3718.

14. SING, A., D. ROST, N. TVARDOVSKAIA, *et al.* 2002. *Yersinia* V-antigen exploits Toll-like receptor 2 and CD14 for interleukin 10-mediated immunosuppression. J. Exp. Med. **196:** 1017–1024.
15. IWASAKI, A. & R. MEDZHITOV. 2004. Toll-like receptor control of the adaptive immune responses. Nat. Immunol. **5:** 987–995.

Comparative Virulence of Phase I and II *Coxiella burnetii* in Immunodeficient Mice

MASAKO ANDOH, KASI E. RUSSELL-LODRIGUE, GUOQUAN ZHANG, AND JAMES E. SAMUEL

Department of Medical Microbiology and Immunology, Texas A&M University System Health Science Center, College Station, Texas 77843-1114, USA

ABSTRACT: *Coxiella burnetii* has two phase variants: highly virulent phase I and avirulent phase II. To examine the differences between the two phase variants in interaction with host response to infection, we performed experimental infection in immunodeficient mice. Experimental *C. burnetii* phase I infection in SCID mice suggested that innate immunity cannot control replication of the bacteria and that acquired immunity is essential for mice to survive infection. In this study, we used SCID and SCIDbg mice to determine whether phase II bacterial infection can be controlled *in vivo*.

KEYWORDS: *Coxiella burnetii*; phase variation; virulence; animal model

INTRODUCTION

Coxiella burnetii, the etiological agent of Q fever, has two phase variants.[1–3] Phase I is a highly virulent variant, replicates in immunocompetent animals, and causes Q fever in humans and pathology in experimental animals. Phase II is an avirulent variant that does not replicate in immunocompetent animals. Because of the difference in virulence, phase I bacteria require biosafety level 3 containment, while phase II bacteria can be cultured under biosafety level 2 conditions. Phase I (RSA493) organisms encode a complete LPS with O side chain, while phase II (RSA439) do not express O side chain and several sugar residues in the core structure because of a major deletion of genes involved with LPS biosynthesis.[4] To examine the differences between the two phase variants in interaction with host response to infection, we performed experimental infection in acquired-immunodeficient mice. Severe combined immunodeficient (SCID) mice, which lack T and B cell functions, are highly susceptible to phase I *C. burnetii*.[5] Experimental *C. burnetii* phase I infection in SCID mice suggested that innate immunity cannot control replication of the bacteria and that acquired immunity is essential for mice to survive infection. In this study, we used SCID and SCIDbg mice, which lack T, B and NK cell functions, to determine whether phase II bacterial infection can be controlled *in vivo*.

Address for correspondence: James E. Samuel, Department of Medical Microbiology and Immunology, Texas A&M University System Health Science Center, 407 Reynolds Building, College Station, Texas 77843-1114, USA. Voice: 979-862-1684; fax: 979-845-3479.
jsamuel@tamhsc.edu

Ann. N.Y. Acad. Sci. 1063: 167–170 (2005).
doi: 10.1196/annals.1355.026

MATERIALS AND METHODS

Bacteria

Two cloned *C. burnetii* strains were used to avoid mixed phase population. *C. burnetii* RSA 493, Nine Mile phase I (NM I) and *C. burnetii* RSA 439, Nine Mile phase II (NM II) were purified and stored at −80°C until use. Numbers of the bacteria were estimated by optical density.[6]

Animals

Five- to six-week-old female SCID, SCIDbg and CB17 (genetic background strain of SCID and SCIDbg mice used in this study) mice were used.

Experimental Infection in Mice

Four mice per group were infected intraperitoneally with 10^4 organisms of NM I or NM II. PBS was as sham infection control.

Evaluation of Infection

Clinical signs and body weight were observed daily. Mice were sacrificed and tissue samples were collected at 28 days post infection (DPI). Spleen weights were measured at necropsy. Histopathology and immunocytochemistry of heart, lung, liver and spleen were done by hematoxylin-eosin staining and anti-*C. burnetii* immunostaining as described previously.[5] Growth of *C. burnetii* was confirmed by detecting the *com1* gene in spleen using a previously described real time PCR method.[7]

RESULTS

Mild Splenomegaly but No Clinical Symptoms in Immunodeficient Mice Infected with NM II

NM II did not cause apparent clinical illness in any mice. No mice lost weight with NM II infection. However, mild splenomegaly was found in SCID and SCIDbg mice but not in CB17 mice at 28 DPI. Spleen weights of mice infected with NM II were: 0.203 ± 0.004 g in SCID mice, 0.164 ± 0.016 g in SCIDbg mice and 0.087 ± 0.012 g in CB17 mice. Spleens of SCID and SCIDbg mice infected with NM II were significantly larger ($P < 0.05$) than CB17 mice. Numbers of bacteria in the spleen of SCID and SCIDbg mice were 1 log greater than the inoculum and were undetectable in CB17 mice. The numbers of NM II bacteria in SCID and SCIDbg were not significantly different. Spleen weights of unchallenged mice were: 0.051 ± 0.005 g in SCID mice, 0.045 ± 0.004 g in SCIDbg mice and 0.083 ± 0.001 g in CB17 mice. Bacterial gene *com1* was undetectable in the spleens of uninfected control mice.

Severe Clinical Symptoms and Splenomegaly in Immunodeficient Mice Infected with NM I

NM I caused severe persistent illness in SCID and SCIDbg mice and mild temporal illness in CB17 mice. In SCID and SCIDbg mice, NM I caused ruffled fur (starting from 9 and 10 DPI, respectively), hunched back (starting from 13 and 14 DPI, respectively) and cachexia (starting from 18 and 21 DPI, respectively). Both mouse strains had severe weight loss. SCID mice survived, but SCIDbg mice were dead in 27.8 ± 0.5 DPI. CB17 mice showed ruffled fur (from 10 to 14 DPI) and slight transient weight loss. Splenomegaly from NM I was severe in SCID and SCIDbg mice and mild in CB17 mice. Spleen weight of mice infected with NM I were: 1.078 ± 0.112 g in SCID mice, 0.695 ± 0.161 g in SCIDbg mice and 0.171 ± 0.012 g in CB17 mice. Spleens of SCID mice infected with NM I were significantly larger ($P < 0.001$) than those of SCIDbg mice. Spleens of both immunodeficient mice infected with NM I were significantly larger ($P < 0.001$) than any spleens from other groups. Numbers of bacteria detected in spleens of SCID and SCIDbg mice were 5 logs greater than the inoculum. Numbers of bacteria in SCID and SCIDbg were not significantly different, but they were significantly higher ($P < 0.05$) than those of CB17 mice.

Localized Histopathology in Mice Infected with NM II

In NM II infection, livers of SCID mice had multiple diffuse granulomas whereas livers of SCIDbg mice had multifocal necrosis with cellular infiltration and granulomas. Livers of CB17 mice had microgranulomas although fewer than SCID mice. In spleens, increased extramedullary hematopoiesis was found in SCID and SCIDbg mice. However, *C. burnetii* antigen was not detected in these lesions. Heart and lungs did not have notable changes from infection with NM II infection compared to unchallenged controls.

Systemic Histopathology in Mice Infected with NM I

In NM I infection, histopathology of SCID and SCIDbg mice were similar with severe diffuse infiltration of macrophages filled with *C. burnetii* antigen. The histopathological changes were found in all organs that we investigated. CB17 mice had small granulomas in liver and spleen. The histopathology in mice infected with NM I in this study was similar to a recent report.[5] However, the lesions of SCIDbg mice were more severe than those of SCID mice. This may be in part because SCIDbg mice died during the course of this experiment and lesions preceded SCID mice pathology.

DISCUSSION

Differences in virulence of phase I and II bacteria were clearly demonstrated in immunodeficient mice. NM II replicated in immunodeficient mice but not in immunocompetent mice, while NM I replicated in all mice tested. Replication of NM II in immunodeficient mice 28 DPI was not as rapid as NM I. This study strongly suggests that innate immunity partially controls phase II infection but that acquired immunity is required for the clearance of the organism. Comparison of SCID and SCIDbg mice challenged with NM I and II showed that NK cells likely have a role in controlling infection. Without NK cells in the absence of acquired immunity, survival time of mice was shorter in NM I infection and histopathology was more severe in NM II infection. However, numbers of bacteria in SCID and SCIDbg mice were not significantly different. The results suggest that NK cells have an accessory role but are not crucial in control of the infection. NK cells likely provide an important supply of IFNγ for activation of macrophages, and activated macrophages are essential for control of phase II infection *in vivo*. Since this experimental challenge lasted only 28 days, it is possible that NM II challenge induce clinical illness in immunodeficient mice with a higher infectious dose or longer experiment time.

Comparison of biological differences of the phase variants has been studied in various ways, but a clear difference of the virulence *in vivo* was only found for pyrogenicity in guinea pigs[8] and may result from LPS O-side-chain differences. In this study, we showed difference of phase I and II *C. burnetii* virulence in pathology for the first time. Since the key components of disease are unclear, *in vivo* study is essential for understanding components of the host-parasite interaction. Further elucidation of virulence of *C. burnetii* and Q fever pathology will benefit from comparison of defined knockout mice.

ACKNOWLEGDMENT

This study was supported by funding from NIH grants AI037744, AI057156 and AI048829.

[*Competing interests statement:* The authors state that they have no competing interests.]

REFERENCES

1. AMANO, K. & J.C. WILLIAMS. 1984. Chemical and immunological characterization of lipopolysaccharides from phase I and phase II *Coxiella burnetii*. J. Bacteriol. **160:** 994–1002.
2. SCHRAMEK, S., R. BREZINA & E. VISACKA. 1983. Different antigenic properties of lipopolysaccharides isolated from *Coxiella burnetii* in phase I and pure phase II. Zentralbl. Bakteriol. Mikrobiol. Hyg. [A]. **255:** 356–360.
3. HACKSTADT, T., M.G. PEACOCK, P.J. HITCHCOCK, *et al.* 1985. Lipopolysaccharide variation in *Coxiella burnetii*: intrastrain heterogeneity in structure and antigenicity. Infect. Immun. **48:** 359–365.
4. HOOVER, T.A., D.W. CULP, M.H. VODKIN, *et al.* 2002. Chromosomal DNA deletions explain phenotypic characteristics of two antigenic variants, phase II and RSA 514 (crazy), of the *Coxiella burnetii* nine mile strain. Infect. Immun. **70:** 6726–6733.
5. ANDOH, M., T. NAGANAWA, A. HOTTA, *et al.* 2003. SCID mouse model for lethal Q fever. Infect. Immun. **71:** 4717–4723.
6. SAMUEL, J.E., M.E. FRAZIER & L.P. MALLAVIA. 1985. Correlation of plasmid type and disease caused by *Coxiella burnetii*. Infect. Immun. **49:** 775–779.
7. BRENNAN, R.E. & J.E. SAMUEL. 2003. Evaluation of *Coxiella burnetii* antibiotic susceptibilities by real-time PCR assay. J. Clin. Microbiol. **41:** 1869–1874.
8. MOOS, A. & T. HACKSTADT. 1987. Comparative virulence of intra- and interstrain lipopolysaccharide variants of *Coxiella burnetii* in the guinea pig model. Infect. Immun. **55:** 1144–1150.

Balb/c Mouse Model and Real-Time Quantitative Polymerase Chain Reaction for Evaluation of the Immunoprotectivity against Q Fever

JINGBO ZHANG, BOHAI WEN, MEILING CHEN, JUN ZHANG, AND DONGSHENG NIU

Beijing Institute of Microbiology and Epidemiology and State Key Laboratory of Pathogen and Biosecurity, Beijing 100071, China

ABSTRACT: The Balb/c mice were infected with *Coxiella burnetii* and samples of blood and major organs from the infected mice were collected on days 1 to 14 after infection. The DNAs extracted from the samples were detected by a developed real-time quantitative PCR specific for *C. burnetii* and high loads of *C. burnetii* were found in spleens, livers, and lungs, particularly in spleens. The Balb/c mice were immunized with whole cell antigen (WCA) of *C. burnetii* and coxiella loads in spleens of mice were assessed by the real-time quantitative PCR on day 7 after challenge with *C. burnetii*. The analysis suggested that phase I whole cells were excellent immunogen that elicited complete protection against coxiella infection by two-booster but not one-booster immunization. The results suggest that the combination of Balb/c model and the real-time quantitative PCR assay is a reliable and sensitive way to evaluate the efficiency of vaccines against Q fever.

KEYWORDS: *Coxiella burnetii*; BALB/c mice; real-time PCR; immunization

INTRODUCTION

Q fever is a worldwide zoonosis caused by *Coxiella burnetii*, an obligate intracellular bacterium. In human, acute Q fever is a flu-like illness, which may be self-limiting or treated with antibiotics.[1] However, chronic Q fever is typically manifested as endocarditis or hepatitis, which is difficult to treat and high in mortality.[1] Therefore, development of efficient vaccines against Q fever has been pursued. Appropriate animal models are necessary for evaluation of protective efficacies of the vaccine candidates and the mice is the most commonly used animal model. BALB/c mouse is intermediately sensitive to lethal challenge of *C. burnetii* and able to generate strong protective immunity after stimulating whole cell antigen (WCA) of *C. burnetii* because of its non-dysfunction in immunity.[2] BALB/c mice infected with

Address for correspondence: Bohai Wen, Beijing Institute of Microbiology and Epidemiology and State Key Laboratory of Pathogen and Biosecurity, 20 Dong-Da-Jie Street, Fengtai, Beijing 100071, China. Voice: +86-10-63820718; fax: +86-10-63815259.
wenbohai@yahoo.com

**Ann. N.Y. Acad. Sci. 1063: 171–175 (2005). © 2005 New York Academy of Sciences.
doi: 10.1196/annals.1355.027**

C. burnetii developed dose-related clinical disease and splenomegaly was used as a major criterion of evaluating vaccinogenic activities of vaccine candidates.[2] However, splenomegaly in the sublethal BALB/c mouse model is not enough for giving a precise evaluation of protective efficacy of vaccine candidates. In this study, a developed real-time quantitative PCR[3] specifically for detecting *C. burnetii* was used to detect loads of *C. burnetii* in spleens of BALB/c mice immunized with WCA of *C. burnetii* after challenge of this pathogen.

MATERIALS AND METHODS

According to the 23S rRNA IVS of *C. burnetii*,[4] a primer pair, CbF (5′-CGGCTGAATTTAAGCGATTTATTTTT-3′) and CbR (5′-CGTAACCACACACG-CATCTCA-3′), and a TaqMan-MGB probe (5′-TGCAATGGGTTCGG-3′) were designed by using Primer Express 2.0 software (PE Applied Biosystems, Foster, CA) and synthesized by Gene Core Biotechnologies (Shanghai, China).[3] Real-time quantitative PCR was performed in 25 μL of volume consisting of 12.5 μL of TaqMan Universal PCR Master Mix (PE Applied Biosystems), 5 μL of primer and probe Mix (2.5 μM each primer and 2.5 μM probe), 2 μL of DNA template, and 5.5 μL of distilled water. The mixture was added in 96-well plate and the plate was incubated in ABI Sequence Detection System for PCR-amplification: one cycle of 50°C for 2 min and 95°C for 10 min to initially activate AmpliTaq Gold DNA polymerase, and then 45 cycles of 95°C for 15 s and 60°C for 1 min to amplify the target DNA.

BALB/c mice (male, 6–8 weeks old) were infected intraperitoneally with 10× 50% infectious dose of *C. burnetii* Xinqiao (phase I) isolated in ticks of China. After infection, three mice each day were sacrificed and their blood, spleens, livers, and hearts were collected for preparation of DNA samples with phenol-chloroform method.[5] The DNA samples were detected by real-time quantitative PCR assay.

Each Balb/c mouse was immunized subcutaneously with 30 μg of WCA of *C. burnetii* emulsified Freund's complete adjuvant. After four weeks, each mouse was given intraperitoneally one booster injection (WCA-1) or two booster injections (WCA-2) at two-week intervals with 15 μg of WCA emulsified in Freund's incomplete adjuvant. Two weeks after booster injection, the mice were intraperitoneally challenged with 10× 50% infectious dose of *C. burnetii* Xinqiao. The mice were sacrificed on day 7 after infection and the splenic samples of mice were collected to prepare DNA samples for real-time quantitative PCR.

RESULTS AND DISCUSSION

The DNA samples extracted from blood of mice infected with *C. burnetii* were detected by real-time quantitative PCR, and the low levels of coxiella load were found on days 1 to 14 and the highest level was on day 7 after infection (FIG. 1). For DNA samples from organ tissues, high levels of coxiella were found in livers and spleens (FIGS. 2 and 3), suggested that *C. burnetii* was well propagated in the macrophages in the two organs, particularly in spleens. In spleens, *C. burnetii* was increased at a great number on days 4 to 7 after infection and the propagation peak was on days 6 and 7 (FIG. 3). The lung was also a site of coxiella infection, but the levels

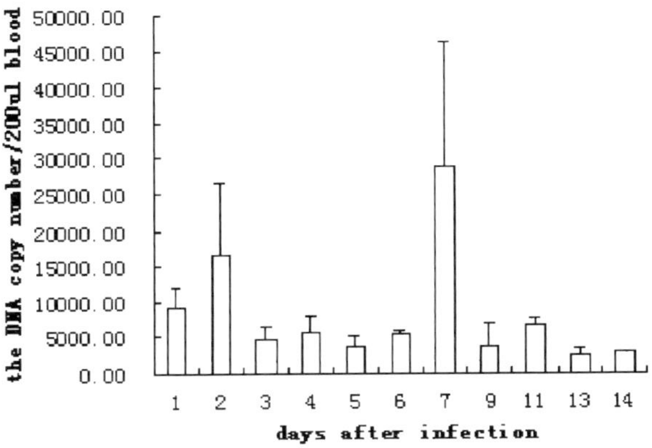

FIGURE 1. The detection of blood samples by real-time PCR.

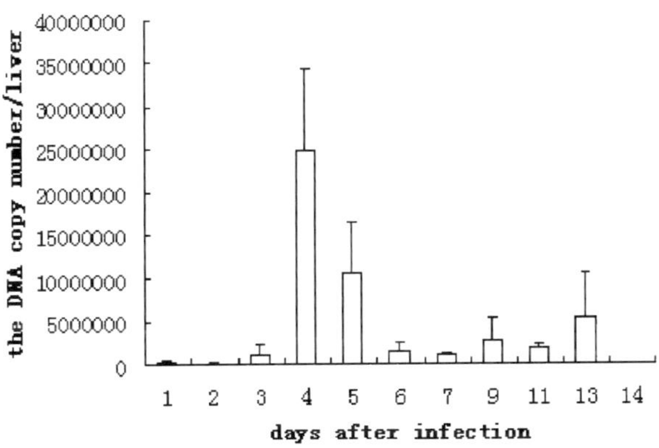

FIGURE 2. The detection of liver samples by real-time PCR.

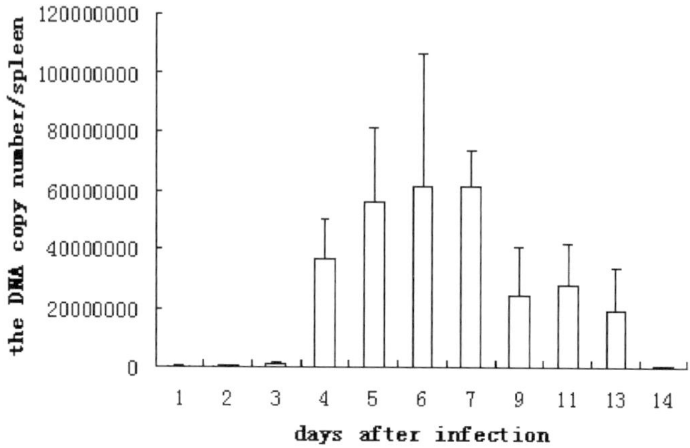

FIGURE 3. The detection of spleen samples by real-time PCR.

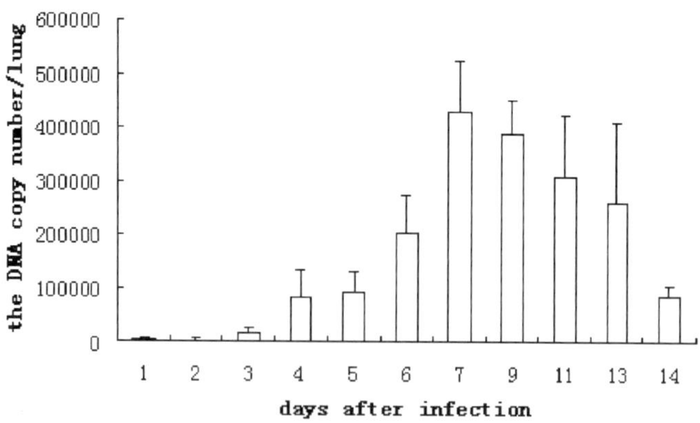

FIGURE 4. The detection of lung samples by real-time PCR.

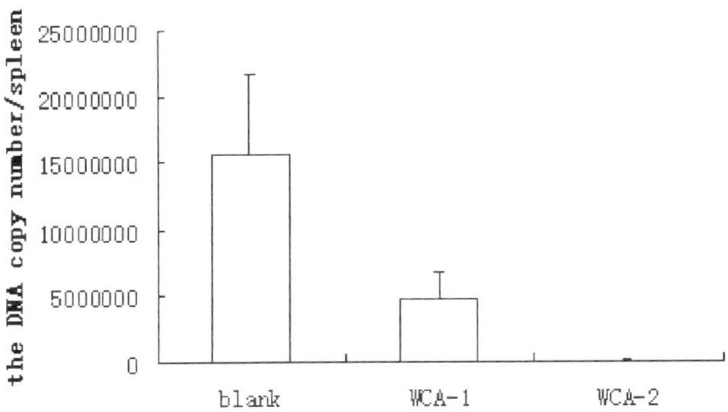

FIGURE 5. The detection of splenic samples from mice immunized with whole cell antigen (WCA) by real-time PCR. Blank, PBS was used for mock-immunization; WCA-1, one-booster immunization; WCA-2, two-booster immunization.

of coxiella load were significantly lower than that in spleens. These results suggest that the spleen of BALB/c mouse is the major organ for coxiella propagation and its burden may reflect the order of severity of infection of *C. burnetii.* Therefore, we used the real-time quantitative PCR to measure coxiella burdens of spleens of mice immunized with WCA of *C. burnetii* on day 7 after challenge of *C. burnetii* for evaluating of immunoprotectivity of the antigen. The results demonstrated that the WCA of *C. burnetii* is an excellent vaccinogen and the protective efficiency of two boosters is markedly better than that of one booster immunization of WCA.

In conclusion, the combination of Balb/c model and the real-time quantitative PCR assay is a reliable and sensitive way to evaluate the efficiency of vaccines against Q fever.

ACKNOWLEDGMENTS

This research was supported by Grant No. 30271214 from the National Natural Science Foundation of China.

[*Conflict of interest statement:* The authors of this research declare that they have no conflict of interest.]

REFERENCES

1. RAOULT, D. & M. MAURIN. 1999. Q fever. Clin. Microbiol. Rev. **12:** 518–553.
2. ZHANG, G., K. KISS, R. SESHADRI, *et al.* 2004. Identification and cloning of immunodominant antigens of *Coxiella burnetii*. Infect. Immun. **72:** 844–852.
3. ZHANG, J.B., B.H. WEN, M.L. CHEN, *et al.* 2005. Detection of *Coxiella burnetii* by real-time quantitative PCR. Chin. J. Zoonoses **21:** 652–655.
4. AFESETH, G., Y.Y. MO & L.P. MALLAVIA. 1995. Characterization of the 23S and 5S rRNA genes of *Coxiella burnetii* and identification of an intervening sequence within the 23S rRNA gene. J. Bacteriol. **177:** 2946–2949.
5. WEN, B.H., R. JIAN, Y. ZHANG, *et al.* 2002. Simultaneous detection of *Anaplasma marginale* and a new *Ehrlichia* species closely related to *Ehrlichia chaffeensis* by sequence analyses of 16S ribosomal DNA in *Boophilus microplus* ticks from Tibet. J. Clin. Microbiol. **40:** 3286–3290.

Hepatitis Associated with *C. burnetii* Isolates

K.E. RUSSELL-LODRIGUE, M.W.J. POELS, G.Q. ZHANG, D.N. MCMURRAY, AND J.E. SAMUEL

Texas A&M University System Health Science Center, Department of Medical Microbiology and Immunology, College Station, Texas 77843-1114, USA

KEYWORDS: ***Coxiella*; isolate; guinea pig; liver; hepatitis; pathology**

INTRODUCTION

Q fever is a zoonotic disease caused by the obligate intracellular, pan-globally distributed bacterium *Coxiella burnetii*. One of the manifestations of infection with *C. burnetii* is acute or chronic hepatitis. Liver biopsy samples from human acute Q fever cases exhibit primarily granulomatous hepatitis with characteristic "doughnut" granulomas, a central vacuole surrounded by a fibrin ring. Though this type of granuloma is often found in Q fever cases, it is not specific to this disease, also occurring in cases of infectious mononucleosis and Hodgkin's disease, among others.[1] Portal triaditis, Kupffer cell hyperplasia, and moderate fatty change have also been described in association with acute Q fever hepatitis.[2] The doughnut granulomas are not found in chronic Q fever hepatitis, which presents primarily as lymphocytic infiltration along portal tracts, nonspecific granulomas, and focal necrosis.[3,4]

A number of *C. burnetii* isolates have been obtained from natural infections of humans and other animals. It has been hypothesized that the clinical expression of Q fever, acute or chronic, relates to unique sequence differences between genomic groups.[5] *C. burnetii* isolates have been separated into six genomic groups based on restriction enzyme banding patterns.[6] The organization of these groups places isolates from ticks and acute human disease (groups I–III) separate from human chronic endocarditis and hepatitis isolates (groups IV and V). Samples isolated from livestock have fallen into multiple groups; isolates from the milk of persistently infected cows are in group I, and isolates causing abortion are in groups III and IV. Group VI isolates collected from feral rodents are considered infectious but avirulent.[7] It has been shown that intraperitoneal inoculation of guinea pigs with group I isolate RSA493 causes a dose-dependent fever and results in pathologic changes primarily associated with the liver[8]; however, hematogenous distribution of the organism after aerosol infection can also lead to hepatic changes. We hypothesize that isolates from different genomic groups will differ in their ability to cause hepatitis in aerosol-challenged guinea pigs.

Address for correspondence: James E. Samuel, Texas A&M University System Health Science Center, Department of Medical Microbiology and Immunology, 414 Reynolds Medical Building, College Station, Texas 77843-1114, USA. Voice: 979-862-1684; fax: 979-845-3479.
jsamuel@tamu.edu

Ann. N.Y. Acad. Sci. 1063: 176–180 (2005). © 2005 New York Academy of Sciences.
doi: 10.1196/annals.1355.068

MATERIALS AND METHODS

Seven- to eight-week old female Hartley guinea pigs were infected via aerosol (Madison Aerosol Chamber; College of Engineering Shops, University of Wisconsin, Madison, WI) with $2{\times}10^6$ phase I *C. burnetii*. Eight isolates from each of four genomic groups were tested: RSA493(group I), RSA334(I), RSA270(I), Q177(IV), Q173(IV), Q212(V), Q217(V), or 7E9-12(VI). Clinical signs of disease were monitored daily, and liver was weighed at necropsy 28 days post infection (p.i.) and collected in 10% buffered formalin for histopathologic evaluation. All slides were evaluated in a blinded fashion. All animal experimentation was performed in AAALAC accredited facilities in accordance with university and federal regulations and was reviewed and approved by the Texas A&M University Laboratory Animal Care Committee.

RESULTS AND DISCUSSION

The characteristic doughnut granulomas of human acute Q fever hepatitis have not been previously described in animal infection experiments and were likewise not seen in guinea pigs infected in this study. RSA 493, RSA334, and RSA270 (group I) liver sections showed a mild hepatitis and severe hepatic lipidosis at death one-week post infection. Only guinea pigs from the RSA493 group were available for evaluation at 28 days post infection; these animals had few pinpoint white to tan foci present on the surface of the liver and histologically exhibited centrilobular hepatocellular degeneration and vacuolization, periportal lymphocyte infiltration, and multiple small granulomas consisting primarily of lymphocytes with few macrophages. Few pinpoint to 4-mm tan to white foci, singly and coalescing, were observed on the liver surface of guinea pigs infected with group IV isolates Q177 and Q173 (FIG. 1a), and periportal lymphocytic infiltration and multiple granulomas of varying sizes were noted histologically. These granulomas were more defined and had a greater amount of histiocytic involvement than those seen in guinea pigs infected with group I isolates. Animals infected with Q173 had the largest and most numerous hepatic granulomas of all animals necropsied from each isolate group (FIG. 1b). Few small granulomas and infiltration of lymphocytes along portal tracts were noted in the livers of group V isolate Q212- and Q217-infected guinea pigs, and the degree of hepatic change indicated that isolates from this group are more hepatovirulent than group I isolates but less than group IV isolates. Necrotic lesions were associated especially with peripheral granulomas in guinea pigs infected with isolates from groups I, IV, and V, and were again most common in animals given group IV isolates. No hepatic granulomas were noted in guinea pigs infected with the group VI isolate 7E9-12. Liver weights did not vary significantly within or between genomic groups.

This study supported the hypothesis of differing abilities of various genomic groups of *C. burnetii* to induce pathologic change in the liver. Group IV isolates produced consistently larger and more numerous hepatic granulomas than other isolates.

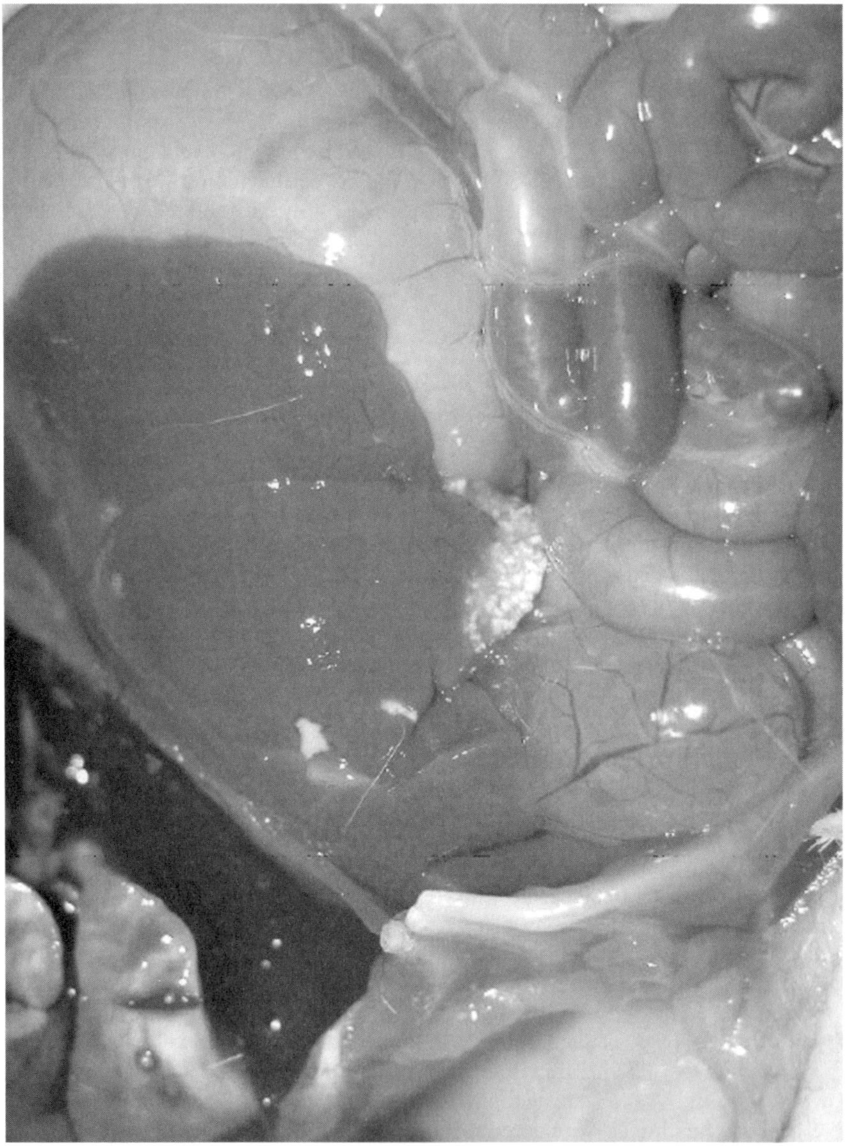

FIGURE 1. **(a)** Pinpoint to 4mm, individual to coalescing, white foci in the liver of a guinea pig 28 days post infection with $2{\times}10^6$ phase I Q173 *C. burnetii.*

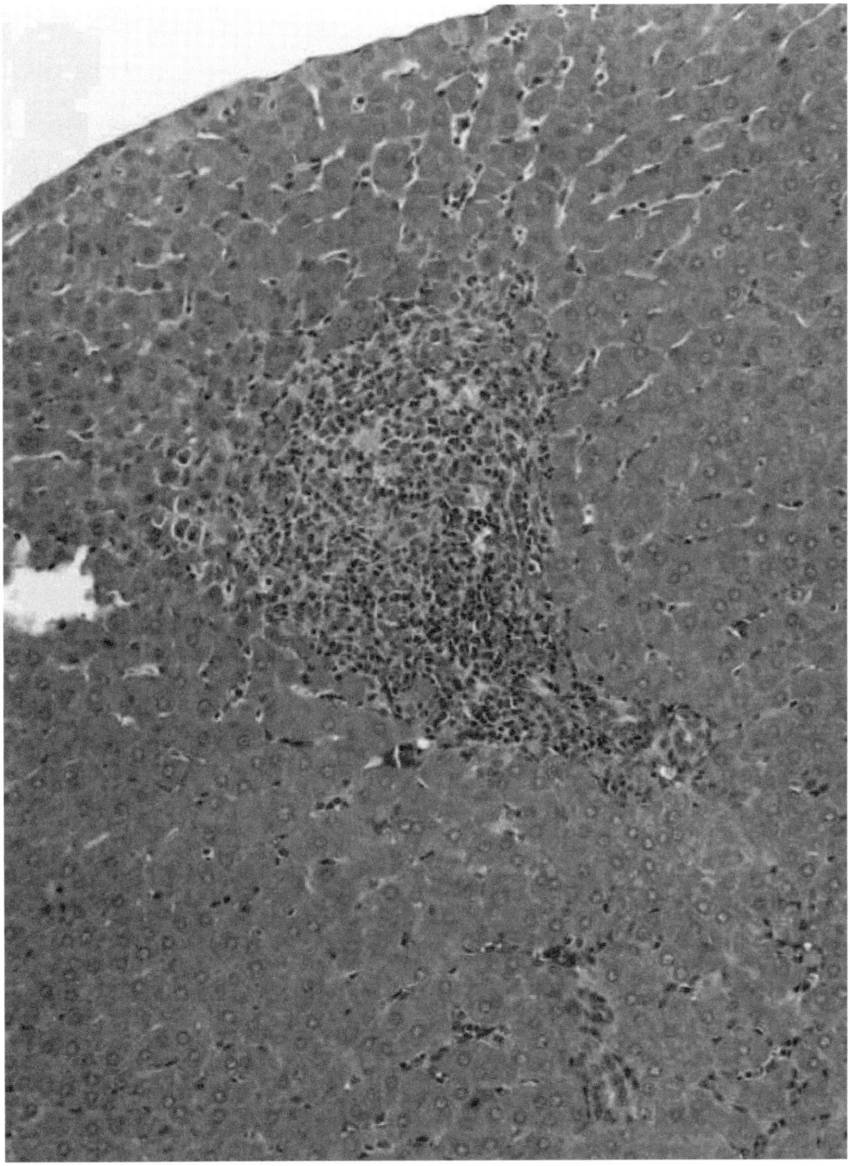

FIGURE 1—*continued.* (**b**) 100× magnification of a single hepatic granuloma from the same guinea pig.

REFERENCES

1. MARRIE, T.J. 1990. Q fever hepatitis. *In* Q Fever. The disease. T.J. Marrie, Ed. **1:** 171–178. CRC Press. Boca Raton, FL.
2. MAURIN, M. & D. RAOULT. 1999. Q fever. Clin. Microbiol. Rev. **12:** 518–553.
3. WESTLAKE, P. *et al.* 1987. The pathology of Q fever hepatitis. A case diagnosed by liver biopsy. J. Clin. Gastroenterol. **9:** 357–363.
4. FOURNIER, P.-E., T.J. MARRIE & D. RAOULT. 1998. Diagnosis of Q fever. J. Clin. Microbiol. **36:** 1823–1834.
5. SAMUEL, J.E., M.E. FRAZIER & L.P. MALLAVIA. 1985. Correlation of plasmid type and disease caused by *Coxiella burnetii*. Infect. Immun. **49:** 775–779.
6. HENDRIX, L.R., J.E. SAMUEL & L.P. MALLAVIA. 1991. Differentiation of *Coxiella burnetii* isolates by analysis of restriction-endonuclease-digested DNA separated by SDS-PAGE. J. Gen. Microbiol. **137:** 269–276.
7. STOENNER, H.G. & D.B. LACKMAN. 1960. The biologic properties of *Coxiella burnetii* isolated from rodents collected in Utah. Am. J. Hyg. **71:** 45–51.
8. LASCOLA, B., H. LEPIDI & D. RAOULT. 1997. Pathologic changes during acute Q fever: influence of route of infection and inoculum size in infected guinea pigs. Infect. Immun. **65:** 2443–2447.

Q Fever Research Group (QRG), Adelaide: Activities-Exit Summary 1980–2004

B. MARMION, R. HARRIS, P. STORM, K. HELBIG, I. PENTTILA, D. WORSWICK AND L. SEMENDRIC

Infectious Diseases Laboratories IMVS, Hanson Institute, School of Pharmacy & Medical Sciences, University of South Australia, Adelaide, South Australia

KEYWORDS: **Q fever vaccine prophylaxis; persistent infection; cytokine dysregulation; immune response gene variation; chronic Q fever**

Q FEVER VACCINE PROPHYLAXIS

1980–1989: The Problem and Vaccine Development

In the early1980s there were 600–800 reported cases of Q fever a year across the country and an uncertain number of mild or subclinical infections indicated by later but limited serological surveys. Q fever notification data for 2003 show high prevalence of infection in northern New South Wales and Queensland; a consistent pattern (FIG. 1). Q fever cases come from the abattoirs and a wide network of associated by-product firms, from the agricultural community raising cattle sheep and goats, from shearing teams, from kangaroo hunters and processors, and sometimes from the general population exposed by proximity to livestock sale yards, feed lots or by visits to farms.

The decision to attempt vaccine prophylaxis was precipitated by a large Q fever outbreak in an abattoir near Adelaide that previously processed bacon pigs but then added feral goats to their program. The vaccine chosen was a highly purified, formalin-inactivated whole cell suspension of the Henzerling strain of *C. burnetii* maintained strictly in Phase1 antigen state by restricted passage in CE yolk sac. The purification and formulation protocol was devised by the (late) Dick Ormsbee (NIH/NIAID, Rocky Mountain Laboratory, Hamilton, Montana USA) and was an advance on earlier whole cell vaccines that were mixtures of Phase 1 and 2 cells (reviewed in ref. 1). CSL Ltd was approached by QRG and Dr Ormsbee and agreed to manufacture the vaccine (= Q Vax, CSL Ltd Melbourne, Vic., Australia) according to the Ormsbee protocol.

The conventional wisdom of the time was that Q fever vaccines were highly reactogenic and prone to cause immune abscess; conclusions based on experience with the older vaccines of larger bacterial mass, used with repeated revaccination and from inadvertent inoculation of subjects immunologically sensitised by previous infection.[1]

Address for correspondence: B.P. Marmion, 14 Birksgate Drive, URRBRAE 5064 South Australia. Voice/fax: 61 8 8379 5514.
chris.nikolaou@imvs.sa.gov.au

Ann. N.Y. Acad. Sci. 1063: 181–186 (2005).
doi: 10.1196/annals.1355.028

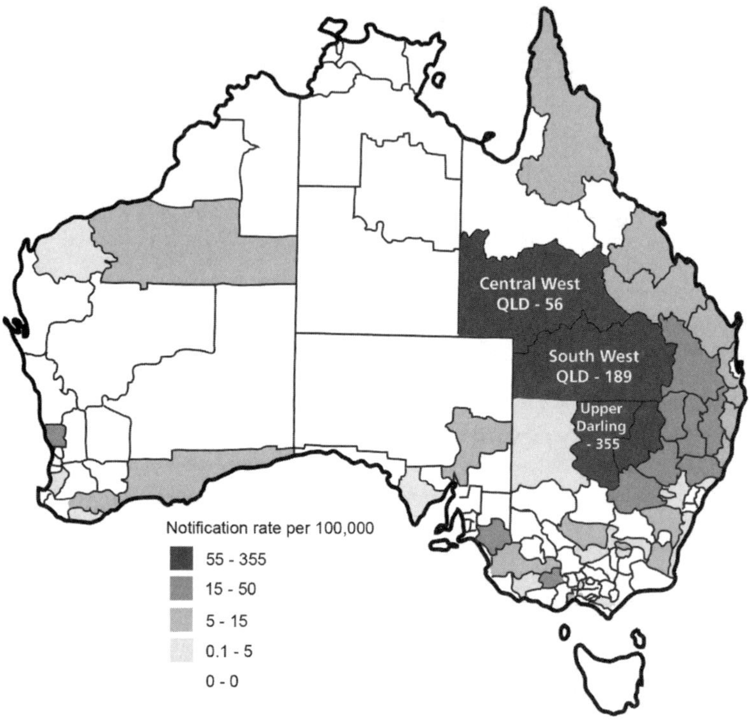

FIGURE 1. Q fever notification rate per 100,000.

The first question to be answered therefore was whether it was possible, with safety, to vaccinate abattoir workers, many of whom had already been infected. This was tested from1980 by open trials of the vaccine in which potential vaccinees were first screened for Q fever antibody and by intradermal skin test for cellular immunity using diluted vaccine. The latter step followed the observations of David Lackman *et al.*, at the Rocky Mountain Laboratory.[1] Only those who were negative in both tests were vaccinated with 30 μg of vaccine subcutaneously (later reduced to 25 μg). The trials involved 4 abattoirs around Adelaide and were gradually extended to others elsewhere in the State. Initial results did not indicate unacceptable reactions relative to the serious nature of the disease prevented. They also suggested a high level of protection.[1,2]

Further work, 1981–1989, charted the brief antibody response to vaccine but demonstrated a prolonged cell-mediated response (CMI) as measured by a CMI surrogate test, lymphocyte stimulation assay, and by measurement of interferon gamma responses.[3–5] In all, > 4000 subjects were involved in the trials.[1,6] There was one immune abscess requiring surgical excision in an individual in whom the pretesting regimen was not followed correctly and a few subjects with a short-term fatigue syndrome. Protection was >95% in the vaccinees and maintained for at least five years.[7] The results of the open trial were confirmed in a blinded, placebo-controlled trial in

Queensland abattoirs in which Q Vax was compared with influenza vaccine.[8] All cases were in the influenza vaccine group. The use of a sequential analysis design in this trial gave a result with a minimum of cases in the unprotected group. Q Vax was licensed for general use by the Federal Health Department in 1989.

1990/3–2000+ Programs Instituted in Abattoirs across the Country

In 1989 Q fever vaccination was recommended for use in meat processing industry by an Expert Committee on occupational zoonoses, but little progress was made until 1993. From that year CSL Ltd, Vaccine Consultants pursued an intensive campaign, visited State Health Departments, large Export Abattoirs and by-products firms to inform and facilitate vaccine programs for existing workers and new recruits and assisted Health Departments to set up clinics and vaccination teams. By 2004 most large abattoirs in States other than Tasmania—which has few Q fever cases—have vaccine programs. FIGURE 2 shows, as an example, the resulting decline in the number of compensation claims for Q fever in the Queensland meat processing industry from 1992 to 2004. (Acute and some chronic Q fever cases are financially compensable in Australia). FIGURE 3 illustrates the decline of Q Fever compensation

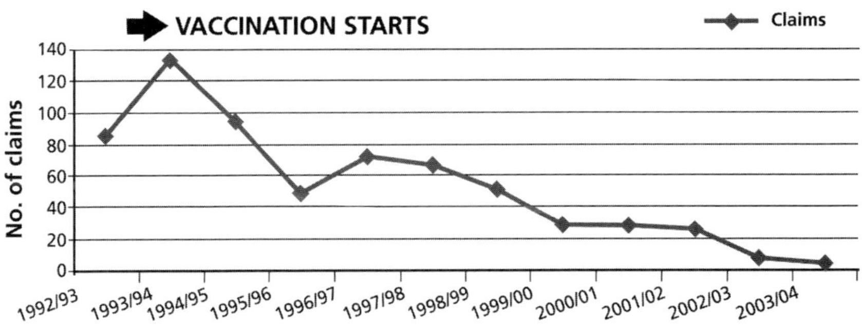

FIGURE 2. Queensland meat industry: Q fever.

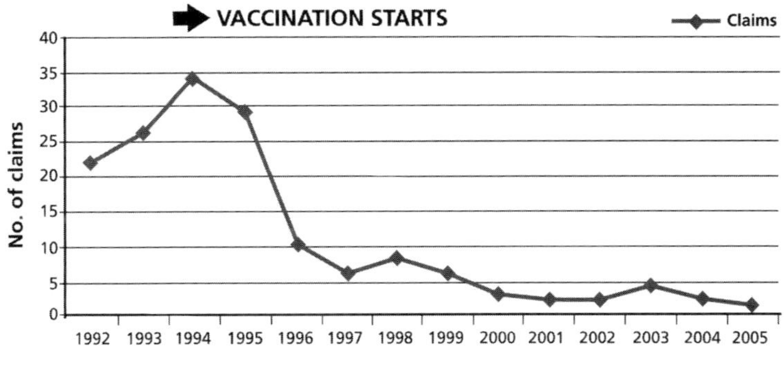

FIGURE 3. AMH Q fever claims (Queensland).

claims in a major meat-processing group with 6 abattoirs—Australian Meat Holdings—over the same period. Absolute numbers of claims are shown, but the curve for rates per 1000 employees follows the same decline as in FIGURE 3. The end result was a marked decline in morbidity and costs for industry and health services.

2000–2005 National Q Fever Management Program

Submissions for financial support to ensure wider use of vaccine were made to the Australian Federal Government in 1999/2000. These were supported by representative bodies in the meat processing and livestock industries and by data from Meat and Livestock Australia Ltd, the Q Fever Research Group and a Health Economics analysis[9] by CSL Ltd. In 2000–2003 the Federal Government allocated ~Aus\$ 18×10^6 to support abattoir programs and to extend vaccination to the agricultural community. The broad objectives and priorities for the Initiative were identified by a Q fever Task Force meeting under the auspices of the Federal Department of Health and were realized via State Immunisation Departments. As a result of very considerable efforts by the latter during 2001–2003, approximately 135,000 doses of vaccine were used. It is a little early to judge the effects in the agricultural community, given their lower attack rates and the lower proportion of the population vaccinated compared with the high risk and high vaccine coverage in the abattoirs. Nevertheless, at present, analysis of Q fever notifications in New South Wales, for example, suggests a general decline in Q fever prevalence (FIG. 4). However varia-

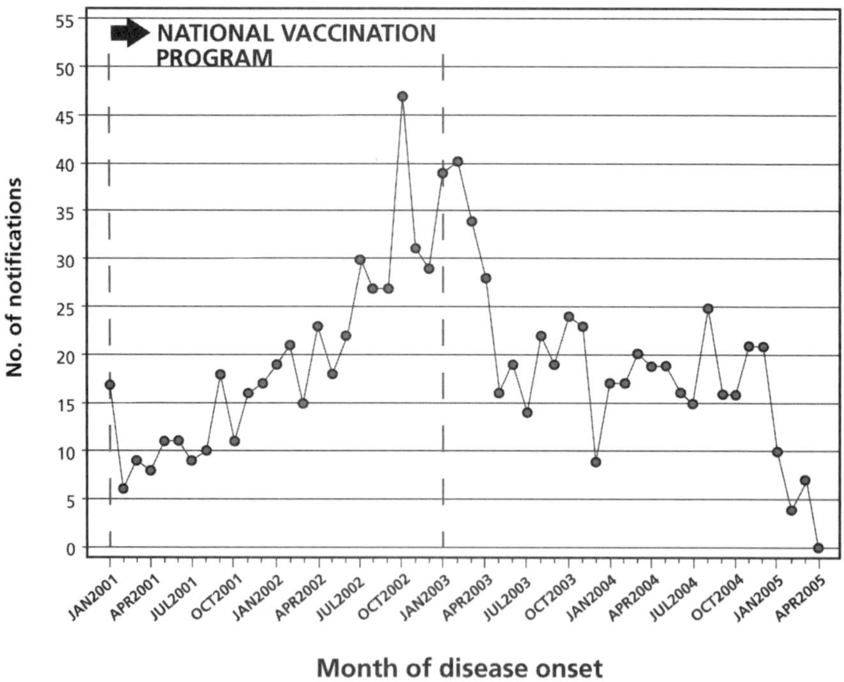

FIGURE 4. Q fever notifications in NSW residents, by month of disease onset, January 2001 to April 2005.

tions in notification data are notoriously multifactorial. The results of the interim analysis are awaited from the Federal Health Department. Longer-term surveillance and focussed studies will be required to confirm the trends.

Conclusions

The inactivated whole cell Q fever vaccine, Q Vax CSL Ltd., is highly protective and has been administered to at least 150 000 subjects, 1980–2004. Reactions due to prior immune sensitization have been minimized by the pretesting regimen aided by use of a trial dose test to resolve ambiguous results.[1,10] Further work is required on the immune response gene background and mechanisms of some rare idiosyncratic systemic reactions in apparently nonimmune subjects, some with existing, unrelated immunological dysfunction. Trial data are also required on optimal dosage levels of vaccine for women and children.

RECENT Q FEVER STUDIES

Cytokine Dysregulation in post-Q Fever Fatigue Syndrome

PENTTILA, I. *et al.* 1998. Cytokine dysregulation in the post-Q fever fatigue syndrome. Q. J. Med. **91:** 549–560. [Relative to controls, PBMC from QFS patients stimulated with Q fever antigens showed up regulated IL-6, increases of IFN-γ and down regulation of IL-2].

Long-Term Persistence of C. burnetii *after Acute Q Fever*

HARRIS, R. *et al.* 2000. Long term persistence of *Coxiella burnetii* in the host after primary Q fever. Epidemiol. Infect. **124:** 543–549.

MARMION, B.P. *et al.* 2005. Long term persistence of *Coxiella burnetii* after acute primary Q fever. Q. J. Med. **98:** 7–20. [PCR assay detected *C. burnetii* genomic sequences in bone marrow of cases of Q fever five and 12 years after infection.]

Immunogenetic Determinants for Chronic Q Fever

HELBIG K. *et al.* 2003. Variation in immune response genes and chronic Q fever. Concepts: Preliminary test with Post-Q fever fatigue syndrome Genes Immun. 2003 4 82-85

HELBIG, K. *et al.* 2005. Analysis of immune response genes in the post Q fever fatigue syndrome, Q fever endocarditis and uncomplicated acute primary Q fever. Q. J. Med. **98:** 565–574. July/August. [Differences in HLA DR genes and polymorphic variants in INFgamma and IL10 control genes within the 3 groups of patients and compared with population control panels.]

ACKNOWLEDGMENTS

Meat and Livestock Aust. Ltd have given generous support to the Q fever Research Group over many years. We thank Dr Heather Gidding (National Centre for Immunisation Research and Surveillance—NCIRS) for her analysis of national Q fever notification data, including FIGURE 1. Mr Geoffrey Yarham (Australian Meat Holdings, QLD) kindly supplied FIGURES 2 and 3. We applaud the major contributions to the control of Q fever by Immunization Teams in the various States, from the mid-1990s onward and particularly during the National Q fever Management Program.

[*Competing interests statement:* The authors declare that they have no competing interests.]

REFERENCES

1. ORMSBEE, R.A. & B.P. MARMION. 1990. Prevention of *Coxiella burnetii* infection: Vaccines and guidelines for those at risk. *In* Q fever. The Disease. T. Marrie, Ed.: 225–248. CRC Press. Boca Raton, FL.
2. MARMION, B.P., R.A. ORMSBEE, M. KYRKOU, *et al.* 1984. Vaccine prophylaxis of abattoir-associated Q fever. Lancet **2:** 1411–1414.
3. WORSWICK, D.A. & B.P. MARMION. 1985. Antibody responses in acute and chronic Q fever and in subjects vaccinated against Q fever. J. Med. Microbiol. **19:** 281–296.
4. IZZO, A.A., B.P. MARMION & D.A. WORSWICK. 1988. Markers of cell mediated immunity after vaccination with an inactivated whole cell Q fever vaccine. J. Infect. Dis. **157:** 781–789.
5. Izzo, A.A. & B.P. Marmion. 1993. Variation in interferon gamma responses to *Coxiella burnetii* antigens with lymphocytes from vaccinated or naturally infected subjects. Clin. Exp. Immunol. **94:** 507–515.
6. MARMION, B.P., R.A. ORMSBEE, M. KYRKOU, *et al.* 1990. Vaccine prophylaxis of abattoir-associated Q fever: eight years experience in Australian abattoirs. Epidemiol. Infect. **104:** 275–287.
7. ACKLAND, J.A., D.A. WORSWICK & B.P. MARMION. 1994. Vaccine prophylaxis of Q fever: a follow up study of Q Vax (CSL Ltd) Med. J. Aust. **160:** 704–708.
8. SHAPIRO, R.A., V. SISKIND, F.D. SCHOFIELD, *et al.* 1990. A randomised, controlled, double-blind, cross-over clinical trial of Q fever vaccine in selected Queensland abattoirs. Epidemiol. Infect. **104:** 267–273.
9. KERMODE, M., K. YONG, S. HURLEY & B.P. MARMION. 2003. An economic evaluation of increased uptake of Q fever vaccination among meat and agricultural industry workers. Aust. NZ J. Pub. Hlth. **27:** 390–398.
10. CSL "Q fever. Your Questions Answered" 1999. MediMedia Communications NSW Australia. 31 pages. Via CSL Ltd. 45 Poplar Rd, Parkville, Vic. 3052 Australia.

Rickettsial Infections

JUAN P. OLANO

Center for Biodefense and Emerging Infectious Diseases, University of Texas Medical Branch, Galveston, Texas, 77555-0609 USA

ABSTRACT: *Rickettsiae* are obligate intracellular α-proteobacteria that primarily target the microvascular endothelium. In the last two decades, new rickettsial pathogens have been associated with human illness around the world. Clinically, the common denominator in all rickettsioses is the development of increased microvascular permeability, leading to cerebral and non-cardiogenic pulmonary edema. With the development of powerful research tools, advances in the understanding of rickettsial pathogenesis have been dramatic. Entry into the host cell is followed by rapid escape into the cytoplasm to avoid phagolysosomal fusion. Spotted fever group rickettsiae induce actin polymerization via a group of proteins called RickA, which promote nucleation of actin monomers via the Arp2/3 complex at one rickettsial pole, propelling the bacteria across the cytoplasm and into neighboring cells. Damage to the host cell is most likely multifactorial. The most extensively studied mechanism is the generation of reactive oxygen species (ROS) and downregulation of enzymes involved in protection against oxidative injury. The significance of ROS-mediated cellular damage *in vivo* is beginning to be elucidated. The main pathogenic mechanism is increased microvascular permeability leading to profound metabolic disturbances in the extravascular compartment. The underlying factors responsible for those changes are beginning to be elucidated *in vitro* and include direct effects of intracellular rickettsiae, cytokines, and possibly activated coagulation factors—all of which most likely modify interendothelial junctions. Our knowledge on rickettsial pathogenesis will continue to expand in the near future as new research tools become available.

KEYWORDS: Rickettsiae; microvascular permeability; reactive oxygen intermediates; alpha proteobacteria

INTRODUCTION

Rickettsiae are small, obligate intracellular, gram-negative, aerobic, coccobacillary α-proteobacteria with a life cycle that includes both vertebrate and invertebrate hosts that can function both as vectors and primary reservoirs. Small mammals function as amplifying hosts and humans are merely accidental hosts. In humans, rickettsiae are responsible for systemic diseases that target the microvascular endothelium leading to highly protean clinical manifestations of which cerebral and

Address for correspondence: Juan P. Olano, M.D., Associate Professor, Department of Pathology, University of Texas Medical Branch, 301 University Blvd., Rt. 0609, Galveston, TX 77555-0609. Voice: 409-772-2870; fax: 409-747-2400.
jolano@utmb.edu

**Ann. N.Y. Acad. Sci. 1063: 187–196 (2005). © 2005 New York Academy of Sciences.
doi: 10.1196/annals.1355.031**

pulmonary edema are the main causes of morbidity and mortality.[1–3] This review will focus on the interactions between rickettsiae and eukaryotic cells. I also summarize important data regarding phylogeny and virulence factors derived from the available genome sequences of selected rickettsiae.

PHYLOGENY

The alpha subdivision of the proteobacteria contains a large number of genera including plant pathogens (*Agrobacterium* and *Rhizobia*), human pathogens (*Brucella, Bartonella*, and *Rickettsia*), and insect endosymbionts (*Wolbachia*).[4] Their life styles represent a wide spectrum including pericellular parasites of plants, facultative intracellular human pathogens, obligate intracellular human pathogens, and plant and insect symbionts. The transition to the intracellular life style that characterizes the *Rickettsiales* most likely occurred far back in evolutionary time as shown by phylogenetic trees that compare available sequences in the α-proteobacteria. Genome sizes in this subdivision range from 1–9 Mb. It is estimated that the ancestral proteobacterium had 3,000–5,000 genes.[4] From this ancient ancestor, intracellular bacteria evolved with invertebrates, animals, and humans by genome reduction. In contrast, soil-growing plant-associated bacteria evolved by genome expansion. Perhaps, one of the most successful symbiotic relationships on the planet occurred approximately 2,000 million years ago when an ancient proteobacterium invaded a eukaryotic cell and eventually evolved into mitochondria.[5,6] In fact, the closest modern relative to mitochondria is *R. prowazekii.*[7,8] Regardless of their life styles, the α-proteobacteria are characterized by their chronic interactions with their hosts or vectors. As such, they have developed exquisite molecular mechanisms responsible for the manipulation of the host cell so that their survival is ensured.

The complete phylogeny of *Rickettsiae* is kingdom, Bacteria; phylum (VII), Proteobacteria (alpha subdivision); class (I), *Rhodospirilli*; order (II), *Rickettsiales*; family, *Rickettsiaceae*; genus, *Rickettsia.*

PATHOGENESIS

For obligate intracellular bacteria, pathogenesis is a concept that involves multiple steps: (1) transmission, (2) entry, (3) initial spread from point of entry to other organs, (4) contact with target cell (adherence and invasion), (5) survival within the host (avoidance of host defenses and adaptation to the host environment), and (6) extension of the niche (modulation of host biology, multiplication and survival). I focus on the steps that involve the interaction between rickettsiae and their eukaryotic host cell.

With the advent of complete rickettsial genome sequences. much more is known about their metabolic capabilities, pathogenesis, and potential virulence factors. However, it is worth mentioning that 49% of the open reading frames (ORFs) in *R. conorii* and 37.3% of the ORFs in *R. prowazekii* correspond to proteins of unknown function and with no homologs in databases.[5,6,9] Simply put, there is a large amount of work to be done in order to understand how these organisms have been so successful in nature and how they induce disease in humans.

In vitro, rickettsiae can be grown in almost any cell line available (epithelial, endothelial, fibroblastic, hematopoietic), implying that their receptor is a ubiquitous protein present in eukaryotic cells. In fact, recent evidence shows that Ku70, a protein that is present in the nucleus, cytoplasm, and lipid raft microdomains in the plasma membrane, might serve as a receptor for *R. conorii.*[10] Ku70 is a multifunctional protein in eukaryotic cells whose main function in the nucleus (along with Ku80) is to serve as part of the DNA-dependent protein (serine/threonine) kinase system. In the cytoplasm, Ku70 functions as an inhibitor of Bax-mediated apoptosis, and in the plasma membrane as a fibronectin binding protein. Ubiquitination seems to be essential for Ku70 to serve as a rickettsial receptor. *In vivo*, rickettsiae target the microvascular endothelium.[3,11,12] Minor secondary targets include cells in the medial layer of arterioles and macrophages. Internalization is active both at the target cell and the bacterium and requires active protein synthesis by the bacterium. The signaling pathways involved in rickettsial entry have been recently characterized and include recruitment of the actin-nucleating complex Arp 2/3 to the site of attachment, and the interaction of several signaling molecules including the small GTPase Cdc42, phosphoinositide 3-kinase, protein tyrosine kinases (specifically the Src family), and focal adhesion kinase (FAK).[13] Potential adhesins have been identified by experiments performed with monoclonal antibodies and include OmpA and OmpB in spotted fever group rickettsiae and OmpB in typhus group rickettsiae.[14–18] Once attached to the host cell, rickettsiae enter the intracellular environment by a process of induced phagocytosis by the "zipper mechanism" in which focal rearrangements of the actin cytoskeleton occur below the site of attachment leading to progressive apposition of the eukaryotic cellular membrane over the bacterium. Once rickettsiae are internalized, escape from the phagosome into the cytosolic compartment takes place after several minutes and is mediated by upregulation of genes coding for proteins with membranolytic activity, namely *tlyC* (hemolysin C) and *pld* (phospholipase D).[19,20] Once in the cytoplasm rickettsiae are not at risk of being destroyed by lethal lysosomal enzymes and the human host has to use other mechanisms to eliminate them. This is successfully done in the majority of cases with the exception of latency in *R. prowazekii* infections and the still controversial evidence of chronic infections caused by *R. helvetica.*[21–23]

Once in the cytoplasm, rickettsiae obtain the necessary nutrients to survive in the intracellular milieu from the host cell. Many of the genes necessary to synthesize certain metabolic products have been replaced by genes encoding for transport systems, including ATP/ADP translocases that probably entered the rickettsial genomes by horizontal transfer from *Chlamydia.*[24–27] Due to their intracellular niche, the "tempo" of rickettsial genome evolution is much slower when compared to extracellular or facultative intracellular organisms. Therefore, horizontal transfers must have occurred more frequently in the early phases in the evolution of these organisms. Furthermore, horizontal gene transfers were probably very common in the early days of life on earth.[28] *Rickettsiae* are capable of producing ATP and most likely do so after depleting the host cell's ATP pool. Such function seems to be so important that there are five copies of the ATP/ADP translocase genes.[8,29] Other important highlights in rickettsial metabolism include the presence of glutamine transporters due to the absence of glutamine synthase, and purine and pyrimidine salvage pathways through the host. However, synthesis of deoxyribonucleotides from ribonucleotide precursors for DNA synthesis is possible since they have the ribonucleotide reductase genes necessary for such conversion. Aminoacid synthesis is very limited and most aminoacids are taken from the host cell's cytoplasm by transporters.[30]

The spotted fever group rickettsiae are capable of polymerizing monomeric actin filaments in the cytoplasm at one of their poles.[31,32] The net result of this action is propulsion of rickettsiae through the cytoplasm and penetration of neighboring cells through the cell membranes. This allows rickettsiae to affect short segments of the microvasculature by invading contiguous endothelial cells without being exposed to the intravascular compartment. The molecular machinery responsible for this action has been elucidated and depends on expression of RickA, a family of proteins that acts through the Arp 2/3 complex, which in turn induces actin polymerization.[33–36] Other examples of actin-based cytoplasmic motility include *Listeria*, *Shigella*, *Burkholderia pseudomallei*, vaccinia virus, and *Mycobacterium marinum.*[37–41] In contrast, the absence of Rick A expression in *R. prowazekii* correlates well with the complete absence of cytoplasmic motility. *R. typhi* induces actin polymerization but the actin tails are short and "hooked" producing inefficient circular movements within the cytoplasm. Since *R. typhi* also lacks Rick A protein expression, the induction of actin polymerization must be due to other still unknown protein(s).

Rickettsiae do not secrete any exotoxins and one of the best studied mechanisms by which they can exert damage to the host cell is oxidative stress. The role of oxygen radicals has been studied extensively *in vitro* and their role *in vivo* is beginning to be elucidated.[42–46] In addition, regulatory oxygenases also seem to play an important role in rickettsial pathogenesis as shown by upregulation of the inducible form of heme oxygenase (HO-1) in *R. rickettsii*–infected endothelial cells and the subsequent upregulation of the cyclooxygenase system.[46] The latter is responsible for increased production of prostaglandins, which in turn, might have dramatic effects on the microvasculature since these substances are well known paracrine homeostatic factors of endothelial cells and the microcirculation.

Adaptation is certainly important for rickettsial organisms since they have to shuttle between vectors (arthropods) and hosts (mammals). Needless to say, the conditions in each of these environments are very different. Five gene copies with homology to *SpoT* genes have been found in rickettsiae.[8,29] The *spoT* gene seems to play an important role when rickettsiae move to their vectors and this same gene probably plays an important role in maintaining *R. prowazekii* and *R. typhi* viable in the feces of the louse and flea vectors, respectively, under very harsh environmental conditions.

In eukaryotic cells, rickettsiae activate NF-κB and one of the results of this activation is the inhibition of apoptosis.[47–49] This effect is mediated via inhibition of apical caspases-8 and -9 and by controlling intracellular levels of the bcl-2 family of proteins, specifically Bid and Bad.[50] Inhibition of apoptosis *in vitro* by intracellular rickettsiae appears logical since they are obligate intracellular organisms and therefore need the cell's nutrients to proliferate. However, *in vivo*, inhibition of apoptosis seems important in the early phases of the disease when rickettsiae start proliferating in the microvascular endothelium. Later in the disease process, when adaptive immunity is in full swing, apoptosis is in fact increased in infected endothelial cells and appears to be the result of perforin and granzyme-mediated apoptotic cell death due to cytotoxic CD8+ T-cells.[51]

Rickettsiae are one of a very selected list of human pathogens that target the microvascular endothelium exclusively. In fact, the hallmark of rickettsial infections in humans is the presence of increased microvascular permeability in all organ systems.[2,12] The main consequence of "leaky" microvessels throughout the body is escape of intravascular fluid into the interstitial space, leading to tissue edema. Such change in vital organs such as the lungs and brain is responsible for most of the morbidity and mortality observed in human infections due to non-cardiogenic pulmonary edema and cerebral edema.[52,53] Understanding the pathogenesis of increased microvascular permeability in rickettsial infections could lead to new avenues of treatment to prevent life-threatening complications. The movement of fluids in and out of the microvascular compartment depends on physical forces across microvessels and chemical modulation of permeability.[54] Physical forces are important in other disease states such as congestive heart failure, protein-losing nephropathies or cirrhosis. However, modulation of the microvascular permeability by chemical mediators is far more powerful than their physical counterparts. Regulation of permeability occurs mostly in precapillary arterioles, capillaries per se, and postcapillary venules, which are the very microvessels that are targeted in rickettsial infections.

Multiple mechanisms by which rickettsiae can induce microvascular permeability have been proposed and they include: (1) endothelial denudation; (2) direct effect as a result of endothelial infection by rickettsiae; and (3) paracrine and autocrine modulation by cytokines, prostaglandins, and products of the coagulation/fibrinolytic cascades. The first mechanism is self explanatory and would explain increased permeability by the mere absence of the endothelial lining in affected microvessels. In these cases, the only structure remaining in the microvessels would be the basement membrane, which would be insufficient to keep the intravascular fluids from leaking into the interstitial space. This mechanism surely happens *in vivo*, but seems to appear late in the disease process when endothelial cells are dying from the presence of massive amounts of intracellular rickettsiae or by apoptotic/necrotic cell death due to CD8+ cytotoxic T-lymphocytes. In fact, circulating endothelial cells have been demonstrated in humans during acute infections.[55]

The second mechanism is beginning to be elucidated. Preliminary experiments in my laboratory have shown that monolayers composed of microvascular endothelial cell lines derived from human brain and dermis increase their permeability *in vitro* as evidenced by decreased transendothelial resistance. These changes are not explained by cell death in the monolayers during the first 24 hours of infection.[56] The molecular mechanisms responsible for these changes are currently being studied, but most likely involve signal transduction pathways affecting the cytoskeleton and ultimately junctional proteins. The role of cytokines is also being studied in my research laboratory and preliminary studies reveal that IL-1-β and TNF-α play an important role in increasing permeability across infected monolayers. IFN-γ on the contrary seems to partially counteract some of the effects of IL-1-β and TNF-α on the infected monolayers at doses of 5 and 10 ng/mL.[56] Even though coagulation abnormalities have been described *in vitro* and *in vivo* during acute rickettsioses,[57,58] autopsy studies performed in humans have not shown disseminated intravascular coagulation and subsequent bleeding as the underlying process responsible for fatalities. However, several products of the coagulation and fibrinolytic cascade could be responsible for increases in permeability across the microcirculation. All these potential mechanisms leading to increased microvascular permeability are by no means mutually exclusive and most likely play additive or synergistic roles *in vitro* and *in vivo*.

Due to the obligate intracellular nature of rickettsial organisms and the absence, until recently, of genetic tools to manipulate the rickettsial genomes, determination of virulence factors has been a slow process. However, due to the availability of complete genome sequences from several rickettsial organisms, the recent reports of successful transformation of rickettsiae, and the discovery of a rickettsia-associated transposon, progress in this area will certainly accelerate exponentially.[59–61] The definition of a virulence factor is highly controversial and a discussion of the topic is beyond the scope of this manuscript. A simple definition of a virulence factor is that of a molecule synthesized by a pathogen that is necessary (although many times not sufficient by itself) to inflict disease in a host. As discussed previously, pathogenesis involves multiple steps and therefore, molecules (proteins, glycoproteins, lipoproteins, etc.) involved in any of those steps are potential virulence factors. Therefore, several virulence factors have already been identified based on *in vivo* and *in vitro* studies and several others are considered potential virulence factors based on genome sequences. A short discussion on this topic follows, but excellent manuscripts on the topic are available.[29,30,62]

Entry into the host cell is mediated by both OmpA and OmpB proteins, both of which are surface exposed and use of monoclonal antibodies against them reduces entry of rickettsiae into the host cells dramatically.[14,16] The role of phospholipase D and hemolysins A and C in phagosomal escape has also been well described.[19,63] Once in the cytoplasm, spotted fever group rickettsiae induce polar actin polymerization via RickA, allowing them to move freely in the cytoplasm and invade neighboring cells.[34,36,64] Factors involved in intracellular survival are probably numerous and examples include InvA, a dinucleoside polyphosphate hydrolase that hydrolyzes toxic dinucleoside oligophosphates within the host cell to produce ATP and therefore favor growth and multiplication.[65,66] An iron-associated superoxide dismutase gene ortholog, *sodB*,[29] was found in *R. typhi* and probably plays a role in neutralizing reactive oxygen intermediates produced in the host cell as part of their response against rickettsial invasion. The molecular machinery necessary for export of proteins outside the bacterium is a sophisticated system that involves several molecules. In rickettsiae, type IV secretion systems play this role and several *virB* orthologs have been found, including inner membrane components (VirB4 and VirB11), periplasmic components (VirB6, VirB8, VirB10), and outer membrane components (VirB3 and VirB9).[29,30] Autotransporters also play a role in moving molecules outside the bacterial cell. As the name implies, proteins are responsible for their own secretion outside the cell. Examples include Sca1-4 and OmpB.[8,29,67]

Rickettsiae are susceptible to few antibiotics including the tetracyclines and chloramphenicol and are highly resistant to beta-lactams and aminoglycosides. Such a narrow susceptibility spectrum is beginning to be understood. A metallo-β-lactamase has been identified in *R. typhi* as well as several penicillin-binding proteins.[29] In addition, multidrug transporters (efflux pumps) have also been found including *emrB*, *bcr*, and 10 other potential ABC transporters. Because of their life cycles, rickettsiae have to adapt to markedly different and sometimes harsh environmental conditions in their arthropod vectors. Such response is called the stringent response and has been studied extensively in other bacteria. Not surprisingly, rickettsiae possess in their genomes several *spoT* genes, Ndk (nucleoside diphosphokinase), and GppA (pppGpp-5′-phosphohydrolase)—all of which play a role in down-regulating transcription and translation by increasing the concentration of GDP 3′-diphosphate and GTP 3′-diphosphate.[29,68]

SUMMARY

Several genes in the published and deposited rickettsial genomes code for proteins with no known function and no matches with other proteins in available databases. Therefore, the potential for research in this area is enormous. With the advent of powerful imaging and molecular techniques, exciting times lay ahead. We now have the capability of genetic manipulation of rickettsiae, eukaryotic cells, and animals in order to perform powerful experiments *in vitro* and *in vivo* to elucidate both the cellular and pathophysiologic alterations leading to the morbidity and mortality associated with these diseases.

ACKNOWLEDGMENTS

This material is based upon work supported by the U.S. Army Research Laboratory and the U.S. Army Research Office under Contract No. DAMD17-02-1-0198.

[*Competing interests statement*: The authors report no competing interests.]

REFERENCES

1. WALKER, D.H., D. RAOULT, J.S. DUMLER, *et al.* 2004. *In* Harrison's Principles of Internal Medicine. Rickettsial Diseases. D.L. Kasper, E. Braunward, A.S. Fauci, *et al.*, Eds.: 999–1008. McGraw-Hill. New York.
2. WALKER, D.H., G.A. VALBUENA & J.P. OLANO. 2003. Pathogenic mechanisms of diseases caused by *Rickettsia*. Ann. NY Acad. Sci. **990:** 1–11.
3. WALKER, D.H. 1997. Endothelial-target rickettsial infection. Lab. Anim. Sci. **47:** 483–485.
4. BATUT, J., S.G. ANDERSSON & D. O'CALLAGHAN. 2004. The evolution of chronic infection strategies in the alpha-proteobacteria. Nat. Rev. Microbiol. **2:** 933–945.
5. KARLBERG, E.O. & S.G. ANDERSSON. 2003. Mitochondrial gene history and mRNA localization: Is there a correlation? Nat. Rev. Genet. **4:** 391–397.
6. ANDERSSON, S.G., O. KARLBERG, B. CANBACK & C.G. KURLAND. 2003. On the origin of mitochondria: a genomics perspective. Philos. Trans. R Soc. Lond. B Biol Sci. **358:** 165–177; discussion 177–179.
7. MULLER, M. & W. MARTIN. 1999. The genome of *Rickettsia prowazekii* and some thoughts on the origin of mitochondria and hydrogenosomes. Bioessays **21:** 377–381.
8. ANDERSSON, S.G., A. ZOMORODIPOUR, J.O. ANDERSSON, *et al.* 1998. The genome sequence of *Rickettsia prowazekii* and the origin of mitochondria. [See comment.] Nature **396:** 133–140.
9. GE, H., Y.Y. CHUANG, S. ZHAO, *et al.* 2003. Genomic studies of *Rickettsia prowazekii* virulent and avirulent strains. Ann. NY Acad. Sci. **990:** 671–677.
10. MARTINEZ, J.J. & P. COSSART. 2005. Identification and characterization of a novel host cell receptor, Ku70, involved in the entry of *Rickettsia conorii* into mammalian cells. Fourth International Conference on Rickettsiae and Rickettsial Diseases, Logrono, Spain, July 18–21, 2005. Trama Impresores SAL.
11. WALKER, D.H. V.L. POPOV & H.M. FENG. 2000. Establishment of a novel endothelial target mouse model of a typhus group rickettsiosis: evidence for critical roles for gamma interferon and CD8 T lymphocytes. Lab. Invest. **80:** 1361–1372.

12. WALKER, D.H. V.L. POPOV, J. WEN & H.M. FENG. 1994. *Rickettsia conorii* infection of C3H/HeN mice. A model of endothelial-target rickettsiosis. Lab. Invest. **70:** 358–368.
13. MARTINEZ, J.J. & P. COSSART. 2004. Early signaling events involved in the entry of *Rickettsia conorii* into mammalian cells. J. Cell Sci. **117:** 5097–5106.
14. LI, H. & D.H. WALKER. 1998. rOmpA is a critical protein for the adhesion of *Rickettsia rickettsii* to host cells. Microb. Pathog. **24:** 289–298.
15. EREMEEVA, M.E., G.A. DASCH & D.J. SILVERMAN. 2000. Interaction of rickettsiae with eukaryotic cells. Adhesion, entry, intracellular growth, and host cell responses. Subcell. Biochem. **33:** 479–516.
16. UCHIYAMA, T. 2003. Adherence to and invasion of Vero cells by recombinant *Escherichia coli* expressing the outer membrane protein rOmpB of *Rickettsia japonica*. Ann. N.Y. Acad. Sci. **990:** 585–590.
17. FENG, H.M., T. WHITWORTH, V. POPOV & D.H. WALKER. 2004. Effect of antibody on the rickettsia-host cell interaction. Infect. Immun. **72:** 3524–3530.
18. LI, H. & D.H. WALKER. 1992. Characterization of rickettsial attachment to host cells by flow cytometry. Infect. Immun. **60:** 2030–2035.
19. RENESTO, P., P. DEHOUX, E. GOUIN, *et al.* 2003. Identification and characterization of a phospholipase D-superfamily gene in rickettsiae. J. Infect. Dis. **188:** 1276–1283.
20. WHITWORTH, T., V.L. POPOV, X.J. YU, *et al.* 2005. Expression of *Rickettsia prowazekii pld* or *tlyC* genes in *Salmonella* induces phagosomal escape. Infect. Immun. **73:** 6668–6673.
21. NILSSON, K., O. LINDQUIST & C. PAHLSON. 1999. Association of *Rickettsia helvetica* with chronic perimyocarditis in sudden cardiac death. Lancet **354:** 1169–1173.
22. NILSSON, K., C. PAHLSON, A. LUKINIUS, *et al.* 2002. Presence of *Rickettsia helvetica* in granulomatous tissue from patients with sarcoidosis. J. Infect. Dis. **185:** 1128–1138.
23. NILSSON, K., A. LIU, C. PAHLSON & O. LINDQUIST. 2005. Demonstration of intracellular microorganisms (*Rickettsia spp.*, *Chlamydia pneumoniae*, *Bartonella spp.*) in pathological human aortic valves by PCR. J. Infect. **50:** 46–52.
24. GREUB, G. & D. RAOULT. 2003. History of the ADP/ATP-translocase-encoding gene, a parasitism gene transferred from a *Chlamydiales* ancestor to plants 1 billion years ago. Appl. Environ. Microbiol. **69:** 5530–5535. [Erratum: Appl. Environ. Microbiol. **70:** 6949.]
25. SCHMITZ-ESSER, S., N. LINKA, A. COLLINGRO, *et al.* 2004. ATP/ADP translocases: a common feature of obligate intracellular amoebal symbionts related to *Chlamydiae* and *Rickettsiae*. J. Bacteriol. **186:** 683–691.
26. AMIRI, H., O. KARLBERG & S.G. ANDERSSON. 2003. Deep origin of plasmid/parasite ATP/ADP translocases. J. Molec. Evol. **56:** 137–150.
27. KOONIN, E.V., K.S. MAKAROVA & L. ARAVIND. 2001. Horizontal gene transfer in prokaryotes: quantification and classification. Annu. Rev. Microbiol. **55:** 709–742.
28. WOESE, C. 1998. The universal ancestor. Proc. Natl. Acad. Sci. USA **95:** 6854–6859.
29. MCLEOD, M.P., X. QIN, S.E. KARPATHY, *et al.* 2004. Complete genome sequence of *Rickettsia typhi* and comparison with sequences of other rickettsiae. J. Bacteriol. **186:** 5842–5855.
30. RENESTO, P., H. OGATA, S. AUDIC, *et al.* 2005. Some lessons from *Rickettsia* genomics. FEMS Microbiol. Rev. **29:** 99–117.
31. HEINZEN, R.A., S.F. HAYES, M.G. PEACOCK & T. HACKSTADT. 1993. Directional actin polymerization associated with spotted fever group *Rickettsia* infection of Vero cells. Infect. Immun. **61:** 1926–1935.
32. TEYSSEIRE, N., C. CHICHE-PORTICHE & D. RAOULT. 1992. Intracellular movements of *Rickettsia conorii* and *R. typhi* based on actin polymerization. Res. Microbiol. **143:** 821–829.
33. HEINZEN, R.A., S.S. GRIESHABER, L.S. VAN KIRK & C.J. DEVIN. 1999. Dynamics of actin-based movement by *Rickettsia rickettsii* in vero cells. Infect. Immun. **67:** 4201–4207.
34. HEINZEN, R.A. 2003. Rickettsial actin-based motility: behavior and involvement of cytoskeletal regulators. Ann. NY Acad. Sci. **990:** 535–547.
35. HARLANDER, R.S., M. WAY, Q. REN, *et al.* 2003. Effects of ectopically expressed neuronal Wiskott-Aldrich syndrome protein domains on *Rickettsia rickettsii* actin-based motility. Infect. Immun. **71:** 1551–1556.

36. JENG, R.L., E.D. GOLEY, J.A. D'ALESSIO, *et al.* 2004. A *Rickettsia* WASP-like protein activates the Arp2/3 complex and mediates actin-based motility. Cell. Microbiol. **6:** 761–769.
37. BREITBACH, K., K. ROTTNER, S. KLOCKE, *et al.* 2003. Actin-based motility of *Burkholderia pseudomallei* involves the Arp 2/3 complex, but not N-WASP and Ena/VASP proteins. Cell. Microbiol. **5:** 385–393.
38. WARD, B.M. & B. MOSS. 2001. *Vaccinia* virus intracellular movement is associated with microtubules and independent of actin tails. J. Virol. **75:** 11651–11663.
39. STAMM, L.M., J.H. MORISAKI, L.Y. GAO, *et al.* 2003. *Mycobacterium marinum* escapes from phagosomes and is propelled by actin-based motility. J. Exp. Med. **198:** 1361–1368.
40. GOLDBERG, M.B. 2001. Actin-based motility of intracellular microbial pathogens. Microbiol. Molec. Biol. Rev. **65:** 595–626.
41. CUDMORE, S., P. COSSART, G. GRIFFITHS & M. WAY. 1995. Actin-based motility of vaccinia virus. Nature **378:** 636–638.
42. SILVERMAN, D.J. & L.A. SANTUCCi. 1988. Potential for free radical-induced lipid peroxidation as a cause of endothelial cell injury in Rocky Mountain spotted fever. Infect. Immun. **56:** 3110–3115.
43. SANTUCCI, L.A., P.L. GUTIERREZ & D.J. SILVERMAN. 1992. *Rickettsia rickettsii* induces superoxide radical and superoxide dismutase in human endothelial cells. Infect. Immun. **60:** 5113–5118.
44. EREMEEVA, M.E. & D.J. SILVERMAN. 1998. Effects of the antioxidant alpha-lipoic acid on human umbilical vein endothelial cells infected with *Rickettsia rickettsii*. Infect. Immun. **66:** 2290–2299.
45. HONG, J.E., L.A. SANTUCCI, X. TIAN & D.J. SILVERMAN. 1998. Superoxide dismutase-dependent, catalase-sensitive peroxides in human endothelial cells infected by *Rickettsia rickettsii*. Infect. Immun. **66:** 1293–1298.
46. RYDKINA, E., S.K. SAHNI, L.A. SANTUCCI, *et al.* 2004. Selective modulation of antioxidant enzyme activities in host tissues during *Rickettsia conorii* infection. Microb. Pathog. **36:** 293–301.
47. CLIFTON, D.R., E. RYDKINA, R.S. FREEMAN & S.K. SAHNI. 2005. NF-kappaB activation during *Rickettsia rickettsii* infection of endothelial cells involves the activation of catalytic IkappaB kinases IKKalpha and IKKbeta and phosphorylation-proteolysis of the inhibitor protein IkappaBalpha. Infect. Immun. **73:** 155–165.
48. CLIFTON, D.R., R.A. GOSS, S.K. SAHNI, *et al.* 1998. NF-kappa B-dependent inhibition of apoptosis is essential for host cell survival during *Rickettsia rickettsii* infection. Proc. Natl. Acad. Sci. USA **95:** 4646–4651.
49. SPORN, L.A., S.K. SAHNI, N.B. LERNER, *et al.* 1997. *Rickettsia rickettsii* infection of cultured human endothelial cells induces NF-kappaB activation. Infect. Immun. **65:** 2786–2791.
50. JOSHI, S.G., C.W. FRANCIS, D.J. SILVERMAN & S.K. SAHNI. 2004. NF-kappaB activation suppresses host cell apoptosis during *Rickettsia rickettsii* infection via regulatory effects on intracellular localization or levels of apoptogenic and anti-apoptotic proteins. FEMS Microbiol. Lett. **234:** 333–341.
51. FENG, H.M. & D.H. WALKER. 2000. Mechanisms of intracellular killing of *Rickettsia conorii* in infected human endothelial cells, hepatocytes, and macrophages. Infect. Immun. **68:** 6729–6736.
52. WALKER, D.H. & J.S. DUMLER. 1997. Rickettsial infections. *In* Pathology of Infectious Diseases. E.E. Lack, Ed.: 789–799. Appleton & Lange, Inc. Stamford, CT.
53. WALKER, D.H. 1998. Rocky Mountain spotted fever and other rickettsioses. *In* Mechanisms of Microbial Disease. G. Medoff, Eds.: 268–274. Williams & Wilkins. Baltimore.
54. LUM, H. & A.B. MALIK. 1996. Mechanisms of increased endothelial permeability. Can. J. Physiol. Pharmacol. **74:** 787–800.
55. GEORGE, F., P. BROUQUI, M.C. BOFFA, *et al.* 1993. Demonstration of *Rickettsia conorii*–induced endothelial injury *in vivo* by measuring circulating endothelial cells, thrombomodulin, and von Willebrand factor in patients with Mediterranean spotted fever. [See comment.] Blood **82:** 2109–2116.

56. KOO, P., M.E. WOODS & J.P. OLANO. 2005. *In vitro* studies of microvascular permeability during *Rickettsia rickettsii* infections. Fourth International Conference on Rickettsiae and Rickettsial Diseases, Logrono, Spain, 2005. Trama Impresores, S.A.L.
57. DAVI, G., C. GIAMMARRESI, S.VIGNERI, *et al.* 1995. Demonstration of *Rickettsia conorii*–induced coagulative and platelet activation *in vivo* in patients with Mediterranean spotted fever. Thromb. Haemost. **74:** 631–634.
58. DAVIDSON, M.G., E.B. BREITSCHWERDT, D.H. WALKER, *et al.* 1990. Vascular permeability and coagulation during *Rickettsia rickettsii* infection in dogs. Am. J. Vet. Res. **51:** 165–170.
59. RACHEK, L.I., A.M. TUCKER, H.H. WINKLER & D.O. WOOD. 1998. Transformation of *Rickettsia prowazekii* to rifampin resistance. J. Bacteriol. **180:** 2118–v2124. [Erratum: J. Bacteriol. 1998. **180:** 4015.]
60. RACHEK, L.I., A. HINES, A.M. TUCKER, *et al.* 2000. Transformation of *Rickettsia prowazekii* to erythromycin resistance encoded by the Escherichia coli *ereB* gene. J. Bacteriol. **182:** 3289–3291.
61. SIMSER, J.A., M.S. RAHMAN, S. DREHER-LESNIC & A.F. AZAD. 2005. *Rickettsia peacockii* transposon, ISRpe1 and disruption of the *rickA* and *sca1*. Fourth International Conference on Rickettsiae and Rickettsial Diseases, Logrono, Spain, 2005. Trama Impresores, SAL.
62. CHAO, C.C., D. CHELIUS, T. ZHANG, *et al.* 2004. Proteome analysis of Madrid E strain of *Rickettsia prowazekii*. Proteomics **4:** 1280–1292.
63. WHITWORTH, T., V.L. POPOV, X.J. YU, *et al.* 2005. Expression of *Rickettsia prowazekii pld* or *tlyC* genes in Salmonella mediates phagosomal escape. Infect. Immun. **73:** 6668–6673.
64. GOUIN, E., C. EGILE, P. DEHOUX, *et al.* 2004. The RickA protein of *Rickettsia conorii* activates the Arp2/3 complex. [See comment.] Nature **427:** 457–461.
65. GAYWEE, J., S. RADULOVIC, J.A. HIGGINS & A.F. AZAD. 2002. Transcriptional analysis of *Rickettsia prowazekii* invasion gene homolog (*invA*) during host cell infection. Infect. Immun. **70:** 6346–6354. [Erratum: Infect. Immun. **71:** 1031.]
66. GAYWEE, J., W. XU, S. RADULOVIC, *et al.* 2002. The *Rickettsia prowazekii* invasion gene homolog (invA) encodes a Nudix hydrolase active on adenosine (5′)-pentaphospho-(5′)-adenosine. Mol. Cell Proteomics **1:** 179–185.
67. OGATA, H., S. AUDIC, P. RENESTO-AUDIFFREN, *et al.* 2001. Mechanisms of evolution in *Rickettsia conorii* and *R. prowazekii*. [See comment.] Science **293:** 2093–2098.
68. OGATA, H., P. RENESTO, S. AUDIC, *et al.* 2005. The genome sequence of *Rickettsia felis* identifies the first putative conjugative plasmid in an obligate intracellular parasite. PLoS Biol. **3:** e248.

The Presence of Eschars, but Not Greater Severity, in Portuguese Patients Infected with Israeli Spotted Fever

RITA DE SOUSA,[a] NAHED ISMAIL,[b] SÓNIA DÓRIA-NÓBREGA,[c] PEDRO COSTA,[d] TIAGO ABREU,[e] ANA FRANÇA,[f] MÁRIO AMARO,[f] PAULA PROENÇA,[g] PAULA BRITO,[h] JOSÉ POÇAS,[h] TERESA RAMOS,[i] GRAÇA CRISTINA,[d] GRAÇA POMBO,[i] LILIANA VITORINO,[j] JORGE TORGAL,[k] FÁTIMA BACELLAR,[a] AND DAVID WALKER[b]

[a]*Centro de Estudos de Vectores e Doenças Infecciosas (CEVDI), National Institute of Health Dr. Ricardo Jorge, Águas de Moura, Portugal*

[b]*Department of Pathology, University of Texas Medical Branch, Galveston, Texas, USA*

[c]*Hospital Amadora-Sintra, Sintra, Portugal*

[d]*Centro Hospitalar do Baixo Alentejo SA, Beja, Portugal*

[e]*Hospital do Espiríto Santo-Évora, Évora, Portugal*

[f]*Hospital Garcia de Orta SA, Almada, Portugal*

[g]*Hospital Distrital de Faro, Faro, Portugal*

[h]*Hospital São Bernardo SA, Setúbal, Portugal*

[i]*Hospital Distrital de Bragança SA, Bragança, Portugal*

[j]*Centro de Genética e Biologia Molecular, Faculdade de Ciências da Universidade de Lisboa, Lisboa, Portugal*

[k]*Departamento de Saúde Pública, Faculdade de Ciências Médicas de Lisboa, Lisboa, Portugal*

ABSTRACT: **In Portugal, Mediterranean spotted fever (MSF) is caused by *R. conorii* Malish and Israeli spotted fever (ISF) strains. It has been suggested that the ISF strain isolated from patients with MSF causes different clinical manifestations compared to those caused by Malish strain, namely the absence of eschar and greater severity. The aim of this study was to analyze the presence or absence of eschar and of fatality in Portuguese patients infected with either Malish or ISF strain. Of 94 patients with a clinical diagnosis of MSF between 1994 to 2004, 47 were infected with Malish strain and 47 with ISF strain. Eschars were reported in 20 patients (49%) infected with Malish strain, and in 17 (39%) with ISF strain. The presence of eschar is not statistically associated to a greater extent with either *R. conorii* strain (*P*=0.346). A total of 22 patients died, 9 infected with Malish strain and 13 infected with ISF strain, and no statistically significant difference was found (*P*=0.330). This study showed that the concepts of absence of the eschar and greater severity in Israeli spotted fever infection should be revised.**

Address for correspondence: Rita de Sousa, Centro de Estudos de Vectores e Doenças Infecciosas (CEVDI), National Institute of Health Dr Ricardo Jorge, Av Liberdade 5, 2965-575 Águas de Moura, Portugal. Voice: +351 265 912 222, fax: +351 265 912 568.
rita.sousa@insa.min-saude.pt

Ann. N.Y. Acad. Sci. 1063: 197–202 (2005).
doi: 10.1196/annals.1355.032

Keywords: ***Rickettsia conorii*; Mediterranean spotted fever; Israeli spotted fever strain; eschars**

INTRODUCTION

Mediterranean spotted fever (MSF) is an acute, febrile tick-borne rickettsiosis caused by *Rickettsia conorii* complex strains. During the past 30 years, different strains of this complex have been isolated from humans and ticks. Although they have some genotypic and phenotypic differences, they are considered the same species.[1] In Portugal, two strains causing MSF, *R. conorii* Malish and ISF strains, were isolated from humans and ticks. The latter strain was isolated in 1997 for the first time in Portugal from patient's blood, whereas previously it had only been found to be present in Israel and Sicily.[2–4] Since 1997, with the isolation of ISF strain, coincidentally or not, an apparent increase of severity of MSF occurred. During the last decade, the number of hospitalizations has increased from fewer than 200 cases per year to more than 400 cases annually.[5] Moreover, the two studies performed in 1997 at the two main hospitals where the severe and fatal cases occurred showed that delayed initiation of appropriate treatment and the co-morbidity condition diabetes were risk factors for severe and fatal outcome, but it was not possible to correlate the severity and fatality with the infective strain.[6,7] It was considered a hypothesis that the ISF strain isolated from patients with MSF causes different or atypical clinical manifestations compared to those caused by *R. conorii* Malish strain, that could lead to a late clinical diagnosis and consequently delay treatment thus leading to a higher number of severe cases. Some authors have reported the absence of eschar and greater severity in patients infected with the ISF strain.[8] Considering these ideas, our aim was to compare the presence or absence of eschar and other clinical features such as fever and rash and the outcome in Portuguese patients infected with either *R. conorii* Malish or ISF strains.

MATERIALS AND METHODS

Samples and Data Collection

Heparinized blood samples and skin biopsies were collected from patients with a clinical diagnosis of MSF during the period from 1994 to 2004. Samples were provided from seven hospitals and sent to Centro de Estudos de Vectores e Doenças Infecciosas (CEVDI) under adequate conditions of refrigeration. The clinical data, age, gender, date of admission to hospital, and clinical signs (fever, rash, eschar) were recorded and analyzed.

Isolation and PCR Detection

The identification of the causative rickettsial strain was established by isolation of the organisms from blood or by PCR on skin biopsies. Isolation of rickettsiae was performed by shell-vial technique as described previously.[9] DNA extracted from each positive culture was tested by PCR using all the primers described by Regnery and colleagues, targeting the following rickettsial genes: *gltA* and *ompA* (a major outer membrane protein). For skin biopsies, a nested-PCR protocol employed external primers CS 415 (5′-GCTATTATGCTTGCGGCTGT-3′) and CS1220 (5′-TGCATTTCTTTCCATTGTGC-3′) and internal primers Rp877p and Rp1258p, which amplify a fragment of *gltA*. For *ompA* Rr190.70p and 190.602n were used as external primers and ompA FW1 (5′-CGCAGCGATAATGCTGAGTA) and ompA RV2 (CACCAAAACCATGATTTGCAG) as internal primers.[10] PCR products were purified by a MiniElute PCR Purification Kit (Qiagen) and sequenced using BigDye terminator cycle sequencing Ready Reaction kit (Applied Biosystems) according to the manufacturer's instructions. Sequences were identified using BLAST software.

Statistical Analysis

Exploratory data analysis was performed by using tables of frequencies and central tendency and dispersion measures for continuous variables. The association between clinical signs and *R. conorii* strains was assessed using the χ^2 test or Fisher's exact test. Student's *t* test was used to compare mean values among strain groups. Mann-Whitney test was used when continuous variables did not show a Gaussian distribution. Statistical analysis was performed using Stata 8.0 software (Stata Press, Texas, USA).

RESULTS

Of 94 patients admitted between January of 1994 and December of 2004 with a clinical diagnosis of MSF, 63 patients had a laboratory-confirmed diagnosis by isolation of *R. conorii* from blood, and 31 patients were diagnosed by PCR on skin biopsies. Forty-seven patients were infected with *R. conorii* Malish strain and 47 with ISF strain. The clinical data analyzed and compared by group of patients infected with *R. conorii* Malish strain or ISF strain showed that the median age for *R. conorii* Malish patients was 64 years and for ISF patients 59 years, with no statistical differences between groups (P=0.304). There was no statistically significant association between gender and infecting strain. Most of the patients were admitted during summer, and the median week of hospitalization for both groups of patients occurred during the 32nd week corresponding to the month of August.

The MSF clinical manifestations analyzed according to the patients' infecting strain are listed in TABLE 1. Fever was present in 82 of the 87 patients with documented body temperature. In the group of patients infected with *R. conorii* Malish strain, 40 (95%) had a documented fever, while 42 (93%) patients infected with ISF strain had fever. No statistically significant association was found in the occurrence of fever (P=0.639) by strain group. The mean patients' temperatures at hospital admission were very similar; for the *R. conorii* Malish group, patients presented with a mean temperature of 38.5°C and ISF group, 38.7°C, with no statistically significant difference (P=0.552) by strain group. Rash was documented in 86 of 89 patients with available data, while 3 patients did not have rash (one was infected with *R. conorii* Malish strain, and 2 patients were infected with ISF strain). Rash was present in 42 (89%) *R. conorii* Malish strain–infected patients and in 44 (94%) of patients infected with ISF strain. In 85 patients with available data, eschars were reported in 37 patients; 20 (49%) of patients infected with *R. conorii* Malish strain had an es-

TABLE 1. MSF clinical manifestations and outcome analyzed according to the patients' infecting strain

Clinical Signs		*R. conorii* Malish *N* (%)	Israeli Spotted Fever Strain *N* (%)	*P* Value
Fever	Yes	40 (95%)	42(93%)	*P*=0.639
	No	2 (5%)	3 (7%)	
Rash	Yes	42 (98%)	44 (96%)	*P*=0.516
	No	1 (2%)	2 (4%)	
Eschar	Yes	20 (49%)	17 (39%)	*P*=0.346
	No	21 (51%)	27 (61%)	
Outcome	Alive	38 (81%)	34 (72%)	*P*=0.330
	Dead	9 (19%)	13 (28%)	

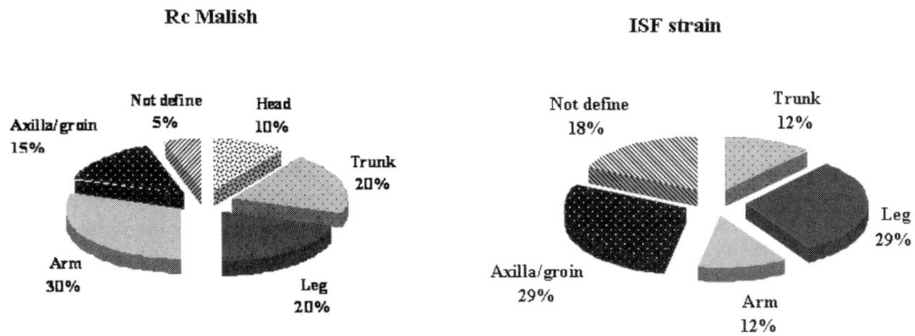

FIGURE 1. Eschar localization by strain.

char, and 17 (39%) of patients with ISF strain. There was no statistically significant association between the presence of an eschar and patients' strain (*P*=0.346). The eschar was found in different parts of the body, such as head, trunk, arm, leg, axilla, and groin, and the distribution was similar in both groups of infected patients (FIG. 1).

The outcome of 94 patients infected with *R. conorii* did not differ significantly between the group of patients infected with *R. conorii* Malish strain and ISF strain (*P*=0.330). Fatal cases occurred in 22 patients, 9 infected with *R. conorii* Malish strain and 13 infected with ISF strain. The comparison by age and outcome did not show statistically significant differences (*P*=0.448) in patients who died with *R conorii* Malish (median age, 63 years) and with ISF strain (median age, 62 years) (FIG. 2).

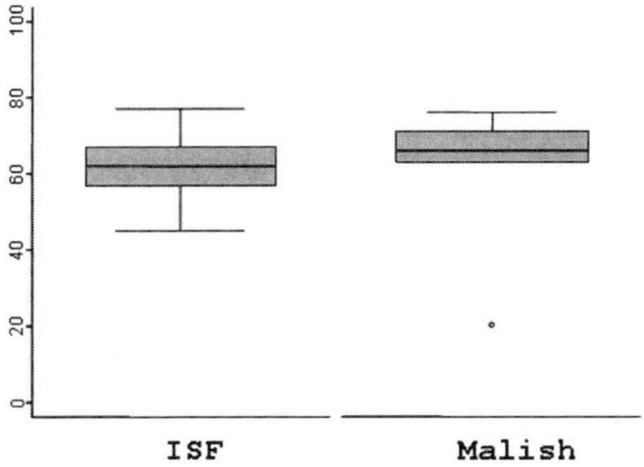

FIGURE 2. Age and outcome in dead patients by strain.

DISCUSSION

The main conclusion of this study is that the triad of fever, rash, and eschar has the same frequency of occurrence in patients infected with *R. conorii* Malish strain or ISF strain, and it is impossible to predict the *R. conorii* strain on clinical grounds.

In this study, it was noteworthy that there was no evidence of an association between presence or absence of eschar in either strain group of Portuguese patients, in contrast with most cases reported from Israel, where a typical eschar is rare or absent in patients infected with ISF.[11] Nevertheless, we could suggest that the contradictory results could be due to differing host responses in different populations (such as children and adults), as the majority of data from Israel is from children and the Portuguese series includes more adults. The identification of the tick bite site is sometimes problematic. The eschar could be hidden in a part of the body such as the axilla, scalp, groin, palpebra, or submammary fold, and it is often difficult for the doctor to detect the eschar because all of the clothes may not be removed for a complete examination of the skin. It was also corroborated that the different strains have the same seasonality as the vector *Rhipicephalus sanguineus* for both strains.

In this study, fatality rates were similar for patients infected with Malish strain and ISF strain, and host factors are probably the most important risk factors for death. This is a large series and is the best evaluation of the comparison of severity for Malish and ISF strains. This fact contrasts with the report of European Society of Clinical Microbiology and Infectious Diseases that described the ISF infections having less than a 1% case fatality rate.[12]

ACKNOWLEDGMENTS

We thank Lígia Cheinho, Teresa Vilares, and Paulo Parreira for technical support.

[*Conflict of interest statement:* The authors of this research declare that they have no conflict of interest.]

REFERENCES

1. WALKER, D.H. *et al.* 1995. Comparative antigenic analysis of spotted fever group rickettsiae from Israel and other closely related organisms. Am. J. Trop. Med. Hyg. **52:** 569–576.
2. BACELLAR, F. *et al.* 1999. Israeli spotted fever rickettsia (*Rickettsia conorii* complex) associated with humam diseases in Portugal. Emerg. Infect. Dis **5:** 835–836.
3. GOLDWASSER, R.A. *et al.* 1974. The isolation of strains of rickettsiae of the spotted fever group in Israel and their differentiation from another members of the group by immunofluorescence methods. Scand. J. Infect. Dis. **6:** 53–62.
4. GIAMMANCO, G. *et al.* 2003. Israeli spotted fever rickettsia in Sicilian *Rhipicephalus sanguineus* ticks. Emerg. Infect. Dis. **9:** 892–893.
5. SOUSA, R.& F. BACELLAR. 2004. Morb-Mortalidade por *R. conorii* em Portugal. Rev. Bras. Parasitol. Vet. **13:** 180–183.
6. AMARO, M. *et al.* 2003. Report of eight cases of fatal and severe Mediterranean spotted fever in Portugal. Ann. N.Y. Acad. Sci. **990:** 331–343.
7. SOUSA, R., *et al.* 2003. Mediterranean spotted fever in Portugal: risk factors for fatal outcome in 105 hospitalized patients. Ann. N.Y. Acad. Sci. **990:** 285–294.
8. YAGUPSKY, P. & B. WOLACH. 1993. Fatal Israeli spotted fever in children. Clin. Infect. Dis. **17:** 850–853.
9. MARRERO, M. & D. RAOULT. 1989. Centrifugation-shell vial technique for rapid detection of Mediterranean spotted fever rickettsia in blood culture. Am. J. Trop. Med. Hyg. **40:** 197–199.
10. REGNERY, R. *et al.* 1991. Genotypic identification of rickettsiae and estimation of inter-species sequence divergence for portions of two rickettsial genes. J. Bacteriol. **173:** 1576-1589.
11. GROSS, E. & P. YAGUPSKY. 1987. Israeli rickettsial spotted fever in children: a review of 54 cases. Acta Trop. **44:** 91–96.
12. BROUQUI, P. *et al.* 2004. Guidelines for the diagnosis of tick-borne bacterial diseases in Europe. Clin. Microbiol. Infect. **10:** 1108–1132.

Similarities and Differences in Host Cell Signaling following Infection with Different *Rickettsia* Species

ELENA RYDKINA,[a] DAVID J. SILVERMAN,[b] AND SANJEEV K. SAHNI[a]

[a]*Hematology-Oncology Unit, Department of Medicine, University of Rochester School of Medicine and Dentistry, Rochester, New York 14642, USA*

[b]*Department of Microbiology and Immunology, University of Maryland School of Medicine, Baltimore, Maryland 21201, USA*

ABSTRACT: Signaling interactions between vascular endothelium and invading rickettsiae provide a unique way of coordinating appropriate physiologic responses, which are important determinants of the ensuing pathogenesis mechanisms such as host defense and inflammation. Two major subgroups of pathogenic *Rickettsia* species, namely the typhus group (TG) and the spotted fever group (SFG), exhibit marked differences in their intracytoplasmic behavior. Using *in vitro* infection of cultured human endothelial cells with *R. rickettsii*, the causative agent of Rocky Mountain SF, we previously identified activation of NF-κB and p38 MAP kinase as essential components of intracellular signaling events responsible for *Rickettsia*-induced transcriptional activation. Our data also suggest that p38 activity does not contribute to NF-κB response, implicating involvement of independent upstream signaling pathways. Since divergent cytopathologies suggest potentially different interactions with host cells, the aim of this study was to compare these responses after endothelial cell infection with *R. conorii*, the agent of Mediterranean SF, and a TG representative *R. typhi*, the agent of endemic typhus.

KEYWORDS: *Rickettsia*; endothelial cells; nuclear factor-κB (NF-κB); mitogen activated protein (MAP) kinase; p38 kinase

INTRODUCTION

Rickettsiae are obligatory intracellular and gram-negative bacteria, which use endothelial cells (EC) as the primary target of *in vivo* infection causing febrile illness in their mammalian hosts.[1] Signaling interactions between vascular endothelium and invading rickettsiae provide a unique way of coordinating appropriate physiologic responses, which are important determinants of the ensuing pathogenesis mechanisms such as host defense and inflammation. Two major subgroups of pathogenic *Rickettsia* species, namely the typhus group (TG) and the spotted fever group (SFG),

Address for correspondence: Elena Rydkina, Ph.D., Department of Medicine: Hematology-Oncology Unit, P.O. Box 610, University of Rochester School of Medicine and Dentistry, Rochester, NY 14642. Voice: 585-275-1043; fax: 585-473-4314.
yelena_rydkina@urmc.rochester.edu

Ann. N.Y. Acad. Sci. 1063: 203–206 (2005).
doi: 10.1196/annals.1355.030

exhibit marked differences in their intracytoplasmic behavior. For example, SFG organisms are known to exploit actin-based motility for intracellular movement and intercellular spread, but TG rickettsiae display either short (*R. typhi*) or no (*R. prowazekii*) actin tails.[2]

A majority of genes expressed by EC in response to inflammatory mediators are regulated by nuclear factor-kappa B (NF-κB).[3] Another set of mechanisms that coordinate signals originating from intracellular and extracellular mediators converge to activate specific mitogen-activated protein (MAP) kinase cascades, the downstream effects of which include the regulation of proteins with diverse cellular functions such as protein kinases, cytoskeletal proteins, and transcription factors like NF-κB.[4] Using *in vitro* infection of cultured human EC with *R. rickettsii*, the causative agent of Rocky Mountain SF, we have previously identified activation of NF-κB and p38 MAP kinase as essential components of intracellular signaling events responsible for *Rickettsia*-induced transcriptional activation.[5,6] Our data also suggest that p38 activity does not contribute to NF-κB response, implicating involvement of independent upstream signaling pathways.[6] Since divergent cytopathologies suggest potentially different interactions with host cells, the aim of this study was to compare these responses after EC infection with *R. conorii*, the agent of Mediterranean SF, and a TG representative *R. typhi*, the agent of endemic typhus.

EC were cultured and infected with different *Rickettsia* species as described previously.[5,6] Viability of *R. conorii* (Malish strain) and *R. typhi* (Wilmington) stocks was determined by plaque assay.[6] These results were confirmed by real-time PCR using primers Rp877p–Rp1258n for *gltA* gene of *Rickettsia* species[8] and an internal probe (TaqMan) with 100% homology to the target gene.

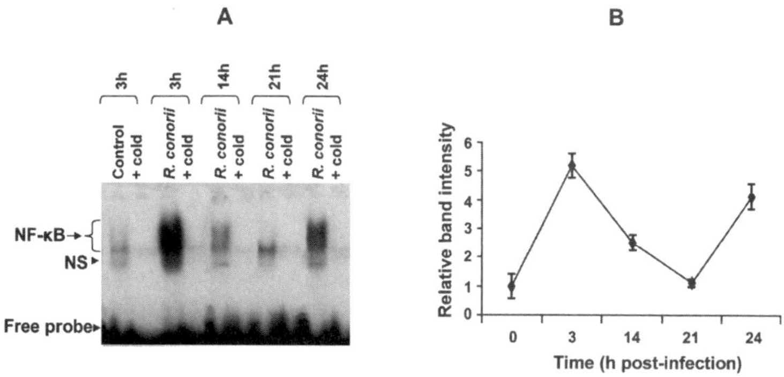

FIGURE 1. Kinetics of *R. conorii*–induced NF-κB activation. EC were incubated with culture medium alone (Control) or with *R. conorii* (~6×10^4 pfu/cm^2) for 3, 14, 21, and 24 h. (**A**) Gel-shift assays using nuclear proteins and γ-[^{32}P]-ATP-labeled consensus NF-κB sequence were performed according to previously published procedures.[5,6] Specificity of the shifted NF-κB complex was demonstrated by inclusion of 10-fold molar excess of unlabeled oligonucleotide (+cold) during DNA-protein binding. (**B**) Quantitiative densitometric analysis of NF-κB response during *R. conorii* infection as a function of time. The values are presented as mean ± standard error of a minimum of three independent experiments. For comparative purposes, the basal levels in uninfected EC (Control) were assigned a value of 1.

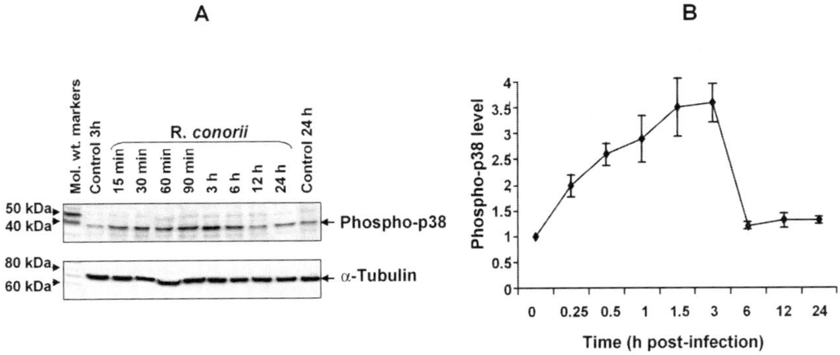

FIGURE 2. *R. conorii*–induced p38 MAP kinase activation. (**A**) Western blot analysis using cellular protein lysates from uninfected controls and infected EC at different times was carried out as described.[6] The results of a representative experiment are shown. (**B**) The quantitative values from volume analysis are presented as mean ± standard error ($N = 3$). For calculations, the average baseline level of p38 phosphorylation in uninfected EC (Control) at 3 and 24 h was assigned a value of 1.

As a marker of activation, DNA-binding activity of NF-κB was monitored by electrophoretic mobility shift assay. Similar to *R. rickettsii*,[5] *R. conorii* infection resulted in a biphasic activation of NF-κB with an early increase in DNA-binding activity (3 h), followed by a later peak at about 24 h (FIG. 1). Antibody supershift assay revealed that activated NF-κB complex was composed of p65-p50 heterodimers and p50 homodimers (not shown). A preliminary study with *R. typhi*, however, indicated only an early activation of NF-κB at 3 h. As for *R. rickettsii* and *R. conorii*, the activated NF-κB species were made of p65-p50 heterodimers and p50 homodimers.

By immunoblotting, we next determined the phosphorylation status of p38 MAPK as an indicator of its activation. The intensity (an average of threefold induction) and time course (maximal response at 1.5–3 h) of increased p38 phosphorylation for *R. conorii* were similar to that of *R. rickettsi*[6] (FIG. 2: A, B). Initial evidence further suggested that *R. typhi* infection of EC triggered somewhat delayed p38 response peaking at about 6 h post-infection. Thus, both spotted fever and typhus species utilize apparently similar signaling mechanisms for endothelial activation, but the intensity and kinetics of host cell responses exhibit distinct variations depending on their intracytoplasmic characteristics.

ACKNOWLEDGMENTS

We thankfully acknowledge the National Institute of Allergy and Infectious Diseases, National Institutes of Health, for financial support through Research Grant AI 40689, and Semion Kiriakidi for excellent technical assistance.

[*Conflict of interest statement:* The authors of this research declare that they have no conflict of interest.]

REFERENCES

1. Walker, D.H. 2004. Ricketts creates rickettsiology, the study of vector-borne obligatory intracellular bacteria. J. Infect. Dis. **189:** 938–955.
2. Heinzen, R.A. 2003. Rickettsial actin-based motility: behavior and involvement of cytoskeletal regulators. Ann. N.Y. Acad. Sci. **990:** 535–547.
3. Yamamoto, Y. & R.B. Gaynor. 2004. IκB kinases: key regulators of the NF-κB pathway. Trends Biochem. Sci. **29:** 72–79.
4. Cowan, K.J. & K.B. Storey. 2003. Mitogen activated protein kinases: new signaling pathways functioning in cellular responses to environmental stress. J. Exp. Biol. **206:** 1107–1115.
5. Clifton, D.R., E. Rydkina, R.S. Freeman & S.K. Sahni. 2005. NF-κB activation during *Rickettsia rickettsii* infection of endothelial cells involves the activation of catalytic IκB kinases IKKα and IKKβ and phosphorylation-proteolysis of the inhibitor protein IκBα. Infect. Immun. **73:** 155–165.
6. Rydkina, E., D.J. Silverman & S.K. Sahni. 2005. Selective activation of p38 stress-activated protein kinase during *Rickettsia rickettsii* infection of human endothelial cells: role in the induction of chemokine response. Cell. Microbiol. **7:** 1519–1530.
7. Roux, V., E. Rydkina, M. Eremeeva & D. Raoult. 1997. Citrate synthase gene comparison, a new tool for phylogenetic analysis and its application for the *Rickettsiae*. Int. J. System. Bacteriol. **47:** 252–261.

Potential Roles for Regulatory Oxygenases in Rickettsial Pathogenesis

SANJEEV K. SAHNI,[a] ELENA RYDKINA,[a] ABHA SAHNI,[a] SURESH G. JOSHI,[a] AND DAVID J. SILVERMAN[b]

[a]*Hematology-Oncology Unit, Department of Medicine, University of Rochester School of Medicine and Dentistry, Rochester, New York 14642, USA*

[b]*Department of Microbiology and Immunology, University of Maryland School of Medicine, Baltimore, Maryland 21201, USA*

ABSTRACT: Clinical and experimental evidence suggests an important role for oxidative stress and associated cellular defense mechanisms in the pathogenesis of vasculopathic rickettsioses. Our laboratory has reported that *R. rickettsii* infection of endothelial cells *in vitro* induces the expression of HO-1, the inducible isoform of the antioxidant defense enzyme heme oxygenase. HO-1 plays a critical role in maintaining the integrity of the vasculature and controls the functioning of the cyclooxygenase (COX) system. This study was undertaken to investigate the expression of COX and HO isozymes during *in vitro* infection of EC with two major representatives of spotted fever group *Rickettsia* species. The mRNA expression of COX-2 was significantly increased in endothelial cells infected with *R. rickettsii* and *R. conorii*, while that of COX-1 remained unaffected. Western blot analysis using total protein lysates from infected endothelial cells and corresponding uninfected controls further confirmed specific induction of COX-2 in response to infection. ELISA measurements on culture supernatants also suggested enhanced secretion of 6-keto $PGF_{1\alpha}$ (stable hydrolysis product of PGI_2 and PGE_2. As a functional consequence of HO-1 upregulation, increased expression of the iron storage protein ferritin following *R. rickettsii* and *R. conorii* infection was also evident. Since products of HO-1 and COX-2 reactions govern a variety of physiologically important functions in the vasculature, further studies to define their regulation in the host cell should provide useful insights into the pathogenesis of rickettsial diseases.

KEYWORDS: cyclooxygenase; endothelial cells; heme oxygenase; *Rickettsia* species; transcriptional regulators

INTRODUCTION

Accruing evidence from *in vitro* and *in vivo* models of infection as well as from patients diagnosed with spotted fever or typhus group rickettsiosis implicates induction of oxidative stress and adaptive regulation of host's superoxide-scavenging and

Address for correspondence: Sanjeev K. Sahni, Hematology-Oncology Unit, Department of Medicine, Box 610, University of Rochester Medical Center, 601 Elmwood Avenue, Rochester, NY 14642. Voice: 585-275-0439; fax: 585-473-4314.
sanjeev_sahni@urmc.rochester.edu

Ann. N.Y. Acad. Sci. 1063: 207–214 (2005).
doi: 10.1196/annals.1355.033

other antioxidant defense mechanisms as one of the major determinants of rickettsial pathogenesis.[1–5] During the last decade, there has also been a growing body of literature documenting the importance of the heme oxygenase (HO) enzyme system in the maintenance of crucial vascular functions and overall integrity of the vasculature. Although the conventional role for HO enzymes, of which HO-1 is highly inducible in many cell types and HO-2 and HO-3 are constitutive, is to catalyze the rate-limiting step in the metabolism of cellular heme to biliverdin, it is becoming increasingly evident that HO converts heme to biologically active products such as biliverdin, bilirubin, ferritin, and carbon monoxide (CO), all of which are capable of modulating crucial cellular functions.[6] More recently described biologic functions of endothelial HO or its reaction products, including regulation of cyclooxygenase (COX) function[7] and control of cell apoptosis[8,9] lend further support to this notion. The most compelling evidence for critically important effects of HO-1 on vascular pathophysiology, however, comes from the description of the first known human case of genetic HO-1 deficiency leading to persistent hemolytic anemia, which is characterized by intravascular hemolysis, abnormal coagulation and/or fibrinolysis with elevated thrombomodulin and von Willebrand factor, severe and persistent endothelial damage, detachment of endothelium in renal glomeruli, and iron deposition in renal and hepatic tissues.[10]

COX isozymes convert arachidonic acid to prostaglandins (PGs) and thromboxanes via PG biosynthetic pathways. Two major isoforms of COX are commonly known as COX-1 and COX-2. While resting cells produce COX-2 at very low levels, its expression is highly induced by pro-inflammatory mediators, mitogenic factors, and stress conditions. COX-1, on the other hand, primarily serves housekeeping functions in many normal physiologic processes.[11] It has also been suggested that induction of oxidative stress and increased expression of COX-2 may be mechanistically linked and we have previously demonstrated that infection of endothelial cells (EC) with *R. rickettsii* triggers the expression of HO-1.[12] In this study, we have conducted simultaneous analysis of the status of COX and HO isoforms during *in vitro* EC infection with *R. rickettsii* and *R. conorii*—two major species of spotted fever rickettsiae known to cause Rocky Mountain spotted fever (RMSF) and Mediterranean SF, respectively. We have also investigated the mRNA expression of the iron-sequestering protein ferritin and the pattern of secretion of prostaglandins by host cells in response to infection. A brief discussion of potential physiological roles of important vasoactive mediators generated as a result of activation of specific isozymes of regulatory oxygenases in determining the pathogenesis of human rickettsial infections is also provided.

MATERIALS AND METHODS

Cell Culture and Infection

Primary cultures of human umbilical vein EC were established and grown as described previously.[12] *R. rickettsii* (Sheila Smith strain) and *R. conorii* (Malish 7) were obtained by lysing heavily infected Vero cells and subsequent purification via density-gradient centrifugation. The titers of infectious stocks were determined by plaque assay.[4] Endothelial cells at passage 2 and 80–90% confluence were infected with about 6×10^4 plaque forming units (pfu) for every cm^2 of culture area.

RNA Isolation, cDNA Probes, and Steady-State mRNA Expression

Total RNA from infected cells and corresponding uninfected controls was isolated and tested for integrity/purity by spectral analysis and ethidium bromide staining on agarose gels. Analysis of mRNA expression of specific genes was carried out by Northern hybridization using an experimental protocol optimized in our laboratory.[13] The double-stranded cDNA probes specific for the coding regions of human COX-1 and COX-2 were obtained from Cayman Chemical Co. (Ann Arbor, MI), while the complementary fragments for HO-1 and HO-2 were generated as described earlier.[12] The probe for heavy-chain ferritin was designed by RT-PCR using the sequence for mRNA of *Rattus norvegicus* ferritin, heavy polypeptide 1 (NCBI: NM 012848). RNA from kidneys from Sprague-Dawley was used for the first strand synthesis and the sequences for PCR primers were: forward (5′-cat caa ccg cca gat caa cct g-3′) and reverse (5′-aga taa agg cag cct gac atg c-3′). The 561 bp PCR product was purified using a gel extraction kit (Qiagen, Valencia, CA) and used as the probe for Northern blotting. All probes were labeled using α-[^{32}P]-dCTP (3000Ci/mmol; Perkin Elmer Life Sciences, Boston, MA) and random-primer labeling kit (Invitrogen, Carlsbad, CA). Unincorporated radioactivity was removed by filtration through Sephadex™ G-50 microspin columns (Amersham Biosciences, Piscataway, NJ).

Preparation of Total Protein Lysates and Western Blotting

Uninfected as well as *Rickettsia*-infected cells at different times were lysed in an SDS-containing buffer supplemented with a mixture of protease inhibitors (Sigma, St. Louis, MO). Protein content of samples was measured by standard Bradford assay and equal amounts of protein were subjected to SDS-PAGE followed by blotting onto nitrocellulose membranes. The membranes were then probed with anti-human COX-2 antibody (Santa Cruz Biotechnology Inc., Santa Cruz, CA) followed by a monoclonal antibody against α-tubulin (Accurate Chemical Corp., Westbury, NY) to ensure equivalent loading of different lanes on the gel. The blots were developed using Western lightning™ detection system (Perkin Elmer Life Sciences, Boston, MA) and high performance chemiluminescence film (Amersham Biosciences, Buckinghamshire, UK).

Prostaglandin Measurements by ELISA

The levels of 6-keto $PGF_{1\alpha}$ and PGE_2 in culture supernatants were determined by high sensitivity, competitive binding-based enzyme-linked immunosorbent assays following instructions provided by the manufacturer (R&D Systems, Minneapolis, MN). The results were calculated from a standard curve created using SOFTmax PRO program capable of generating four-parameter logistic curve-fit.

Densitometry and Statistics

The optimum autoradiographic exposures of blots were scanned in the grayscale mode using an HP ScanJet scanner at a resolution setting of 600 dpi. Band intensities

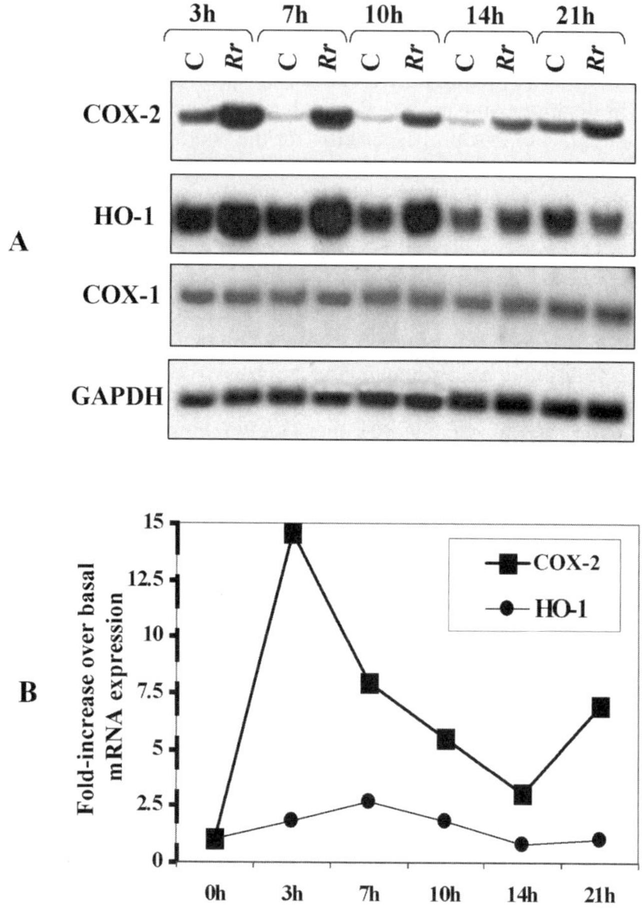

FIGURE 1. Expression of mRNA for COX and HO isoenzymes after host cell infection with SFG rickettsiae. (**A**) Total RNA from uninfected [C] and *R. rickettsii*-infected [*Rr*] endothelial cells at different time-points was subjected to DMSO-glyoxal denaturing electrophoresis on agarose gels and electrotransferred to nylon membranes. Species-specific hybridization with ^{32}P-labeled COX-2, HO-1, COX-1, and GAPDH probes was followed by extensive washing of the blots and exposure to Kodak X-OMAT™ imaging film. (**B**) The results of COX-2 (*filled rectangles*) and HO-1 (*filled spheres*) mRNA expression were quantitated as described in *Materials and Methods*. For each condition, the signal intensity of COX-2 or HO-1 mRNA was normalized to that of the housekeeping gene GAPDH. Relative fold-increases in the signal intensity over basal expression in untreated conditions were then calculated for each time point. The data represent average values from a minimum of four independent observations. Simultaneous analysis of cells infected with *R. conorii* yielded similar results.

were quantified using ImageQuant, Version 3.3 (Molecular Dynamics, Sunnyvale, CA). Statistical analysis was conducted using SigmaStat, Version 3.0.1 or Microsoft® Excel 2002-SP2.

RESULTS AND DISCUSSION

Consistent with our previous observations,[4,12] indirect immunofluorescent staining using specific antibody against SFG rickettsiae confirmed that incubation with *R. rickettsii* and *R. conorii* at about 6×10^4 pfu/ cm^2 (4 to 5 organisms per cell) resulted in the infection of >50% and 80% of EC with an average of 3–4 rickettsiae at 3 and 6 h, respectively. By Northern blot (FIG. 1A) and semiquantitative PCR analyses (not shown), unstimulated EC expressed consistent basal levels of COX-1 mRNA (~2.9 kb) and low but detectable levels of COX-2 mRNA (~4.4 kb) at all time points of this study. Endothelial cell infection with both *Rickettsia* species had no significant effect on COX-1, while COX-2 expression displayed robust induction of more than 5- to 10-fold at 3 h in comparison to uninfected controls (FIG. 1A). Interestingly, COX-2 mRNA levels higher than the matching controls were sustained at later times (7, 10, and 14 h), followed by a secondary peak at 21 h post-infection (FIGS. 1A and 1B), apparently coinciding with the previously described biphasic nature of NF-κB activation.[13] Although corresponding analysis of HO isozymes demonstrated increased expression of the 1.8 kb HO-1 mRNA at 3 and 7 h, the mean induction of about three- to fourfold over basal steady-state expression was not as dramatic as that for COX-2. Similar to COX-1 however, the levels of both 1.9 and 1.3 kb transcripts of the constitutive isoform HO-2 remained relatively unaltered (not shown).

Since it has been established that enhanced mRNA expression does not inevitably result in translation into protein in all cellular events, we carried out immunoblotting for COX-2 on isolated protein lysates. Representative data in FIGURE 2 shows that EC infected with *R. rickettsii* and *R. conorii* contain higher amounts of COX-2 protein in comparison to simultaneously cultured but uninfected cells. Using a human COX-2 specific antibody as the primary probe and rhodamine-conjugated secondary antibody, we also performed immunofluorescent staining on cells fixed at different

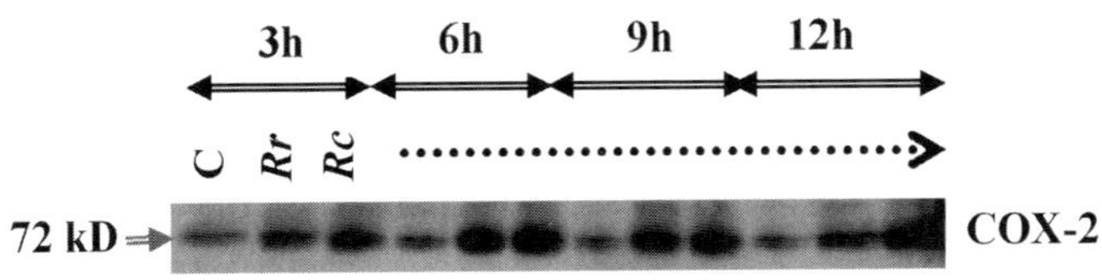

FIGURE 2. Effect of *R. rickettsii* and *R. conorii* infection on the production of COX-2 protein in endothelial cells (EC). For Western blot analysis, lysates were harvested from uninfected [C], *R. rickettsii*–infected [*Rr*], and *R. conorii*–infected [*Rc*] EC at 3, 6, 9, and 12 h post-infection. Total cellular protein preparations (25 μg for each experimental sample) were loaded onto a 10% SDS–polyacrylamide gel, electrophoresed under denaturing conditions, and transferred onto nitrocellulose membrane. Immunoblots were probed using an anti-human COX-2 specific antibody and developed with a chemiluminescence-based detection system. The representative blot demonstrates increased expression of COX-2 protein (72 kD) during *in vitro* infection of host EC with SFG rickettsiae.

times after infection to confirm this finding. Furthermore, quantitative measurements by enzyme immunoassays also indicated pronounced increase in the secretion of prostaglandin metabolites 6-keto $PGF_{1\alpha}$ and PGE_2 into culture media by infected EC (data not shown).

An effective mechanism to control the free iron released by HO-1–mediated cleavage of heme from participating in redox reactions is its sequestration within ferritin, a multimeric protein composed of 24 symmetrically arranged subunits named heavy (H) and light (L) chains. Due to the very high capacity for storing free intracellular iron, upregulation of ferritin genes is accompanied by increased activity of HO-1 in many instances.[14] Considering that H-ferritin manifests the ferroxidase activity to oxidize Fe^{2+} into Fe^{3+} to allow storage of iron and thus, may serve as an effective anti-oxidant molecule and contribute to the cytoprotective effects of HO-1, we have initially investigated the status of H-ferritin expression at the mRNA level. Results presented in FIGURE 3 clearly suggest enhanced transcription of H-ferritin during *in vitro* infection of EC with both *R. rickettsii* and *R. conorii*. It is important to emphasize, however, that further detailed studies are necessary to evaluate any changes in ferritin synthesis in response to infection, keeping in mind the potential relevance of post-transcriptional or translational modifications.

Based on the evidence summarized above, we conclude that: (1) two specific isoforms of regulatory oxygenases activated during EC infection with SFG rickettsiae are COX-2 and HO-1; (2) HO-1 expression is associated with the regulation of ferritin, which is known to perform potent anti-oxidant and anti-apoptotic functions in the vasculature; and (3) it is likely that induced secretion of vasoactive PGs by infected cells is dependent on the activity of COX-2. Given the current status of the knowledge on the versatility of HO-generated products in the vascular system (for example anti-inflammatory, anti-apoptotic, anti-proliferative properties of CO and potent anti-oxidant functions of bilirubin[6–10]) and recognition of PGs as pleiotropic

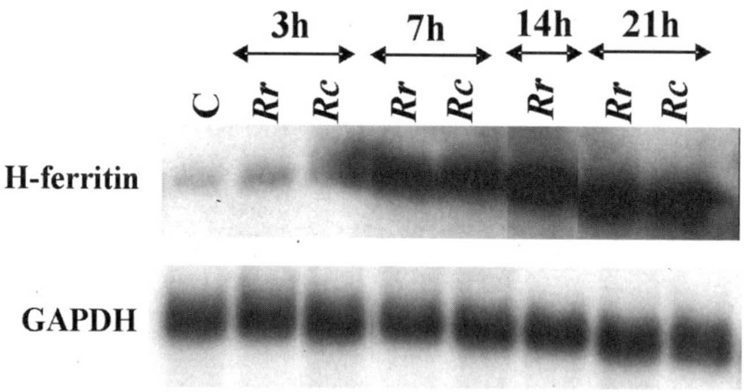

FIGURE 3. Northern blot analysis of H-ferritin mRNA during *Rickettsia* infection. Total RNA (5 µg) isolated from endothelial cells infected with either *R. rickettsii* [*Rr*] or *R. conorii* [*Rc*] and those left uninfected [C] were processed as described in legend to FIGURE 1. Employing conditions optimized for cross-species hybridization, the blot was first probed with rat H-ferritin cDNA probe. Subsequent stripping and reprobing of the blot with a 1.0 kb human GAPDH probe confirmed that comparable amounts of RNA had been applied to each lane. Shown are the results of a typical experiment (*N*=2).

modulators of immune response(s) and vascular permeability,[11] it can be expected that cytoprotective and/or inflammatory roles of HO and COX enzyme systems play an important role in the pathogenesis of rickettsial diseases. Although the demonstration of increased PG synthesis and secretion during interactions of typhus rickettsiae with host cells suggests a commonality in responses triggered by SF and typhus groups of organisms,[15] the likelihood of possible differences in the intensity and signaling mechanisms also exists due to unique variations in their intracellular growth and motility characteristics.[1] Another recently described novel function of COX-2 derived PGE_2 is to support replication of intracellular pathogens.[16,17] Therefore, *in vitro* culture systems amenable to targeted manipulation(s) and well-established animal models of rickettsial infections should be exploited to assess the effectiveness of targeting PG production in blocking processes linked to rickettsial multiplication and possibility of interplay between HO and COX systems. Continuation of this line of investigation to enhance our understanding of the mechanisms underlying host cell responses, physiological implications of bioactive reaction products, and possible roles in the progression of infection will not only advance our understanding of rickettsial pathogenesis, but may also identify new diagnostic and therapeutic targets.

ACKNOWLEDGMENTS

We thank Li Hua Rong, Loel C. Turpin, and Semion Kiriakidi for technical assistance; and Teresa Sherman and Keith Nehrke, Ph.D., for providing anti-ferritin cDNA probe. This work was supported in part by U.S. Public Health Service Grants AI 40689 and HL 30616 from the National Institutes of Health, Bethesda, MD.

[*Conflict of interest statement:* The authors of this research declare that they have no conflict of interest.]

REFERENCES

1. Eremeeva, M.E., G.A. Dasch & D.J. Silverman. 2000. Interaction of rickettsiae with eukaryotic cells: adhesion, entry, intracellular growth, and host cell responses. Subcell. Biochem. **33:** 479–516.
2. Walker, D.H., G.A. Valbuena & J.P. Olano. 2003. Pathogenic mechanisms of diseases caused by *Rickettsia*. Ann. N.Y. Acad. Sci. **990:** 1–11.
3. Eremeeva, M.E., Z. Liang, C. Paddock *et al.* 2003. *Rickettsia rickettsii* infection in the pine vole, *Microtus pinetorum*: kinetics of infection and quantitation of antioxidant enzyme gene expression by RT-PCR. Ann. N.Y. Acad. Sci. **990:** 468–473.
4. Rydkina, E., S.K. Sahni, L.A. Santucci *et al.* 2004. Selective modulation of antioxidant enzyme activities in host tissues during *Rickettsia conorii* infection. Microb. Pathog. **36:** 293–301.
5. Walker, D.H. 1990. The role of host factors in the severity of spotted fever and typhus group rickettsioses. Ann. N.Y. Acad. Sci. **590:** 10–19.
6. Otterbein, L.E, M.P. Soares, K. Yamashita & F.H. Bach. 2003. Heme oxygenase-1: unleashing the protective properties of heme. Trends Immunol. **24:** 449–455.
7. Abraham, N.G. & R. Olszanecki. 2003. Cyclooxygenase activity is regulated by the heme oxygenase system in microvessel endothelial cells. Adv. Exp. Med. Biol. **525:** 59–66.

8. SOARES, M.P., A. USHEVA, S. BROUARD *et al.* 2002. Modulation of endothelial cell apoptosis by heme oxygenase-1-derived carbon monoxide. Antioxid. Redox. Signal. **4:** 321–329.
9. PHAM, C.G., C. BUBICI, F. ZAZZERONI *et al.* 2004. Ferritin heavy chain upregulation by NF-κB inhibits TNFα-induced apoptosis by suppressing reactive oxygen species. Cell **119:** 529–542.
10. YACHIE, A., Y. NIIDA, T. WADA *et al.* 1999. Oxidative stress causes enhanced endothelial cell injury in human heme oxygenase-1 deficiency. J. Clin. Invest. **103:** 129–135.
11. DAVIDGE, S.T. 2001. Prostaglandin H synthase and vascular function. Circ. Res. **89:** 650–660.
12. RYDKINA, E., A. SAHNI, D.J. SILVERMAN & S.K. SAHNI. 2002. *Rickettsia rickettsii* infection of cultured human endothelial cells induces heme oxygenase 1 expression. Infect. Immun. **70:** 4045–4052.
13. CLIFTON, D.R., E. RYDKINA, R.S. FREEMAN & S.K. SAHNI. 2005. NF-κB activation during *Rickettsia rickettsii* infection of endothelial cells involves the activation of catalytic IκB kinases IKKα and IKKβ and phosphorylation-proteolysis of the inhibitor protein IκBα. Infect. Immun. **73:** 155–165.
14. BALLA, J., G.M. VERCELLOTTI, K. NATH *et al.* 2003. Haem, haem oxygenase, and ferritin in vascular endothelial cell injury. Nephrol. Dial. Transplant. **18:** v8–v12.
15. WALKER, T.S., J.S. BROWN, C.S. HOOVER & D.A. MORGAN. 1990. Endothelial prostaglandin secretion: effects of typhus rickettsiae. J. Infect. Dis. **162:** 1136–1144.
16. ZHU, H., J.P. CONG, D. YU *et al.* 2002. Inhibition of cyclooxygenase 2 blocks human cytomegalovirus replication. Proc. Natl. Acad. Sci. USA **99:** 3932–3937.
17. YONEDA, H., K. MIURA, H. MATSUSHIMA *et al.* 2003. Aspirin inhibits *Chlamydia pneumoniae*–induced NF-kappa B activation, cyclo-oxygenase-2 expression, and prostaglandin E2 synthesis and attenuates chlamydial growth. J. Med. Microbiol. **52:** 409–415.

Growth of Typhus Group and Spotted Fever Group Rickettsiae in Insect Cells

TSUNEO UCHIYAMA

Department of Virology, Institute of Health Biosciences, University of Tokushima Graduate School, 3-18-15 Kuramoto, Tokushima 770-8503, Japan

ABSTRACT: To analyze the host dependency of rickettsial growth, NIAS-AeAl-2 insect cells (AeAl2) derived from mosquito were first used in this study. It was demonstrated that typhus group rickettsiae (TGR) grew well in AeAl2 cells, but spotted fever group rickettsiae (SFGR) failed. To elucidate the inhibitory process of the growth of SFGR in AeAl2 cells, the adherence and invasion were first analyzed. SFGR possessed abilities to adhere to and invade AeAl2 cells as well as TGR in contrast to their inability of the growth in the cells. Morphologically, generation of microvilli could not be observed on AeAl2 cells inoculated with either group of rickettsiae. On the contrary, Vero cells inoculated with rickettsiae generated a great number of microvilli that adhered to rickettsiae and engulfed them into the cells. The roles of rickettsial major outer membrane protein A and B (rOmpA and rOmpB) were later investigated using *E. coli* expressing either rOmpA or rOmpB on their surface. Bacteria expressing either one of the major outer membrane proteins of rickettsiae as well as bacteria not expressing these proteins showed adherence to and invasion of AeAl2 cells. Thus, it is yet to be elucidated whether these major outer membrane proteins have any roles in these steps.

KEYWORDS: adherence; growth; insect cells; invasion; rickettsiae; spotted fever group; typhus group

INTRODUCTION

The vectors of spotted fever group rickettsiae (SFGR) are ticks classified as *Arachnoidea*. Those of typhus group rickettsiae (TGR), on the other hand, are lice and fleas that belong to *Insecta*. Until recently, the host dependency of the growth of SFGR and TGR in the cells derived from arthropod had not been well documented. As for tick cells, several reports about the kinetics of rickettsiae in these cells had been published.[1,2] For insect cells, it was reported very recently by Rovery and colleagues that the transcription of *spoT* gene paralogs were suppressed during the infection of *R. conorii* in *Aedes albopictus* (C6/36) cells at 10°C for 38 days. The temperature was then shifted to 37°C followed by a rapid upregulation of *spoT1* gene expression.[3] NIAS-AeAl-2 (AeAl2) cells are fibroblast-like cells derived from neo-

Address for correspondence: Tsuneo Uchiyama, Department of Virology, Institute of Health Biosciences, University of Tokushima Graduate School, 3-18-15 Kuramoto, Tokushima 770-8503, Japan. Voice: +81-88-633-9232; fax: +81-88-633-7080.
uchiyama@basic.med.tokushima-u.ac.jp

Ann. N.Y. Acad. Sci. 1063: 215–221 (2005).
doi: 10.1196/annals.1355.034

natal larval body of mosquito *Aedes albopictus* and susceptible to Chilo iridescent virus.[4] The cells have been used to analyze the growth of obligate intracellular parasitic microorganisms, such as *Wolbachia*, and the cytotoxicity of parasporal inclusions from bacteria, such as *Bacillus thuringiensis*, but have not been used for rickettsial growth.[5,6]

SFGR possess two major surface antigen proteins, rOmpA and rOmpB.[7–9] Only one major surface antigen protein SPA or SLP is present in TGR, which is highly homologous and cross-reactive with rOmpB of SFGR.[10-13] These proteins are heat-modifiable and heat-labile.[7–9,13] Although the functions of these major surface proteins are yet to be well characterized, it is suggested that at least the proteins are related to the protective immunity.[7,8,14–16] It is also reported that the infection is inhibited when the recombinant rOmpA and rOmpB or antibodies to these proteins were added at the time of inoculation of the rickettsiae.[17] A role of rOmpB in the steps of adherence and invasion of host cells by rickettsiae was examined by using a recombinant *Escherichia coli* expressing rOmpA or rOmpB on the surface (unpublished observation).[18] Single expression of rOmpA or rOmpB on the surface of *E. coli* added an ability to the recombinant *E. coli* to adhere to and invade host Vero cells.

In this study, adherence, invasion, and growth were analyzed by using AeAl2 insect cells and Vero mammalian cells inoculated with TGR, SFGR, and *E. coli* expressing rOmpA or rOmpB on the surface.

MATERIALS AND METHODS

Cells

Vero cells were used for preparation of rickettsial stocks for infection. The AeAl2 cell line was a generous gift of H. Urakami.

Rickettsial Strains

R. japonica, strain YH, *R. conorii*, strain Malish 7, and *R. montanensis*, strain Tick, as SFGR and *R. prowazekii*, strain Breinl, and *R. typhi*, strain Wilmington, as TGR were propagated in Vero cells. Rickettsiae were then purified as described previously and used for infection.[13]

Growth Kinetics of Rickettsiae in AeAl2 Cells

AeAl2 cell monolayers in a 12-well plate were inoculated at a multiplicity of infection (MOI) of 0.1 pfu/cell with these rickettsiae and incubated in IPL-41 medium (Gibco BRL, Grand Island, NY) containing 10% fetal bovine serum (FBS) at 28°C. The medium was changed every three days and the yields of rickettsiae were plaque-assayed on Vero cell monolayers.

Adherence of Vero and AeAl2 Cells by Rickettsiae

Vero and AeAl2 cells were inoculated with the rickettsiae at a multiplicity of infection (MOI) of 0.1 pfu/cell and incubated for 5, 10, 20, 60, 120, or 180 min at 21°C in MEM and IPL-41 medium, respectively, containing 10% FBS. Adhered and unadhered rickettsiae were plaque-assayed on Vero-cell monolayers.

Recombinant E. coli *Expressing rOmpA or rOmpB*

Recombinant *E. coli* transduced with ether gene for rickettsial major outer membrane protein, rOmpA or rOmpB, was cultivated in LB medium containing 50 μg/mL carbenicillin as described previously.[18] Recombinant proteins were induced by the addition of 1 mM isopropyl-β-D-thiogalactopyranoside. The induced *E. coli* expressing the recombinant proteins or uninduced ones were used for examining adherence to and invasion of AeAl2 cells.

Adherence to and Invasion of AeAl2 Cells by Rickettsiae and the Recombinant E. coli

Confluent monolayers of AeAl2 cells were prepared on coverslips in a 12-well plate (Iwaki Glass Co., Chiba, Japan) in IPL-41 medium containing 10% FBS. The purified rickettsiae or induced bacteria were suspended in IPL-41 medium containing 10% FBS and was inoculated at an multiplicity of infection of 10 pfu/cell in a well and incubated at 28°C for 60 min. The cells on a coverslip were washed with PBS thoroughly, fixed with methanol, and stained by Giménez staining. The stained cells were observed under a light microscope.

For scanning electron microscopy (SEM), AeAl2 cells grown on coverslips were also inoculated with the rickettsiae or recombinant bacteria. After incubation at 28°C for 60 min, the cells were washed thoroughly with PBS, fixed with 1% isotonic glutaraldehyde and 1% osmium tetroxide, dehydrated with serial dilution of ethanol, followed by critical-point drying. The coverslips were mounted on aluminum blocks, metal-vapor–deposited, and observed under a Hitachi S-800 scanning electron microscope. For transmission electron microscopy (TEM), AeAl2 cells were grown in 12-well plates directly. The inoculation procedure was the same as that for the light microscopy and SEM. After inoculation and incubation for 60 min, the cells were washed with PBS and processed for observation as described previously.[19] Thin sections of the samples were observed under a JEOL JEM-1200EXII transmission electron microscope.

RESULTS

Growth of TGR and SFGR in AeAl2 Cells

As shown in FIGURE 1, TGR grew well in AeAl2 cells as well as in Vero cells (data of Vero cells were not shown). On the other hand, SFGR did not grow in AeAl2 cells contrary to their growth in Vero cells (data of Vero cells were not shown). Rickettsial infectivity decreased to an undetectable level up to 7 days of infection.

Adherence of Vero Cells and AeAl2 Cells by TGR and SFGR

Since the growth of SFGR in AeAl2 cells was restricted, the adherence step was analyzed if it was completed. As shown in FIGURE 2, adherence of AeAl2 cells by

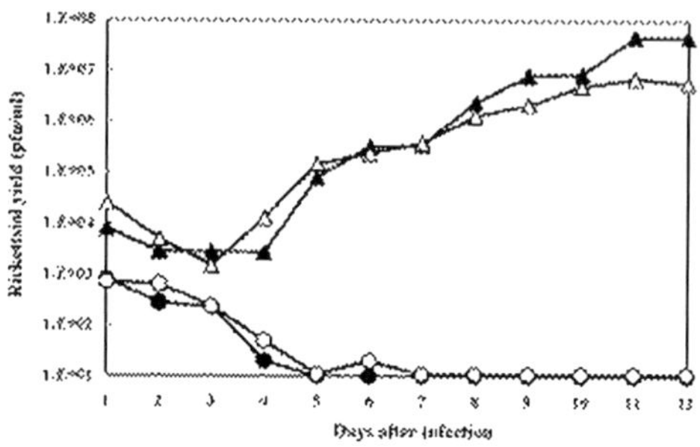

FIGURE 1. Growth of TG and SFG rickettsiae in AeAl2 cells: (*closed circle*) *R japonica*, (*open circle*) *R. montanensis*, (*closed triangle*) *R. prowazekii*, (*open triangle*) *R typhi*.

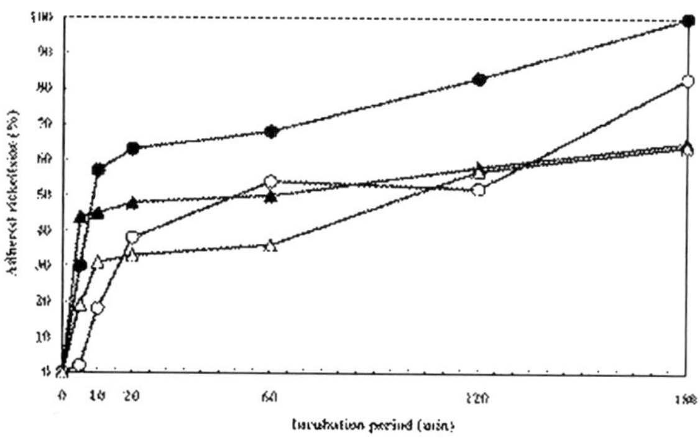

FIGURE 2. Adherence of Vero and AeAl2 cells by *R. japonica* and *R. typhi*: (*closed circle*) adherence of Vero cells by *R. japonica*, (*open circle*) adherence of AeAl2 cells by *R. japonica*, (*closed triangle*) adherence of Vero cells by *R. typhi*, (*open triangle*) adherence of AeAl2 cells by *R. typhi*.

R. japonica was successfully completed as well as those in other combinations of rickettsiae and host cells.

Morphological Studies on the Adherence to and Invasion of AeAl2 Cells by the Rickettsiae

Giménez staining of the inoculated AeAl2 cells with ether group of rickettsiae showed the cells adhered and/or invaded by rickettsiae (data not shown). SEM of the inoculated AeAl2 cells by either group of rickettsiae demonstrated the adherence and invasion of the host cells by the rickettsiae independent of their group (FIG. 3). The rickettsiae under the process of evacuating from phagosomes to the cytoplasm after being engulfed by AeAl2 cells were demonstrated by TEM (data not shown). Microvilli increased in number after adherence of Vero cells by either group of rickettsiae (FIGS. 3C and 3D). On the other hand, the increase of microvilli did not occur after adherence of AeAl2 cells by rickettsiae (FIGS. 3A and 3B).

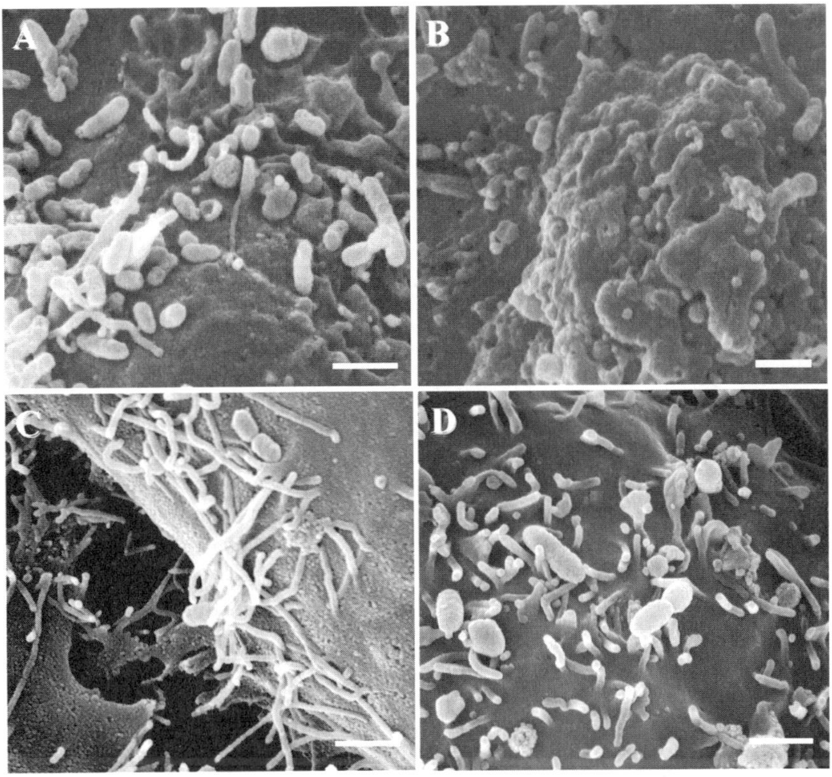

FIGURE 3. SEM of AeAl2 cells inoculated with *R. typhi* (**A**) and *R. japonica* (**B**) and of Vero cells inoculated with *R. typhi* (**C**) and *R. japonica* (**D**) for 60 min at 28°C. Bars: 1 μm.

Adherence to and Invasion of AeAl2 Cells by the Recombinant Bacteria

As both groups of rickettsiae adhered to and invaded AeAl2 cells independent of their growth, the role of the major surface antigen proteins, rOmpA and rOmpB, were examined by using recombinant *E. coli* expressing these proteins on their surface. *E. coli* expressing either of the proteins adhered to and invaded the cells, although *E. coli* without expressing these proteins also adhered to and invaded the cells unexpectedly (data not shown).

DISCUSSION

The vectors for TGR belong to *Insecta*, while those for SFGR belong to *Arachnoidea*. As expected from the host-vector dependency of rickettsiae, SFGR did not grow in AeAl2 insect cells, while TGR grew well in the cells. However, in the recent report by Rovery and colleagues, they mentioned that *R. conorii* grew well in C6/36 cells at 37°C, but not at 10°C.[3] There is a discrepancy between the restriction of the growth at 28°C shown here and the upregulation of the growth at 37°C by their experiments although both the cells derived from *Aedes albopictus*. As 37°C is rather a high temperature for the physiological growth of insect cells and may be so for the growth of rickettsiae in insect cells in nature, growth kinetics of the rickettsiae in each cell line at a temperature such as 28°C should be compared.

In order to clarify where the restriction of the growth of SFGR in AeAl2 cells occurred, the first step of rickettsial infection, that is, adherence and invasion, was analyzed by means of plaque assay and electron microscopy. As shown in FIGURES 2 and 3, SFGR adhered to and invade AeAl2 cells as effectively as other combinations of rickettsiae and host cells. Thus, it is suggested that the restriction occurred after these steps. Further analyses of the steps after the internalization of the rickettsiae into AeAl2 cells should be performed.

To elucidate the role of two major surface antigen proteins of rickettsiae in the adherence and invasion of AeAl2 cells by both group of rickettsiae, recombinant *E. coli* expressing these proteins were analyzed for their ability to adhere to and invade the cells. A previous study using the recombinant proteins and antibodies to these proteins suggested that both the rOmpA and rOmpB have some roles in the adherence of rickettsiae to Vero cells.[17] It also suggests the importance of native conformation of these proteins for the effective function as an adhesin. Li and colleagues reported that purified rOmpA and monoclonal antibodies against rOmpA of *R. rickettsii* showed inhibition of rickettsial adherence.[20] When the recombinant *E. coli* containing *ompA* or *ompB* gene were used, they adhered to and invaded Vero cells only after induction of these proteins (unpublished observations).[18] Unexpectedly, however, even *E. coli* that did not express these proteins possessed the ability of adherence and invasion of AeAl2 cells as well as those expressing these proteins, so that the molecular species that are associated with these steps may be rOmpA, rOmpB, and/or other molecules. This issue is yet to be clarified.

The manner of entry of AeAl2 cells by rickettsiae was not similar to that of Vero cells where the induction of microvilli and their adherence to rickettsiae was marked (FIG. 3).[18] The rickettsiae were adhered to the cell surface rather directly and then engulfed. Thus, the system for adherence and invasion of AeAl2 cells by rickettsiae might be different from that of Vero cells. Further studies on the functions of rOmpA, rOmpB, and the other outer membrane proteins will elucidate the more precise mechanism of internalization of rickettsiae into the host cells including mammalian cells and arthropod cells.

[*Conflict of interest statement:* The author of this research declares that there is no conflict of interest.]

REFERENCES

1. POLICASTRO, P.F., U.G. MUNDERLOH, E.R. FISCHER & T. HACKSTADT. 1997. *Rickettsia rickettsii* growth and temperature-inducible protein expression in embryonic tick cell lines. J. Med. Microbiol. **46:** 839–845.
2. MUNDERLOH, U.G., S.F. HAYES, J. CUMMINGS & T.J. KURTTI. 1998. Microscopy of spotted fever Rickettsia movement through tick cells. Microsc. Microanal. **4:** 115–121.
3. ROVERY, P., P. RENESTO, N. CRAPOULET, *et al.* 2005. Transcription response of *Rickettsia conorii* exposed to temperature variation and stress starvation. Res. Microbiol. **156:** 211–218.

4. MITSUHASHI, J. 1981. A new continuous cell line from larvae of the mosquito *Aedes albopictus* (*Diptera*, *Culicidae*). Biomed. Res. **2:** 599–606.
5. NODA, H., T. MIYOSHI & Y. KOIZUMI. 2002. *In vitro* cultivation of *Wolbachia* in insect and mammalian cell lines. In Vitro Cell. Dev. Biol. Animal **38:** 423–427.
6. MIZUKI, A., M. OHBA, T. AKAO, *et al.* 1999. Unique activity associated with non-insecticidal *Bacillus thuringiensis* parasporal inclusions: *in vitro* cell-killing action on human cancer cells. J. Appl. Microbiol. **86:** 477–486.
7. ANACKER, R.L., R.H. LIST, R.E. MANN, *et al.* 1985. Characterization of monoclonal antibodies protecting mice against *Rickettsia rickettsii*. J. Infect. Dis. **151:** 1052–1060.
8. ANACKER, R.L., G.A. MCDONALD, R.H. LIST & R.E. MANN. 1987. Neutralizing activity of monoclonal antibodies to heat-sensitive and heat-resistant epitopes of *Rickettsia rickettsii* surface proteins. Infect. Immun. **55:** 825–827.
9. LI, H., B. LENZ & D.H. WALKER. 1988. Protective monoclonal antibodies recognize heat-labile epitopes on surface proteins of spotted fever group rickettsiae. Infect. Immun. **56:** 2587–2593.
10. CARL, M., M.E. DOBSON, W.-M. CHING & G.A. DASCH. 1990. Characterization of the gene encoding the protective paracrystalline-surface layer protein of *Rickettsia prowazekii*: presence of a truncated identical homolog in *Rickettsia typhi*. Proc. Natl. Acad. Sci. USA **87:** 8237–8241.
11. HAHN, M.-J., K.-K. KIM, I.-S. KIM & W.-H. CHANG. 1993. Cloning and sequence analysis of the gene encoding the crystalline surface layer protein of *Rickettsia typhi*. Gene **133:** 129–133.
12. GILMORE, R.D., JR., W. CIEPLAK, JR., P.F. POLICASTRO & T. HACKSTADT. 1991. The 120 kilodalton outer membrane protein (rOmp B) of *Rickettsia rickettsii* is encoded by an unusually long open reading frame: evidence for protein processing from a large precursor. Mol. Microbiol. **5:** 2361–2370.
13. UCHIYAMA, T., T. UCHIDA, J.W. WEN & D.H. WALKER. 1994. Demonstration of heat-labile and heat-stable epitopes of *Rickettsia japonica* on ultrathin sections. Lab. Invest. **71:** 432–437.
14. VISHWANATH, S., G.A. MCDONALD & N.G. WATKINS. 1990. A recombinant *Rickettsia conorii* vaccine protects guinea pigs from experimental boutonneuse fever and Rocky Mountain spotted fever. Infect. Immun. **58:** 646–653.
15. MCDONALD, G.A., R.L. ANACKER & K. GARJIAN. 1987. Cloned gene of *Rickettsia rickettsii* surface antigen: candidate vaccine for Rocky Mountain spotted fever. Science **235:** 83–85.
16. MCDONALD, G.A., R.L. ANACKER, R.E. MANN & L.J. MILCH. 1988. Protection of guinea pigs from experimental Rocky Mountain spotted fever with a cloned antigen of *Rickettsia rickettsii*. J. Infect. Dis. **158:** 228–231.
17. UCHIYAMA, T. 1999. Role of major surface antigens of *Rickettsia japonica* in the attachment to host cells. *In* Rickettsiae and Rickettsial Diseases at the Turn of the Third Millennium. D. Raoult & P. Brouqui, Eds.: 182–188. Elsevier. Paris.
18. UCHIYAMA, T. 2003. Adherence to and invasion of Vero cells by recombinant *Escherichia coli* expressing the outer membrane protein rOmpB of *Rickettsia japonica*. Ann. N.Y. Acad. Sci. **990:** 585–590.
19. UCHIYAMA, T. & T. UCHIDA. 1988. Ultrastructural study on Japanese isolates of spotted fever group rickettsiae. Microbiol. Immunol. **32:** 1163–1166.
20. LI, H. & D. H. WALKER. 1998. rOmp A is a critical protein for the adhesion of *Rickettsia rickettsii* to host cells. Microb. Pathog. **24:** 289–298.

Genome Comparison Analysis of Molecular Mechanisms of Resistance to Antibiotics in the *Rickettsia* Genus

J.M. ROLAIN AND D. RAOULT

Unité des Rickettsies, CNRS UMR 6020, IFR 48, Faculté de Médecine, Université de la Méditerranée, 27 Bd Jean Moulin, 13385 Marseille Cedex 05, France

ABSTRACT: In this study we describe molecular mechanisms of resistance to several classes of antibiotics within drug targets by *in silico* genome comparisons for bacteria of the genus *Rickettsia*. Apart from the mutations in the *rpoB* gene in naturally rifampin-resistant *Rickettsia* species previously reported by our team, we found that typhus group (TG) rickettsiae had a triple amino acid difference in the highly conserved region of the L22 ribosomal protein as compared to the spotted fever group rickettsiae (SFG), which could explain the natural resistance of SFG rickettsia to erythromycin. We found also that the genome of *R. conorii* contains an aminoglycoside 3′-phosphotransferase. Finally, either *folA* gene (encoding dihydrofolate reductase) and/or *folP* gene (encoding dihydropteroate synthase) was missing in the genome of rickettsial strains explaining the natural resistance to cotrimoxazole. Finally, multiple genes encoding for pump efflux were found especially in the genome of *R. conorii* that could be involved in resistance to antibiotics. Five specific ORFs related to antibiotic resistance have been identified in the genome of *R. felis* including a streptomycin resistance protein homologue, a class C beta-lactamase, a class D beta-lactamase, a penicillin acylase homologue, and an ABC-type multidrug transporter system. For the first time, using this approach, an experimental beta-lactamase activity has been shown for this bacterium. We believe that whole genome sequence analysis may help to predict several phenotypic characters, in particular resistance to antibiotics for obligate intracellular bacteria.

KEYWORDS: *Rickettsia; in silico*; antibiotic resistance; genome analysis

INTRODUCTION

All members of the genus *Rickettsia* are obligate gram-negative intracellular bacteria. The genus comprises typhus group rickettsiae, which includes *R. prowazekii,* the agent of epidemic typhus, and *R. typhi,* the agent of murine typhus and spotted fever group (SFG) rickettsiae.[1] The number of recognized SFG rickettsioses has recently increased due to the introduction of cell culture and molecular biological test-

Address for correspondence: D. Raoult, Unité des rickettsies, IFR 48, CNRS UMR 6020, Université de la Méditerranée, Faculté de medicine, 27 boulevard Jean Moulin, 13385 Marseille cedex 5, France. Voice: 330491385517; fax: 330491830390.
Didier.Raoult@medecine.univ-mrs.fr

**Ann. N.Y. Acad. Sci. 1063: 222–230 (2005). © 2005 New York Academy of Sciences.
doi: 10.1196/annals.1355.035**

ing methods.[2] Eight new species pathogenic for humans (or new diseases) have been described since 1991: *Rickettsia japonica* in Japan, *Rickettsia honei* on Flinders Island (between Australia and Tasmania), *Rickettsia africae* in Africa and the West Indies, *R. felis* in 2001,[3] *Rickettsia slovaca* in Europe,[4] *Rickettsia aeschlimannii* in Africa and Europe, *Rickettsia helvetica* in Europe and Asia, *Rickettsia heilongjangensis* in Asia, and *R. parkeri* in the United States.[5] Two new subspecies were also reported: *Rickettsia conorii* subsp. *caspia* in Russia, Africa, and Kosovo, and *Rickettsia sibirica mongolotimonae* in China, Europe, and Africa.[6,7]

Several methods of evaluation of susceptibility to antibiotics have been used for bacteria of the genus *Rickettsia.* The plaque assay and a colorimetric assay[8] have been the most used for evaluating antiinfectives for this group of organisms. However, because of the technical difficulties in working with these agents, susceptibility testing will probably be confined to relatively few laboratories. Furthermore, it is evident that when *in vivo* techniques, such as suppression of lethality in chicken embryos, are compared with *in vitro* techniques, such as the plaque assay, results may be somewhat discrepant.[9] The two assays (plaque assay and colorimetric assay) depend on the induction of cytopathic effects and plaque formation in cell cultures by the rickettsiae, but some rickettsiae do not normally cause cytopathic effects in primary cultures.[8,10] Recently, Ives and colleagues[11] described a new assay that uses immunofluorescence staining, which avoids the problem of a lack of cytopathic effects. Very recently we have developed a new quantitative PCR DNA assay using the Lightcycler system for the evaluation of antibiotic susceptibilities of three rickettsial species including *R. felis*, a rickettsial species that does not induce plaque in cell cultures.[10] This latter assay appears to be more sensitive and reproducible and has been successfully adapted to evaluate susceptibility to antibiotics of numerous other intracellular bacteria including *Coxiella burnetii*,[12,13] *Tropheryma whipplei*,[14] or bacteria of the genus *Anaplasma* and *Ehrlichia.*[15] All the results of susceptibility to the different classes of antibiotics for bacteria of the genus *Rickettsia* are summarized in TABLE 1. Overall, doxycycline and fluoroquinolone compounds are consistently active against all rickettsial strains whereas beta-lactam compounds, aminoglycosides, and cotrimoxazole are not.[8,10] Among the macrolide compounds, typhus group rickettsia were susceptible to erythromycin (minimum inhibitory concentrations [MICs]) from 0.125 to 0.5 μg/mL) whereas SFG rickettsia were not susceptible to erythromycin (MICs from 2 to 8 μg/mL). Susceptibility to rifampin varied, with typhus group rickettsia and most SFG rickettsiae being susceptible, while a cluster including *R. massiliae, R. montanensis, R. rhipicephali, R. aeschlimannii,* and strain Bar 29 were more resistant (MICs from 2 to 4 μg/mL).

In this study we have investigated the resistance mechanisms of bacteria of the genus *Rickettsia* to antibiotics by *in silico* comparison for the presence of known antibiotic resistance determinants known to be target genes involved in molecular resistance in other bacteria. These genes were retrieved from available genomes at the KEGG Encyclopedia website (http://www.genome.jp/kegg/kegg2.html) for *R. conorii* strain Malish 7, *R. typhi* strain Wilmington, and *R. prowazekii* strain Madrid E or from ongoing genome sequence for *R. felis*. When necessary, the nucleotide sequence of genes and/or amino acid sequences were compared and aligned to look at possible mutations known to be associated with antibiotic resistance using the CLUSTALW program supported by the Infobiogen website (www.infobiogen.fr).

TABLE 1. Antibiotic susceptibility of rickettsiae as determined using *in vitro* cell models [8,10]

Organism	Blm	Dox	Chm	Sxt	Rif	Ery	Cla	Amg	Qui
Spotted Fever Group									
R. conorii subgroup *R. conorii* subsp. *conorii, caspia* and *israelensis, R. rickettsii, R. sibirica, R. australis, R. akari, R. japonica, R. honeï, R. africae; R. sibirica mongo-lotimonae, R. bellii, R. canada, R. helvetica, R parkeri, R. felis*	R	S	S	R	S	R	S	R	S
R. massiliae subgroup *R. massiliae, R. aeschlimanii, R. montanensis, R. rhipicephali*	R	S	S	R	R	R	S	R	S
Typhus Group									
R. typhi and *R. prowazekii*	R	S	S	R	S	S	S	R	S

Abbreviations: Amg, aminoglycosides; Blm, beta-lactams; Chm, chloramphenicol; Cla, clarithromycin; Dox, doxycycline; Ery, erythromycin; Qui, quinolones; R, resistant; Rif, rifampin; S, susceptible.

RESISTANCE TO BETA-LACTAM ANTIBIOTICS

Beta-lactam compounds act on penicillin binding protein (PBP), which is involved in cell wall synthesis. Resistance is most often due to the presence of beta-lactamases, but mutations in PBPs resulting in reduced affinity for beta-lactam antibiotics are also commonly observed. Resistance is less frequently due to changes in the cell wall or active efflux. The inactivation of *ampG* by mutation or deletion confers non inducible and microconstitutive beta-lactamase phenotypes to the bacterial cell.[16] The relative resistance of intracellular bacteria to this class of antibiotics was mainly linked to the poor penetration of beta-lactam compounds in cells.[17] However, even if MICs for amoxicillin are not achievable in humans, it is possible to inhibit the growth of rickettsiae with concentrations ranging from 128 to 256 μg/mL.[8]

Five specific ORFs related to antibiotic resistance have been identified in the genome of *R. felis* including a class C beta-lactamase, a class D beta-lactamase, a penicillin acylase homologue, and an ABC-type multidrug transporter system.[18] For the first time, using this approach, we were able to demonstrate experimentally the presence of beta-lactamase activity for this bacterium.[18] Interestingly we have also found two genes encoding for beta-lactamases in the genome of *R. conorii* but without activity (unpublished observation) and none in the genome of *R. prowazekii* and *R. typhi*, whereas these three bacteria possess PBPs and *ampG* genes.

RESISTANCE TO MLS ANTIBIOTICS

Macrolides are composed of lactone compounds with 14 members (erythromycin and clarithromycin), 15 members (azithromycin), or 16 members (josamycin, spiramycin). Macrolide, lincosamide, and streptogramin (MLS) antibiotics are chemically distinct inhibitors of protein synthesis.[19] Macrolides inhibit protein synthesis by stimulating dissociation of the peptidyl-tRNA molecule from the ribosomes during elongation.[19] The first mechanism of macrolide resistance described was due to posttranscriptional modifications of the 23S rRNA by the adenine-N^6 methyltransferase.[20] These enzymes add one or two methyl groups to a single adenine (A2058 in *E. coli*) in the peptidyltransferase region of domain V of 23S rRNA common to the binding of MLS_B antibiotics. Modification of the ribosomal target confers cross-resistance to MLS_B antibiotics and remains the most frequent mechanism of resistance. In general, genes encoding these methylases have been designated *erm* (erythromycin ribosome methylation).[19] We did not find these encoding genes in the genomes of bacteria of the genus *Rickettsia.* Two other mechanisms of resistance to macrolides have been described: target site modification and active efflux of the antibiotic from the cell. These alternative mechanisms of resistance confer resistance to only one or two of the antibiotic classes of the MLS_B complex. Antibiotic target-site modification occurs by mutations especially at bases G2057, A2058, and A2059 in domain V of 23S rRNA and confer resistance to several MLS_B antibiotics by altering the binding site.[21] We have recently shown that such a resistance mechanism was correlated with resistance to macrolides in the *Anaplasma/Ehrlichia* genus.[15] In certain bacterial species, macrolide resistance can be due to mutations in ribosomal proteins L4 (encoded by *rplD* gene) and L22 (encoded by *rplV* gene).[22,23] Interestingly, we found three amino acid differences between TG rickettsia and SFG rickettsia (7 SFG rickettsial strains) in the highly conserved region at the C terminus of the L22 protein (FIG. 1).[24] A number of different antibiotic resistance genes code for efflux proteins, which pump the antibiotic out of the cell or the cellular membrane, keeping intracellular concentrations low and ribosomes free from antibiotic. Many of these proteins (*mefA, mefE*) have homology to the major facilitator superfamily (MFS), the resistance/nodulation/division (RND) superfamily (AcrAB-TolC, *Mex, MtrD, AmrB*), or the ATP binding cassette (ABC) transporter (*msrA, lmrA*).[19] Similarly, we found that the genome of *R. conorii* contains 6 encoding genes for RND superfamily and 20 encoding genes similar to that of ABC transporters whereas

		C terminus of the L22 protein	Erythromycin susceptibility
TG rickettsia[1]	60	IANAENNLGLDIDRLIITKATVGK**SV**VMKR**I**MPRAKGRATRINKFFSNLYITVTEK	S
SFG rickettsia[2]	60	VANAENNLGLDIDRLIITKATVGK**AL**VMKR**V**MPRAKGRATRINKFFSNLDITVTEK	R
S. pneumoniae	58	VANAENNFGLDKANLVVSEATANEGPTMKRFRPRAKGSASPINKRTAHITVAVAEK	V
S. aureus	54	LANAEHNYDMNTDELVVKEAYANEGPTLKRFRPRAQGRASAINKRTSHITIVVSDG	V
E. coli	54	IANAEHNDGADIDDLKVTKIFVDEGPSMKRIMPRAKGRADRILKRTSHITVVVSDR	V
H. influenzae	54	IANAEHNDGADIDDLKVAKIFVDEGPSMKRVMPRAKGRADRILKRTSHITVVVSDR	V

FIGURE 1.

R prowazekii and *R. typhi* did not contain RND superfamily encoding genes and fewer encoding genes for ABC transporter (4 and 12, respectively). This difference may be also involved in the difference of susceptibility to macrolide compounds between these two subgroups.

RESISTANCE TO AMINOGLYCOSIDES

Aminoglycosides such as gentamicin, tobramycin, amikacin, and streptomycin, bind to the ribosomes and thus interfere with protein synthesis. Resistance to these antimicrobials is widespread with more than 50 aminoglycoside-modifying enzymes already described. These enzymes are classified as aminoglycoside acetyltransferases (AAC), aminoglycoside nucleotidyltransferases (ANT), and aminoglycoside phosphotransferases (APH). Besides aminoglycoside-modifying enzymes, efflux systems homologous to resistance nodulation division family[25,26] and rRNA mutations in the 16S rRNA gene or the *rpsL* gene encoding ribosomal protein S12 have been described.[27,28]

In the genome of *R. conorii* we have found one gene encoding for a protein similar to an aminoglycoside 3′-phosphotransferase and a streptomycin resistance protein homologue in the genome of *R. felis,* whereas genomes of *R. typhi* and *R. prowazekii* does not contain such encoding genes. Sequence alignment of the available genomes did not show any amino acid substitution in ribosomal protein S12, es-

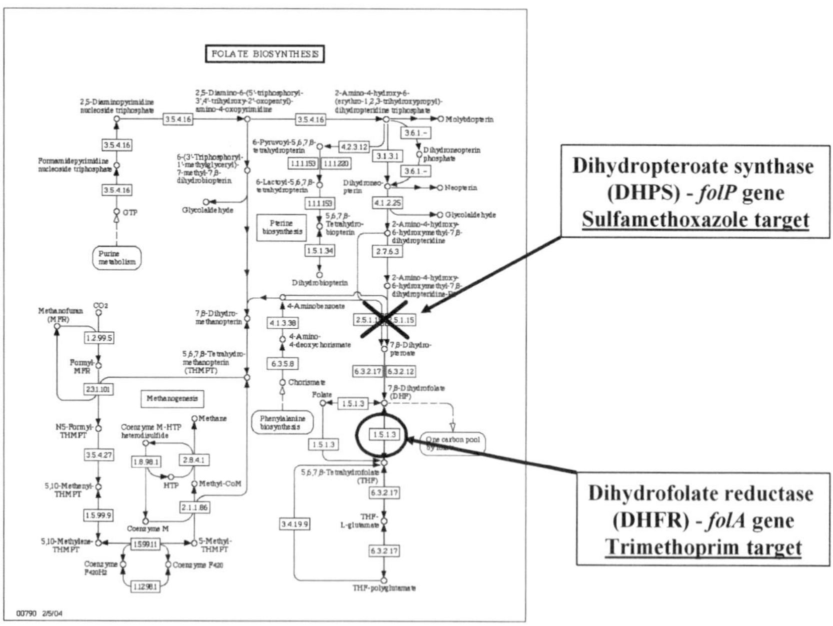

FIGURE 2.

pecially at codons 43, 88, or 93 known to confer resistance to streptomycin in *Mycobacterium tuberculosis*.[27] Similarly, we did not find any nucleotide substitutions in loop 530 and 915 of 16S rRNA, known to confer resistance to aminoglycoside compounds.[27] Thus, the mechanism of resistance to aminoglycosides in rickettsiae remains unexplained, except for *R. felis* and *R. conorii*.

RESISTANCE TO RIFAMPIN

The molecular mechanism of rifampin activity involves inhibition of DNA-dependent RNA polymerase. Rifampin binds to the beta-subunit of the RNA polymerase and results in transcription inhibition. Genetic studies conducted in the early 1980s recorded that *E. coli* strains resistant to rifampin had missense mutations and short deletions in the *rpoB* gene.[29,30] Moreover, 17 mutational alterations affecting 14 amino acid residues in the *E. coli* RNA polymerase beta-subunit that mediate rifampin resistance have been described.[31] Resistance to rifampin can also be due to an efflux system.[32,33] Typhus group rickettsiae are naturally susceptible to rifampin,[8] but rifampin-resistant strains of *R. typhi*[34] and *R. prowazekii*[35] have been selected *in vitro* after random mutagenesis. The rifampin mutant *rpoB* strain of *R. typhi* had three nucleotide substitutions, which resulted in amino acid changes at residues 151, 201, and 271,[34] whereas rifampin-resistant mutant of *R. prowazekii* had a single point mutation that results in an arginine-to-lysine change at position 546 of the RNA polymerase beta subunit.[35] Although TG rickettsiae are naturally susceptible to rifampin, experimental studies have delineated a cluster of naturally rifampin-resistant spotted fever group species.[8] A single point mutation resulting in a phenylalanine-to-leucine change at position 973 of the *Rickettsia conorii rpoB* sequence and present in all the rifampin-resistant species was absent in all the rifampin-susceptible species and explains such phenotypic difference.[36]

RESISTANCE TO TRIMETHOPRIM AND SULFAMETHOXAZOLE

Sulfamethoxazole is a structural analog of *p*-aminobenzoic acid (PABA) and a competitor of PABA in the synthesis of dihydropteroic acid, the first step in the synthesis of dihydrofolic acid. Sulfamethoxazole binds to the enzyme coding dihydropteroate synthase (DHPS), which catalyzes this reaction. Trimethoprim is an analog of dihydrofolic acid, an essential component in the synthesis of amino acids and nucleotides that competitively inhibits the enzyme dihydrofolate reductase (DHFR) in the folate pathway. The sequential enzymatic blockade by sulfamethoxazole and trimethoprim is responsible for the very strong synergistic effect observed between the two compounds.

Resistance to sulfamethoxazole is mainly due to mutations in the structural gene for DHPS (*folP*) gene,[37,38] but acquisition of genes (*sul1* and *sul2*) mediated by transposons and plasmids and expressing dihydropteroate synthases highly resistant to sulfonamide have been found.[39]

Resistance to trimethoprim can be caused by a number of mechanism including overproduction of the host DHFR, mutations in the structural gene for DHFR (*folA* gene),[40,41] and the acquisition of a gene (*dfr*) encoding a resistant DHFR enzyme.[42]

The mechanism of greatest clinical importance is the production of plasmid-encoded, trimethoprim-resistant forms of dihydrofolate reductase. For the bacteria of the genus *Rickettsia*, the resistance to these compounds is linked to the absence of such encoding genes (*folA* and/or *folP*) in their genomes. Indeed, the genomes of the TG rickettsia (*R. typhi* and *R. prowazekii*) do not contain *folA* and *folP* gene whereas *R. felis, R. conorii, R. sibirica,* and *R. rickettsii* had only the *folA* gene (FIG. 2). This is in accordance with the fact that isolation of SFG rickettsiae from ticks by use of cotrimoxazole in the culture medium to prevent overgrowth of bacterial contaminants was possible.[43] Moreover, Ruiz Beltran and Herrero Herrero reported that cotrimoxazole was ineffective in the treatment of rickettsioses.[44]

CONCLUSIONS

Genome analysis may help to predict possible molecular mechanisms of resistance for fastidious and intracellular bacteria for which transformation assays are usually not suitable.

[*Competing interests statement:* The authors state that they have no competing financial interests.]

REFERENCES

1. RAOULT, D. & V. ROUX. 1997. Rickettsioses as paradigms of new or emerging infectious diseases. Clin. Microbiol. Rev. **10:** 694–719.
2. RAOULT, D. 2004. A new rickettsial disease in the United States. Clin. Infect. Dis. **38:** 812v813.
3. RAOULT, D., B. LA SCOLA, M. ENEA, *et al.* 2001. A flea-associated Rickettsia pathogenic for humans. Emerg. Infect. Dis. **7:** 73–81.
4. RAOULT, D., P. BERBIS, V. ROUX, *et al.* 1997. A new tick-transmitted disease due to *Rickettsia slovaca.* Lancet **350:** 112–113.
5. PADDOCK, C.D., J.W. SUMNER, J.A. COMER, *et al.* 2004. *Rickettsia parkeri*: a newly recognized cause of spotted fever rickettsiosis in the United States. Clin. Infect. Dis. **38:** 805–811.
6. RAOULT, D., P. BROUQUI & V. ROUX. 1996. A new spotted-fever-group rickettsiosis. Lancet **348:** 412.
7. PRETORIUS, A.M. & R.J. BIRTLES. 2004. *Rickettsia mongolotimonae* infection in South Africa. Emerg. Infect. Dis. **10:** 125–126.
8. ROLAIN, J.M., M. MAURIN, G. VESTRIS & D. RAOULT. 1998. *In vitro* susceptibilities of 27 Rickettsiae to 13 antimicrobials. Antimicrob. Agents Chemother. **42:** 1537–1541.
9. RAOULT, D., P. ROUSSELLIER, V. GALICHER, *et al.* 1986. *In vitro* susceptibility of *Rickettsia conorii* to ciprofloxacin as determined by suppressing lethality in chicken embryos and by plaque assay. Antimicrob. Agents Chemother. **29:** 424–425.
10. ROLAIN, J.M., L. STUHL, M. MAURIN & D. RAOULT. 2002. Evaluation of antibiotic susceptibilities of three rickettsial species including *Rickettsia felis* by a quantitative PCR DNA assay. Antimicrob. Agents Chemother. **46:** 2747–2751.
11. IVES, T.J., E.L. MARSTON, R.L. REGNERY & J.D. BUTTS. 2001. *In vitro* susceptibilities of Bartonella and Rickettsia spp. to fluoroquinolone antibiotics as determined by immunofluorescent antibody analysis of infected Vero cell monolayers. Int. J. Antimicrob. Agents **18:** 217–222.
12. BRENNAN, R.E. & J.E. SAMUEL. 2003. Evaluation of *Coxiella burnetii* antibiotic susceptibilities by real- time PCR assay. J. Clin. Microbiol. **41:** 1869–1874.

13. BOULOS, A., J.M. ROLAIN, M. MAURIN & D. RAOULT. 2004. Evaluation of antibiotic susceptibilities against *Coxiella burnetii* by real time PCR. Int. J. Antimicrob. Agents **23:** 169–174.
14. BOULOS, A., J.M. ROLAIN & D. RAOULT. 2004. Antibiotic susceptibility of *Tropheryma whipplei* in MRC5 cells. Antimicrob. Agents Chemother. **48:** 747–752.
15. BRANGER, S., J.M. ROLAIN & D. RAOULT. 2004. Evaluation of antibiotic susceptibilities of *Ehrlichia canis, Ehrlichia chaffensis,* and *Anaplasma phagocytophilum* by real-time PCR. Antimicrob. Agents Chemother. **48:** 4822–4828.
16. CHAHBOUNE, A., M. DECAFFMEYER, R. BRASSEUR & B. JORIS. 2005. Membrane topology of the *Escherichia coli AmpG* permease required for recycling of cell wall anhydromuropeptides and *AmpC* beta-lactamase induction. Antimicrob. Agents Chemother. **49:** 1145–1149.
17. MAURIN, M. & D. RAOULT. 1996. Optimum treatment of intracellular infection. Drugs **52:** 45–59.
18. OGATA, H., P. RENESTO, S. AUDIC, *et al.* 2005. The genome sequence of *Rickettsia felis* identifies the first putative conjugative plasmid in an obligate intracellular parasite. PLOS Biology. In press.
19. ROBERTS, M.C., J. SUTCLIFFE, P. COURVALIN, *et al.* 1999. Nomenclature for macrolide and macrolide-lincosamide-streptogramin B resistance determinants. Antimicrob. Agents Chemother. **43:** 2823–2830.
20. WEISBLUM, B. 1995. Erythromycin resistance by ribosome modification. Antimicrob. Agents Chemother. **39:** 577–585.
21. VESTER, B. & S. DOUTHWAITE. 2001. Macrolide resistance conferred by base substitutions in 23S rRNA. Antimicrob. Agents Chemother. **45:** 1–12.
22. CANU, A., B. MALBRUNY, M. COQUEMONT, *et al.* 2002. Diversity of ribosomal mutations conferring resistance to macrolides, clindamycin, streptogramin, and telithromycin in *Streptococcus pneumoniae.* Antimicrob. Agents Chemother. **46:** 125–131.
23. TAIT-KAMRADT, A., T. DAVIES, M. CRONAN, *et al.* 2000. Mutations in 23S rRNA and ribosomal protein L4 account for resistance in pneumococcal strains selected *in vitro* by macrolide passage. Antimicrob. Agents Chemother. **44:** 2118–2125.
24. ROLAIN, J.M. & D. RAOULT. 2005. Prediction of resistance to erythromycin in the genus Rickettsia by mutations in L22 ribosomal protein. J. Antimicrob. Chemother. **56** (2): 396–398.
25. SOBEL, M.L., G.A. MCKAY & K. POOLE. 2003. Contribution of the MexXY multidrug transporter to aminoglycoside resistance in *Pseudomonas aeruginosa* clinical isolates. Antimicrob. Agents Chemother. **47:** 3202–3207.
26. POOLE, K. 2001. Multidrug efflux pumps and antimicrobial resistance in *Pseudomonas aeruginosa* and related organisms. J. Mol. Microbiol. Biotechnol. **3:** 255–264.
27. RAMASWAMY, S. & J.M. MUSSER. 1998. Molecular genetic basis of antimicrobial agent resistance in *Mycobacterium tuberculosis*: 1998 update. Tuber. Lung Dis. **79:** 3–29.
28. KATSUKAWA, C., A. TAMARU, Y. MIYATA, *et al.* 1997. Characterization of the *rpsL* and *rrs* genes of streptomycin-resistant clinical isolates of *Mycobacterium tuberculosis* in Japan. J. Appl. Microbiol. **83:** 634–640.
29. LISITSYN, N.A., E.D. SVERDLOV, E.P. MOISEYEVA, *et al.* 1984. Mutation to rifampicin resistance at the beginning of the RNA polymerase beta subunit gene in *Escherichia col.* Mol. Gen. Genet. **196:** 173–174.
30. OVCHINNIKOV, Y.A., G.S. MONASTYRSKAYA, V.V. GUBANOV, *et al.* 1981. The primary structure of *Escherichia coli* RNA polymerase. Nucleotide sequence of the *rpoB* gene and amino-acid sequence of the beta-subunit. Eur. J. Biochem. **116:** 621–629.
31. JIN, D.J. & C.A. GROSS. 1988. Mapping and sequencing of mutations in the *Escherichia coli rpoB* gene that lead to rifampicin resistance. J. Mol. Biol. **202:** 45–58.
32. CHANDRASEKARAN, S. & D. LALITHAKUMARI. 1998. Plasmid-mediated rifampicin resistance in *Pseudomonas fluorescens.* J. Med. Microbiol. **47:** 197–200.
33. VAN BAMBEKE, F., E. BALZI & P.M. TULKENS. 2000. Antibiotic efflux pumps. Biochem. Pharmacol. **60:** 457–470.
34. TROYER, J.M., S. RADULOVIC, S.G. ANDERSSON & A.F. AZAD. 1998. Detection of point mutations in *rpoB* gene of rifampin-resistant *Rickettsia typhii.* Antimicrob. Agents Chemother. **42:** 1845–1846.

35. RACHEK, L.I., A.M. TUCKER, H.H. WINKLER & D.O. WOOD. 1998. Transformation of *Rickettsia prowazekii* to rifampin resistance. J. Bacteriol. **180:** 2118–2124.
36. DRANCOURT, M. & D. RAOULT. 1999. Characterization of mutations in the rpoB gene in naturally rifampin-resistant *Rickettsia* species. Antimicrob. Agent Chemother. **43:** 2400–2403.
37. VEDANTAM, G. & B.P. NICHOLS. 1998. Characterization of a mutationally altered dihydropteroate synthase contributing to sulfathiazole resistance in *Escherichia coli.* Microb. Drug Resist. **4:** 91–97.
38. SWEDBERG, G., S. RINGERTZ & O. SKOLD. 1998. Sulfonamide resistance in *Streptococcus pyogenes* is associated with differences in the amino acid sequence of its chromosomal dihydropteroate synthase. Antimicrob. Agents Chemother. **42:** 1062–1067.
39. SKOLD, O. 2001. Resistance to trimethoprim and sulfonamides. Vet. Res. **32:** 261–273.
40. MASKELL, J.P., A.M. SEFTON & L.M. HALL. 2001. Multiple mutations modulate the function of dihydrofolate reductase in trimethoprim-resistant *Streptococcus pneumoniae.* Antimicrob. Agents Chemother. **45:** 1104–1108.
41. ADRIAN, P.V. & K.P. KLUGMAN. 1997. Mutations in the dihydrofolate reductase gene of trimethoprim-resistant isolates of *Streptococcus pneumoniae.* Antimicrob. Agents Chemother. **41:** 2406–2413.
42. FLUIT, A.C., M.R. VISSER & F.J. SCHMITZ. 2001. Molecular detection of antimicrobial resistance. Clin. Microbiol. Rev. **14:** 836–871.
43. KELLY, P.J., D. RAOULT & P.R. MASON. 1991. Isolation of spotted fever group rickettsias from triturated ticks using a modification of the centrifugation-shell vial technique. Trans. R. Soc. Trop. Med. Hyg. **85:** 397–398.
44. RUIZ BELTRAN, R. & J.I. HERRERO HERRERO. 1992. Deleterious effect of trimethoprim-sulfamethoxazole in Mediterranean Spotted Fever (letter). Antimicrob. Agents Chemother. **36:** 1342–1344.

Cloning and Sequence Analysis of the 22-kDa Antigen Genes of *Orientia tsutsugamushi* Strains Kato, TA763, AFSC 7, 18-032460, TH1814, and MAK 119

HONG GE,[a] MIN TONG,[a] ANDREW LI,[b] RAJAN MEHTA,[b] AND WEI-MEI CHING[a]

[a]*Rickettsial Diseases Department, Infectious Diseases Directorate, Naval Medical Research Center, Silver Spring, Maryland 20910, USA*

[b]*Thomas Jefferson High School for Science and Technology Mentorship Program, Alexandria, Virginia 22312, USA*

ABSTRACT: The 22-kDa protein antigen is one of several antigens recognized by sera from scrub typhus patients infected with *Orientia tsutsugamushi*. The 22-kDa protein genes from six *O. tsutsugamushi* strains (Kato, TA763, AFSC 7, 18-032460, TH1814, MAK119) were cloned and their sequences were determined and compared to each other and to the Karp strain sequence listed in GenBank. The sequence alignment revealed that the promoter regions of these seven strains were highly conserved. However, the ORFs exhibited some variation. The phylogenetic analysis of the DNA sequences indicated that among the seven strains assessed, Kato and TA763 were the most closely related, while Karp and TH1814 were the most distantly related. The information gained from this analysis will facilitate our selection of *O. tsutsugamushi* strains from which antigens should be derived to be included in a multivalent vaccine candidate for scrub typhus.

KEYWORDS: *Orientia tsutsugamushi*; scrub typhus; 22-kDa antigen; vaccine

INTRODUCTION

Many different serotypes of *Orientia tsutsugamushi*, the causative agent of scrub typhus, have been documented. The identification of protective antigens, which may be responsible for the different serotypes, is crucial to the understanding of homotypic and heterotypic immunity to *O. tsutsugamushi* and to the development of a scrub typhus vaccine. Western blot analysis of *O. tsutsugamushi* cell lysates with patient sera has identified at least five protein antigens of molecular mass 110, 56, 47, 35, and 22 kDa. Among these antigens, the variable 56-kDa protein antigen is the most

Address for correspondence: Dr. Hong Ge, Rickettsial Diseases Department, Infectious Diseases Directorate, Naval Medical Research Center, Silver Spring, Maryland 20910, USA. Voice: 301-319-7439; fax: 301-319-3015.
geh@nmrc.navy.mil

Disclaimer: This work was supported by Work Unit Number A0311. The views expressed in this article are those of the author and do not necessarily reflect the official policy or position of the Department of the Navy, Department of Defense, nor the U.S. Government.

Ann. N.Y. Acad. Sci. 1063: 231–238 (2005).
doi: 10.1196/annals.1355.036

abundant and is recognized by almost all scrub typhus patients' sera.[1] The 47-kDa antigen is believed to be the most conserved antigen, while the 56-kDa and 110-kDa protein antigens exhibit considerable variations. The sequences of 22-kDa antigens are not available from strains other than prototype Karp strain.

It has been shown that the 22-kDa protein contains B- and T- cell epitopes and that a recombinant 22- kDa protein could induce antigen-specific proliferation of T-cells from mice immunized with whole cell *O. tsutsugamushi.*[2] Many studies have demonstrated that protective immunity to scrub typhus is led by specific T cells; especially Th1 cells. These results suggest that it may be beneficial to include 22-kDa antigen in a multicomponent vaccine candidate. Therefore, we amplified 22-kDa genes from six strains (Kato, TA763, AFSC 7, 18-032460, TH1814, MAK119) and compared their sequences to each other and to that of the Karp strain. The information obtained in this study from the different strains will facilitate our selection of strains to be included in the development of a multivalent vaccine against scrub typhus.

MATERIALS AND METHODS

Purification of Genomic DNA, PCR Amplification, Cloning and Fast-Screening of the 22-kDa Gene

The genomic DNAs were purified from *O. tsutsugamushi*–infected mouse spleens. Cell pellet was resuspended in ATL lysis buffer (Qiagen, Valencia, CA). After proteinase K digestion and RNase treatment according to manufacturer instructions, DNA was extracted by phenol-chloroform-isoamyl alcohol three times and precipitated with ethanol-sodium acetate. Purified *O. tsutsugamushi* genomic DNAs from six strains (Kato, TA763, AFSC 7, 18-032460, TH1814, MAK 119) were used as templates for PCR. The primers were designed for amplification of the entire 22-kDa gene based on the published sequence of Karp strain (forward: 5′ TAA GTC GAC ATA CTA TAT CAT CTA CAC AGA AGT TG 3′ and reverse: 5′ TAA GGC ATA TGT ATT CTA CTA TAG CTT GGG GT 3′). The PCR yielded a 1,211 bp fragment that was cloned into pPCR-Script Amp SK+ vector and the positive clones were selected with the Epicentre® Colony Fast-Screen™ Kit (Madison, WI).

Sequencing, Sequence Alignment, and Phylogenetic Analysis of the Amplified 22-kDa Gene

The positive clones were sequenced on the ABI 370 analyzer (Foster City, CA). The inserted sequences from three colonies of each strain were determined. The chromatography was manually examined to resolve any discrepancies in sequencing. The confirmed sequences of six strains were aligned for comparison with that of the Karp strain and phylogenetic trees were constructed by CLUSTALW comparison (version 1.82).

RESULTS

Sequence alignment of seven 22-kDa genes (six determined in this study and the published sequence of Karp strain) demonstrated that the promoter regions were

```
Kato                TAAGTCGACATACTATATCATCTACACAGAAGTTGAGTAAAAAATTGCAGCTATGTATTT 60
TA763               TAAGTCGACATACTATATCATCTACACAGAAGTTGAGTAAAAAGCTACAGCTATGTATTT 60
AFSC7               TAAGTCGACATACTATATCATCTACACAGAAGTTGAGTAAAAAACTGCAGCTATGTATTT 60
Karp                TAAGTCGACATACTATATCATCTACACAGAAGTTGAGTAAAAAACTGCAGCTATGTATTT 60
18-032460           TAAGTCGACATACTATATCATCTACACAGAAGTTGAGTAAAAAGCTACAGCTATATATTT 60
TH1814              TAAGTCGACATACTATATCATCTACACAGAAGTTGAGTAAAAAACTGCAGCTATGTATTT 60
MAK119              TAAGTCGACATACTATACCATCTACACAGAAGTTGAGTAAAAAACTGCAGCTATGTATTT 60
                    ***************** *************************  * ******* *****

Kato                CATTAGCAACTTTTATATTACGTTGCATCCTATATGCTTCACGATTAAAAATATAATTCA 120
TA763               CATTAGCAACTTTTATATTACGTTGCATCCTATATGCTTCACGATTAAAAATATAATTCA 120
AFSC7               CATTAGCAACTTTTATATTACGTTGCATCCTATATGCTTCACGATTAAAAATATAATTCA 120
Karp                CATTAGCAACTTTTATATTACGTTGCATCCTATATGCTTCACGATTAAAAATATAATTCA 120
18-032460           CATTAGCAACTTTTATATTACGTTGCATCCTATATGCTTCACGATTAAAAATATAATGCA 120
TH1814              CATTAGCAACTTTTATATTACGTTGCATCCTATATGCTTCACGATTAAAGATATAATTCA 120
MAK119              CATTAGCAACTTTTATATTACGTTGCATCCTATATGCTTCACGATTAAAAATATAATTCA 120
                    ************************************************* ******* **

Kato                TAGCCTGTTTTAATA-TTTAGCTAACTAAAAGAAATATTTTGTAAGATAATACAGTATAT 179
TA763               TAGCCTGTTTTAATA-TTTAGCTAACTAAAAGAAATATTTTGTAAGATAATACAGTATAT 179
AFSC7               TAGCCTGTTTTAATA-TTTAGCTAACTAAAAGAAATATTTTGTAAGATAATACAGTATAT 179
Karp                TAGTCTGTTTTAATA-TTTAGCTAACTAAA-GAAATATCCTGCAAGATAATACAGTATGT 178
18-032460           TAGTCTGTTTTAATAATTTAGCTAACTAAA-GAAATATCTTGCAAGATAATACAGTATAT 179
TH1814              TAGCCTGTTTTAATA-TTTAGCTAACTAAAAGAAATATTTTGTAAGATAATATAGTATAT 179
MAK119              TAGCCTGTTTTAATA-TTTAGCTAACTAAAAGAAATATTTTGTAAGATAATACAGTATAT 179
                    *** *********** ************** *******  ** ********* ***** *
                                                            -75
Kato                GTATAATCATGATATATGATAGAGGATCAATACAACTGAAACAATATTAGTTATTGATAA 239
TA763               GTATAATCATGATATATGATAGAGGATCAATACAACTGAAACAATATTAGTTATTGATAA 239
AFSC7               GTATAATCATGATATATGATAGAGGATCAATACAACCGAAACAATATTAGTTATTGATAA 239
Karp                GTATAATCATGATATATGATAAATGATCAATATAACTGAAATAATATTAGTTATTGATAA 238
18-032460           GTATAATTATTATATGTGATAGAGTATCAATACAATTGAAATAATATTAGTTATTGATAA 239
TH1814              GTATAATCATGATATATGATAGAGGATCAATACAACTGAAACAATATTAGTTATTGATAA 239
MAK119              GTATAATCATGATATATGATAGAGGATCAATACAACTGAAACAATATTAGTTATTGATAA 239
                    ******* ** **** ***** *  ******* **  **** ******************
                                                                           start
Kato                CTGCATAATATTTAAGTATATTTTTAAGTATTACTAATATTATAAGGAATTATCTTTATG 299
TA763               CTGCATAATATTTAAGTATATTTTTAAGTATCACTAATATTATAAGGAATTATCTTTATG 299
AFSC7               CTGCATAATATTTAAGTATATTTTTAAGTATTACTAATATTATAAGGAATTATCTTTATG 299
Karp                CTGCATAATATTTAAGTATATTTTTAAGTATTACTAATATTATAAGGAATTATCTTTATG 298
18-032460           CTGCATAATATTTAAGTATATTTTTAAGTATTACTAATATTATAAGGAATTATCTTTATG 299
TH1814              CTGCATAATATTTAAGTATATTTTTAAGTATTACTAATATTATAAGGAATTATCTTTATG 299
MAK119              CTGCATAATATTAGAGTATATTTTTAAGTATTACTAATATTATAAGGAATTATCTTTATG 299
                    ************  ***************** ****************************

Kato                AGTAAAGAAGCAACAGAACTCAAAGAAAATATGAATAAAGCAATGGAGTCTGCATCGCAA 359
TA763               AGTAAAGAAGCAACAGAACTCAAAGAAAATATGAATAAAGCAATGGAGTCTGCATCGCAA 359
AFSC7               AGTAAAGAAGCAACAGAACTCAAAGAAAGTATGGATCAAGCAATGAAGTCTGCATCGCAA 359
Karp                AGTAAAGAAGCAACAGAACTCAAAGAAAGTATGGATCAAGCAATGAAGTCTGCATCGCAA 358
18-032460           AGTAAAGAAGCAACAGAACTCAAAGAAAGTATGGATCAAGCAATGAAGTCTGCATCGCAA 359
TH1814              AGTAAAGAAGCAACAGATCTCAAAGAAAATATGAATAAAGCAATGGAGTCTGCATCCCAA 359
MAK119              AGTAAAGAAGCAACAGATCTCAAAGAAAATATGAATAAAGCAATGGAGTCTGCATCCCAA 359
                    ***************** ********** **** ** ******** ********** ***

Kato                AATTCAAGTATTTCAGCTGAACAAAAATTACAACTTGAAAACGAAAAAAAGGAACTGCAA 419
TA763               AATTCAAGTATTTCAGCTGAACAAAAAGCACAACTTGAAAATGAAAAAAAGGAACTGCAA 419
AFSC7               AATTCAAGTATTTCAGCTGAACAAAAATTACAACTTGAAAAAGAAAAAAAGGAACTGCAA 419
Karp                AATTCAAGCATTTCAGCTGAACAAAGATCACAACTTGAAAAAGAAAAAAAGGAACTGCAA 418
18-032460           AATTCGAGTATTTCAGCTGAACAAAAATTACAACTTGAAAACGAAAAAAAGGAACTGCAA 419
TH1814              AGTTCAAGCCTTTCAGCTAAACAAAGATCAGAACTTGAAACTGAAAAAAATGAACTGCAA 419
MAK119              AGTTCAAGCCTTTCAGCTAAACAAAAATCAGAACTTGAAACTGAAAAAAATGAACTGCAA 419
                    * *** **  ******** ****** *  * *********  ******** *********
```

FIGURE 1. The alignment of 22-kDa genes from seven *O. tsutsugamishi* strains.

```
Kato          GGACAAATTAGCGATATTACTGGAAAAGATGAACAATCTCAACAAACTACAATGGATAAA 479
TA763         GGCCAAATTAGCGATATTGCTGGAAAAGATGAACAAACCCAACAAACTACAATGGATAAA 479
AFSC7         GGCCAAATTGGCGATATCACTGGGAAAGATGAACAAACCCAACAAACTACAATGAATAAA 479
Karp          GGCCAAATTGGCGATATCACTGGGAAAGATGAACAAACCCAACAAACTACAATGAATAAA 478
18-032460     GGCCAAATTGGCGATATCACTGGGAAAGATGAACAAACCCAACAAACTACAATGAATAAA 479
TH1814        AGCCAAATTAGCGCTATTACTGGAAAAGATAAACAATCTCAAGAAACTACAATGGCTAAA 479
MAK119        AGCCAAATTAGCGCTATTACTGGAAAAGATAAACAATCTCAAGAAACTACAATGGCTAAA 479
               * ****** *** ***  **** ****** ***** * *** ***********  ****

Kato          TTGAAAGAATGGATGTTAAAGATCAAGGAATTTATCACAAGTAAGGATTTTTCAGAGCTA 539
TA763         TTAAAAGAATGGATGTTAAAGATCAAGGAATTTATCACAAGTAATGATTTTTCAAAGCTA 539
AFSC7         TTAAAAGAATGGATGTTAAAGATCAAGGATTTTCTTACAAGTGATGATTTTTCAAAGCTA 539
Karp          TTAAAAGAATGGATGTTAAAGATCAAGGATTTTCTTATAAGTGATGATTTTTCAAAGCTA 538
18-032460     TTAAAAGAATGGATGTTAAAGATCAAGGATTTTCTTACAAGTGATGATTTTTCAAAGCTA 539
TH1814        TTGAAAGAATGGATGTTAAAGATCAAGGAATTTATTACAAGTCAGGATTTTTCCAATCTA 539
MAK119        TTGAAAGAATGGATGTTAAAGATCAAGGAATTTATTACAAGTCAGGATTTTTCCAATCTA 539
              ** ************************** *** * * **** * ********  * ***

Kato          GTAGATAGCGTAGTAAAATTTGTACAAACTGCAGTCAAAGTTTCCACAGAAATGGCACAA 599
TA763         GTAGATAGCGCAGTGCAATTTGTACAAACAGCAGTCAAAGTTTCCGCAGAAATGGTGCAG 599
AFSC7         GTAGATAGCGCAGTAAAATTTGTACAAACTGCAGTTAAGGTTTCCACAGAAATGATGCAG 599
Karp          GTAGATAGCGCAGTAAAATTTGTACAAACTGCAGTTAAGGTTTCCACAGAAATGATGCAG 598
18-032460     GTAGATAGCGCAGTAAAATTTGTACAAACTGCAGTTAAGGTTTCCACAGAAATGATGCAG 599
TH1814        GTAGATAGTGCAGTAAAATTTGTACAAACTGCAGTTAAGGTCTCTACAGAAATGATGAAG 599
MAK119        GTAGATAGTGCAGTAAAATTTGTACAAACTGCAGTTAAGGTCTCTACAGAAATGATGAAG 599
              ******** * ***  ************* ***** ** ** **  ********    *

Kato          GCCTTTACAGGCATGAAAGATAAAGGAATAATGGGAGTAGCTGCAGGCATACAAACTGTT 659
TA763         GCTTTTACAGGCATGAAAGAGAAAGGAATAATGGGTGTAGCTGCAGGCATAAAAACTGTT 659
AFSC7         GCCTTTACAGGCATGAAAGAGAAAGGAATAATGGGTGTAGCTGCAGGCATACAAACTGTT 659
Karp          GCCTTTACAGGCATGAAAGAGAAAGGAATAATGGGTGTAGCTGCAGGCATACAAACTGTT 658
18-032460     GCTTTTACAGGCATGAAAGAGAAAGGAATAATGGGAGTAGCTGCAGGAATACAAACTGTT 659
TH1814        GCTTTTACAGGCATGAAAGAGAAAGGAATAATGGGTGTAGCTGAAGGCATACAAACTGTT 659
MAK119        GCTTTTACAGGCATGAAAGAGAAAGGAATAATGGGTGTAGCTGAAGGCATACAAACTGTT 659
              ** ***************** ************** ******* *** *** ********

Kato          ACTAGTGGATTCCAAGATATAACCCAAGGTGTGAGCAAGATGGTTGAAGCTGGAGAAGCA 719
TA763         ACTAGTGGATTCCAAGATATAACCCAAGGTGTGAGCAGGATGGTTGAAGCTGGAGAAGCA 719
AFSC7         ACTAGTGGATTTCAAAATATAACACAAGGGGTGAGCAATATGATTGAAGCTGGAGAAGCA 719
Karp          ACTAGTGGATTTCAAAATATAACACAAGGGGTGAGCAATATGATTGAAGCTGGAGAAGCA 718
18-032460     ACTACTGGATTCCAAAGTATAACCCAAGGTGTGAGCAATATGATTGAAGCTGGAGAAGCA 719
TH1814        ACTACTGGATTCCAAAGTATAACCCAAGGTGTGAGCAATATGATTGAAGCTGGAGAAGCA 719
MAK119        ACTACTGGATTCCAAAGTATAACCCAAGGTGTGAGCAATATGATTGAAGCTGGAGAAGCA 719
              **** ****** ***  ****** ***** *******  *** *****************

Kato          GCAGTAAAGCACTTTTCTTCTTCTGGAGATAAAATGGGAAAGAAATTTTTAGGAGCAGAG 779
TA763         GCAGCAAAGCACTTTTCTTCTTCTGGAGATAAAAT---AAAAGAAATTTTAGGAGCAGAG 776
AFSC7         GCAGTAAAACACTTTTCTTCTCCTAGAGATAAAAT---AAAAGAAGCTTTAGGAGCAGAA 776
Karp          GCAGTAAAACACTTTTCTTCTCCTAGAGATAAAAT---AAAAGAAGCTTTAGGAGCAGAA 775
18-032460     GCAGCAAAGCACTTTTCTTCTCCTGGCGATAAAAT---AAAAGAAGCTTTAGGAGCAGAG 776
TH1814        GCAGCAAAGCACTTTTCTTCTCCTGGCGATAAAAT---AAAAGAAGCTTTAGGAGCAGAG 776
MAK119        GCAGCAAAGCACTTTTCTTCTCCTGGCGATAAAAT---AAAAGAAGCTTTAGGAGCAGAG 776
              **** *** ************ ** * ********   ***  **  ************
```

FIGURE 1 — *continued.*

```
Kato          GGATTAGCTAAACTTCAAGCTGCTAGCGCTGGATTACAAAATAATGCTAGTATAGCATCA 839
TA763         GGATTAGCTAAACTTCAAGCTGCTAGCGCTGGATTACAGAGTAATGCTAGTATAGCATCA 836
AFSC7         GGACTAGCTAAACTTCAAGCTGCTAGCGCTGGATTACAAAATAATGCTAGTATAGCATCA 836
Karp          GGATTAGCTAAACTTCAAGCTGCTAGCGCTGGATTACAAAATAATGCTAGTATAGCATCA 835
18-032460     GGACTAGCTAAACTTCAAGCTGCTAGCGCTGGATTACAAAGTAATGCTAGTATAGCATCA 836
TH1814        GGACTAGCTAAAACTTCAGCTGCTAGTGCTGGATTACAAAATAATGCTAGTATAGCATCA 836
MAK119        GGACTAGCTAAACTTCAAGCTGCTAGTGCTGGATTACAAAATAATGCTAGTATAGCATCA 836
              *** ********  *  ********* *********** * *******************

Kato          CCTTCAGCTAGTAGTGTATCAACTCCAACAGCAGCGCGC------ACACAACAGAAAGAC 893
TA763         CCTTCAGCTAGTAGTGTATCAACTCCAACAGCAGCGCGCTCAACAACACCACAGAAAGAC 896
AFSC7         TCTTCAGCTAGT---GTATCAACTCCAACAGCAGCACGC------CCACAACAGAAAGAC 887
Karp          TCTTCAGCTAGT---GTATCAACTCCAACAGCAGCGCGC------ACACAACAGAAAGAC 886
18-032460     TCTTCAGCTAGT---GTATCAACTCCAACAGCAGCACGCTCC---CCACAACAGAAAGAC 890
TH1814        TCTTCAGCTAGT---GTATCAACTCCAACAGCAGCACGT------ACACAACAGAAAGAC 887
MAK119        TCTTCAGCTAGT---GTATCAACTCCAACAGCAGCACGT------ACACAACAGAAAGAC 887
               ***********   ******************** **        *** **********

                             stop
Kato          ---TCTATAGCAAGATAAAACA-GTATGATAACACTAGAATAGGATAATTTTAAGCGTGT 949
TA763         AGTTCTATAGCAAGATAAAACA-GTATTATAACACTAGGATAGGATAATTTTAAGCGTGT 955
AFSC7         ---TCTATAGCAAGATAAAACAAGTATTCTAACGCTAGAATAGAATAATTTTAAGCGCGT 944
Karp          AGTTCTATAGCAAGATAAAACA-GTATTATAACGCTAGAATAGAATAATTTTAAGCGCGT 945
18-032460     ---TCTATAGCAAGATAAAACA-GTATGATAACACTAGAATAGGATAATTTTAAGCGTGT 946
TH1814        AGTTCTATAGCAAGATAAAACA-GTATGATAACACTAGAATAGGATAATTTTAAGCGTGT 946
MAK119        AGTTCTATAGCAGGATAAA-CA-GTATGATAACACTAGAATAGGATAATTTTAAGCGTGT 945
                 ********* ****** ** ****  **** **** **** ************* **

Kato          TAGCCAAGAAAAAAGAAAAA---AACAGATATAAGAAAAAATTAAGTTTAAAGT-TAAAA 1005
TA763         TTG-------AGAGAAAAAA---CATAGATATAAGAAAAAATTAAGTTTAAAGTCTAAAA 1005
AFSC7         GTTAGCGAAGAAAGAAAAAAAAAACATAGATATAAGAAAAAATTAAGTTTAAAGT-TAAAA 1003
Karp          GTTAGCGAAGAAAGAAAAAA--ACATAGATATAAGAAAAAATTAAGTTTAAAGT-TAAAA 1002
18-032460     TT---------GAGAAAAAA---CATAGATATAAGAAAAAATTAAGTTTAAAGT-TAAAA 993
TH1814        TG---------GAGAAAAAA---CATAGATATAAGAAAAAATTAAGTTTAAAGT-TAAAA 993
MAK119        TG---------GAGAAAAAA---CATAGATATAAGAAAAAATTAAGTTTAAAGT-TAAAA 992
                          *  *****    * **************************** *****

Kato          TAACTTGCAACTCAATTAATCTAGTAGATATGTTTTAATCTTTACGAAGATTAAATAAAT 1065
TA763         TAACTTGCAACTCAATTAATCTAGTAAATATGTTTTAATCTTTACGAAGATTAAATAAAT 1065
AFSC7         TAACTTGCAACTCAATTAATCTAGTAGATATGTTTTAATCTTTACGAAGATTAAATAAAT 1063
Karp          TAACTTGCAACTCAATTAATCTAGTAGATATGTTTTAATCTTTACGAAGATTAAATAAAT 1062
18-032460     TAACTTGCAACTCAATTAATCTAGTAGATATGTTTTAATCTTTACGAAGATTAAATAAAT 1053
TH1814        AAACTTGCAACTCAATTAATCTAGTAAATATGTTTTAATCTTTACGAAGGAAAATAAAT 1053
MAK119        AAACTTGCAACTCAATTAATCTAGTAAATATGTTTTAATCTTTACGAAGATTAAATAAAT 1052
               ************************* **********************   ********

Kato          TAAGTATAAAGGATACTTTTGCTTACCCCAAGCTATAGTAGAATAATACATATGCCTTA 1124
TA763         TAAGTATAAAGGATACTTTTGCTTACCCCAAGCTATAGTAGAATAATACATATGCCTTA 1124
AFSC7         TAAGTATAAAGGATACTTTTGCTTACCCCAAGCTATAGTAGAATAATACATATGCCT-- 1120
Karp          TAAGTATAAAGGATACTTTTGCTTACCCCAAGCTATAGTAGAATAATACATATGCCTTA 1121
18-032460     TAAGTATAAAGGATACTTTTGCTTACCCCAAGCTATAGTAGAATAATACATATGCCTT- 1111
TH1814        TAAGTATAAAGGATACTTTTTCTTACCCCAAGCTATAGTAGAATAATACATAT-CCTTA 1111
MAK119        TAAGTATAAAGGATACTTTTGCTTACCCCAAGCTATAGTGGAATAATACATATGCCTTA 1111
              ******************** ****************** ************* ***
```

FIGURE 1 — *continued.*

highly conserved, while the open reading frames (ORFs) showed sequence variations scattered all over the region (FIG. 1). In the promoter regions, the different strains' upstream sequences between –1 to –75 bp before the ATG start codon were almost identical except for two nucleotides of MAK119 (242, 243) and one nucleotide of TA763 (261). However, there were quite a lot of single nucleotide differences throughout the entire ORF among these seven strains. In addition, there were five triple nucleotide insertions or deletions within the 150 bp region before the stop codon relative to Karp 22-kDa sequence. Using the Karp strain sequence as the reference, percentages of sequence homology observed among these strains if the insertions and deletions were not counted were as follows: AFSC7, 99.46%; 18-032460, 98.13%; TA763, 96.25%; Kato, 96.07%; MAK119, 95.27%; TH1814, 95.18%. The alignment for the deduced protein sequences of seven strains was performed as well (FIG. 2). Although amino acid variations were found scattered throughout the whole ORF, the results indicated that the 22-kDa protein is relatively conserved. Their relationships to Karp strain were similar to those seen in DNA sequence comparisons. The percentages of protein sequence homology among these

```
Kato          MSKEATELKENMNKAMESASQNSSISAEQKLQLENEKKELQGQISDITGKDEQSQQTTMD
TA763         MSKEATELKENMNKAMESASQNSSISAEQKAQLENEKKELQGQISDIAGKDEQTQQTTMD
AFSC7         MSKEATELKESMDQAMKSASQNSSISAEQKLQLEKEKKELQGQIGDITGKDEQTQQTTMN
18-032460     MSKEATELKESMDQAMKSASQNSSISAEQKLQLENEKKELQGQIGDITGKDEQTQQTTMN
TH1814        MSKEATDLKENMNKAMESASQSSSLSAKQRSELETEKNELQSQISAITGKDKQSQETTMA
MAK119        MSKEATDLKENMNKAMESASQSSSLSAKQKSELETEKNELQSQISAITGKDKQSQETTMA
Karp          MSKEATELKESMDQAMKSASQNSSISAEQRSQLEKEKKELQGQIGDITGKDEQTQQTTMN
              ******:***.*::**:****.**:**:*: :**.**:***.**. *:***:*:*:***

Kato          KLKEWMLKIKEFITSKDFSELVDSVVKFVQTAVKVSTEMAQAFTGMKDKGIMGVAAGIQT
TA763         KLKEWMLKIKEFITSNDFSKLVDSAVQFVQTAVKVSAEMVQAFTGMKEKGIMGVAAGIKT
AFSC7         KLKEWMLKIKDFLTSDDFSKLVDSAVKFVQTAVKVSTEMMQAFTGMKEKGIMGVAAGIQT
18-032460     KLKEWMLKIKDFLTSDDFSKLVDSAVKFVQTAVKVSTEMMQAFTGMKEKGIMGVAAGIQT
TH1814        KLKEWMLKIKEFITSQDFSNLVDSAVKFVQTAVKVSTEMMKAFTGMKEKGIMGVAEGIQT
MAK119        KLKEWMLKIKEFITSQDFSNLVDSAVKFVQTAVKVSTEMMKAFTGMKEKGIMGVAEGIQT
Karp          KLKEWMLKIKDFLISDDFSKLVDSAVKFVQTAVKVSTEMMQAFTGMKEKGIMGVAAGIQT
              **********:*: *.***:****.*:*********:** :******:******* **:*

Kato          VTSGFQDITQGVSKMVEAGEAAVKHFSSSGDKMGKKFLGAEGLAKLQAASAGLQNNASIA
TA763         VTSGFQDITQGVSRMVEAGEAAAKHFSSSGDKI-KEILGAEGLAKLQAASAGLQSNASIA
AFSC7         VTSGFQNITQGVSNMIEAGEAAVKHFSSPRDKI-KEALGAEGLAKLQAASAGLQNNASIA
18-032460     VTTGFQSITQGVSNMIEAGEAAAKHFSSPGDKI-KEALGAEGLAKLQAASAGLQSNASIA
TH1814        VTTGFQSITQGVSNMIEAGEAAAKHFSSPGDKI-KEALGAEGLAKTSAASAGLQNNASIA
MAK119        VTTGFQSITQGVSNMIEAGEAAAKHFSSPGDKI-KEALGAEGLAKLQAASAGLQNNASIA
Karp          VTSGFQNITQGVSNMIEAGEAAVKHFSSPRDKI-KEALGAEGLAKLQAASAGLQNNASIA
              **:***.******.*:******.*****. **: *: ******** .*******.*****

Kato          SPSASSVSTPTAAR--TQQKDS-IAR
TA763         SPSASSVSTPTAARSTTPQKDSSIAR
AFSC7         SSSAS-VSTPTAAR--PQQKDS-IAR
18-032460     SSSAS-VSTPTAAR--SPQQKDSIAR
TH1814        SSSAS-VSTPTAAR--TQQKDSSIAR
MAK119        SSSAS-VSTPTAAR--TQQKDSSIAG
Karp          SSSAS-VSTPTAAR--TQQKDSSIAR
              *.*** ********  . *:.. **
```

FIGURE 2. The alignment of amino acids of 22-kDa protein genes from seven *O. tsutsugamishi* strains.

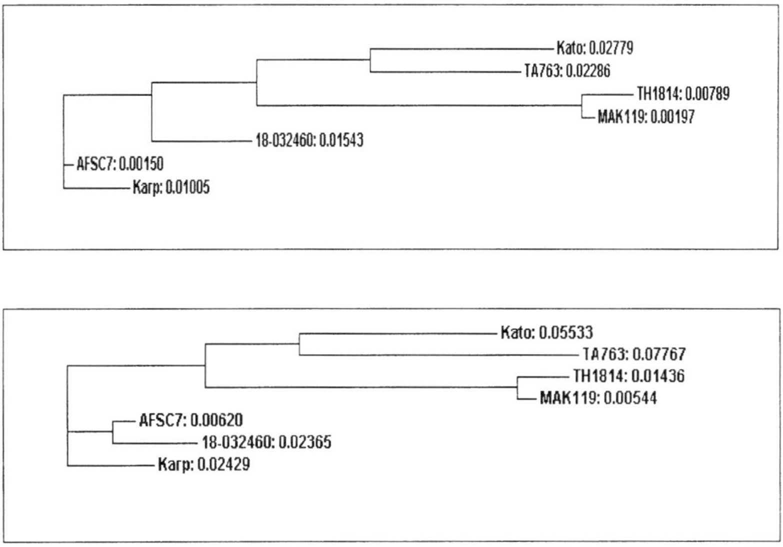

FIGURE 3. The phylogenetic trees for the ORFs of 22-kDa genes (*top*) and protein sequence (*bottom*).

strains compared to Karp strain were 98.02%, 93.07%, 86.14%, 86.14%, 84.65%, and 84.65% in AFSC7, 18-032460, Kato, TA763, TH1814, and MAK119, respectively, if insertions or deletions were excluded.

Phylogenetic trees were constructed using DNA sequences of the ORF (611 bp) and the translated protein sequences of 22-kDa genes by CLUSTALW method (FIG. 3a and b). The lengths of tree lines were proportional to the distances among strains. These distances were also labeled by bootstrap values after the strain names. Based on the DNA sequences of 22-kDa ORF (FIG. 3a), the strains of Kato and TA763 were grouped into the same cluster, while the strains of TH1814 and MAK119, and the strains of AFSC7 and Karp were grouped into two separate clusters. The distance of ORF between strains calculated in this method suggested that the most divergent strains were Karp and TH1814, while Kato and TA763 were the most closely related strains (FIG. 3a). The protein sequence of 22-kDa protein was analyzed by CLUSTALW 1.82 as well (FIG. 3b). Overall, the phylogenetic trees from DNA and protein sequences look similar. But in protein analysis, the 18-032460 instead of Karp was grouped into the same cluster with AFSC7 and the most divergent strains were 18-032460 and TA763.

DISCUSSION

O. tsutsugamushi isolates are antigenically heterogeneous.[3] Therefore, the development of a multivalent vaccine against *O. tsutsugamushi* that provides heterologous protection has been a major concern. The 22-kDa antigen gene, a possible scrub typhus vaccine component, was first cloned and expressed using the template from Karp strain.[2] However, knowing the 22-kDa sequences from other strains is essential in determining the level of disparity that exists among the various strains of *O. tsutsugamushi*. In this study, we sequenced and analyzed 22-kDa genes from six *O. tsutsugamushi* strains. The results from DNA and protein sequence analysis provided the first sequence comparison and phylogenetic relationship among these *O. tsutsugamushi* strains based on the 22-kDa antigen. The data also extended the earlier findings of the 22-kDa gene from Karp strain and will be helpful in the design and development of scrub typhus vaccines.

The search of the BLAST database for the 22-kDa DNA or protein sequence did not retrieve any sequences with significant homology. There is no conserved domain found on this protein as well. Therefore, the function of this 22-kDa protein remains unknown. However, previous study[2] showed that native 22-kDa protein were reactive with immune serum against homologous strains. The recombinant Karp 22-kDa protein was recognized by polyclonal rabbit antibodies raised against whole-cell lysate. Moreover, the computational analysis of amino acid sequence revealed several potential T-cell epitopes on this protein and this recombinant protein induced a strong proliferation of a T cell line that produced IL-2 and IFN-γ.[2] All this information has strengthened the idea of including the 22-kDa protein as one of the protective antigens in multicomponent scrub typhus vaccine candidates. Therefore, we cloned the 22-kDa gene from *O. tsutsugamushi* Karp into a DNA vaccine plasmid VR1012 (pKp22) and evaluated its protective efficacy in a lethal-challenge mouse model. To our surprise, the preliminary results suggested that pKp22 not only did not provide any protection but it also inhibited the protective effect of other scrub typhus vaccine candidates (Ching and colleagues, unpublished data). We do not understand these results, however we still believe that the phylogenetic relationships based on the sequences of 22-kDa genes are very valuable in selecting *O. tsutsugamushi* strains to generate components for vaccine purpose. We are in the process of determining 22-kDa sequences from additional strains of *O. tsutsugamushi*.

[*Competing interests statement:* The authors declare that they have no competing interests.]

REFERENCES

1. Ching, W.-M., H. Wang, C. Eamsila, *et al.* 1998. Expression and refolding of truncated recombinant major outer membrane protein antigen (r56) of *Orientia tsutsugamushi* and its use in enzyme-linked immunosorbent assays. Clin. Diagn. Lab. Immunol. **5:** 519–526.
2. Hickman, C.J., C.K. Stover, S.W. Joseph & E.V. Oaks. 1991. Molecular cloning and sequence analysis of a *Rickettsia tsutsugamushi* 22 kDa antigen containing B- and T-cell epitopes. Microb. Pathog. **11:** 19–31.
3. Seong, S.Y., M.S. Choi & I.S. Kim. 2001. *Orientia tsutsugamushi* infection: overview and immune responses. Microbes Infect. **3:** 11–21.

Nitric Oxide as a Mediator of Increased Microvascular Permeability during Acute Rickettsioses

MICHAEL E. WOODS,[a] GARY WEN,[a] AND JUAN P. OLANO[a,b]

[a]*Department of Pathology,* [b]*Center for Biodefense and Emerging Infectious Diseases, University of Texas Medical Branch, 301 University, Galveston, Texas 77555-0609, USA*

ABSTRACT: Rickettsiae primarily infect the microvascular endothelium, leading to changes in microvascular permeability that result in potentially severe pulmonary and cerebral edema. The mechanisms responsible for these changes are not well understood. One potential mechanism of increased vascular permeability is the anti-rickettsial nitric oxide response described by Walker and colleagues. We hypothesized that anti-rickettsial levels of nitric oxide adversely affects microvascular permeability *in vitro*. To this end we sought to describe the effects of exogenous nitric oxide on the proliferation of intracellular rickettsiae while monitoring the transendothelial electrical resistance as a measure of endothelial barrier integrity. It was determined that the addition of the NO-donor DETA NONOate at certain levels results in a dose-dependent change in electrical resistance across the monolayer while effectively limiting the number of intracellular rickettsiae in human microvascular endothelial cells. The data presented support the idea that nitric oxide produced by infected endothelial cells may be contributing to the changes in vascular permeability that occur during acute rickettsioses. Future experiments aim to elaborate on these results in a model that more clearly depicts the *in vivo* response as well as to describe the changes that occur with respect to interendothelial junctions.

KEYWORDS: Rickettsiae; nitric oxide; vascular permeability; transendothelial resistance; ECIS

INTRODUCTION

Rickettsial diseases represent some of the most severe bacterial infections known to man including epidemic typhus and Rocky Mountain spotted fever. These diseases, caused by *Rickettsia prowazekii* and *Rickettsia rickettsii*, respectively, are the result of their widespread involvement of the endothelial cells lining the microvasculature throughout the body. In severe cases, non-cardiogenic pulmonary edema and cerebral edema are the most feared complications as a result of interstitial pneumonitis and meningoencephalitis.[1] Changes in microvascular permeability

Address for correspondence: Juan P. Olano, Department of Pathology, University of Texas Medical Branch, 301 University, Galveston, Texas 77555-0609, USA. Voice: (409) 772-2870; fax (409) 747-2400.
jpolano@utmb.edu

**Ann. N.Y. Acad. Sci. 1063: 239–245 (2005). © 2005 New York Academy of Sciences.
doi: 10.1196/annals.1355.037**

have been described during rickettsiosis in a mouse model of infection, but these studies are very limited and do not provide an explanation for rickettsiae-induced permeability.[2]

A topic of intense investigation has been mechanisms of immunity to rickettsiae. Specifically, it has been shown that endothelial cells are capable of controlling rickettsiae through a nitric oxide–dependent mechanism. This response, a result of inducible nitric oxide synthase (iNOS) upregulation, is itself dependent on cytokine stimulation of the endothelium by certain pro-inflammatory cytokines, namely TNF-α, IFN-γ, IL-1β, and RANTES.[3,4] The antibacterial properties of nitric oxide (NO) have been well described, as has the critical role of NO as a mediator of vascular tone, platelet coagulation, and endothelial cell function.[5–9] The apparent conundrum presented by this set of facts presents us with an opportunity to better understand the pathogenesis of rickettsial diseases as well as the role of the host immune response in the pathogenesis of the acute rickettsioses.

We sought to better understand the effects of nitric oxide on rickettsiae-infected endothelial cells and how these effects in turn affect the integrity of an endothelial monolayer. We hypothesized that anti-rickettsial levels of nitric oxide are sufficient to negatively affect the integrity of an endothelial monolayer *in vitro*. To this end, we monitored transendothelial electrical resistance after the addition of a nitric oxide donor to confluent, rickettsiae-infected human microvascular endothelial cells. We also examined the ability of the NO donor DETA NONOate to control proliferation of intracellular rickettsiae using real-time PCR.

MATERIALS AND METHODS

Reagents

MCDB 131 was purchased from Gibco (Carlsbad, CA). Fetal calf serum (FCS) was purchased from Hyclone (Logan, UT). Epidermal growth factor was purchased from Chemicon (Temecula, CA) Heparin, sulfanilamide, and naphthylethylenediamine were purchased from Sigma (St. Louis, MO). DETA NONOate was purchased from Cayman Chemicals (Ann Arbor, MI). iQ SYBR Green Supermix was obtained from BioRad (Hercules, CA).

Cell Culture

The human microvascular endothelial cell line, HMEC-1 (courtesy of Mr. Francisco Candal, CDC, Atlanta, GA), was cultured in MCDB131 + 10% FCS + 100 μg/mL heparin + 10 ng/mL EGF in 5% CO_2 at 37°C. All experiments were performed between passages 20–25, and cells were fed with MCDB131 + 1% FCS.

Rickettsiae

Rickettsiae conorii (Malish 7) strain was kindly obtained from Drs. David Walker and Hui-Min Feng. A 10% yolk sac suspension was cultured in Vero cells (ATCC, Manassas, VA) twice and purified using renografin density gradient centrifugation. Rickettsiae were frozen at –80°C in sucrose-phosphate-glutamate buffer and their titer was determined by plaque assay on Vero cells.

Electric Cell-Substrate Impedance Sensing

HMEC-1 were cultured on 8W10E gold-coated electrodes connected to the 1600R ECIS System (Applied Biophysics, Troy, NY). The cells were cultured until a steady level of resistance was reached. The cells were then infected with 10 MOI of *R. conorii* (Malish 7) and treated with the nitric oxide donor DETA NONOate at 0, 100, and 500 μM. The cells were monitored for 120 h with electrical resistance measurements being taken every 2 minutes. Experiments were performed in sets of four and standard deviation was determined at 6-h time points and plotted as a measure of statistical difference.

Real-Time PCR

HMEC-1 were cultured in a 24-well plate until confluent. The cells were then infected with 10 MOI of *R. conorii* and administered DETA NONOate at 0, 100, and 500 μM. At 24-h time points the monolayer was washed with warm phosphate buffered saline and DNA was extracted using the Qiagen DNeasy Tissue Kit (Valencia, CA). Relative gene copy numbers were determined for the rickettsial citrate synthase gene, *gltA*, and the human gene for glyceraldehyde phosphate dehydrogenase, *gapdh*. The primers for *gltA* were as follows: forward primer CS-5 (GAGAGAAATTATATCCAAATGTTGAT) and reverse primer CS-6 (AGGGTCTTCGTGCATTTCTT).[10] The primers for h*gapdh* were as follows: forward primer hGAPDH-145(S) (CAATGACCCCTTCATTGACC) and reverse primer hGAPDH-250(AS) (GACAAGCTTCCCGTTCTCAG). iQ SYBR Green Supermix was utilized at the appropriate concentration with primers at 200 nM. One microliter of DNA from each sample was added to 24 microliters of Supermix cocktail. Real-time PCR was performed on an iCycler iQ Real-Time PCR Detection System using the following protocol: 2 min at 95°C followed by 40 cycles of 95°C for 15 seconds, 50°C for 30 seconds and 60°C for 30 seconds. relative copy numbers of *gltA* were determined by the ΔΔ method.[11]

Nitrite Determination

Nitrite levels were determined using the Greiss assay as previously described.[3]

RESULTS

Effect of Exogenous Nitric Oxide on Endothelial Permeability

HMEC-1 cells, cultured on 8W10E gold-coated electrodes, were infected with *R. conorii* at an MOI of 10 and demonstrated a level of integrity consistent with controls for the first 3 days of infection. After 72 h we saw a statistically significant drop in resistance as compared to uninfected controls. Conversely and perhaps most surprisingly, when the endothelial cells were infected with *R. conorii* and also treated with the nitric oxide donor DETA NONOate at 100 μM we saw no statistically significant drop in electrical resistance over the course of the 5-day experiment as compared to uninfected controls. Future experiments are needed to determine if this trend would continue past 5 days. Finally, administration of DETA NONOate at

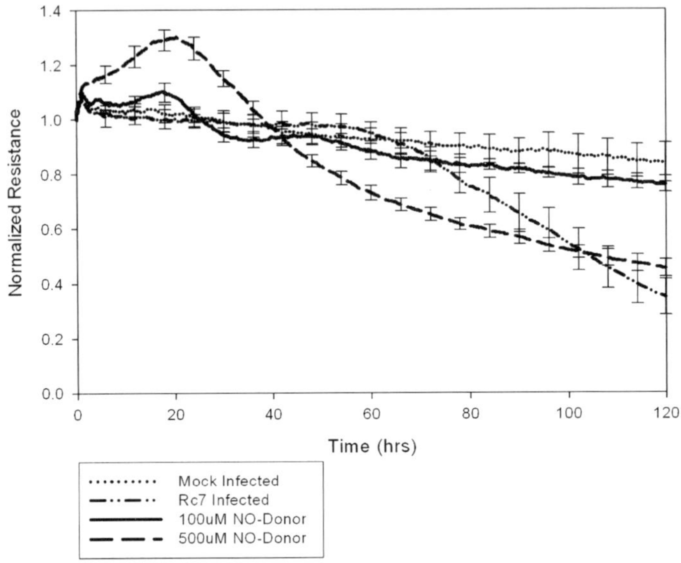

FIGURE 1. Exogenous nitric oxide influences the integrity of endothelial monolayers infected with *R. conorii*. Addition of the NO donor DETA NONOate at 100 μM extended the life span of the infected monolayers for at least two more days. Conversely when administered at 500 μM we saw a marked increase in electrical resistance within the first 24 h followed by a slow and steady decrease in resistance, indicating an increase in microvascular permeability. *R. conorii*–infected, non-NO–stimulated endothelial cells maintained their level of resistance for the first 3 days of infection at which time they began to undergo cell death and subsequent loss of monolayer integrity.

500 μM demonstrated a profound effect on the integrity of the endothelial monolayer. We saw a significant increase in resistance during the first 24 h of infection and stimulation followed by a slow and steady decline in endothelial integrity as determined by a drop in resistance (FIG. 1). Taken together these findings support the hypothesis that nitric oxide can affect the integrity of rickettsiae-infected endothelial monolayers.

Effect of Exogenous Nitric Oxide on Rickettsial Gene Copy Number

HMEC-1 were cultured in 24-well plates and DNA was extracted at 24, 48, and 72 h of infection and/or stimulation with DETA NONOate. Rickettsial gene copy numbers were normalized to human *gapdh* and copy numbers of rickettsiae between samples were compared using the ΔΔ method. We saw no significant change in the numbers of rickettsiae between cells stimulated with and without DETA NONOate for the first 48 hours. However after 72 h we saw nearly 23 times as many rickettsiae in those cells not stimulated with nitric oxide as compared to those treated at either 100 or 500 μM (TABLE 1). Intriguingly we saw no significant difference between the ability of either dose of DETA NONOate to control rickettsiae as compared to the other.

TABLE 1. Exogenous nitric oxide limits the proliferation of intracellular *R. conorii*

	R. conorii/R. conorii + DETA NONOate (100 μM)	*R. conorii/R. conorii* + DETA NONOate (500 μM)
24 h	1.76±0.98 ×	1.15±0.17 ×
48 h	3.34±1.99 ×	2.00±0.90 ×
72 h	23.5±8.99 ×	23.45±10.54 ×

The effect is not noticed until 3 days after infection when there were significantly fewer rickettsiae as measured by real-time PCR for the rickettsial citrate synthase gene, *gltA*. Relative gene copy number was normalized to h*gapdh* and compared using the ΔΔ method. Data indicate fold change in relative copy numbers compared to untreated, infected cells.

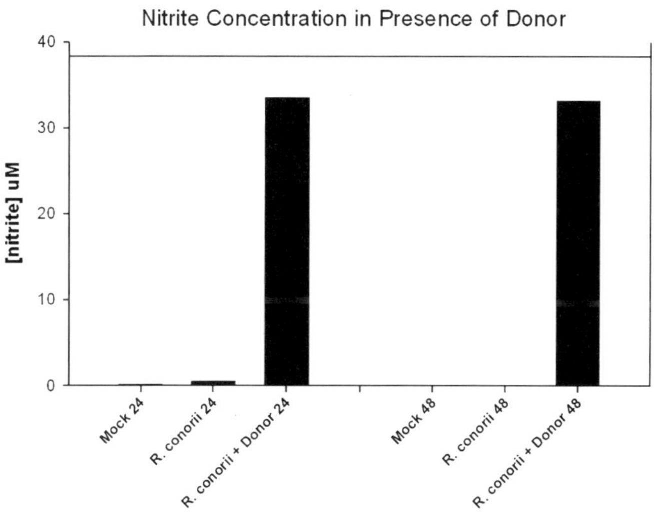

FIGURE 2. Introduction of the NO donor DETA NONOate releases nitric oxide into the environment that is subsequently converted to nitrite. Nitrite was detected within 24 h of addition of the donor molecule and remained at high levels.

Confirmation of the Presence of Nitric Oxide By-Products in Cell Culture Supernatants

To confirm that we have introduced NO into the system we tested the cell culture supernatants using the Greiss reaction. We were able to detect high levels of nitrite, a by-product of NO metabolism, at 24 h after addition of DETA NONOate. The levels maintained themselves through at least the next day of the experiment (FIG. 2).

DISCUSSION

The mechanisms leading to increased microvascular permeability during rickettsial infection have not been extensively studied. There is considerable evidence supporting the role of reactive oxygen species (ROS) as a mechanism of cell damage in response to rickettsiae infection. Work by our lab suggests that the presence of ROS may have little effect on rickettsiae-induced changes in tight junction or adherens junction assembly. Instead, the accumulation of ROS may eventually lead to cell death resulting in changes in permeability at late stages of infection. To more accurately reflect the changes that take place in an *in vivo* environment we have decided to pursue a mechanism shown to be an important anti-rickettsial response and that supports the idea that increased microvascular permeability induced by rickettsiae is in part due to an immunopathological mechanism. Nitric oxide is a well known regulator of vascular tone, vascular remodeling, and interendothelial junction assembly. Previous work has also shown that both mouse and human endothelial cells are able to mount an effective anti-rickettsial response when stimulated by certain pro-inflammatory cytokines. How does this response occur in an animal and what effect will that have on the function of the microvasculature?

By introducing NO into this system of rickettsiae-infected microvascular endothelial cells we have been able to expand on the role of NO itself as not only an antibacterial effector molecule, but also as a potent regulator of vascular permeability. These studies have revealed that NO is very effective at limiting the number of intracellular rickettsiae. The mechanism of this inhibition however is not well understood at this time. Likewise we have shown that certain lower levels of NO donors can effectively extend the life span of endothelial monolayers and has relatively little effect on the barrier function of the monolayer. Conversely, higher levels of the NO donor produce dramatic changes in the integrity of the monolayer by first stabilizing the monolayer and then causing a slow and steady loss of barrier function. Without knowing the degree of NO release in infected endothelial cells *in vivo* at this time we are unable to make conclusions about the definite role of NO as a mechanism leading to increased microvascular permeability. The data presented do at least acknowledge the possibility that this might be the case. However, it also supports the notion that NO may purely be a defense mechanism and that there are other stimuli responsible for the loss of barrier properties. As stated previously, a true NO response by way of the iNOS enzyme is dependent on cytokine stimulation of the endothelium. It is likely that cytokine stimulation of the endothelium would cause changes in vascular permeability independent of NO production and would present a challenge in interpreting results in a system this complex, as suggested by preliminary data from our laboratory (J.P. Olano, personal communication). We expect future experiments using primary mouse brain endothelial cells to better describe the true importance of NO as not only an anti-rickettsial defense mechanism but also as a contributor to disease pathogenesis. In particular, we are interested in the effects of NO on the tight junctions that are distributed ubiquitously throughout the brain.

ACKNOWLEDGMENTS

This material is based upon work supported by the U.S. Army Medical Research and Material Command under Grant DAMD17-02-01-0198 (J.P.O.) and the NIH

T32 Training Grant in Biodefense AI 060549 (M.E.W.). The content of the information presented here does not reflect the position or the policy of the government, and no official endorsement should be inferred.

[*Competing interests statement:* The authors have no competing interests.]

REFERENCES

1. Walker, D.H., V.L. Popov, J. Wen & H.M. Feng. 1994. *Rickettsia conorii* infection of C3H/HeN mice. A model of endothelial-target rickettsiosis. Lab. Invest. **70:** 358–368.
2. Walker, D.H., G.A. Valbuena & J.P. Olano. 2003. Pathogenic mechanisms of diseases caused by Rickettsia. Ann. N.Y. Acad. Sci. **990:** 1–11.
3. Walker, D.H., V.L. Popov, P.A. Crocquet-Valdes, *et al.* 1997. Cytokine-induced, nitric oxide-dependent, intracellular antirickettsial activity of mouse endothelial cells. Lab. Invest. **76:** 129–138.
4. Feng, H.M. & D.H. Walker. 2000. Mechanisms of intracellular killing of *Rickettsia conorii* in infected human endothelial cells, hepatocytes, and macrophages. Infect. Immun. **68:** 6729–6736.
5. Kubes, P. & D.N. Granger. 1992. Nitric oxide modulates microvascular permeability Am. J. Physiol. **262:** H611–H615.
6. Hinder, F., M. Booke, L.D. Traber & D.L. Traber. 1997. Nitric oxide and endothelial permeability J. Appl. Physiol. **83:** 1941–1946.
7. Hofmann, F., A. Ammendola & J. Schlossmann. 2000. Rising behind NO: cGMP-dependent protein kinases. J. Cell Sci. **113:** 1671–1676.
8. Chakravortty, D. & M. Hensel. 2003. Inducible nitric oxide synthase and control of intracellular bacterial pathogens. Microbes Infect. **5:** 621–627.
9. Albrecht, E.W., C.A. Stegeman, P. Heeringa, *et al.* 2003. Protective role of endothelial nitric oxide synthase. J. Pathol. **199:** 8–17.
10. Horta, M.C., M.B. Labruna, L.A. Sangioni, *et al.* 2004. Prevalence of antibodies to spotted fever group rickettsiae in humans and domestic animals in a Brazilian spotted fever-endemic area in the state of Sao Paulo, Brazil: Serologic evidence for infection by *Rickettsia rickettsii* and another spotted fever group *Rickettsia* Am. J. Trop. Med. Hyg. **71:** 93–97.
11. Olano, J.P., G. Wen, H.M. Feng, *et al.* 2004. Histologic, serologic, and molecular analysis of persistent ehrlichiosis in a murine model. Am. J. Pathol. **165:** 997–1006.

Cloning and Expression of 51-kDa Antigenic Protein of *Neorickettsia ristícii* NR-JA1

MYEONG-KYU PARK, EUN-HA KIM, MAE-RIM CHO, YING-HUA YI, MI-JIN LEE, DEVENDRA H. SHAH, JIN-HO PARK, BAE-KEUN PARK,[a] SEONG-KUG EO, JOHN-HWA LEE, AND JOON-SEOK CHAE

Bio-Safety Research Institute and College of Veterinary Medicine, Chonbuk National University, Jeonju 561-756, Korea

[a]College of Veterinary Medicine, Chungnam National University, Yousung-gu, Taejeon 305-764, Korea

ABSTRACT: *Neorickettsia* (*Ehrlichia*) *risticii* is a causative agent of acute diarrheal syndrome in horses, commonly known as Potomac horse fever. Korean isolate of *N. risticii* NR-JA1 was cultivated in mouse macrophage cell line P388D1. A complete ORF of p51 antigenic protein gene was amplified and cloned into pQE32 and pcDNA3.1 vectors and the resultant clones were named as pQE32/Nr-51 and pcDNA3.1/Nr-51, respectively. Recombinant p51 (rp51) protein antigen was expressed in *E. coli* (pQE32/Nr-51) and cos-7 cell line (pcDNA3.1/Nr-51). The rp51 protein showed immunoreactivity with anti-mouse p51 antibodies. BALB/c mice were inoculated with recombinant plasmid DNA (pcDNA3.1/Nr-51). The serum samples collected from these BALB/c mice showed IgG ELISA titers of 1:128. In a Western immunoblot assay, these serum samples showed a strong reactivity to rp51 expressed in cos-7 cell line transfected with pcDNA3.1/Nr-51. The results of this preliminary indicate that *N. risticii* p51 protein is an immmuno-dominant antigen and may be a good target for the development of serological or a molecular diagnostic test and possibly an improved recombinant DNA based vaccine against Potomac horse fever.

KEYWORDS: **Potomac horse fever; *Neorickettsia risticii*; NR-JA1**

INTRODUCTION

Potomac horse fever (PHF) is an equine disease caused by a monocytotropic rickettsia, *Neorickettsia* (formerly *Ehrlichia*) *risticii*.[1] The disease was first observed in 1979 in the areas along the Potomac River in Maryland and Virginia. Since then, it has been diagnosed in most parts of the USA, Canada, Europe and other parts of the world.[2] With a fatality rate of 5 to 30%, PHF remains a significant problem for horse owners.

Humoral immunity is considered important in the host defense against PHF. Infected horses and mice develop a strong immunoglobulin G antibody response and

Address for correspondence: Joon-Seok Chae, Bio-Safety Research Institute and College of Veterinary Medicine, Chonbuk National University, Jeonju 561-756, Korea.
jschae@chonbuk.ac.kr

Ann. N.Y. Acad. Sci. 1063: 246–251 (2005).
doi: 10.1196/annals.1355.038

protection against *N. risticii* infection.[3,4] Passive transfer of horse antisera to *N. risticii* or mouse antibodies to *N. risticii* (antiserum or purified immunoglobulin G) protected mice against *N. risticii* challenge infection, strongly indicating that antibody mediates the immunity.[3,5]

Molecular analysis of *N. risticii* strain (strain 25-D) indicated the presence of nine major component antigens (indicated by molecular mass: 110, 70, 68, 55, 51, 50, 49, 33, and 28 kDa), all of which are apparent surface antigens, as determined by ^{125}I surface labeling.[6] However, it has been demonstrated that the strain-specific antigens from different *N. risticii* isolates vary in their sizes and sequences.[7] A 51-kDa protein (p51) is the major antigen recognized in horses with PHF.[8] P51 has been found in all *N. risticii* strains identified to date. Based on a search of the GenBank database, it is not found in any other bacteria.[7,9] Moreover, p51 is predicted to be an outer membrane protein by PSORT analysis (http://psort.nibb.ac.jp/), indicating that it may be an important protein for *N. risticii*. However, the information regarding whether the P51 protein is expressed by the organisms isolated from cultures and if this protein can be used as diagnostic or immunoprophylactic antigen, is relatively scarce. We have recently isolated *N. risticii* NR-JA1 from cercaria from stream-water snails. This report presents the results of our preliminary studies on immunologic properties of *in vitro* and *in vivo* expressed p51 protein gene from Korean strain of *N. risticii* NR-JA1.

MATERIALS AND METHODS

Amplification and Cloning of p51 Gene from N. risticii *NR-JA1*

The genomic DNA was extracted from *N. risticii* NR-JA1 using DNeasy Tissue kit (Qiagen, USA). A complete ORF (1,544 bp) of p51 gene was amplified using the primer sets shown in TABLE 1. The 5′ end of each primer was modified to contain *BamH*-I and either *Kpn*-I or *Xba*-I restriction endonuclease sites to facilitate directional cloning in pQE32 vector (Quiagen, USA) and pcDNA3.1 (+) vector (Invitrogen, USA). The PCR conditions included an initial denaturing period of 5 min at 95°C followed by 35 cycles of 95°C for 1.5 min, 48°C for 1.5 min, 72°C for 2 min, and a final extension at 72°C for 7 min. A 1,544 bp PCR product was purified and cloned in to pQE32 and pcDNA3.1 (+) vectors as per the protocols provided by the manufacturer. The resultant plasmids were named as pQE32/Nr-51 and pcDNA3.1/Nr-51, respectively.

TABLE 1. Primers used for PCR amplification of *N. risticii* p51 gene

Primer[a]	Nucleotide Sequence (5′ to 3′)	Position[b]
S4-*Bam*HI	5′-**GGA TCC** CAT GTA TAA ACT TAG CAA GAT ATT ACT TTT GAC GGC G-3′	898–933
Nr51 *Kpn* I	5′-GG**G GTA CC**T TAG TAC GAC ACC TTC AC-3′	2433–2416
Nr51 *Xba* I	5′-GC**T CTA GA**T TAG TAC GAC ACC TTC AC-3′	2433–2416

[a]The restrictions sites in each primer are shown in boldface. [b]Positions are based on 51-kDa gene sequence of *N. risitcii* (GenBank accession no. U85784).

In Vitro *Expression of Recombinant p51*

The recombinant p51 was expressed in chemically competent *E. coli* M15 cells transformed with pQE32/Nr-51 as well as in cos-7 cell line transfected with pcDNA3.1/Nr-51. The expressed protein in both the systems was detected by SDS-PAGE. Subsequently, rp51 protein was purified using standard procedures and stored at –20°C until further use.

In Vivo *Expression of rp51 DNA for Immunization Studies in Mice*

Two groups (*N*=6) of 6-week-old male BALB/c mice were used for immunization studies. Group I received 50 µg of pcDNA3.1 which served as a negative control, while Group II was inoculated intramuscularly with 50 µg of recombinant plasmid DNA, pcDNA3.1/Nr51. Both the groups received booster immunization 14 days after first immunization. The blood samples were collected 3 days post booster immunization and the serum samples were subjected to Western immunoblot analysis and ELISA assay for titration of antibody response against rp51 protein antigen.

RESULTS

Cloning and in Vitro *Expression of rp51 Protein*

A complete ORF of 51 kDa protein antigen gene of *N. risticii* NR-JA1 isolate cultivated in mouse macrophage cell line P388D1 was amplified to obtain 1,544 bp PCR product (FIG. 1). The PCR product cloned into pQE32 and pcDNA3.1 vectors were named as pQE32/Nr-51 and pcDNA3.1/Nr-51, respectively. SDS-PAGE anal-

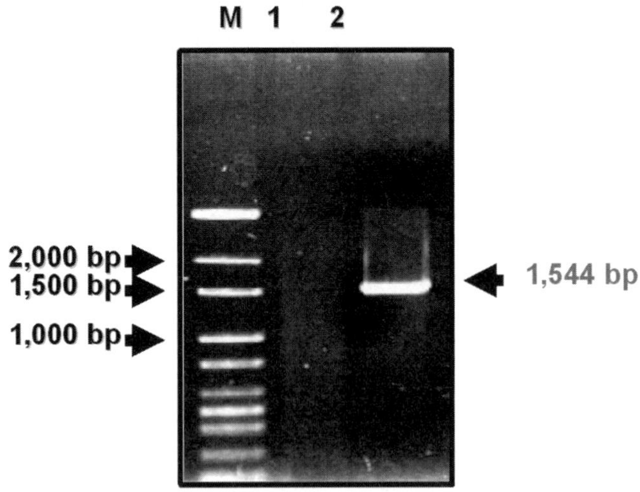

FIGURE 1. PCR amplicon of *E. risticii* p51 protein gene (1,544 bp). M, DNA size marker; lane 1, negative control; lane 2, *E. risticii* NR-A1.

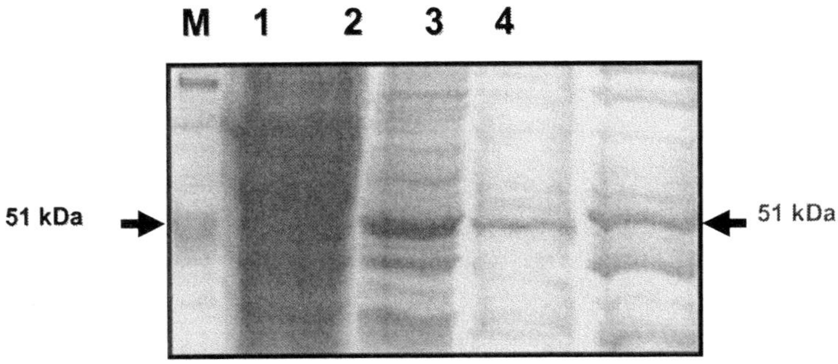

FIGURE 2. Recombinant p51 protein was analyzed through SDS-PAGE. Lane 1 to 3 represent the protein profiles of the non-induced, induced, and purified proteins, from *E. coli* cells transformed with pQE32/Nr-51. Lane 4 shows cos-7 cell extract transfected with pcDNA3.1/nr51.

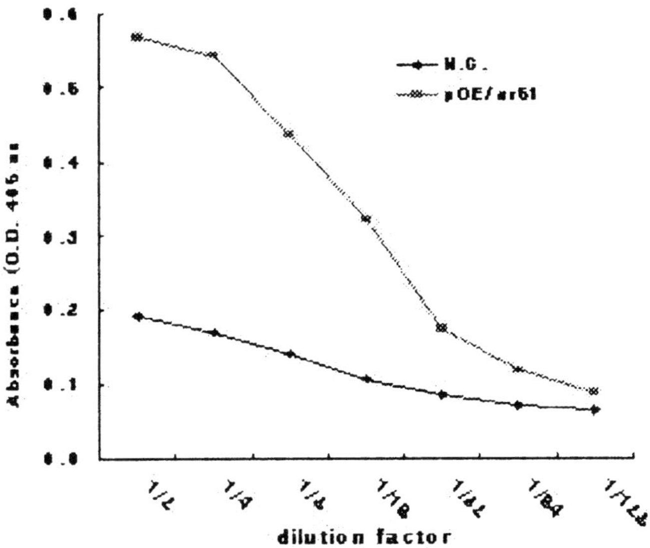

FIGURE 3. Serum IgG antibody responses of BALB/C mice to recombinant plasmid pcDNA3.1/Nr-51.

ysis of rp51 protein expressed in *E. coli* (pQE32/Nr-51) as well as cos-7 cell line (pcDNA3.1/Nr-51) revealed a characteristic band of 51 kDa (FIG. 2).

In Vivo *Expression and Experimental Immunization of Mice*

Mice were injected intradermally with the recombinant plasmid pcDNA3.1/Nr-51 to allow *in vivo* expression of p51 protein. Serum samples from mice immunized with pcDNA3.1/Nr-51 were analyzed by ELISA, which showed a serum IgG antibody titer of 1:128 (FIG. 3). Moreover, the serum samples collected from BALB/c

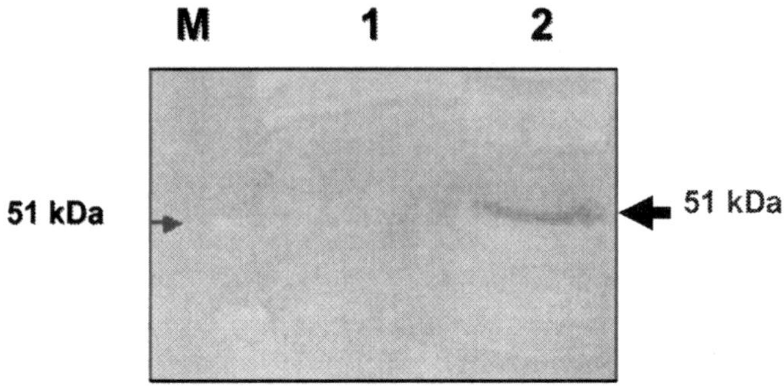

FIGURE 4. Western immunoblot reactivity of the p51 protein antigen purified from cos-7 cell transfected with pcDNA3.1/Nr51. Mouse anti-pcDNA3.1/Nr51 polyclonal serum was used.

mice inoculated with pcDNA3.1/Nr-51 also showed strong immunoreactivity with pcDNA3.1/Nr-51 protein antigen expressed in cos-7 cell lines (FIG. 4). Western blot analysis revealed that mouse anti-p51 serum as well as a serum sample collected from *N. risticii* infected horse strongly reacted with both purified recombinant p51 and 51-kDa native proteins of *N. risticii* NR-JA1 cultured in P388D1 cells (data not shown).

DISCUSSION

The 51-kDa antigen of *N. risticii* is one of the major proteins against which infected horses develop antibodies early in the infection.[8] Antibodies against major antigens of *N. risticii* have also been implicated in the protective immune response against experimental infection.[7,9] Thus, in order to characterize the immunogenic properties of *N. risticii* NR-JA1, we performed cloning, expression, and immunization studies with 51-kDa protein antigen. We found that rp51 protein was expressed *in vitro* (in *E. coli* and cos-7 cell line) as well as *in vivo* (in a mouse model). Moreover, *N. risticii* NR-JA1 strain cultured in P388D1 cells also expressed native p51 protein, indicating that p51 is a naturally expressed protein in *N. risticii.* The mice injected with recombinant p51 plasmid (pcDNA3.1/Nr-51) also showed strong antibody titers when analyzed by ELISA using purified recombinant p51 antigen. Hence, the finding of our study should provide an insight into the understanding immunogenic potential of p51 antigen. It appears that p51 antigenic protein may be a good target for the development of effective diagnostic or immunoprophylactic agent, not only because of its immunogenic potential but also because the p51 gene is present only in *N. risticii* and has been found consistently in all *N. risticii* strains identified to date.[3,4] Moreover, p51 predicted to be an outer membrane protein by PSORT analysis (http://psort.nibb.ac.jp/). Therefore it appears that p51 antigen could be a potential target for the development of improved serological or molecular diagnostic methods and possibly a recombinant DNA vaccine against PHF.

ACKNOWLEDGMENTS

This work was supported by grant No. (R01-2001-00246) from the Basic Research program of the Korea Science & Engineering Foundation and partially supported by the Brain Korea 21 Project in E007.

[*Competing interests statement:* The authors report that they have no competing interests.]

REFERENCES

1. DUMLER, J.S., A.F. BARBET, C.P. BEKKER, *et al.* 2001. Reorganization of genera in the families Rickettsiaceae and Anaplasmataceae in the order Rickettsiales: Unification of some species of Ehrlichia with Anaplasma, Cowdria with Ehrlichia and Ehrlichia with Neorickettsia, descriptions of six new species combinations and designation of *Ehrlichia equi* and "HGE agent" as subjective synonyms of *Ehrlichia phagocytophila*. Int. J. Syst. Evol. Microbiol. **51:** 2145–2165.
2. RIKIHISA, Y. 2004. Rickettsial diseases. *In* Equine Internal Medicine, 2nd edit. S.M. Reed, W.M. Bayly & D.C. Sellon, Eds.: 96–109. W.B. Saunders. Philadelphia, PA.
3. RIKIHISA, Y., R. WADA, S.M. REED & S. YAMAMOTO. 1993. Development of neutralizing antibody in horses infected with *Ehrlichia risticii*. Vet. Microbiol. **36:** 139–147
4. VEMULAPALLI, R., B. BISWAS & S.K. DUTTA. 1995. Pathogenic, immunologic, and molecular differences between two *Ehrlichia risticii* strains. J. Clin. Microbiol. **33:** 2987–2993.
5. KAYLOR, P.S., T.B. CRAWFORD, T.F. MCELWAIN & G.H. PALMER. 1991. Passive transfer of antibody to *Ehrlichia risticii* protects mice from ehrlichiosis. Infect. Immun. **59:** 2058–2062.
6. DUTTA, S.K., B. SHANKARAPPA, S.R. THAKER & B.L. MATTINGLY-NAPIER. 1990. DNA restriction endonuclease cleavage pattern and protein antigen profile of *Ehrlichia risticii*. Vet. Microbiol. **25:** 29–38.
7. DUTTA, S.K., R. VEMULAPALLI & B. BISWAS. 1998. Association of deficiency in antibody response to vaccine and heterogeneity of *Ehrlichia risticii* strains with Potomac horse fever vaccine failure in horses. J. Clin. Microbiol. **36:** 506–512.
8. VEMULAPALLI, R., B. BISWAS & S.K. DUTTA. 1998. Studies with recombinant proteins of *Ehrlichia risticii*: identification of strain-specific antigen as a protective antigen. Vet. Parasitol. **76:** 189–202.
9. KANTER, M., J. MOTT, N. OHASHI, *et al.* 2000. Analysis of 16S rRNA and 51-kilodalton antigen gene and transmission in mice of *Ehrlichia risticii* in virgulate trematodes from *Elimia livescens* snails in Ohio. J. Clin. Microbiol. **38:** 3349–3358.

Activity of Telithromycin against Thirteen New Isolates of *C. burnetii* Including Three Resistant to Doxycycline

JEAN-MARC ROLAIN, FRÉDÉRIC LAMBERT, AND DIDIER RAOULT

Unité des rickettsies, IFR 48, CNRS UMR 6020, Université de la Méditerranée, Faculté de medicine, 13385 Marseille cedex 5, France

ABSTRACT: In this study we have evaluated the *in vitro* activity of antibiotics against 13 new isolates of *Coxiella burnetii* using a real-time quantitative PCR assay. MICs against doxycycline ranged from 1 to 8 μg/mL, telithromycin from 0.5 to 2 μg/mL , and all strains had MICs ≥ 8 μg/mL for erythromycin. We report that strains resistant to doxycycline exist either in humans or animals.

KEYWORDS: *Coxiella burnetii*; Q fever; telithromycin; doxycycline

Q fever is a worldwide zoonosis caused by *Coxiella burnetii,* a strict intracellular bacteria that is considered a potential biological weapon.[1,2] There are two clinical forms of the disease: acute and chronic. The main clinical presentations of acute Q fever are febrile pneumonia or hepatitis. Endocarditis is the main clinical manifestation of chronic Q fever and represents one of the most problematic disease for eradication. For acute Q fever, antibiotics with a bacteriostatic activity are sufficient to shorten the duration of the disease. Chronic Q fever is a severe disease that can relapse despite years of antibiotic treatment. In this case, a bactericidal activity is required to eradicate *C. burnetii* infection. Tetracyclines remain the first-line antibiotics to treat acute Q fever with fluoroquinolones being used as an alternative.[2] Among macrolide compounds, erythromycin is not currently considered a safe alternative in acute Q fever treatment[3] owing to reports of therapeutic failures with this antibiotic, probably due to heterogeneous susceptibility to erythromycin among different *C. burnetii* strains.[4,5] Conversely, telithromycin, a new ketolide compound, was shown to be very effective when evaluated against reference strains of *C. burnetii.*[6] The current recommended regimen for therapy of Q fever endocarditis is the association of doxycycline and hydroxychloroquine for 18 to 36 months.[7,8] Doxycycline level in serum should be monitored and posology adapted in order to obtain a serum concentration of at least 5 μg/mL.[9]

C. burnetii is very fastidious and thus evaluation of antibiotic susceptibility has been rarely reported for clinical isolates except from our lab using the shell vial

Address for correspondence: D. Raoult, CNRS UMR 6020, Université de la Méditerranée, Faculté de medicine, 27 boulevard Jean Moulin, 13385 Marseille cedex 5, France. Voice: 33049138551; fax: 330491830390.

Didier.Raoult@medecine.univ-mrs.fr

**Ann. N.Y. Acad. Sci. 1063: 252–256 (2005). © 2005 New York Academy of Sciences.
doi: 10.1196/annals.1355.039**

method.[2,10] The shell vial technique was the most widely used method[11] and *in vitro* MICs against doxycycline usually ranged from 1 to 4 μg/mL.[5,6,11–13] Recent developments in molecular biology, especially the use of quantitative real-time PCR, make it possible to test clinical isolates routinely with increased rapidity and sensitivity.[14–16] Interestingly, MICs obtained using this more sensitive method were slightly higher than previous results obtained with reference strains.[15] This has been recently confirmed when testing new isolates with MICs against doxycycline ranging from 1 to 8 μg/mL, for which we found a correlation between ratio of doxycycline to MIC and rapid decline of antibody levels during treatment of Q fever endocarditis.[14] Especially, we have reported for the first time a human isolate of *C. burnetii* resistant to doxycycline (MIC=8 μg/mL) in a patient with Q fever endocarditis who died during the course of the treatment.[14] We therefore undertook to examine in the present study the bacteriostatic activity of doxycycline and telithromycin comparatively to erythromycin using a modified real-time Lightcycler® PCR assay previously described.[14,15] We selected thirteen new isolates of *C. burnetii* obtained either from patients with acute (three isolates) and with chronic Q fever (eight isolates including the resistant isolate previously reported[14]) or from animals (two isolates) and against the Q212 and Nine Mile reference strains. For each isolate, the number of DNA copies at day 0 and at day 15 were recorded and compared using a Student's *t* test. Growth ratio for each strain was calculated as log (number of DNA copies at day 15)/log (number of DNA copies at day 0). MIC was defined as the first antibiotic concentration allowing inhibition of growth of the bacterium as measured by comparison of number of DNA copies at day 15 with antibiotic versus day 0 and day 15 without antibiotic.

For the 13 new isolates, the mean of growth ratio was of 1.38 ± 0.09 [range 1.24–1.52] and estimated doubling time was of 80 h (range 72–90), whereas the estimated doubling time was of 15 h and 37 h for Q212 and Nine Mile strains, respectively. Results of MICs for the three antibiotics are summarized in TABLE 1. MICs against doxycycline ranged from 1 to 8 μg/mL, telithromycin from 0.5 to 2 μg/mL and all strains had MICs ≥ 8 μg/mL for erythromycin. There was no difference in MICs for the 13 strains according to their origin.

As previously described, real-time quantitative PCR assay was more sensitive than IFA for evaluation of antibiotic susceptibility.[14] Moreover, the method allows the precisely counting of the number of bacteria during a particular period of time. This is of major importance for evaluation of antibiotic susceptibility since it is necessary to obtain a sufficient growth of bacteria before ending the experiment. Especially of interest, we show that fresh clinical isolates grow more slowly compared to a reference strain and need to be cultivated for at least 15 days in the antibiotic assay. Several *in vitro* cell subcultures may lead to an adaptation of the strain to cell culture and a more rapid growth as reported for bacteria of the genus *Rickettsia.*[17] In this study, we did find any differences of susceptibility to antibiotics relative to the origin of the isolates as suggested in the past.[18]

However, we have found a wide heterogeneity of susceptibility to doxycycline as recently described[14] and we report that strains resistant to doxycycline exist either in human or in animal. This resistance is worrying as doxycycline is the reference treatment. Because antibiotic pressure on *C. burnetii* in humans is believed to be low, it is possible that decreased susceptibility to doxycycline was linked to antibiotic pressure in livestock[19] and/or in plant agriculture.[20] This may select resistant strains

TABLE 1. MICs of antibiotics against 13 strains of *C. burnetii*

		MICs (µg/mL)		
Strain	Origin	Doxycycline (µg/mL)	Erythromycin (µg/mL)	Telithromycin (µg/mL)
1	Endocarditis	1	>8	0.5
2	Endocarditis	1	>8	1
3	Endocarditis	1	>8	1
4	Endocarditis	4	8	0.5
5	Endocarditis	4	>8	0.5
6	Human placenta	4	>8	2
7	Mouse	4	>8	0.5
8	Endocarditis	4	>8	0.5
9	Endocarditis	4	>8	1
10	Acute Q fever (blood)	4	>8	1
11	Endocarditis[a]	8	>8	2
12	Goat	8	>8	0.5
13	Acute Q fever (blood)	8	>8	0.5

[a]This patient died during the course of the treatment (see ref. 14).

and alternative antibiotic treatment may be important. Horizontally acquired DNA integrated into a natural isolate of *Chlamydia suis,* a pathogen of pigs, has been recently reported suggesting that this phenomenon may occur within any other obligate intracellular bacterium.[21] The mechanism of resistance for our isolates is not known and further studies are needed to understand the exact molecular support of resistance. Finally, we confirm that erythromycin was not effective *in vitro* against all isolates of *C. burnetii* and should not be used for acute Q fever, New macrolide compounds, especially telithromycin, had better *in vitro* efficacy and could be useful as a safe alternative therapy. Indeed, using a standard regimen of telithromycin of 800 mg/day, the mean serum concentration is 2 µg/mL and thus as compared to the MICs found in our study, the ratio would be greater than 1.

In conclusion, our results may have consequences for the treatment of Q fever if strains resistant to doxycycline emerge. New drugs such as telithromycin may play a major role in the treatment of Q fever. Surveillance of susceptibility to doxycycline of new isolates should be assessed in order to detect resistant isolates. We now evaluate routinely the susceptibility to doxycycline of each new isolate using the real-time quantitative assay and currently we are able to give this result in about 3 months, a delay compatible with adjustment of posology during the course of treatment for chronic Q fever. The molecular mechanism of resistance to doxycycline in these strains should be evaluated to develop new molecular tools for rapid detection of resistant strains.

We believe that the role of the new macrolides for which no antibiotic resistance was detected, such as clarithromycin and telithromycin, should be further investigated and that clinical trials are warranted.

ACKNOWLEDGMENTS

This work was supported by the INSERM program of research in microbiology 2003.

[*Competing interests statement:* The authors state that they have no competing interests.]

REFERENCES

1. MADARIAGA, M.G., K. REZAI. G.M. TRENHOLME & R.A. WEINSTEIN. 2003. Q fever: a biological weapon in your backyard. Lancet Infect. Dis. **3:** 709–721.
2. MAURIN, M. & D. RAOULT. 1999. Q fever. Clin. Microbiol. Rev.**12:** 518–553.
3. RAOULT, D. 2003. Use of macrolides for Q fever. Antimicrob. Agents Chemother. **47:** 446.
4. MAURIN, M. & D. RAOULT. 1993. *In vitro* susceptibilities of spotted fever group rickettsiae and *Coxiella burnetii* to clarithromycin. Antimicrob. Agents Chemother. **37:** 2633–2637.
5. RAOULT, D., H. TORRES & M. DRANCOURT. 1991. Shell-vial assay: Evaluation of a new technique for determining antibiotic susceptibility, tested in 13 isolates of *Coxiella burnetii*. Antimicrob. Agents Chemother. **35:** 2070–2077.
6. ROLAIN, J.M., M. MAURIN, A. BRYSKIER & D. RAOULT. 2000. *In vitro* activities of telithromycin (HMR 3647) against *Rickettsia rickettsii, Rickettsia conorii, Rickettsia africae, Rickettsia typhii, Rickettsia prowasekii, Coxiella burnetii, Bartonella henselae, Bartonella quintana, Bartonella bacilliformis,* and *Ehrlichia chaffeensis*. Antimicrob. Agents Chemother. **44:** 1391-–1393.
7. RAOULT, D., P. HOUPIKIAN, H. TISSOT DUPONT, *et al.* 1999. Treatment of Q fever endocarditis: comparison of two regimens containing doxycycline and ofloxacin or hydroxychloroquine. Arch. Int. Med. **159:** 167–173.
8. HOUPIKIAN, P., G. HABIB, T. MESANA & D. RAOULT. 2002. Changing clinical presentation of Q fever endocarditis. Clin. Infect. Dis. **34:** E28–E31.
9. ROLAIN, J.M., M.N. MALLET & D. RAOULT. 2003. Correlation between serum levels of doxycycline and serology evolution in patients treated for *Coxiella burnetii* endocarditis. J. Infect. Dis. **9:** 1322–1325.
10. RAOULT, D., G. VESTRIS & M. ENEA. 1990. Isolation of 16 strains of *Coxiella burnetii* from patients by using a sensitive centrifugation cell culture system and establishment of strains in HEL cells. J. Clin. Microbiol. **28:** 2482–2484.
11. GIKAS, A., I. SPYRIDAKI, E. SCOULICA, *et al.* 2001. *In vitro* susceptibility of *Coxiella burnetii* to linezolid in comparison with its susceptibilities to quinolones, doxycycline, and clarithromycin. Antimicrob. Agents Chemother. **45:** 3276–3278.
12. GIKAS, A., I. SPYRIDAKI, A. PSAROULAKI, *et al.* 1999. *In vitro* susceptibility of *Coxiella burnetii* to trovafloxacin in comparison with susceptibilities to pefloxacin, ciprofloxacin, ofloxacin, doxycycline, and clarithromycin. Antimicrob. Agents Chemother. **42:** 2747–2748.
13. ROLAIN, J.M., M. MAURIN & D. RAOULT. 2001. Bacteriostatic and bactericidal activities of moxifloxacin against *Coxiella burnetii*. Antimicrob. Agents Chemother. **45:** 301–302.
14. ROLAIN, J.M., A. BOULOS, M.N. MALLET & D. RAOULT. 2005. Correlation between ratio of doxycycline to MIC and rapid decline of antibody levels during treatment of Q fever endocarditis. Antimicrob. Agents Chemother. In press.
15. BOULOS, A., J.M. ROLAIN, M. MAURIN & D. RAOULT. 2004. Evaluation of antibiotic susceptibilities against *Coxiella burnetii* by real time PCR. Int. J. Antimicrob Agents **23:** 169–174.
16. BRENNAN, R.E. & J.E. SAMUEL. 2003. Evaluation of Coxiella burnetii antibiotic susceptibilities by real- time PCR assay. J. Clin. Microbiol. **41:** 1869–1874.

17. ROLAIN, J.M., M. MAURIN, G. VESTRIS & D. RAOULT. 1998. *In vitro* susceptibilities of 27 Rickettsiae to 13 antimicrobials. Antimicrob. Agents Chemother. **42:** 1537–1541.
18. YEAMAN, M.R. & O.G. BACA. 1990. Unexpected antibiotic susceptibility of a chronic isolate of *Coxiella burnetii*. Ann. NY Acad. Sci. **590:** 297–305.
19. MCEWEN, S.A. & P.J. FEDORKA-CRAY. 2002. Antimicrobial use and resistance in animals. Clin. Infect. Dis. **34:** S93–S106.
20. VIDAVER, A.K. 2002. Uses of antimicrobials in plant agriculture. Clin. Infect. Dis. **34:** S107–100.
21. DUGAN, J., D.D. ROCKEY, L. JONES & A.A. ANDERSEN. 2004. Tetracycline resistance in *Chlamydia suis* mediated by genomic islands inserted into the chlamydial inv-like gene. Antimicrob. Agents Chemother. **48:** 3989–3995.

Effect of Antibiotic Treatment in Patients with DEBONEL/TIBOLA

V. IBARRA, J.R. BLANCO, A. PORTILLO, S. SANTIBÁÑEZ, L. METOLA, AND J.A. OTEO

Área de Enfermedades Infecciosas, Hospitales San Millán-San Pedro-de La Rioja, Logroño, (La Rioja), Spain

ABSTRACT: DEBONEL/TIBOLA is a tick-borne acute/sub-acute infection transmitted in our environment by *Dermacentor marginatus* and mainly caused by *Rickettsia slovaca*. The aim of our study was to know the effect of starting early treatment in the course of the DEBONEL/TIBOLA.

KEYWORDS: DEBONEL/TIBOLA; azithromycin; early treatment; Spain; doxycycline

INTRODUCTION

DEBONEL/TIBOLA is a tick-borne acute/subacute infection transmitted in our environment by *Dermacentor marginatus* and mainly caused by *Rickettsia slovaca.*[1] Up to now, no treatment has been officially established. Different antibiotics have been used for the treatment of this disease and some authors have recommended that only those patients who show progressive symptoms be treated.[2] The aim of our study was to investigate the effect of starting early treatment in the course of the DEBONEL/TIBOLA.

MATERIAL AND METHODS

Patients who were diagnosed with DEBONEL/TIBOLA (N=34) in our hospital from January 2001 to December 2004 were studied. All patients were treated early with antibiotics. The mean time from the onset of symptoms to the start of treatment was three days (range was 1 to 5 days). Doxycycline (100 mg twice a day for 14 days) was administered to all adult patients (N=24). Ten patients (9 children and a pregnant) were treated with azithromycin (10 mg/kg once a day for 5 days). Disease durations for these patients were evaluated.

Address for correspondence: José A. Oteo, Área de Enfermedades Infecciosas, Hospitales San Millán-San Pedro-de La Rioja, Avda. Viana, N° 1, 26001 Logroño (La Rioja), Spain. Voice: 34 941 297275; fax: 34 941 297267.

jaoteo@riojasalud.es

Ann. N.Y. Acad. Sci. 1063: 257–258 (2005). © 2005 New York Academy of Sciences.
doi: 10.1196/annals.1355.040

TABLE 1. Evolution of the 34 patients included in this study

Antibiotic treatment	Number of patients (N=34)	Days with fever	Days for improvement of lymphadenopathy	Diameter of alopecia greater than 0.5 cm (cm)
Doxycycline	7 (1[a])	—	7	No
	6	—	7	Yes (1)
	2	—	15	No
	1	—	4	No
	1	—	7	Yes (1.5)
	1	—	15	Yes (1.5)
	1	2	2	Yes (1.5)
	1	2	15	No
	4	2	7	No
Azithromycin	6 (1[a])	—	7	No
	1	—	5	Yes (1)
	1	—	7	Yes (2)
	1	1	7	Yes (1)
	1	2	7	No

[a]Two out of the 34 patients presented with a tick bite outside of the scalp region. —, No fever.

RESULTS AND DISCUSSION

A quick improvement of the signs and symptoms was observed in all cases. Eight patients had fever, which disappeared 48 hours after beginning the treatment. For most patients (88%) the painful lymphadenopathy improved within 7 days. Twenty three out of 34 patients (68%) fully recovered. Twelve patients (35%) developed persistent alopecia at the site of the bite after healing of the local reaction. These patients had an alopecia area of 0.5–2.0 cm in diameter that lasted three months. Data are shown in TABLE 1.

In conclusion, doxycycline and azithromycin are safe and effective for the treatment of DEBONEL/TIBOLA. Nevertheless, data for the course of the diseases for patients without antibiotic treatment were not available. According to our experience, starting early treatment in the course of the infection is recommended.

ACKNOWLEDGMENTS

This study was supported in part by grants from the Fondo de Investigación Sanitaria (FIS PI021810 and G03/057), Ministerio de Sanidad y Consumo, Spain.

[*Competing interests statement:* The authors have no competing interests.]

REFERENCES

1. OTEO, J.A., V. IBARRA, J.R. BLANCO, *et al.* 2004. *Dermacentor*-borne necrosis erythema and lymphadenopathy. A new tick-borne disease. Clin. Microbiol. Infect. **10:** 327–333.
2. LAKOS, A. 2002. Tick-borne lymphadenopathy (TIBOLA). Wien. Klin. Wochenschr. **114:** 648–654.

Structural Features of Lipopolysaccharide from *Rickettsia Typhi*

The Causative Agent of Endemic Typhus

MARCELA FODOROVA, PAVOL VADOVIC, LUDOVIT SKULTETY, KATARINA SLABA, AND RUDOLF TOMAN

Laboratory for Diagnosis and Prevention of Rickettsial and Chlamydial Infections, Institute of Virology, SAS, 845 05 Bratislava, Slovakia

ABSTRACT: *Rickettsia typhi* causes endemic typhus, a relatively mild, acute febrile illness characterized by headache and macular rash. It is maintained in rodents and transmitted to humans by flea *Xenopsylla cheopis*. *R. typhi* contains a lipopolysaccharide thought to display a noticeable antigenic activity. We examined its structural features and it appears that the O-specific chain of the *R. typhi* LPS is composed mainly of the alternating Glc and QuiNAc residues linked by 1→4 bonds.

KEYWORDS: *Rickettsia typhi*; lipopolysaccharide; composition; structure; endemic typhus

INTRODUCTION

Rickettsia typhi causes endemic typhus. The disease is a relatively mild, acute febrile illness characterized by headache and macular rash. It is maintained in rodents and transmitted to humans by flea *Xenopsylla cheopis*.[1] It is known that *R. typhi* contains a lipopolysaccharide (LPS), which is thought to display a noticeable antigenic activity.[2] However, its immunoreactive epitopes have been unknown thus far.

MATERIALS AND METHODS

Cultivation and purification of the *R. typhi* was accomplished as described.[3] Crude LPS was isolated and purified as described[4] for the *Coxiella burnetii* LPS. The polymer was investigated for its chemical composition and structure by methylation-linkage analysis in combination with gas chromatography (GC), GC-mass spectrometry (GC-MS), and electrospray ionization–MS (ESI-MS) techniques.

Address for correspondence: Rudolf Toman, Institute of Virology, SAS, Dubravska cesta 9, 845 05 Bratislava, Slovakia. Voice: 421-2-59302418; fax: 421-2-54774284.
virutoma@savba.sk.

Ann. N.Y. Acad. Sci. 1063: 259–260 (2005). © 2005 New York Academy of Sciences.
doi: 10.1196/annals.1355.041

RESULTS AND DISCUSSION

SDS-PAGE of the *R. typhi* LPS gave a "ladder-like" banding pattern typical for LPSs having a regular structure of the O-specific chain. Sugar analysis of the LPS gave glucose (Glc), quinovosamine (QuiN), and glucosamine (GlcN) in the molar ratio 1.4:1:0.3. Surprisingly, no heptose was found, which is a common sugar constituent of the core regions of enterobacterial LPSs. Colorimetric assays showed the presence of 3-deoxy-D-*manno*-oct-2-ulosonic acid (Kdo) and phosphate. After mild acid hydrolysis and lipid A removal, the remaining polysaccharide (PS) was dephosphorylated and subjected to methylation-linkage analysis. The major peaks in GC-MS represented 4-substituted Glc and QuiN, and terminal Glc and QuiN. Small peaks of 4-substituted and terminal GlcN were found, too. The ESI-MS spectrum of the dephosphorylated PS (negative mode) was dominated by the ion at m/z 1455 corresponding to a Hex_8 glycoform with the composition $GlcNAc_2$•Glc_3•$QuiNAc_3$. Its MS/MS gave ions from which the sequence of the octasaccharide GlcNAc-GlcNAc-QuiNAc-Glc-QuiNAc-Glc-QuiNAc-Glc was established.

In conclusion, it appears that the O-specific chain of the *R. typhi* LPS is composed mainly of the alternating Glc and QuiNAc residues linked by 1→4 bonds.

ACKNOWLEDGMENTS

We thank Ludmila Hasikova and Margita Benkovicova for technical help. This work was supported in part by grant No. 2/3021/25 of the Scientific Grant Agency of Ministry of Education of the Slovak Republic and the Slovak Academy of Sciences.

[*Competing interests statement:* The authors state that they have no competing interests.]

REFERENCES

1. Azad, A.F., S. Radulovic, J.A. Higgins, *et al.* 1997. Flea-borne rickettsioses: ecologic considerations. Emerg. Infect. Dis. **3:** 319–317.
2. Schramek, S., R. Brezina & J. Kazar. 1977. Some biological properties of an endotoxic lipopolysaccharide from the typhus group rickettsia. Acta Virol. **21:** 439–441.
3. Amano, K.I., J.C. Williams & G.A. Dasch. 1998. Structural properties of lipopolysaccharides from *Rickettsia typhi* and *Rickettsia prowazekii* and their chemical similarity to the lipopolysaccharide from *Proteus vulgaris* OX19 used in the Weil-Felix test. Infect. Immun. **66:** 923–926.
4. Skultety L., R. Toman & V. Patoprsty. 1998. A comparative study of lipopolysaccharides from two *Coxiella burnetii* strains considered to be associated with acute and chronic Q fever. Carbohyd. Polymers **35:** 189–194.

Analysis of Immunoprotectivity of the Recombinant OmpA of *Rickettsia heilongjiangensis*

YANMEI JIAO, BOHAI WEN, MEILING CHEN, DONGSHENG NIU, JUN ZHANG, AND LING QIU

Beijing Institute of Microbiology and Epidemiology and State Key Laboratory of Pathogen and Biosecurity, Beijing 100071, China

ABSTRACT: A truncated gene *ompA* was amplified from *Rickettsia heilongjiangensis* isolated in China and a 56-kDa truncated OmpA protein was expressed in *E. coli* cells transformed with the *ompA*-recombined expression plasmid. High levels of serum antibodies to *R. heilongjiangensis* and proliferation of the splenic cells were found in mice immunized with the truncated OmpA. After challenge with *R. heilongjiangensis* or *R. rickettsii*, fever and pathological damages of the guinea pigs immunized with the truncated OmpA were significantly slighter as compared with those of nonimmunized guinea pigs. These results suggest that the truncated OmpA of *R. heilongjiangii* is immunogenic for effectively inducing humoral and cell-mediated immune responses against homologous and heterologous species in the spotted fever group.

KEYWORDS: *Rickettsia heilongjiangensis*; outer membrane protein A; immunity

INTRODUCTION

Rickettsia heilongjiangensis was first isolated from *Dermacentor sylvarum* ticks collected around Suifenhe in Heilongjiang Province of China in 1982 and later this pathogen was isolated from patients in this area of China.[1] Recently, *R. heilongjiangensis* was also identified in ticks and in samples of patients in the Russian Far East suspected of having spotted fever.[2,3]

The major immunodominant surface-exposed proteins of SFG rickettsiae, outer member protein A (OmpA) and B (OmpB), are the principal rickettsial vaccine candidate antigens.[4,5] OmpA, a characteristic component of SFG rickettsiae, contains a large domain of nearly identical, hydrophilic, tandem repeat units.[6] In this study, a gene fragment encoding a nonrepeat and hydrophilic fragment of the OmpA protein was amplified from *R. heilongjiangensis* and a truncated OmpA protein was expressed in *E. coli* cells transformed with the *ompA*-recombined expression plasmid.

Address for correspondence: Bohai Wen, Beijing Institute of Microbiology and Epidemiology and State Key Laboratory of Pathogen and Biosecurity, 20 Dong-Da-Jie Street, Fengtai, Beijing 100071, China. Voice: +86-10-63820718; fax: +86-10-63815259.
wenbohai@yahoo.com

Ann. N.Y. Acad. Sci. 1063: 261–265 (2005).
doi: 10.1196/annals.1355.042

MATERIALS AND METHODS

Based on the published *ompA* gene sequence of *R. heilongjiangensis* (GenBank accession number: AY280710.1), a primer pair, $P_{5218–5236}$ (5′-ATGGGATCCAAT-AGCCTAGCCTTTAATA-3′) and $P_{6792–6774}$ (5′-TTGGTACCACCTTGCTGAGC-GAAATA-3′), was designed, with the added *Bam*HI and *Kpn*I restriction sites being underlined.

The amplified *ompA* fragment and prokaryotic expression plasmid pQE30 were digested with DNA endonucleases, *Bam*HI and *Kpn*I, respectively, and the digested DNA fragments, *ompA* and pQE30, were ligated with each other according to a standard method. *E. coli* M15 was transformed with the ligation mixture and the transformed colonies were screened on Luria-Bertani medium (LB) containing ampicillin and kanamycin.

E. coli M15 harboring the recombinant plasmid was propagated in LB liquid media containing ampicillin and kanamycin at 37°C with shaking and induced to express the target gene by isopropyl-β-D-thiogalactopyranoside (IPTG).[7]

The expressed truncated OmpA was purified from the debris of transformed *E. coli* by affinity chromatography with nickel-nitrilotriacetic acid (Ni-NTA) resin (Qiagen GmbH, Hilden, Germany) under native conditions according to the manufacturer's protocols and was used to immunize animals.[7] For primary immunization, 25 μg and 75 μg of truncated OmpA emulsified in Freund's adjuvant were injected into each mouse and guinea pig, respectively, by subcutaneous route. After 4 weeks, each mouse or guinea pig was intraperitoneally boosted two times at 10-day intervals with 25 μg and 75 μg of truncated OmpA emulsified in Freund's incomplete adjuvant, respectively. PBS emulsified in the same Freund's adjuvant was used to inject mice or guinea pigs as a mock-immunization.

Eight days after the second booster, 3 mice in each group were killed and spleens were ground into single-cell suspensions in RPMI 1640 medium supplemented with 10% fetal bovine serum for splenic cell proliferation assay.[7] The splenic cells *in vitro* were stimulated with the truncated OmpA, and levels of cell proliferation responses were measured by an MTT (3-[4,5-dimethylthiazol-2-yl]-2,5-diphenyltetrazolium bromide) test.

Twenty-eight days after the last booster injections, the guinea pigs were intraperitoneally challenged with 1.3×10^7 cells of *R. rickettsii* or *R. heilongjiangensis*.

RESULTS AND DISCUSSION

Using recombinant protein technology based on the recognized protective antigens of SFG rickettsiae may provide a rational approach to development of subunit vaccines against spotted fever. OmpA, a major surface antigen of SFG rickettsiae, is highly homologous among different species of SFG rickettsiae and its cross-protection has been well demonstrated.[4–6]

In this study, we chose $ompA_{5218–6792}$ located at the nonrepeated region of the *ompA* gene of *R. heilongjiangensis* as a target fragment. The truncated *ompA* gene (1575 bp) was amplified from the genomic DNA of *R. heilongjiangensis* by PCR and the truncated OmpA recombinant protein was expressed in *E. coli* cells transformed by the *ompA*-recombined plasmid (FIG. 1).

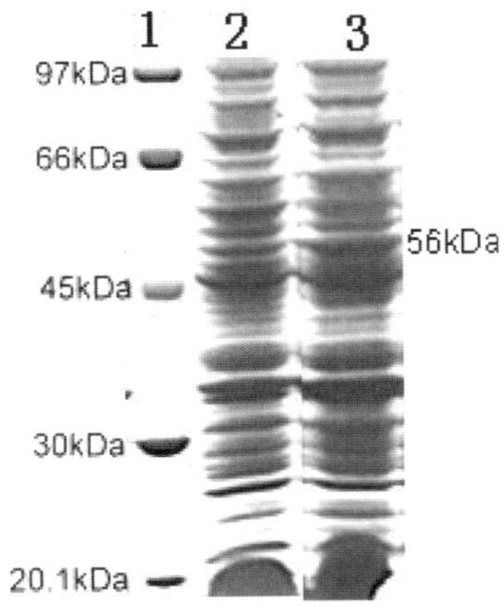

FIGURE 1. SDS-PAGE analysis of *E. coli* cells transformed with pQE30/*ompA*: lane 1, protein marker; lane 2, uninduced pQE30/*ompA*/*E. coli*; lane 3, pQE30/*ompA*/*E. coli* induced by IPTG.

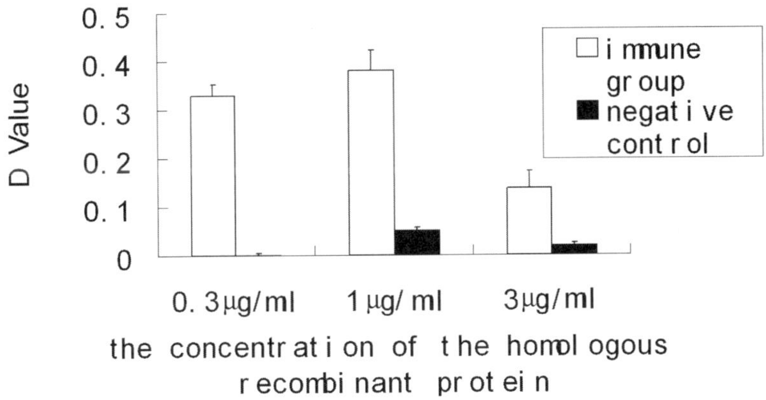

FIGURE 2. Splenic cell proliferation responses to recombinant OmpA. Immunized group: the splenic cells from the mice immunized with truncated OmpA. Negative control: the splenic cells from the mice mock-immunized with PBS.

The proliferation level of splenic cells from mice immunized with OmpA was significantly higher than that of mice injected with PBS ($P < 0.05$) (FIG. 2). The titers of IgG antibodies to *R. heilongjiangensis* in sera from mice and guinea pigs immunized with the truncated OmpA were 1:640 and 1:1280, respectively, detected by immunofluorescence assay (IFA) on day 8 after the second booster immunization. These results indicate that the truncated OmpA is a good immunogen.

The guinea pigs developed fever on day 2 after challenge with the rickettsial agents. However, the fever of guinea pigs mock-immunized with PBS was signifi-

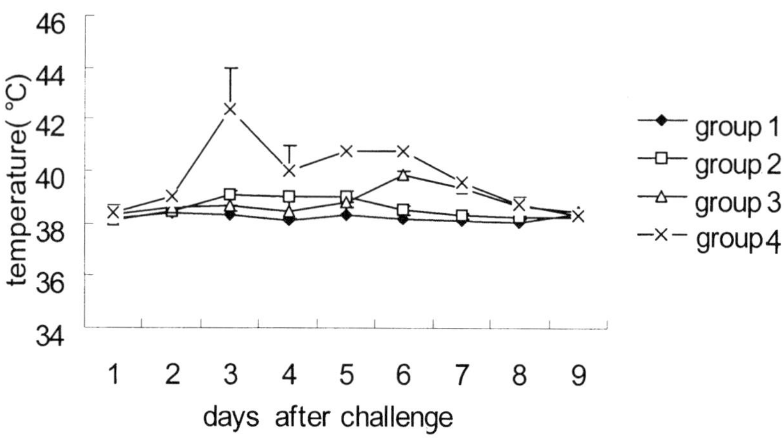

FIGURE 3. Changes of guinea pig temperature. Group 1: OmpA-immunized guinea pigs challenged with *R. heilongjiangii*. Group 2: PBS-immunized guinea pigs challenged with *R. heilongjiangensis*. Group 3: OmpA-immunized guinea pigs challenged with *R. rickettsii*. Group 4: PBS-injected guinea pigs challenged with *R. rickettsii*.

cantly higher than that of those immunized with the truncated OmpA ($P < 0.05$) on days 3 to 7 after challenge with *R. heilongjiangensis* or *R. rickettsii* (FIG. 3). Ballooning degeneration of liver tissue, severe interstitial pneumonia with severe edema and fibrosis of lung tissues, and coagulation necrosis and degeneration of cardiac muscle were observed in guinea pigs mock-immunized with PBS, examined on day 10 after challenge with the rickettsial agents. However, no prominent pathologic change was found in guinea pigs immunized with the truncated OmpA.

The resulting data in this study suggest that the truncated OmpA of *R. heilongjiangensis* is immunogenic for effectively inducing humoral and cell-mediated immunoresponses against homologous and heterologous species in the spotted fever group.

[*Competing interests statement:* The authors state that they have no competing interests.]

REFERENCES

1. LOU, D., Y.M. WU, B. WANG *et al.* 1989. Confirmation of patients with tick-borne spotted fever caused by *Rickettsia heilongjiangensis*. Chin. J. Epidemiol. **10:** 128–132.
2. MEDIANNIKOV, O.Y., Y. SIDELNIKOV, L. IVANOV *et al.* 2004. Acute tick-borne rickettsiosis caused by *Rickettsia heilongjiangensis*. Emerg. Infect. Dis. **10:** 810–817.
3. SEXTON, D.J. & D.H. WALKER. 1999. Spotted fever group rickettsioses. *In* Tropical Infectious Diseases: Principles, Pathogens, and Practice, pp. 579–584. Churchill Livingstone. Philadelphia.
4. CROCQUET-VALDES, P.A., C.M. DÍAZ-MONTERO, H-M. FENG *et al.* 2002. Immunization with a portion of rickettsial outer membrane protein A stimulates protective immunity against spotted fever rickettsiosis. Vaccine **20:** 979–988.

5. VISHWANATH, S., G.A. MCDONALD & N.G. WATKINS. 1990. A recombinant *Rickettsia conorii* vaccine protects guinea pigs from experimental boutonneuse fever and Rocky Mountain spotted fever. Infect. Immunol. **58:** 646–653.
6. ANDERSON, B.E., G.A. MCDONALD, D.C. JONES & R.L. REGNERY. 1990. A protective protein antigen of *Rickettsia rickettsii* has tandemly repeated, near-identical sequences. Infect. Immunol. **58:** 2760–2769.
7. YU, Y., B.H. WEN, B.G. WEN *et al.* 2005. Induction of protective immunity against scrub typhus with a 56-kilodalton recombinant antigen fused with 47-kilodalton antigen of *Orientia tsutsugamushi* Karp. Am. J. Trop. Med. Hyg. **72:** 458–464.

Short- and Long-Term Immune Responses of CD-1 Outbred Mice to the Scrub Typhus DNA Vaccine Candidate: p47Kp

GUANG XU,[a] SUCHISMITA CHATTOPADHYAY,[a] JU JIANG,[a] TEIK-CHYE CHAN,[a] CHIEN-CHUNG CHAO,[a] WEI-MEI CHING,[a,b] AND ALLEN L. RICHARDS[a,b]

[a]*Rickettsial Diseases Department, Naval Medical Research Center, Silver Spring, Maryland, USA*

[b]*Department of Preventive Medicine and Biometrics, Uniformed Services University of Health Sciences, Bethesda, Maryland, USA*

ABSTRACT: *Orientia tsutsugamushi* is an obligate intracellular bacterium that is the causative agent of scrub typhus. To develop an effective vaccine to prevent or ameliorate scrub typhus, knowledge of the protective immune response to *O. tsutsugamushi* needs to be ascertained. Our laboratory has demonstrated that the DNA vaccine vector pVR1012 carrying the *O. tsutsugamushi* Karp strain 47-kDa protein gene (p47Kp) consistently provides outbred mice protection against homologous challenge.

KEYWORDS: CD-1 mice; immunization; p47Kp; scrub typhus; vaccine

INTRODUCTION

The host immune response to *Orientia tsutsugamushi*, an obligate intracellular bacterium that is the causative agent of scrub typhus, is believed to be mediated by both the humoral and cellular arms of the immune system, with greater importance associated with the latter.[1,2] To develop an effective vaccine to prevent or ameliorate scrub typhus, knowledge of the protective immune response to *O. tsutsugamushi* needs to be ascertained. Our laboratory has demonstrated that the DNA vaccine vector pVR1012 carrying the *O. tsutsugamushi* Karp strain 47-kDa protein gene (p47Kp) consistently provides outbred mice protection against homologous challenge (W-M. Ching *et al.*, unpublished data). To assist in characterizing the immune response to this successful immunization strategy, we have evaluated the induction of antigen-specific antibody, and IFNγ, IL-4, and IL-13 secreting spleen cells derived from p47Kp-immunized mice at 4, 8, and 12 weeks and 6 months after immunization.

Address for correspondence: Allen L. Richards, Rickettsial Diseases Department, Naval Medical Research Center, 503 Robert Grant Avenue, Silver Spring, MD 20910-7500. Voice: 301-319-7668; fax: 301-319-9458.
richardsa@nmrc.navy.mil

Ann. N.Y. Acad. Sci. 1063: 266–269 (2005).
doi: 10.1196/annals.1355.043

METHODS

Seven- to eight-week-old female Swiss CD-1 outbred mice were inoculated intramuscularly with 100 μg of p47Kp once, twice, or three times at 4-week intervals before spleens were collected and processed. Spleen cells from immunized mice were evaluated for the presence of IFNγ, IL-4, and IL-13 secreting cells induced by *in vitro* stimulation with recombinant 47-kDa antigen from the Karp strain of *O. tsutsugamushi* (Kp r47) using cytokine-specific ELISpot assays. These immune responses were measured at 4 weeks and 6 months after the last immunization. The number of IFNγ, IL-4, and IL-13 producing mouse spleen cells were determined by ELISpot assays that utilized cytokine-specific monoclonal antibodies. Spleen cells (0.5 and 1.0×10^6 cells/well) were incubated with 1.0 μg/well of Kp r47 for 48 h. After washing, detection antibodies were added, the plates were incubated overnight, and then phosphatase-labeled streptavidin was added for 2 h. Following washing, the colored spots produced after adding BCIP/NBT phosphatase substrate were measured using the CLT ImmunoSpot Analyzer (Cellular Technology Ltd., Cleveland, OH). Sera from blood collected at 3 and 7 weeks and 6 months after immunization were assessed for antigen-specific IgG by ELISA similar to the procedure described previously,[2] except that 0.3 μg/well of Kp r47 antigen and an anti-mouse IgG antibody conjugated to HRP (KPL, Gaithersburg, MD) were used.

RESULTS

Mice immunized for 4, 8, or 12 weeks with a single dose of p47Kp induced a greater number of antigen-specific IFNγ producing cells than those from control mice immunized with vector alone (FIG. 1A). However, mice immunized for 8 weeks with two doses or 12 weeks with three doses of p47Kp produced a much greater number of antigen-specific IFNγ producing cells than the single immunizations (FIG. 1A). In addition to IFNγ producing spleen cells, IL-4 and IL-13 secreting cells were detected, especially from mice with two- and three-dose immunizations with p47Kp (FIG. 1A). Similar ELISpot results were obtained 6 months following the last immunization injection (FIG. 1B).

Antibody levels were either not detectable or very low at 3 weeks after immunization. However, antigen-specific antibody levels at 7 weeks ranged from a geometric mean titer of 635 for a single immunization to ≥6400 for three immunizations. Similar antibody levels were seen at 6 months (data not shown).

CONCLUSIONS

In addition to a strong antibody response, these results demonstrate that IFNγ and to a lesser extent IL-4 and IL-13 secreting spleen cells are induced *in vitro* in an antigen-specific manner following immunization of outbred CD-1 mice with the scrub typhus DNA vaccine candidate p47Kp. Moreover, CD-1 mice similarly immunized have been shown to be protected from homologous challenge (W-M. Ching *et al.*, unpublished data). Last and more importantly, this study shows that the strong antigen-specific immune responses to p47Kp were still observable 6 months

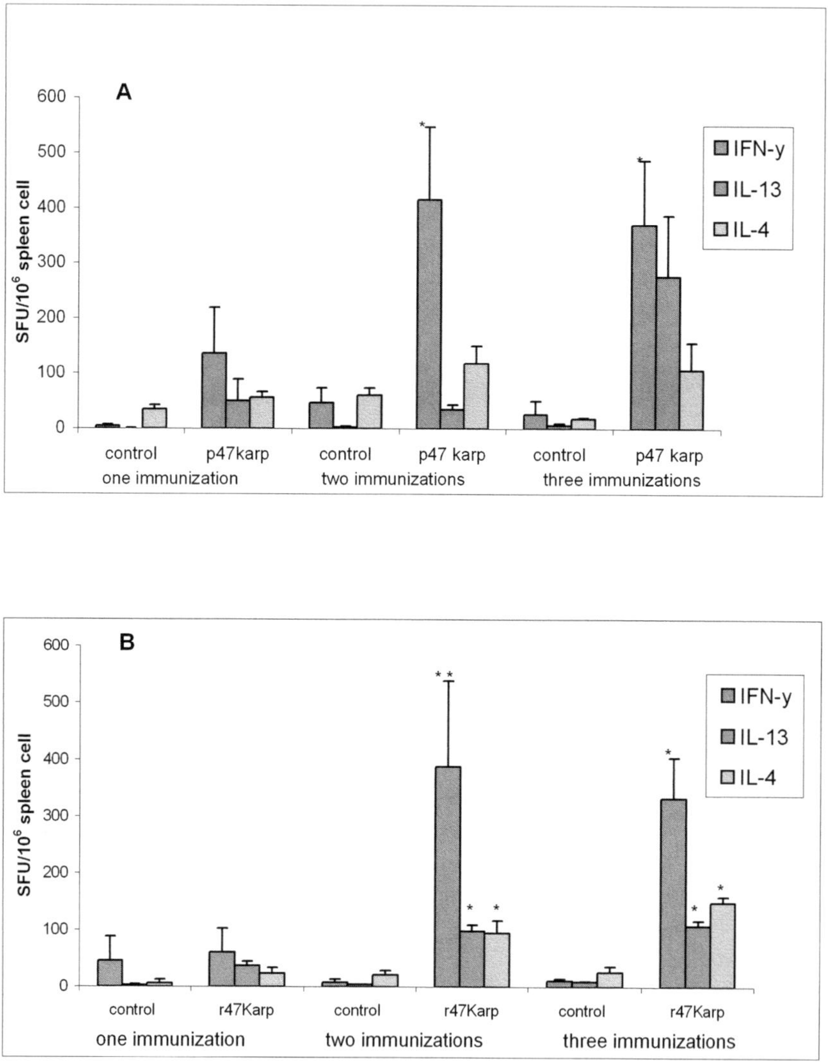

FIGURE 1. Antigen-specific spleen cell cytokine responses following multiple immunizations (1–3) at 4-week intervals. Spot forming units (SFU) are the number of cytokine producing cells reported for 1×10^6 spleen cells. Results are derived from spleen cells of mice that were immunized at **(A)** 4 weeks and **(B)** ~6 months earlier. Data shown represent the mean values plus SDs of 3 mice. Student's *t*-tests were used to calculate *P* values: $*P < 0.05$; $**P < 0.07$.

following immunization, suggesting that memory lymphocytes were generated by this vaccine candidate.

ACKNOWLEDGMENTS

This work was supported by Work Unit Number 6000.RAD1.B998.J.A0310.

DISCLAIMER

The opinions and assertions contained herein are the private ones of the authors and are not to be construed as official or reflecting the views of the Navy Department or the Department of Defense at large. The experiments reported herein were conducted according to the principles set forth in the "Guide for the Care and Use of Laboratory Animals" (1996, Institute of Laboratory Animals Resources, National Research Council, National Academy Press, Washington, D.C.).

[*Competing interests statement:* The authors state that they have no competing interests.]

REFERENCES

1. Jerrells, T.R. & C.E. Eisemann. 1983. Role of T-lymphocytes in production of antibody to antigens of *Rickettsia tsutsugamushi* and other *Rickettsia* species. Infect. Immunol. **41:** 666–674.
2. Chattopadhyay, S., J. Jiang, T-C. Chan *et al.* 2005. Successful induction of humoral and cellular immune responses in cynomolgus monkeys to the scrub typhus vaccine candidate, Kp r56. Infect. Immunol. **73:** 5039–5047.

Bartonellae as Elegant Hemotropic Parasites

RICHARD J. BIRTLES

Disease Ecology Unit, Centre for Comparative Infectious Diseases, Faculty of Veterinary Science, University of Liverpool, Leahurst, Cheshire CH64 7TE, United Kingdom

ABSTRACT: *Bartonella* species are hemotropic bacterial parasites of a wide range of mammals that occasionally cause disease in humans. The low prevalence of clinical manifestations compared to the high prevalence of infection underlines the elegance of these parasites that carefully exploit their hosts in a manner that optimizes their transmission. Recent research efforts have begun to determine the strategies involved in this exploitation, and significant progress has been made in unraveling an unusually complex natural cycle. Studies aimed at determining bacterial attributes involved in parasitism characterized several "virulence" factors and explored their modes of action. These efforts have provided an intriguing foundation on which future efforts aimed at comprehending these sophisticated parasites can be soundly based.

KEYWORDS: *Bartonella*; bacteria; host; infection; parasitism; pathogen

BARTONELLAE AS HUMAN PATHOGENS

Bartonella species are Gram-negative bacteria that share a specific evolutionary history with the genera *Brucella*, *Agrobacterium*, *Rhizobium*, and related taxa within the class Alphaproteobacteria. Like many of their phylogenetic neighbors, bartonellae are facultative intracellular bacteria, a characteristic that manifests in the laboratory as the ability to invade, replicate, and persist within a number of different mammalian cell lines as well as in axenic media.

Several *Bartonella* species are now well established as human pathogens. Two species, *Bartonella bacilliformis* and *Bartonella quintana*, have long been associated with disease, the former causing Carrión's disease among the inhabitants of the Andean Cordillera in South America and the latter causing trench fever among troops during World War I and World War II. However, *Bartonella* species have attained their current level of notoriety following the identification of new species within the genus and the implication of these, and the established species, in a wider range of syndromes. One of these newly identified species, *Bartonella henselae*, has become the most medically important member of the genus, associated with lymphadenopathy (cat scratch disease), ocular infections, and an increasing number of other manifestations.[1] *B. henselae* infections are zoonoses, with the domestic cat and other felids serving as reservoir hosts for the bacterium. In these reservoirs, *B. henselae* infections

Address for correspondence: Richard J. Birtles, Disease Ecology Unit, Centre for Comparative Infectious Diseases, Faculty of Veterinary Science, University of Liverpool, Leahurst, Chester High Road, Cheshire CH64 7TE, United Kingdom. Voice: +44-151-794-6122; fax: +44-151-794-6005. richard.birtles@liverpool.ac.uk

Ann. N.Y. Acad. Sci. 1063: 270–279 (2005).
doi: 10.1196/annals.1355.044

are maintained primarily as chronic bacteremia, usually in the absence of overt clinical signs.[2] The most important means of infection transmission between animals is *Ctenocephalides felis*, the cat flea.[2] *B. quintana* has reemerged as an important agent of endocarditis and recurrent protracted bacteremia and fever, primarily among those living under poor socioeconomic conditions, including the inner-city homeless of industrialized countries and refugees in central Africa. Unlike *B. henselae*, *B. quintana* is not a zoonotic agent, but rather humans serve as a reservoir; asymptomatic carriage of the bacterium by humans is becoming increasingly recognized.[3] Infections are transmitted by the human-specific ectoparasite, the body louse, *Pediculus humanus corporis*.[3] Carrión's disease appears to be becoming more prevalent and more widespread across western South America than previously recognized. Over 11,000 cases of the disease were reported in 2004.[4] The disease itself is biphasic, manifesting as a severe hemolytic anemia (Oroya fever) or as multifocal angiomatous lesions, most frequently on the skin (verruga peruana). However, asymptomatic carriage of *B. bacilliformis* is also common in regions where the disease is endemic, an observation that, along with the failure to identify other reservoirs, points to the bacterium being maintained solely by humans. *Lutzomyia* sand flies are considered its principal vector.[5]

BARTONELLAE AS HEMOTROPIC PARASITES

Comparison of the epidemiologies and physiopathologies of the medically important bartonellae reveals common traits. All induce hemotropic infections in their mammalian reservoir host, which, on the whole, appear not to cause immediate detriment to the host. Only when "accidentally" introduced into the wrong host, or when encountering immunocompromised individuals among a reservoir host population, is infection more likely to result in acute clinical manifestation. Finally, all agents are transmitted between mammalian hosts by hematophagous arthropods. Together, these observations provide an insight into the natural cycle of bartonellae that, although occasional pathogens, are probably better considered as parasites that have evolved to elegantly exploit their hosts. Given that their transmission is ultimately reliant on a viable and healthy host, bartonellae will not have evolved mechanisms that overly burden their hosts such that transmission is jeopardized. Thus, although several bartonella "virulence" factors have been characterized, they are perhaps better considered as mechanisms by which bartonella parasitism is mediated.

DIVERSITY OF HOSTS AND HOST-SPECIFICITY

One of the most obvious indicators of the success of bartonellae as parasites is the diversity of mammals that are known to be exploited by them. *Bartonella* infections have been encountered in virtually all species surveyed, which to date have extended to members of seven different orders of mammalia including carnivores, primates, ungulates, rodents, lagomorphs, insectivores, and bats.[6,7] The exceptional species that do not seem prone to infection are horses, some mustelids (unpublished observations), and spring hares (*Pedetes capensis*),[8] although why these animals should be resistant to bartonellae is unclear. Among susceptible hosts, the rates of exposure and infection are remarkably high; a probably accurate generalization would be that the majority of individuals will be infected at some time in their lives. Adaptation by bartonellae to exploit such a diversity of mammals has generally resulted in some degree of host-specificity. All 20 or so well-characterized and validated *Bartonella* species described to date are only capable of parasitizing only a limited number of mammal species.[6] For example, *B. bacilliformis* and *B. quintana* naturally infect only humans, and *B. henselae* infects a wider range of felid hosts. *B. alsatica* only exploits rabbits, although some of the other small mammal–associated species have a broader, but nonetheless ultimately limited, host range including both arvicoline and murid rodents and insectivorous shrews.[9] Some hosts are prone to infection by different *Bartonella* species; cats are parasitized by *B. clarridgeiae* and *B. koehlerae* as well as *B. henselae*, and communities of European woodland rodents such as wood mice (*Apodemus sylvaticus*) and bank voles (*Clethrionomys glareolus*) can maintain at least four different *Bartonella* species.[9,10] Phylogenetic inference of the evolutionary relationships among *Bartonella* species have indicated that those species associated with a particular mammalian host are not specifically related. Furthermore, there is no apparent congruence between the phylogeny of bartonellae and that of the specific hosts they parasitize.[8] These observations suggest that the adaptation of bartonellae to specific hosts was not an ancient occurrence, but rather members of different lineages have been able to adapt to their current hosts far more recently, a hypothesis that may indicate that the basis for host-specificity is not particularly complex.

DISSECTION OF THE NATURAL CYCLES OF BARTONELLAE

Research efforts using different *Bartonella* species have not only suggested many commonalities among their natural cycles, but also that these cycles are surprising complex. Many of the mammal-associated stages of this progression were very elegantly demonstrated using rats experimentally infected with the rat-associated species, *B. tribocorum*,[11] but other stages have been far less well characterized. The current paradigm for the natural cycle of bartonellae is presented in FIGURE 1 and can broadly be divided into several stages, as discussed below:

Host Inoculation and Seeding of the Bloodstream

This stage of the bartonella life cycle appears to be the most complicated, comprising at least three different steps. Current opinion is that vascular endothelial cells serve as a primary niche for bartonellae prior to them entering the bloodstream. The passage of infecting bartonellae from the site of inoculation has yet to be elucidated. Indeed, whether the vascular endothelium closest to the site of inoculation is parasitized or whether remote sites are selected or arbitrarily infected is unknown. Most of the cellular microbiological studies of bartonellae have focused on their interaction with endothelial cells. This enthusiasm is based on the unique ability of bartonellae among bacteria to induce vasoproliferation, as observed clinically among verruga peruana patients and occasionally among immunocompromised people infected with *B. henselae* and *B. quintana*. However, it is clear that such manifestations are extremely rare among normal reservoir host populations. For example, *B. henselae*–

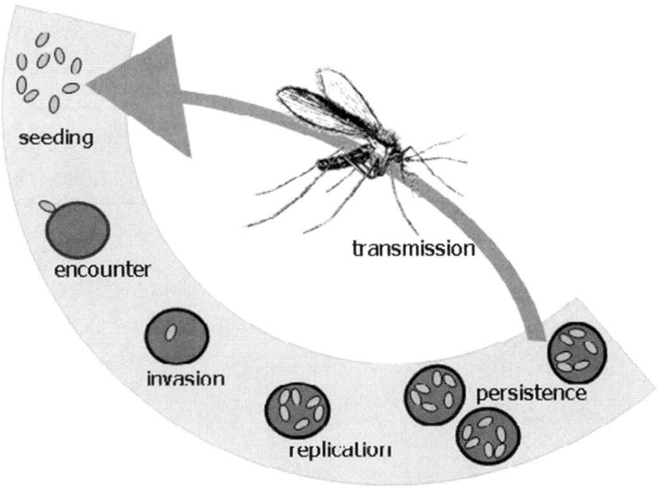

FIGURE 1. Current paradigm of the course of bartonella natural cycle in the mammalian reservoir host. Following inoculation, bacteria are eventually seeded into the bloodstream, where they encounter, associate with, and then invade erythrocytes. Within erythrocyes, bartonellae replicate and then persist throughout the life span of their host cell, facilitating their uptake by bloodsucking arthropods that serve as their vectors.

associated feline angioproliferative lesions have not been reported and pathological examination of tissues from over 100 naturally infected woodland rodents in the United Kingdom has not revealed any evidence of angiogenic lesions on the skin or in internal organs (unpublished observations). Given these observations, it appears unlikely that the induction of angiogenesis is an essential, and thus deliberate, part of the parasitic strategy of bartonellae.

The modeling of exploitation of vascular endothelial cells by bartonellae *in vitro* using cocultures has demonstrated peri- and intracellular parasitism and associated cytoskeletal rearrangements,[12] cell and bacterial proliferation,[13–15] inhibition of apoptosis,[16] and activation of various signal transduction pathways resulting in proinflammatory responses.[17,18] Some bartonella virulence factors associated with subversion of endothelial cell function have been discovered and characterized. Several genes homologous to members of the type IV secretion system–encoding *vir* locus of *Agrobacterium tumefaciens* were encountered and characterized in *B. henselae*;[19,20] then, exploration of their regulation demonstrated that expression was induced in intracellular bacteria.[21] Subsequently, the complete locus was characterized in *B. tribocorum* and experiments demonstrated that mutants in which the locus had been disrupted were unable to induce bacteremia in an experimental rat model[22] or mediate physiological changes in endothelial cell cocultures.[23] Most recently, exploration of the genes downstream of the *vir* locus has demonstrated that they code for effector proteins that are translocated into endothelial cells by the VirB-D4 apparatus.[24] A family of nonfimbrial adhesions, which mediate binding to host cells or extracellular matrix proteins, have been identified in *B. henselae* and *B. quintana*, comprising BadA[25] and VompA-D.[26] The essential role of BadA in interactions with endothelial cell cultures was demonstrated using a mutant in which *badA* was disrupted. This mutant was observed to be unable to bind extracellular matrix proteins or adhere to endothelial cells, and endothelial cells infected with the mutant did not produce proinflammatory cytokines.[25] Finally, as discussed in depth in a separate paper in this journal, the heat-shock protein GroEL is actively secreted by bartonellae and has a role in mediating endothelial cell activation and proliferation.[15]

The period of time that bartonellae are maintained within the endothelial cell bed is uncertain; however, one hypothesis can be drawn from the observation that seeding of the bloodstream from this niche appears to be an orchestrated process. In the *B. tribocorum*–rat model system, the period of blood sterility that is established soon after experimental inoculation comes to an abrupt end after about five days with the release of large numbers of bacteria into the bloodstream.[11] Additional orchestrated releases follow this initial episode at regular, five-day intervals, which may reflect reinfection of the endothelial bed by bacteria released during the previous episode.[11] If this is the case, then the association between bartonellae and specific endothelial cells is relatively short lived.

Exploitation of Erythrocytes

The colonization of erythrocytes is, perhaps, the most intriguing parasitic strategy evolved by bartonellae. The dynamics of erythrocyte exploitation by bartonellae has been measured in several experimentally infected animals, including mice, cats, and rats,[11,27,28] and monitoring of bacteremia in captive, naturally infected rodents has yielded results that generally match those observed in experimentally infected animals, although occasionally far more prolonged infections are encountered (see FIG. 2). All studies have demonstrated that bacteremia can be extremely chronic, lasting, for example, several weeks in rodents and several months in cats—a feature that clearly facilitates uptake of bartonellae by blood-feeding arthropods. However, infections are not maintained at the same intensity throughout this period, but rather the concentration of bartonellae in the blood rises rapidly during the initial stages of the bacteremia and then gradually declines over the remainder of the infection period (FIG. 3). The peak infection intensities appear to vary between hosts. Monitoring of naturally acquired infections has revealed that, in humans infected with *B. quintana*, up to 1 in 20,000 erythrocytes[3] are infected, whereas woodland rodent–associated bartonellae induce far more intense infections, parasitizing as many as 1 in 250 erythrocytes (FIG. 3). Why this marked variation occurs is unclear; more intense infections will favor transmission, but this benefit must be weighed against the cost on host well-being caused by the possible compromised functionality of parasitized erythrocytes.

The dynamics of bartonella bacteremia has been further dissected using a *B. tribocorum*–Wistar rat experimental system[11] in which the interaction between circulating biotinylated erythrocytes and green fluorescent protein–expressing bacteria was quantified using flow cytometry. The study demonstrated that bartonellae associated with and entered mature erythrocytes, and then bacteria replicated until reaching an apparent ceiling of about eight bacteria per cell. After this replicative period, the number of intracellular bacteria remained static for the remaining life span of the erythrocyte, which did not appear to be shortened as a result of infection.[11]

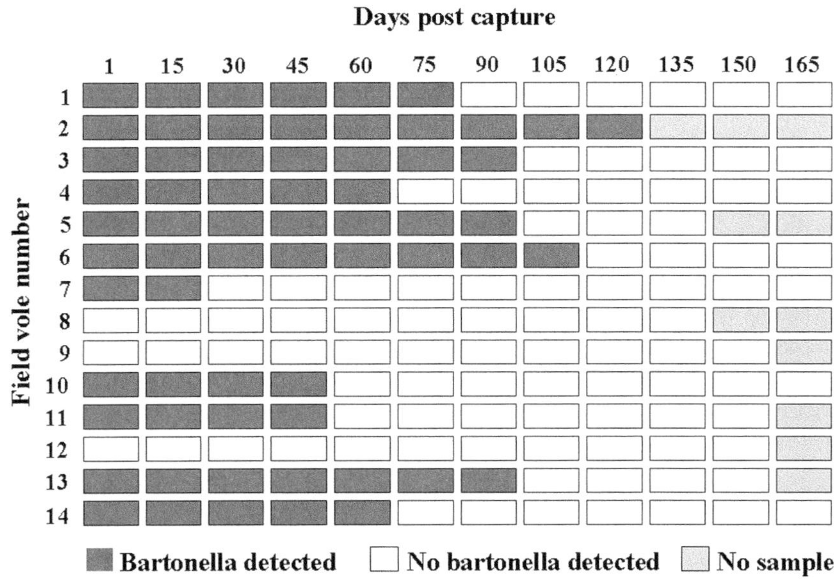

FIGURE 2. Longevity of bartonella bacteremia in 14 naturally infected field voles (*Microtus agrestis*). Voles were captured at field sites in northern England, treated to remove all ectoparasites, and then held in isolation. Blood samples collected at weekly intervals from the tail tip were tested for the presence of bartonellae using a genus-specific polymerase chain reaction.[38] Bacteremia could be detected for up to 120 days after ectoparasite removal. Note that animals that were not bacteremic when ectoparasites were removed did not subsequently become bacteremic, and no evidence of recurrent bacteremia was observed among infected animals.

Despite a good knowledge of the dynamics of bartonella parasitism of erythrocytes, very little is known about the molecular mechanisms that underlie this exploitation. Some characterization of erythrocyte receptors and bartonella ligands has been attempted, yielding somewhat conflicting results, although there does appear to be a carbohydrate component to the receptor.[29] Molecular studies have identified two genetic loci that encode proteins that appear to have a role in erythrocyte association. The first of these loci, the *ial* locus, comprising two genes *ialA* and *ialB*, was identified by its ability to confer an erythrocyte-invading phenotype on *E. coli* cells into which it had been introduced.[30] Subsequently, disruption of *ialB* in *B. bacilliformis* resulted in a 50% reduction in erythrocyte invasion efficiency.[31] IalA is a putative cytoplasmic nudix hydrolase and IalB is an inner membrane–associated protein, so how either functions in erythrocyte invasion is unclear.[30,31] The second locus comprises an operon that shares colinearity and very high similarity with the *trw* operon on the broad host range antibiotic resistance plasmid R388 that encodes a type IV secretion system.[32] Disruption of one of the genes within the operon, *trwE*, in *B. tribocorum* resulted in a mutant unable to cause intraerythrocytic bacteremia in experimentally infected rats. However, bartonella Trw apparatus may well not act as a secretion system because bartonella genomes lack *trwB*, the gene that encodes a coupling protein

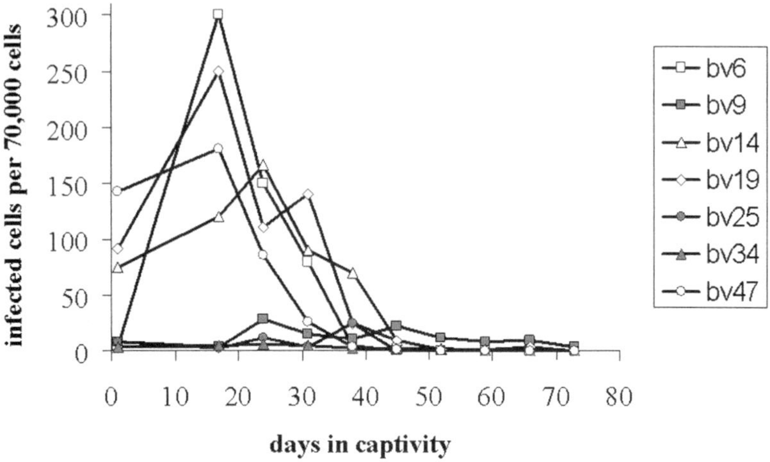

FIGURE 3. Quantification of intensity of bartonella bacteremia in 7 naturally infected field voles. Voles were handled as described in FIGURE 2. The proportion of infected erythrocytes was determined by microscopic examination of Giemsa-stained blood smears prepared from weekly blood collections. Four animals demonstrated dynamics akin to those observed following experimental inoculations, involving a dramatic rise in infection intensity followed by a gradual decline over a 3- or 4-week period. However, 3 animals maintained very protracted low-intensity bacteremia.

essential for effector molecule delivery by the R388 Trw secretion system. An alternative role for bartonella Trw as a producer of highly variable pili has been proposed.[32] This hypothesis is supported by the presence of numerous highly variable tandem repeats of some of the genes that putatively encode cell surface–expressed components of the type IV pilus. The presence of these tandem repeats provides bartonellae with the means to synthesize elongated or structurally diverse pili that might mediate different cell tropisms (including that for erythrocytes) or antigenic variation.[32]

A role for antigenic variation in the prolongation of bartonella infections has yet to be identified and, indeed, given that parasitism of erythrocytes affords bartonellae immunological privilege, the influence of host response on bartonella parasitism is unclear. Some reservoir hosts, such as cats, mount a significant humoral response, although bacteremia persists in the face of this.[27] However, in other hosts, particularly small mammals, specific antibodies are only very rarely detected.[33] Thus, although studies involving experimentally infected rodents have indicated a role for antibodies in the abrogation of bacteremia,[34] the validity of extrapolation of these data to their naturally infected counterparts is debatable.

Arthropod Interaction

Arthropods play an essential role in the natural cycle of all *Bartonella* species, serving as vectors and possibly reservoir hosts. Very little is known about the nature of arthropod exploitation or the underlying molecular mechanisms. An experimental model of *B. quintana* infection of its natural vector, the human body louse (*Pediculus humanus corporis*), has been described and has been used to demonstrate that bartonellae maintain a lifelong extracellular infection of the louse midgut.[35] There was no evidence that bartonellae invaded midgut epithelial cells or other parts of the louse body. Infection did not appear to induce any symptoms in the lice, with the survival rate of infected lice being no different to that of uninfected lice. Furthermore, bartonellae could not be detected in either eggs or larvae produced by infected lice, indicating that vertical transmission did not occur. Viable bartonellae were, however, present in fecal material shed by infected lice.[35] Studies on *B. henselae*–infected cat fleas (*Ctenocephalides felis*) have revealed similar findings. In an early study, bacteria were fed to fleas using an artificial feeding device and were monitored in the midgut for up to nine days, during which time they multiplied. Viable *B. henselae* could also be detected in flea feces for the same time period.[36] The results of these studies suggest that, just as with their mammalian hosts, bartonellae are able to establish prolonged infections of their arthropod vectors. Furthermore, given that infections appear to be limited to the midgut, transmission of bartonella from arthropods to mammals is not a direct process, but rather is mediated by infected fecal material. Such a strategy seems somewhat inefficient; however, given that the arthropod vectors exploited by bartonellae share an obligate and intimate relationship with their hosts, the extremely frequent contacts between them provide ample opportunities for deposition of infected feces onto the host skin. Moreover, arthropod bites generally induce irritation of the skin, provoking the scratching that may result in the introduction of infected fecal material into the host's body.

CONCLUSIONS

Recent advances in our understanding of bartonella parasitism have been greatly facilitated by the development of useful infection models, the introduction of effective molecular tools, and the availability of complete genome sequence data for *B. henselae* and *B. quintana*.[37] These resources are now being increasingly exploited by a small but expanding community of enthusiastic and ambitious scientists to explore the molecular basis of bartonella parasitism. These efforts have yielded significant progress in unraveling not only the bacterial attributes that mediate this parasitism, but also their modes of action, and this momentum will undoubtedly lead to more discoveries in the near future. It is important, however, to interpret results in the context of bartonellae as elegantly adapted parasites rather than opportunistic pathogens and, to this end, data drawn from naturally infected hosts will be useful in supporting observations made during laboratory-based studies.

ACKNOWLEDGMENTS

I would like to thank colleagues in the Disease Ecology Unit for their collaboration in the study of the dynamics of bartonella bacteremia in naturally infected field voles and for instructive and entertaining discussion on the ecological aspects of bartonella parasitism.

[*Competing interests statement*: The author states that there is no conflict of interest.]

REFERENCES

1. Chomel, B.B., H.J. Boulouis & E.B. Breitschwerdt. 2004. Cat scratch disease and other zoonotic *Bartonella* infections. J. Am. Vet. Med. Assoc. **224:** 1270–1279.
2. Birtles, R.J. 2005. Bartonellosis. *In* Arthropod-Borne Infectious Diseases of the Dog and Cat. Manson Pub. London.
3. Brouqui, P., A. Stein, H.T. Dupont *et al.* 2005. Ectoparasitism and vector-borne diseases in 930 homeless people from Marseilles. Medicine **84:** 61–68.
4. Ministerio de Salud, Peru [http://www.minsa.gob.pe/portal/].
5. Ihler, G.M. 1996. *Bartonella bacilliformis*: dangerous pathogen slowly emerging from deep background. FEMS Microbiol. Lett. **144:** 1–11.
6. Boulouis, H.J., C.C. Chang, J.B. Henn *et al.* 2005. Factors associated with the rapid emergence of zoonotic *Bartonella* infections. Vet. Res. **36:** 383–410.
7. Concannon, R., K. Wynn-Owen, V.R. Simpson & R.J. Birtles. 2005. Molecular characterisation of haemoparasites infecting bats (Microchiroptera) in Cornwall, United Kingdom. Parasitology **131:** 489–496.
8. Pretorius, A.M., L. Beati & R.J. Birtles. 2004. Diversity of bartonellae associated with small mammals inhabiting Free State province, South Africa. Int. J. Syst. Evol. Microbiol. **54:** 1959–1967.
9. Birtles, R.J., T.G. Harrison & D.H. Molyneux. 1994. *Grahamella* in woodland mammals in the UK: isolation, prevalence, and host-specificity. Ann. Trop. Med. Parasitol. **88:** 317–327.
10. Holmberg, M., J.N. Mills, S. McGill *et al.* 2003. *Bartonella* infection in sylvatic small mammals of central Sweden. Epidemiol. Infect. **130:** 149–157.
11. Schulein, R., A. Seubert, C. Gille *et al.* 2001. Invasion and persistent intracellular colonization of erythrocytes: a unique parasitic strategy of the emerging pathogen *Bartonella*. J. Exp. Med. **193:** 1077–1086.
12. Dehio, C., M. Meyer, J. Berger *et al.* 1997. Interaction of *Bartonella henselae* with endothelial cells results in bacterial aggregation on the cell surface and the subsequent engulfment and internalisation of the bacterial aggregate by a unique structure, the invasome. J. Cell Sci. **110:** 2141–2154.
13. Garcia, F.U., J. Wojta, K.N. Broadley *et al.* 1990. *Bartonella bacilliformis* stimulates endothelial cells *in vitro* and is angiogenic *in vivo*. Am. J. Pathol. **136:** 1125–1135.
14. Kempf, V.A., M. Schaller, S. Behrendt *et al.* 2000. Interaction of *Bartonella henselae* with endothelial cells results in rapid bacterial rRNA synthesis and replication. Cell. Microbiol. **2:** 431–441.
15. Minnick, M.F., L.S. Smitherman & D.S. Samuels. 2003. Mitogenic effect of *Bartonella bacilliformis* on human vascular endothelial cells and involvement of GroEL. Infect. Immunol. **71:** 6933–6942.
16. Kirby, J.E. & D.M. Nekorchuk. 2002. *Bartonella*-associated endothelial proliferation depends on inhibition of apoptosis. Proc. Natl. Acad. Sci. USA **99:** 4656–4661.
17. Fuhrmann, O., M. Arvand, A. Gohler *et al.* 2001. *Bartonella henselae* induces NF-kappaB-dependent upregulation of adhesion molecules in cultured human endothelial cells: possible role of outer membrane proteins as pathogenic factors. Infect. Immunol. **69:** 5088–5097.
18. Kempf, V.A., B. Volkmann, M. Schaller *et al.* 2001. Evidence of a leading role for VEGF in *Bartonella henselae*–induced endothelial cell proliferations. Cell. Microbiol. **3:** 623–632.
19. Padmalayam, I., K. Karem, B. Baumstark & R. Massung. 2000. The gene encoding the 17-kDa antigen of *Bartonella henselae* is located within a cluster of genes homologous to the *virB* virulence operon. DNA Cell Biol. **19:** 377–382.
20. Schmiederer, M. & B. Anderson. 2000. Cloning, sequencing, and expression of three *Bartonella henselae* genes homologous to the *Agrobacterium tumefaciens virB* region. DNA Cell Biol. **19:** 141–147.

21. SCHMIEDERER, M., R. ARCENAS, R. WIDEN *et al.* 2001. Intracellular induction of the *Bartonella henselae virB* operon by human endothelial cells. Infect. Immunol. **69:** 6495–6502.
22. SCHULEIN, R. & C. DEHIO. 2002. The VirB/VirD4 type IV secretion system of *Bartonella* is essential for establishing intraerythrocytic infection. Mol. Microbiol. **46:** 1053–1067.
23. SCHMID, M.C., R. SCHULEIN, M. DEHIO *et al.* 2004. The VirB type IV secretion system of *Bartonella henselae* mediates invasion, proinflammatory activation, and antiapoptotic protection of endothelial cells. Mol. Microbiol. **52:** 81–92.
24. SCHULEIN, R., P. GUYE, T.A. RHOMBERG *et al.* 2005. A bipartite signal mediates the transfer of type IV secretion substrates of *Bartonella henselae* into human cells. Proc. Natl. Acad. Sci. USA **102:** 856–861.
25. RIESS, T., S.G. ANDERSSON, A. LUPAS *et al.* 2004. *Bartonella* adhesin A mediates a proangiogenic host cell response. J. Exp. Med. **200:** 1267–1278.
26. ZHANG, P., B.B. CHOMEL, M.K. SCHAU *et al.* 2004. A family of variably expressed outer-membrane proteins (Vomp) mediates adhesion and autoaggregation in *Bartonella quintana*. Proc. Natl. Acad. Sci. USA **101:** 13630–13635.
27. ABBOTT, R.C., B.B. CHOMEL, R.W. KASTEN *et al.* 1997. Experimental and natural infection with *Bartonella henselae* in domestic cats. Comp. Immunol. Microbiol. Infect. Dis. **20:** 41–51.
28. BOULOUIS, H.J., F. BARRAT, D. BERMOND *et al.* 2001. Kinetics of *Bartonella birtlesii* infection in experimentally infected mice and pathogenic effect on reproductive functions. Infect. Immunol. **69:** 5313–5317.
29. WALKER, T.S. & H.H. WINKLER. 1981. *Bartonella bacilliformis*: colonial types and erythrocyte adherence. Infect. Immunol. **31:** 480–486.
30. MITCHELL, S.J. & M.F. MINNICK. 1995. Characterization of a two-gene locus from *Bartonella bacilliformis* associated with the ability to invade human erythrocytes. Infect. Immunol. **63:** 1552–1562.
31. COLEMAN, S.A. & M.F. MINNICK. 2001. Establishing a direct role for the *Bartonella bacilliformis* invasion-associated locus B (IalB) protein in human erythrocyte parasitism. Infect. Immunol. **69:** 4373–4381.
32. SEUBERT, A., R. HIESTAND, F. DE LA CRUZ & C. DEHIO. 2003. A bacterial conjugation machinery recruited for pathogenesis. Mol. Microbiol. **49:** 1253–1266.
33. KOSOY, M.Y., R.L. REGNERY, T. TZIANABOS *et al.* 1997. Distribution, diversity, and host specificity of *Bartonella* in rodents from the southeastern United States. Am. J. Trop. Med. Hyg. **57:** 578–588.
34. KOESLING, J., T. AEBISCHER, C. FALCH *et al.* 2001. Cutting edge: antibody-mediated cessation of hemotropic infection by the intraerythrocytic mouse pathogen *Bartonella grahamii*. J. Immunol. **167:** 11–14.
35. FOURNIER, P.E., M.F. MINNICK, H. LEPIDI *et al.* 2001. Experimental model of human body louse infection using green fluorescent protein–expressing *Bartonella quintana*. Infect. Immunol. **69:** 1876–1879.
36. HIGGINS, J.A., S. RADULOVIC, D.C. JAWORSKI & A.F. AZAD. 1996. Acquisition of the cat scratch disease agent *Bartonella henselae* by cat fleas (Siphonaptera:Pulicidae). J. Med. Entomol. **33:** 490–495.
37. ALSMARK, C.M., A.C. FRANK, E.O. KARLBERG *et al.* 2004. The louse-borne human pathogen *Bartonella quintana* is a genomic derivative of the zoonotic agent *Bartonella henselae*. Proc. Natl. Acad. Sci. USA **101:** 9716–9721.
38. TELFER, S., K.J. BOWN, R. SEKULES *et al.* 2005. Disruption of a host-parasite system following the introduction of an exotic host species. Parasitology **130:** 661–668.

Production of Recombinant Protein Pap31 and Its Application for the Diagnosis of *Bartonella bacilliformis* Infection

A. TAYE,[a,b] H. CHEN,[a,b] K. DUNCAN,[a,b] Z. ZHANG,[a,b] L. HENDRIX,[c] J. GONZALEZ,[b] AND W. CHING[a,b]

[a]*Rickettsial Diseases Department, Naval Medical Research Center, Silver Spring, Maryland 20910-7500, USA*

[b]*Department of Preventive Medicine and Biometrics, Uniformed Services University of Health Sciences, Bethesda, Maryland, USA*

[c]*Texas A&M University System Health Science Center, College Station, Texas, USA*

ABSTRACT: Tropical bartonellosis is a highly fatal epidemic and endemic infectious disease that occurs throughout the communities of the Andes Mountains in South America. The disease is caused by the facultative intracellular bacteria, *Bartonella bacilliformis*. The emergence of bartonellosis in new geographic areas and an increase in the number of reported cases suggest the need for a rapid test for epidemiologic study and investigation of the disease burden. The objective of this research is to develop a rapid serologic diagnostic test using recombinant antigens to overcome the limitations of the current standard IFA technique for laboratory diagnosis. Western blot analysis with patient sera of whole cell lysate separated on a 2D gel identified Pap31 as a dominant antigen. PCR primers were designed according to the sequence of ATCC strain 35685 to amplify the gene coding for Pap31 from a local isolate (HOSP 800-09, Peru). The amplicon was subsequently cloned into pET24a, adding the T7 tag, and expressed in *E. coli*. Patient sera with different IFA titers confirmed the diagnostic band of 31 kDa on a Western blot of SDS-PAGE. The performance of affinity-purified recombinant Pap31 (rPap31) was also evaluated in an ELISA format with 137 patient sera of known IFA titers. The range of ELISA reading from positive sera did not overlap with the range of those from negative sera, suggesting the potential application of rPap31 in both ELISA for high throughput regional hospital settings and in the construction of handheld rapid tests for rural clinical sites.

KEYWORDS: *Bartonella bacilliformis*; Pap31; ELISA; infection

Bartonella bacilliformis, a small (0.2–0.5 × 1.0 μm), motile, pleomorphic coccobacillus, is the etiological agent of Oroya fever for the acute phase and verruga peruana for the chronic phase of Carrión's disease. The disease is endemic in high-altitude regions of the Colombian, Ecuadorian, and Peruvian Andes. The acute phase is char-

Address for correspondence: Wei-Mei Ching, Rickettsial Diseases Department, Infectious Diseases Directorate, Naval Medical Research Center, 503 Robert Grant Avenue, Silver Spring, MD 20910-7500. Voice: 301-319-7438; fax: 301-319-7460.
chingw@nmrc.navy.mil

**Ann. N.Y. Acad. Sci. 1063: 280–285 (2005). © 2005 New York Academy of Sciences.
doi: 10.1196/annals.1355.045**

acterized by hemolytic anemia, fever, pallor, and transient immunosuppression.[1] The chronic phase is characterized by cutaneous vascular lesions. Without antibiotics, mortality rates of 40–88% have been reported.[2,3] Early diagnosis of the disease is very important for effectiveness of therapy. Furthermore, despite endemicity in South America, bartonellosis is becoming an increasingly important health issue with the recent rise in reported cases and the emergence into new locations, increasing the potential threat to overseas travelers.[4]

A number of techniques are currently available for the diagnosis of *B. bacilliformis* exposure and infection. However, they all suffer from being nonspecific, extremely laborious, expensive, or time-consuming. These limitations are especially acute when the required tests are conducted by facilities with limited resources. Laboratory culture of *B. bacilliformis* is hampered by the bacterium's fastidious nature. It requires two to five weeks to culture and identify the isolate. Peripheral blood smears and histopathologic studies are the most frequently used methods of diagnosis. However, the sensitivity of this method is only 36% when compared to bacterial isolation.[2] PCR amplification of various *B. bacilliformis* specific genes has been demonstrated to be useful. While these molecular techniques offer high sensitivity and specificity, PCR assays require equipment and expertise not widely available in endemic areas.

Serological assays using whole-cell antigen or recombinant 65-kDa antigen in ELISA or Western blot have been reported, but suffered from lack of specificity. The current gold standard method, indirect fluorescence assay (IFA), uses irradiated whole-cell antigen preparation from cocultivated Vero cells.[5] The method is sensitive, but costly, and requires expertise to achieve reproducible results. Because *B. bacilliformis* is the causative agent of Oroya fever and verruga peruana, where mortality can be exceptionally high, improved methods to detect *B. bacilliformis* exposure are needed over existing procedures. We have identified a protein antigen, Pap31, a homologue of a bacteriophage-associated protein in *Bartonella henselae* (also called HbpA), that is an excellent candidate for a diagnostic reagent.[6] The Pap31 protein, from the virulent Peruvian strain of *B. bacilliformis*, is found to be a highly expressed antigen in growing cultures of *B. bacilliformis*. Furthermore, the protein is immunologically dominant, making it an ideal antigen for use in enzyme-linked immunosorbent assays (ELISA) and in immunoblotting assays. The Pap31 has been sequenced and a recombinant Pap31 can be produced in bulk. The use of this single protein antigen permits the use of ELISA, Western blot methods, or rapid lateral flow assay for the diagnosis of *B. bacilliformis* infection. All these methods are preferable over currently available regimens.

MATERIALS AND METHODS

Identification of Pap31 as the Immunodominant Antigen

Bartonella bacilliformis strain ATCC KC583 was grown on 5% rabbit blood agar plates at 28°C in the absence of CO_2. After 10–14 days, the bacteria were harvested with BHI medium (3.5 mg/mL). Total bacterial proteins (30 μg) were separated via 2D gel electrophoresis. The gel was either stained with SYPRO (Bio-Rad Laboratories, CA) or electrotransferred onto a polyvinylidene difluoride (PVDF) membrane.

Seroreactive protein antigens were detected by immunoblotting with a patient serum. The corresponding 5 protein spots were cut out for N-terminal amino acid sequencing.

Cloning, Expression, and Purification of Recombinant Pap31 (rPap31)

Primers for rPap31 were designed according to the ATCC strain 35685 (KC583) sequence determined by L. Hendrix. The sequence has just been submitted to GenBank (accession number DQ207957) (forward primer: gcagcatatgttatgatcccgcaagaaata; reverse primer: ctaaaggcacaaccacaacgcattcttaag). The rPap31 gene segment was amplified using the genomic DNA of a local strain HOSP 800-09 as the template. PCR product was inserted between the NdeI and EcoRI sites of the expression vector pET24a (pET24a-pap31). The rPap31 protein was expressed in *E. coli* BL21 (DE3) after induction with 1 mM IPTG. The Pap31 gene segment in pET24a was recloned

A

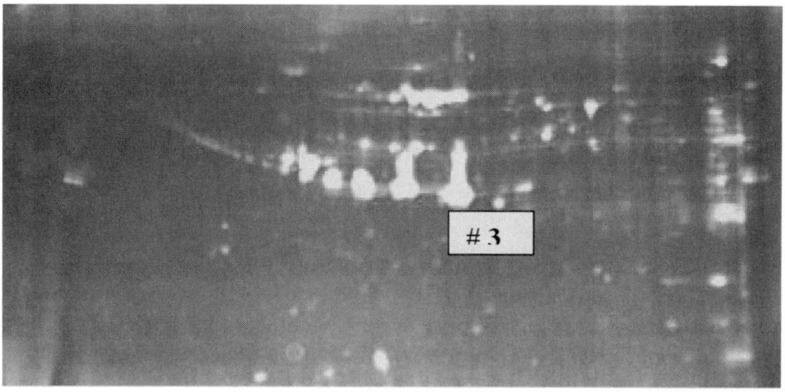

B

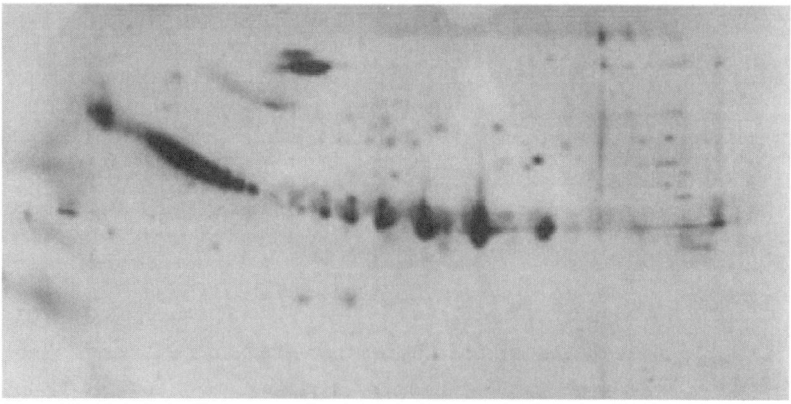

FIGURE 1. Two-dimensional gel electrophoresis and Western blot analysis of proteins from *Bartonella bacilliformis* whole-cell lysate. (**A**) Total protein stained by SYPRO in a pH range of 3–7. (**B**) Western blot analysis of the protein shown in *panel A* staining with serum from a *B. bacilliformis*–infected patient.

by GenWay Biotech Incorporated (San Diego, CA) to attach a T7 tag to the N-terminus of the rPap31 gene insert. The rPap31 was expressed as an inclusion body, which was washed and solubilized with 8 M urea in the presence of 1% Triton X-100 and 2 mM DTT in 50 mM Tris HCl, pH 8.0. The polypeptide was refolded by dialysis against 0.1 mM EDTA/12% glycerol in 50 mM Tris-HCl, pH 8.0, at 4°C. The refolded protein was further purified using the T7-tag affinity column in the presence of 2 M urea.

Evaluation of rPap31 for Serological Reactivity

Sera were collected from Peruvian patients with acute or chronic phase bartonellosis in 2000. Western blot analysis and ELISA were carried out as previously described.[7]

RESULTS AND DISCUSSION

Under 2D gel electrophoresis of the lyzed whole-cell total protein, 4 to 5 moieties migrated near, but not identically, to the Pap31 protein (FIG. 1). All spots were cut out of the gel and subjected to amino acid sequencing. Of the 5 dominant proteins, spot no. 3 yielded the longest amino acid sequence, closely resembling that of *B. henselae* Pap31. Western blot analysis with IFA-positive patient sera proved that it was the immunodominant antigen. For the IFA test, sera with titers greater than 128 were designated as positive and those with 128 and below as negative for bartonella infection. For the Western blot, the diagnostic band is at 30.3 kDa, the size of our recombinant protein antigen, rPap31 (FIG. 2). Patient sera were diagnosed as positive if reactive with a band of this size. Diagnosis was confirmed by comparing

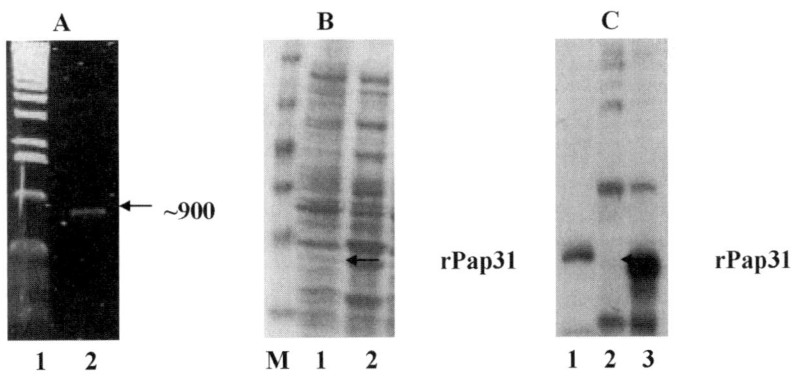

FIGURE 2. Cloning and expression of recombinant Pap31 (rPap31). **(A)** Amplification of the Pap31 gene by PCR: lane 1, 1-kb ladder; lane 2, PCR product. **(B)** Expression of the recombinant antigen rPap31 in *E. coli* BL21 (DE3) by vector pET24a-Pap31: lane 1, uninduced; lane 2, induced. **(C)** Confirmation of the seroreactivity of rPap31 by Western blot analysis with patient serum: lane 1, *B. bacilliformis* cell lysate; lane 2, BL21 (DE3) carrying pET24a; lane 3, BL21 (DE3) carrying pET24a-Pap31.

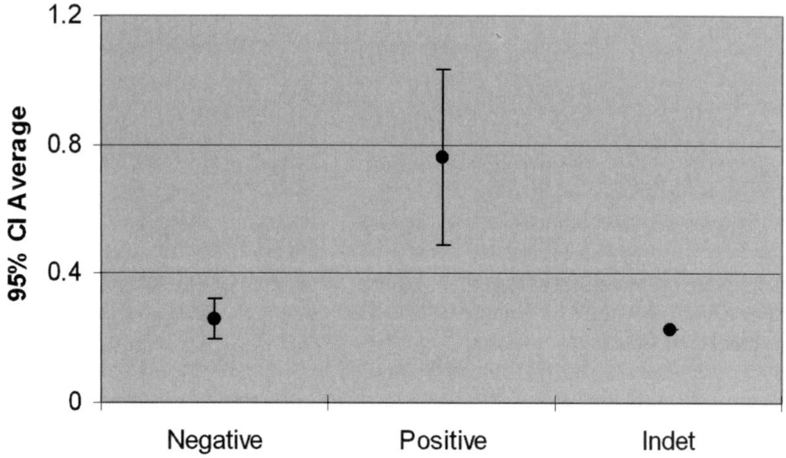

FIGURE 3. ELISA results versus IFA results for 137 sera: mean and 95% CI of ELISA OD by IFA result. Samples with IFA titers equal to or higher than 256 were considered as positive. Indetermined ("Indet") means that, after repeated testing (5 times) by IFA, the sample cannot be given as a clear positive or a clear negative.

the membrane with those incubated with the negative control serum and the positive control patient serum. The rPap31 exhibited both high sensitivity and specificity in ELISA (FIG. 3). Among the 137 samples tested, 107 were IFA-negative, 29 were IFA-positive, and 1 was indetermined.

The ELISA OD range (95% confidence interval) of the IFA negatives did not overlap with those of the IFA positives. The rPap31 is easy to purify and store, and can go through several freeze-thaw cycles without losing its antigenicity. The protein would be well suited for use in any antibody-based assay, including ELISA, Western blotting, and rapid immunochromatographic assays.

ACKNOWLEDGMENTS

This work was supported by Work Unit Number 6000.RAD1.J.A0310. The views expressed in this article are those of the authors and do not necessarily reflect the official policy or position of the Department of the Navy, Department of Defense, nor the U.S. Government.

[*Competing interests statement:* The authors declare that they have no conflicting financial interests.]

REFERENCES

1. GROOT, H. 1951. Human bartonellosis or Carrion's disease. *In* Clinical Tropical Medicine, pp. 615–640. Mosby. St. Louis.

2. SCHULTZ, M. 1968. A history of bartonellosis (Carrion's disease). Am. J. Trop. Med. Hyg. **17:** 503–515.
3. GRAY, G.C., A.A. JOHNSON, S.A. THORTON *et al.* 1990. An epidemic of Oroya fever in the Peruvian Andes. Am. J. Trop. Med. Hyg. **42:** 215–221.
4. KOSEK, M., R. LAVARELLO, R.H. GILMAN *et al.* 2000. Natural history of infection with *Bartonella bacilliformis* in a nonendemic population. J. Infect. Dis. **182:** 865–872.
5. CHAMBERLIN, J., L. LAUGHLIN, S. GORDON *et al.* 2000. Serodiagnosis of *Bartonella bacilliformis* infection by indirect fluorescence antibody assay: test development and application to a population in an area of bartonellosis endemicity. J. Clin. Microbiol. **38:** 4269–4271.
6. CHENOWETH, M.R., C.E. GREENE, D.C. KRAUSE & F.C. GHERARDINI. 2004. Predominant outer membrane antigens of *Bartonella henselae*. Infect. Immunol. **72:** 3097–3105.
7. CHING, W.M., H. WANG, C. EAMSILA *et al.* 1998. Expression and refolding of truncated recombinant major outer membrane protein antigen (r56) of *Orientia tsutsugamushi* and its use in enzyme-linked immunosorbent assays. Clin. Diagn. Lab. Immunol. **5:** 519–526.

Bartonella bacilliformis GroEL: Effect on Growth of Human Vascular Endothelial Cells in Infected Cocultures

LAURA S. SMITHERMAN AND MICHAEL F. MINNICK

Division of Biological Sciences, University of Montana, Missoula, Montana 59812, USA

ABSTRACT: *Bartonella* are the only bacteria known to induce angioproliferative lesions of the human vasculature and liver during infection. Previous work from our lab suggests that GroEL participates in the mitogenic response observed in HUVEC cultures supplemented with the soluble fraction of *Bartonella bacilliformis*. Work in this study shows that exposure to high concentrations of the fraction is actually cytotoxic for HUVECs. To analyze this phenomenon, live *B. bacilliformis*–HUVEC cocultures were employed to study the effect of excess bacterial GroEL on the host cell during active infection. Four *B. bacilliformis* strains were generated to produce varying levels of GroEL. HUVEC cocultures with LSS100, a strain that synthesizes markedly greater quantities of GroEL relative to others, significantly accelerates apoptosis of the cocultured HUVECs relative to other strains. Acceleration of apoptosis can be inhibited by Z-VAD-FMK, a pan-caspase inhibitor. Time course data show that, at 18 h of infection, both LSS100 and control strains significantly inhibit spontaneous apoptosis of cocultured HUVECs, as previously reported for other *Bartonella* species. However, by 48 h, LSS100 significantly increases apoptosis of the host cell. We hypothesize that intracellular *Bartonella* GroEL functions as an Hsp60 analogue, a eukaryotic orthologue known to accelerate pro-caspase 3 activation by enhancing its vulnerability to upstream activator caspases. These data suggest another strategy whereby *Bartonella* may regulate host cell growth.

KEYWORDS: *Bartonella*; GroEL; apoptosis; endothelial cells

INTRODUCTION

A frequent manifestation of bartonellosis in humans is the production of angioproliferative lesions of the skin (bacillary angiomatosis and verruga peruana) and liver (bacillary peliosis hepatis).[1] Such vascular lesions can be life-threatening to the patient, and data suggest that they are induced by a consortium of stimuli, including *Bartonella*-derived mitogens for endothelial cells,[2–4] inhibition of endothelial cell apoptosis by the bacterium,[5,6] plus induction of host cell cytokines, growth factors, and a proinflammatory response.[7–9]

Address for correspondence: Michael F. Minnick, Division of Biological Sciences, 32 Campus Drive #4824, University of Montana, Missoula, MT 59812-4824. Voice: 406-243-5972; fax: 406-243-4184.
mike.minnick@mso.umt.edu.

Ann. N.Y. Acad. Sci. 1063: 286–298 (2005). © 2005 New York Academy of Sciences.
doi: 10.1196/annals.1355.046

Recent data from our laboratory suggest that GroEL participates in increased *in vitro* proliferation of human umbilical vein endothelial cells (HUVECs) exposed to culture supplements consisting of the soluble fraction of *Bartonella bacilliformis*.[10] Experiments showed that (1) final HUVEC numbers correlated with GroEL levels in the culture supplement, (2) mitogenicity of the fraction can be increased if the *Bartonella* source culture is subjected to temperature upshift, and (3) mitogenicity of the fraction can be inhibited if it is pretreated with anti–*B. bacilliformis* GroEL antiserum. Whether GroEL is a mitogen for HUVECs or serves as a chaperonin to the actual *Bartonella* mitogen(s) (or both) is unknown. Interestingly, *B. bacilliformis* GroEL was found to be actively secreted, and the chaperonin was detectable in both soluble and inner/outer membrane fractions of the bacterium.[10]

In addition to serving as major antigens during bacterial infection,[11] GroEL homologues from other pathogens have been reported to alter the growth rates of cultured human cells. For example, *Chlamydia pneumoniae* GroEL is mitogenic for human vascular smooth muscle cells in culture.[12] *Actinobacillus actinomycetemcomitans* GroEL is mitogenic for cultured epithelial cells at low concentration, but is cytotoxic at higher concentrations or upon prolonged exposure.[13–15]

The purpose of this study was to examine the effect of *B. bacilliformis* on HUVEC cocultures and to study the consequences of excess bacterial GroEL during an active infection *in vitro*.

MATERIALS AND METHODS

Bacterial Strains, Cell Lines, and Tissue Culture

Bacterial strains used in this study are listed in TABLE 1. *B. bacilliformis* was cultivated on heart infusion agar/blood plates (HIAB) as previously described.[10] *E. coli* was grown overnight at 37°C in Luria Bertani medium supplemented with appropriate antibiotics as needed. HUVECs were purchased and routinely cultured in EGM at 37°C, 5% CO_2, and 100% relative humidity, per the supplier's instructions (Clonetics, Walkersville, MD). HUVEC use was restricted to tissue culture passages 1–4 to minimize variability between experiments.

B. bacilliformis–*HUVEC Tissue Cocultures*

The effect of *B. bacilliformis* infection and overexpression of GroEL on HUVEC growth and morphology was examined in cocultures. Gelatin-coated, 96-well plates containing EGM were seeded with ~2000 HUVECs per well, and plates were incubated for 4 h to allow for adherence. Cultures were infected by adding 1.6×10^8 bacteria suspended in EGM to each well and incubating for 3 h. Unbound bacteria were subsequently removed by thoroughly rinsing three times with M199 containing 20% fetal calf serum (M199-FCS). The wells were brought to a final volume of 100 µL M199-FCS. HUVECs were cultured and assayed for cell numbers at 96 h postinfection. Digital micrographs were obtained by staining cells with Hema-Quik Stain (Fisher Scientific, Pittsburgh, PA) and visualizing with a Zeiss Axioskop photomicroscope (Zeiss, Thornwood, CA) interfaced with Image-Pro Plus 3.0 software (Media Cybernetics, Silver Spring, MD).

TABLE 1. Bacterial strains and plasmids used in this study

Strain/plasmid	Relevant genotype/description	Source/reference
B. bacilliformis		
KC583	Neotype strain	ATCC (27)
JB584	Transformation-competent strain	(20)
LSS100	JB584 containing pGRO1	(10)
LSS001	JB584 containing pBBR1-MCS2	(10)
LSS200	JB584 containing pGRO1Δ	This study
E. coli		
DH5α	Host for plasmid propagation	Gibco-BRL (Grand Island, NY)
Plasmids		
pBBR1MCS-2	*B. bacilliformis* shuttle vector, Km^r	(20, 28)
pGRO1	pBBR1MCS-2 with cloned *B. bacilliformis groESL* operon	(10)
pGRO1Δ	pGRO1 with 1002-bp deletion in *groEL* and 4 intervening *Xho*I linkers	This study

Growth and Apoptosis Assays

B. bacilliformis cell lysates were prepared by harvesting bacteria into ice-cold phosphate-buffered saline (PBS; pH 7.4) containing 0.1-mm glass beads and lysing for 3 min with a Fastprep FP120 disrupter (Thermo Savant, Holbrook, NY). Particulates were removed from the lysate by centrifuging at 16,000*g* for 5 min followed by ultracentrifugation at 100,000*g* for 60 min. HUVECs were typically seeded at 1000 cells per well in EGM or M199-FCS media with lysate supplements of 0–300 μg protein/mL. Heat-treated lysates were prepared by treating for 7 min at 100°C. HUVEC numbers were measured using an acid phosphatase assay[16] calibrated with linear standard curves of enzyme activity as a function of viable, adherent HUVEC numbers (0–36,000 cells by hemocytometer) as previously described.[10] Standard curves for the assays encompassed all OD_{405} values reported in this study.

Apoptosis was examined using 96-h cocultures infected with *B. bacilliformis* LSS001 or LSS100, in the presence or absence of the pan-caspase inhibitor, Z-VAD-FMK, at a final concentration of 50 μM. Negative control cultures were treated with equal volumes of solvent (100% ethanol) minus the inhibitor. Briefly, HUVECs were incubated for 3 h at 37°C with *B. bacilliformis* and 50 μM Z-VAD-FMK. Cocultures were subsequently rinsed three times with M199-FCS and cultured an additional 96 h in M199-FCS containing Z-VAD-FMK (50 μM). Final HUVEC numbers were quantified using an acid phosphatase assay as described above. Apoptosis was also quantified by assaying DNA fragmentation in *B. bacilliformis*/HUVEC cocultures incubated for 18 h, 48 h, and 96 h postinfection using a Cell Death Detection ELISA per the manufacturer's instructions (Roche Applied Science, Indianapolis, IN). Supernatants were also assayed to assess the extent of secondary necrosis in the cultures.

Sodium Dodecyl Sulfate–Polyacrylamide Gel Electrophoresis (SDS-PAGE) and Immunoblot Analysis

Protein concentrations of samples were determined with a BCA assay kit (Pierce, Rockford, IL) and a bovine serum albumin standard. SDS-PAGE was done by standard protocol[17] using protein samples solubilized in Laemmli sample buffer and polyacrylamide gels (12.5% acrylamide; w/v). SDS-PAGE gels were fixed and stained with Coomassie brilliant blue by standard protocol[17] or were immediately transferred to nitrocellulose (0.45-μm pore size; Osmonics, Minnetonka, MN) for immunoblot analysis.[18] Immunoblots were developed as previously described,[10] using rabbit anti–*B. bacilliformis* GroEL antiserum (1:1000 dilution), horseradish peroxidase–conjugated goat anti-rabbit IgG antibody (1:2000 dilution) (Sigma Chemical, St. Louis, MO), H_2O_2 as a substrate, and 4-chloronapthol as the chromogen. Images were digitized with a Scanmaker 9800XL and ScanWizard Pro software (Microtek, Carson, CA).

DNA Cloning, Manipulation, and Gene Expression

Plasmids used in this study are listed in TABLE 1. The pGRO1 plasmid contains a functional *B. bacilliformis groESL* operon[10] and was mutagenized by digestion with *Pml*I to remove an internal 1002-bp fragment of *groEL*. The resulting DNA was purified from crystal violet–stained agarose gels (1% agarose; w/v) with a GeneClean II kit (QBiogene, Vista, CA), and then ligated to 10-mer *Xho*I linkers (Promega, Madison, WI) using T4 DNA ligase and standard protocol.[17] The resulting plasmid, pGRO1Δ, was sequenced using an ABI 3100 automated sequencer (Applied Biosystems, Foster City, CA) as previously described[19] and was found to contain an intact *groES* gene, 36 residual bases at the 5′ end of *groEL*, a 1002-bp deletion, and 4 copies of the *Xho*I linker, resulting in a nonsense mutation immediately downstream. Transformation of *B. bacilliformis* was done by electroporation as previously described.[20]

Graphical and Statistical Analyses

Graphs were generated with Sigmaplot 8.0 software (SPSS, Chicago, IL). Statistical significance was determined by a Student's *t* test or one-way analysis of variance using Instat 3.0 software (GraphPad, San Diego, CA). A P value of <0.05 was considered significant. Mean values ± standard deviations (SD) are reported in this study.

RESULTS AND DISCUSSION

In a previous study, we discovered that HUVEC numbers in 96-h cultures correlated with the quantity of *B. bacilliformis* lysate initially added to the tissue culture, with maximal numbers resulting from a supplement of 10 μg lysate protein/mL medium.[10] However, assays in this study did not examine lysate doses greater than 50 μg/mL. In the same study, we found that *B. henselae* cell lysates possessed significantly less mitogenicity for HUVECs than *B. bacilliformis* lysates at a 10 μg/mL dose.[10] Subsequent studies with *B. henselae* lysates actually showed a dose-

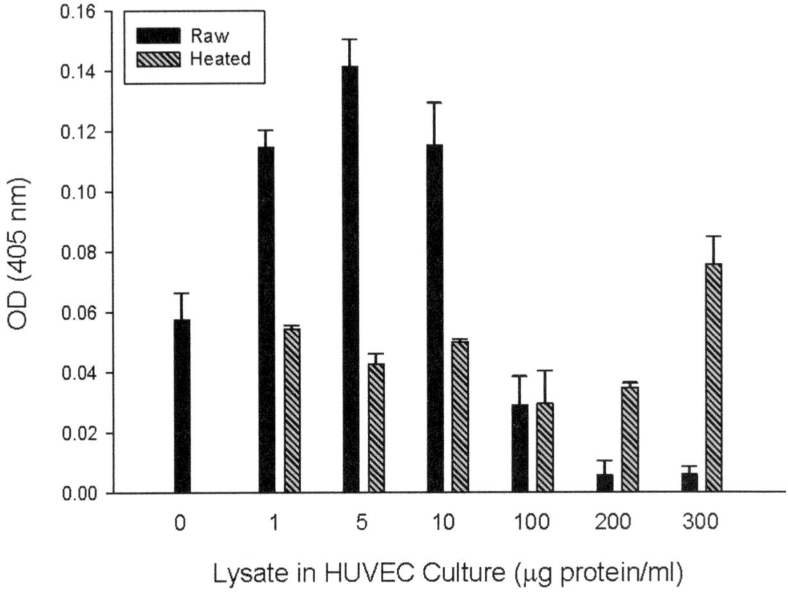

FIGURE 1. Dose response of HUVECs cultured 96 h in EGM supplemented with a range of *B. bacilliformis* KC583 cell lysate concentrations as indicated, showing mitogenic activity at 1–10 μg/mL and inhibition of growth at 100–300 μg/mL dosages. Data represent the average of 3 experiments ± SD. [Raw, raw lysate; heated, lysate pretreated at 100°C for 7 min.]

dependent inhibition of HUVEC growth in response to the supplement (Smitherman and Minnick, unpublished data). To determine if *B. bacilliformis* lysates are also inhibitory at higher doses, we assayed HUVEC growth in EGM medium (Clonetics) supplemented with a broad range of lysate concentrations. As before, resulting data show that a *B. bacilliformis* lysate is significantly mitogenic ($P \leq 0.001$) at doses ranging from 1–10 μg lysate/mL culture, resulting in a 2- to 3-fold increase in HUVEC numbers relative to heat-treated controls. A dosage of 100 μg/mL was neither mitogenic nor inhibitory for HUVECs, and treatment with heat-treated or raw lysates at this concentration produced indistinguishable results. Further analysis showed that the lysate significantly inhibited ($P \leq 0.006$) HUVEC growth when used at 200 and 300 μg/mL doses, with 83% and 92% reductions relative to their respective heat-treated controls. Data also suggest that a heat-resistant mitogen, perhaps LPS, may be active at very high doses (200–300 μg/mL; see FIG. 1).

Since the results in FIGURE 1 were similar to those observed with *A. actinomycetemcomitans*, a bacterium whose GroEL is mitogenic for cultured epithelial cells at low doses, but cytotoxic at higher doses,[13,14] we explored the possibility that *B. bacilliformis* GroEL might be involved in inhibiting HUVEC growth at the higher lysate dosages. To that end, we generated 4 *B. bacilliformis* strains that produce different levels of GroEL. JB584 was chosen as the parental strain because of its

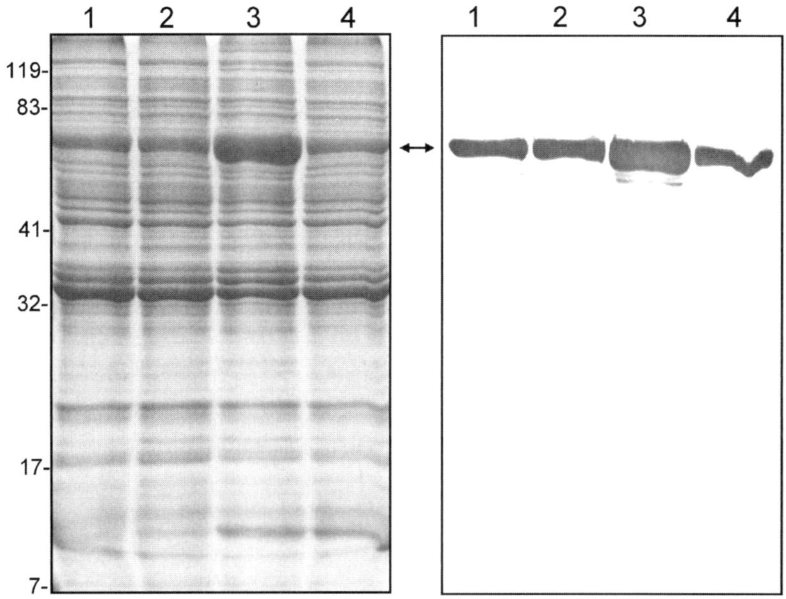

FIGURE 2. Differential GroEL synthesis in 4 *B. bacilliformis* strains. (**A**) Coomassie blue–stained SDS-PAGE analysis of the total protein profiles for strains JB584, LSS001, LSS100, and LSS200 (lanes 1–4, respectively). (**B**) The corresponding immunoblot developed with rabbit anti–*B. bacilliformis* GroEL antiserum. All lanes contain 30 μg total protein. GroEL is indicated by a *double arrow*. Molecular mass values from protein standards are given to the left in kDa.

amenability to transformation and genetic manipulation,[20] and it was electroporated with pBBR1MCS-2 shuttle vector to produce a negative control strain, designated LSS001. JB584 was also transformed with pGRO1, a high copy-number plasmid containing the *B. bacilliformis groESL* operon, to generate strain LSS100. In order to examine the respective effect of GroES and GroEL on HUVEC growth, the *groEL* gene of pGRO1 was deleted to create pGRO1Δ, a construct transformed into JB584 to produce strain LSS200. FIGURE 2 shows the SDS-PAGE analysis of the total protein profiles of the 4 resulting strains grown on HIAB plates, plus the corresponding immunoblot developed with rabbit anti–*B. bacilliformis* GroEL. These data clearly show that *B. bacilliformis* LSS100 produces substantially more GroEL *in vitro*, and densitometry analysis of immunoblots containing total protein profiles (FIG. 2B) reveals approximately a 2-fold increase in the protein relative to the other 3 strains.

The effect of these 4 *B. bacilliformis* strains on the growth of HUVECs in coculture was examined at 96 h postinfection. Data show a significant increase in cell numbers for HUVECs cocultured with strains JB584 (31% increase; $P < 0.0001$) or LSS001 (34% increase; $P < 0.0001$) compared to uninfected controls (FIG. 3). However, strain LSS100, producing roughly twice the amount of GroEL as compared to the other strains (FIG. 2), causes a marked and significant reduction in HUVEC numbers

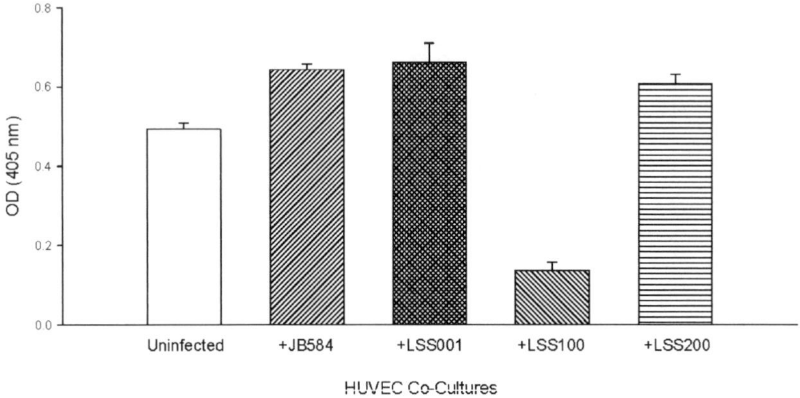

FIGURE 3. Number of HUVECs in M199-FCS medium following a 96-h coculture with *B. bacilliformis* strains JB584, LSS001, LSS100, or LSS200. Data represent the average of 6 experiments ± SD.

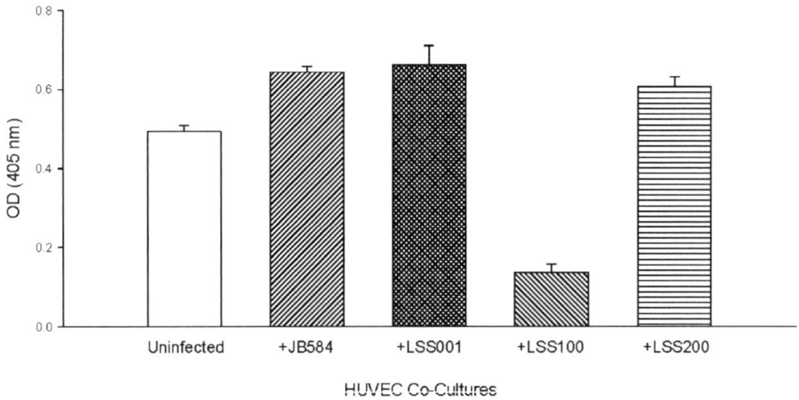

FIGURE 4. Immunoblot showing GroEL levels in infected HUVECs cultivated in M199-FCS, following a 96-h coculture with the indicated *B. bacilliformis* strains. Lane 1, uninfected HUVECs (no detectable GroEL); lanes 2–5, HUVECs infected with JB584, LSS001, LSS100, or LSS200, respectively. The GroEL protein is arrowed.

(79% less than JB584-infected cocultures and 72% less than uninfected HUVECs; $P < 0.0001$ for both) (FIG. 3).

To ensure that GroEL levels in LSS100 were also elevated during tissue culture infections, large-scale HUVEC cocultures (5 mL) were prepared and harvested at 96 h. The total protein profiles (HUVEC plus *Bartonella*) were analyzed on immunoblots probed with anti–*B. bacilliformis* GroEL antiserum. These data show that GroEL cannot be detected in uninfected HUVECs and is markedly greater in the LSS100 infection as compared to cocultures with the other *Bartonella* strains (e.g., a 4-fold increase over the JB584-infected cocultures by densitometry) (FIG. 4). Taken as a whole, the data suggest that the decrease in HUVECs observed in the LSS100-infected cocultures is due to an elevated quantity of GroEL since infection with LSS200 (containing a deletion mutation in the cloned *groEL* and otherwise isogenic) abrogates the inhibitory effect on growth and restores cell numbers to levels that are similar to JB584 or LSS001 cocultures. In fact, differences between HUVEC cocultures infected with JB584 and LSS001, or LSS200 (FIG. 3), are not significantly different from one another ($P > 0.05$). The data also suggest that GroES is not responsible for the inhibitory effect seen in an LSS100 infection, as both the *groES* gene and the *groESL* operon promoter are intact in the pGRO1Δ plasmid harbored by LSS200 (FIG. 3). Nevertheless, these data do not rule out the possibility that a GroES-GroEL complex could be involved in the activity.

The morphology of the 96 h–infected HUVEC cocultures was subsequently examined by microscopy following fixing and staining with Hema-Quik (Fisher Scientific). HUVECs infected with JB584, LSS001, or LSS200 were indistinguishable from one another by visual inspection of their gross cellular morphology (FIG. 5), although infected cells were for the most part more vacuolated and granulated than uninfected HUVECs. Similar changes in morphology have been previously reported for HUVECs infected with *B. henselae* and *B. quintana*[2] or *B. bacilliformis*.[21,22] Unlike the other cocultures, HUVECs infected with LSS100 consistently showed cell shrinkage, chromatin condensation, and membrane blebbing, all characteristics of cells undergoing apoptosis (FIG. 5), and DAPI and TUNEL staining qualitatively supported this observation (not shown).

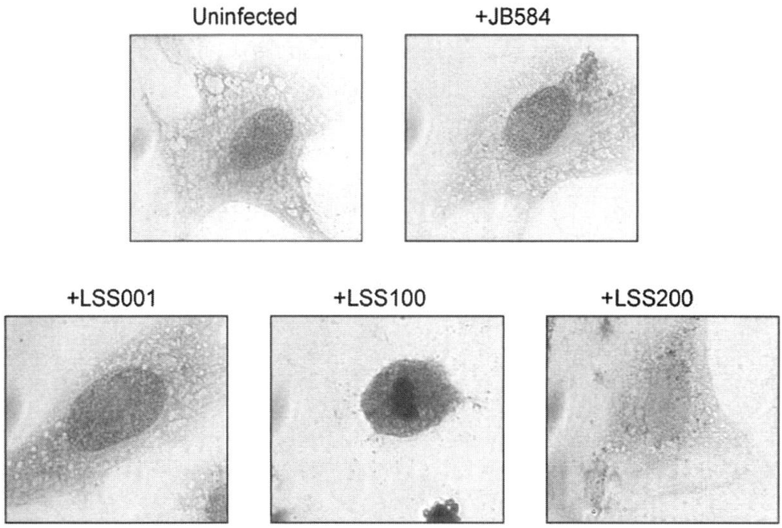

FIGURE 5. Micrographs showing representative cell morphologies of infected HUVECs following a 96-h coculture with 4 *B. bacilliformis* strains including JB584, LSS001, LSS100, and LSS200. An uninfected HUVEC is provided for comparison. Cells were visualized using Hema-Quik Stain (Fisher Scientific) and are shown at 1000× magnification. Note the marked apoptosis in +LSS100 cells.

To investigate whether apoptosis was occurring in response to the elevated intracellular GroEL levels, HUVEC cocultures infected with LSS001 or LSS100 were incubated for 96 h in the presence of the pan-caspase inhibitor, Z-VAD-FMK, or an equal volume of its respective solvent (100% ethanol) as a negative control (FIG. 6). Results show that infection with LSS001 significantly increases HUVEC numbers relative to the respective uninfected control cultures incubated with ethanol (14.9% increase) or Z-VAD-FMK (30.4% increase) ($P < 0.0001$ for both). However, infection with LSS100 in the presence of ethanol results in a marked and significant decrease (84.9%; $P < 0.0001$) relative to the uninfected control. Overall, these results are similar to those observed in the absence of ethanol (FIG. 3). When Z-VAD-FMK is included in the LSS001 cocultures, HUVEC numbers increase slightly, but significantly (8.1%; $P < 0.008$), relative to the respective negative control, likely reflecting inhibition of spontaneous apoptosis. Perhaps most notable was the marked and significant increase (549%; $P < 0.0001$) in HUVEC numbers in the LSS100 cocultures treated with Z-VAD-FMK relative to the ethanol control. In fact, the inhibitor restored HUVEC numbers in these particular cocultures to levels similar to what is observed in uninfected host cells. Taken together, data in FIGURE 6 suggest that the LSS100 strain, with its overproduction of GroEL during infection of the cultured host cells, can trigger HUVEC apoptosis by 96 h postinfection, and that the process can be inhibited by treatment with Z-VAD-FMK.

To unequivocally demonstrate HUVEC apoptosis and to examine the process over time, we measured histone-associated DNA fragments from LSS001– and

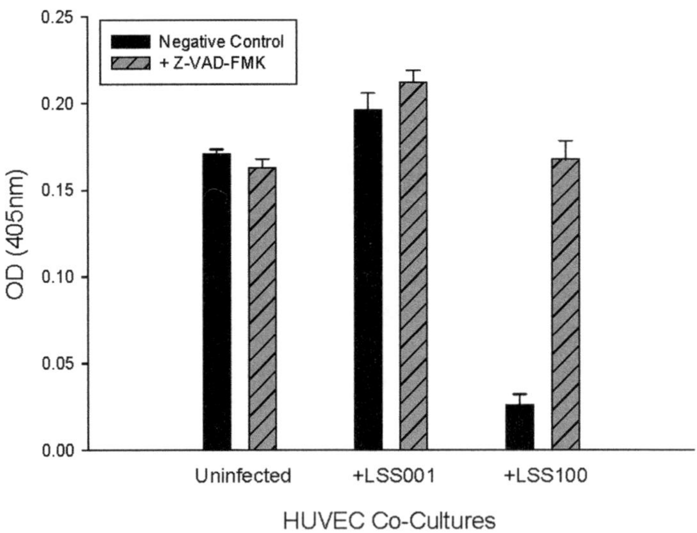

FIGURE 6. Z-VAD-FMK inhibits the reduction of HUVEC numbers observed with a *B. bacilliformis* LSS100 coculture. HUVEC numbers at 96 h of coculture in M199-FCS medium plus the indicated *B. bacilliformis* strain together with Z-VAD-FMK (50 μM) or an equal volume of solvent (100% ethanol) as a negative control are shown. Data represent the average of 6 experiments ± SD.

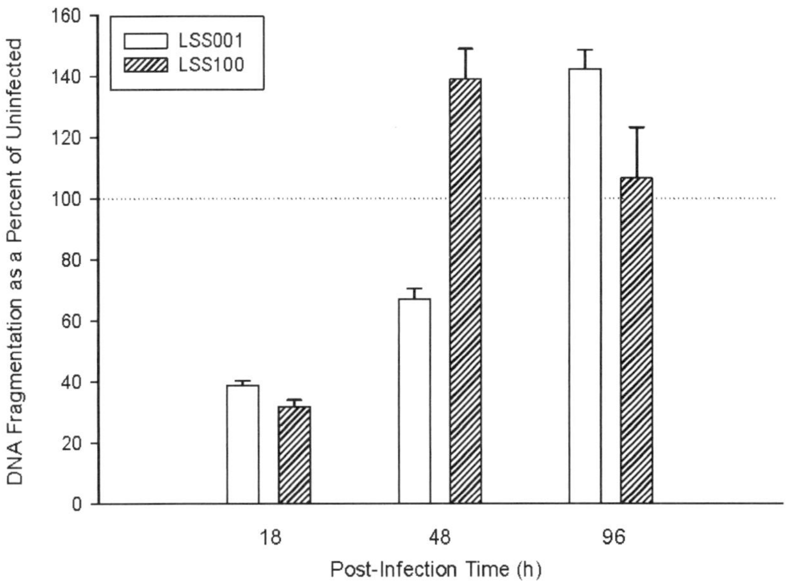

FIGURE 7. HUVEC DNA fragmentation during a *B. bacilliformis* LSS001 and LSS100 coculture as determined by ELISA (Roche). Results from cocultured HUVECs at 18 h, 48 h, and 96 h are shown as a percentage of uninfected HUVECs, with the 100% line outlined. Data represent the average of 3 experiments ± SD (3 independent determinations were done per experiment).

LSS100–HUVEC cocultures by assaying with an ELISA at three postinfection time points (FIG. 7). At 18 h, both LSS001 and LSS100 cocultures significantly suppress spontaneous host cell apoptosis (39% and 32% of the apoptosis observed in uninfected HUVECs; $P < 0.0001$); and LSS100 causes a slight, but significantly greater suppression of apoptosis than LSS001 ($P = 0.011$). To our knowledge, these are the first data showing that *B. bacilliformis* can interfere with spontaneous apoptosis of HUVECs, as previously reported for *B. henselae*–HUVEC cocultures.[5,23] As the *Bartonella* infection proceeds, the LSS100 cocultures show a significant increase in HUVEC apoptosis at 48 h relative to uninfected HUVECs (139% increase; $P = 0.0032$) and over 200% greater apoptosis than cocultures infected with LSS001 ($P = 0.0003$). In marked contrast, LSS001 cocultures maintained a significant inhibition of spontaneous apoptosis (~67% of what is observed in uninfected cells; $P = 0.0004$). Interestingly, although the LSS001 strain continues to inhibit spontaneous apoptosis of HUVECs at 48 h, the level of inhibition is roughly half that observed in the 18-h cocultures (FIG. 7). This last observation may be due to an accumulation of GroEL in the cell as the bacterium replicates over time. Assays on culture supernatants from both 18- and 48-h infections contained only trace amounts (<0.07 OD_{405} units) of fragmented DNA (not shown), suggesting that secondary necrosis was not a major factor at these time points. At 96 h, both strains enhance apoptosis as compared to uninfected HUVECs, and culture supernatants suggest that secondary necrosis occurs in both the uninfected cells and those cocultured with LSS100. On the contrary, supernatants from LSS001 cocultures showed only trace amounts of DNA, suggesting that secondary necrosis is not occurring (not shown). Taken as a whole, the data suggest that (a) both strains inhibit host cell apoptosis within the first 18 h of infection, (b) overproduction of GroEL by LSS100 markedly enhances apoptosis by 48 h, and (c) both strains enhance HUVEC apoptosis by 96 h.

Previous work has shown that the type IV secretion system (VirB) of *B. henselae* is essential to rearrangement of the host cell cytoskeleton during infection, activation of a proinflammatory response via NF-κB, inhibition of HUVEC apoptosis, and mediation of a cytotoxic/cytostatic effect when HUVECs are cocultured with bacteria at high titer.[23] Interestingly, VirB is not involved in *Bartonella* mitogenicity for HUVECs. Based upon our results, it is tempting to speculate that accumulation of secreted GroEL during the high titer *B. henselae* infection may have contributed to the observed HUVEC cytotoxicity in that study. Whether *Bartonella* GroEL is actually secreted by VirB is unknown, but recent data showing that GroEL is a substrate for the type IV secretion system in *Brucella*, a closely related pathogen, suggests that it is at least a possibility.[24]

Hsp60, a eukaryotic analogue of GroEL released by the mitochondria, has been shown to accelerate pro-caspase 3 activation by enhancing its vulnerability to upstream activator caspases. As such, Hsp60 constitutes an important regulator of apoptotic cell death.[25,26] Hsp60 activation of caspase 3 is apparently dependent upon an excess (16-fold) of the chaperonin, whereas equimolar amounts of Hsp60 are inefficient at stimulating caspase 3 maturation. Based upon these observations and results of this study, we hypothesize that intracellular infection of HUVECs by *Bartonella* is accompanied by release of GroEL and that the protein eventually accumulates in the cytosol to a threshold level that stimulates caspase 3 maturation and apoptosis. Normally, this process would require considerable time and increase in bacterial load as infection progresses. In contrast, infection by a GroEL-overproducing strain, like LSS100, dramatically increases the kinetics of this process and the resulting apoptosis.

To reconcile the different activities that we have ascribed to GroEL, it is important to note that the previous study that implicates the protein as a participant in HUVEC mitogenicity was done using cell cultures exposed to soluble fractions of *B. bacilliformis*,[10] whereas the current study examines the effects of GroEL synthesis by the pathogen during active infection. Undoubtedly, HUVEC surface receptors for GroEL are different from those located within the confines of the cell and may contribute to the different effects observed. Previous studies with *Chlamydia pneumoniae* have shown that GroEL binds the TLR-4 of human vascular smooth muscle cell and is a potent mitogen.[12] In eukaryotes, extracellular Hsp60 binds to TLR-2, TLR-4, CD91, and CD36,[6] and it is conceivable that extracellular binding of *Bartonella* GroEL to these or other receptors might enhance endothelial cell proliferation. Alternatively or in addition, GroEL could serve as a chaperonin that protects or maintains proper folding of some uncharacterized bacterial mitogen(s) in the cell lysate. We do not believe the mitogenic/extracellular[10] and the apoptotic/intracellular effects (this study) are mutually exclusive. It is even conceivable that accumulation of *Bartonella* GroEL during an intracellular infection and subsequent induction of apoptosis could provide a host cell escape route for the bacterium. Regardless, our data suggest that GroEL released by *Bartonella* during intracellular infection may represent another strategy for regulating host cell growth.

ACKNOWLEDGMENTS

This work was supported by Public Health Service Grant No. AI52101 to M. F. Minnick, who was also supported by Public Health Service Grant No. AI053111. Automated nucleotide sequencing was done at the Murdock Sequencing Facility at the University of Montana–Missoula. We are grateful to Sonja Best for helpful discussions and suggestions.

[*Conflict of interest statement:* The authors of this research declare that they have no conflict of interest.]

REFERENCES

1. Koehler, J.E. 1996. *Bartonella* infections. Adv. Pediatr. Infect. Dis. **11:** 1–27.
2. Conley, T., L. Slater & K. Hamilton. 1994. *Rochalimaea* species stimulate human endothelial cell proliferation and migration *in vitro*. J. Lab. Clin. Med. **124:** 521–528.
3. Garcia, F.U., J. Wojta, K.N. Broadley *et al.* 1990. *Bartonella bacilliformis* stimulates endothelial cells *in vitro* and is angiogenic *in vivo*. Am. J. Pathol. **136:** 1125–1135.
4. Maeno, N., H. Oda, K. Yoshiie *et al.* 1999. Live *Bartonella henselae* enhances endothelial cell proliferation without direct contact. Microb. Pathog. **27:** 419–427.
5. Kirby, J.E. & D.M. Nekorchuk. 2002. *Bartonella*-associated endothelial proliferation depends on inhibition of apoptosis. Proc. Natl. Acad. Sci. USA **99:** 4656–4661.
6. Sreedhar, A.S. & P. Csermely. 2004. Heat shock proteins in the regulation of apoptosis: new strategies in tumor therapy—a comprehensive review. Pharmacol. Ther. **101:** 227–257.
7. Fuhrmann, O., M. Arvand, A. Göhler *et al.* 2001. *Bartonella henselae* induces NF-κB-dependent upregulation of adhesion molecules in cultured human endothelial cells: possible role of outer membrane proteins as pathogenic factors. Infect. Immun. **69:** 5088–5097.
8. Kempf, V.A., B. Volkmann, M. Schaller *et al.* 2001. Evidence of a leading role for VEGF in *Bartonella henselae*–induced endothelial cell proliferations. Cell. Microbiol. **3:** 623–632.
9. Resto-Ruiz, S.I., M. Schmiederer, D. Sweger *et al.* 2002. Induction of a potential paracrine angiogenic loop between human THP-1 macrophages and human microvascular endothelial cells during *Bartonella henselae* infection. Infect. Immun. **70:** 4564–4570.
10. Minnick, M.F., L.S. Smitherman & D.S. Samuels. 2003. Mitogenic effect of *Bartonella bacilliformis* on human vascular endothelial cells and involvement of GroEL. Infect. Immun. **71:** 6933–6942.
11. Zügel, U. & S.H. Kaufmann. 1999. Role of heat shock proteins in protection from and pathogenesis of infectious diseases. Clin. Microbiol. Rev. **12:** 19–39.
12. Sasu, S., D. LaVerda, N. Qureshi *et al.* 2001. *Chlamydia pneumoniae* and chlamydial heat shock protein 60 stimulate proliferation of human vascular smooth muscle cells via toll-like receptor 4 and p44/p42 mitogen–activated protein kinase activation. Circ. Res. **89:** 244–250.
13. Goulhen, F., A. Hafezi, V.J. Uitto *et al.* 1998. Subcellular localization and cytotoxic activity of the GroEL-like protein isolated from *Actinobacillus actinomycetemcomitans*. Infect. Immun. **66:** 5307–5313.
14. Zhang, L., S.L. Pelech, D. Mayrand *et al.* 2001. Bacterial heat shock protein-60 increases epithelial cell proliferation through the ERK1/2 MAP kinases. Exp. Cell Res. **266:** 11–20.
15. Zhang, L., S. Pelech & V-J. Uitto. 2004. Long-term effect of heat shock protein 60 from *Actinobacillus actinomycetemcomitans* on epithelial cell viability and mitogen-activated protein kinases. Infect. Immun. **72:** 38–45.

16. CONNOLLY, D.T., M.B. KNIGHT, N.K. HARAKAS *et al.* 1986. Determination of the number of endothelial cells in culture using an acid phosphatase assay. Anal. Biochem. **152:** 136–140.
17. AUSUBEL, F.M., R. BRENT, R.E. KINGSTON *et al.* 1995. Current Protocols in Molecular Biology. Wiley. New York.
18. TOWBIN, H., T. STAEHELIN & J. GORDON. 1979. Electrophoretic transfer of proteins from polyacrylamide gels to nitrocellulose sheets: procedure and some applications. Proc. Natl. Acad. Sci. USA **76:** 4350–4354.
19. CARROLL, J.A., S.A. COLEMAN, L.S. SMITHERMAN & M.F. MINNICK. 2000. Hemin-binding surface protein from *Bartonella quintana*. Infect. Immun. **68:** 6750–6757.
20. BATTISTI, J.M. & M.F. MINNICK. 1999. Development of a system for genetic manipulation of *Bartonella bacilliformis*. Appl. Environ. Microbiol. **65:** 3441–3448.
21. GARCIA, F.U., J. WOJTA & R.L. HOOVER. 1992. Interactions between live *Bartonella bacilliformis* and endothelial cells. J. Infect. Dis. **165:** 1138–1141.
22. VERMA, A., G.E. DAVIS & G.M. IHLER. 2001. Formation of stress fibres in human endothelial cells infected with *Bartonella bacilliformis* is associated with altered morphology, impaired migration and defects in cell morphogenesis. Cell. Microbiol. **3:** 169–180.
23. SCHMID, M.C., R. SCHULEIN, M. DEHIO *et al.* 2004. The VirB type IV secretion system of *Bartonella henselae* mediates invasion, proinflammatory activation and antiapoptotic protection of endothelial cells. Mol. Microbiol. **52:** 81–92.
24. WATARAI, M., S. KIM, J. ERDENEBAATAR *et al.* 2003. Cellular prion protein promotes *Brucella* infection into macrophages. J. Exp. Med. **198:** 5–17.
25. SAMALI, A., J. CAI, B. ZHIVOTOVSKY *et al.* 1999. Presence of a pre-apoptotic complex of pro-caspase-3, Hsp60, and Hsp10 in the mitochondrial fraction of Jurkat cells. EMBO J. **18:** 2040–2048.
26. XANTHOUDAKIS, S., S. ROY, D. RASPER *et al.* 1999. Hsp60 accelerates the maturation of pro-caspase-3 by upstream activator proteases during apoptosis. EMBO J. **18:** 2049–2056.
27. BRENNER, D.J., S.P. O'CONNOR, D.G. HOLLIS *et al.* 1991. Molecular characterization and proposal of a neotype strain for *Bartonella bacilliformis*. J. Clin. Microbiol. **29:** 1299–1302.
28. KOVACH, M.E., P.H. ELZER, D.S. HILL *et al.* 1995. Four new derivatives of the broad-host-range vector pBBR1MCS, carrying different antibiotic-resistance cassettes. Gene **166:** 175–176.

Occurrence of *Bartonella henselae* and *Bartonella quintana* among Human Immunodeficiency Virus–Infected Patients

M. PAPE,[a] P. KOLLARAS,[b] K. MANDRAVELI,[a] A. TSONA,[b] S. METALLIDIS,[b] P. NIKOLAIDIS,[b] AND S. ALEXIOU-DANIEL[a]

[a]*Department of Microbiology, School of Medicine, Laboratory of Infectious Diseases, AHEPA University Hospital of Thessaloniki, Thessaloniki, Greece*

[b]*First Internal Medicine Department, Infectious Diseases Division, AHEPA University Hospital of Thessaloniki, Thessaloniki, Greece*

ABSTRACT: The purpose of this study was to determine the seroprevalence against *Bartonella henselae* and *Bartonella quintana* among a risk group, patients with HIV infection, and to identify the epidemiological factors involved. Our data indicate that the prevalence of Bartonella infection among HIV-infected patients is much greater than that in the healthy population of the same area and that Bartonella infection should be considered in the differential diagnosis for patients with HIV disease.

KEYWORDS: *Bartonella henselae*; *Bartonella quintana*; HIV; infection

INTRODUCTION

Bartonella infection can be difficult to diagnose, especially when it presents with nonspecific symptoms, such as fever. Since immunocompetent patients are a potential risk group of infection by this bacteria, the purpose of this study was to determine the seroprevalence against *Bartonella henselae* and *Bartonella quintana* among a risk group, patients with HIV infection, and to identify the epidemiological factors involved.[1]

MATERIALS AND METHODS

Samples

Between October 2004 and April 2005, serum samples from 253 HIV patients from northern Greece were collected. The epidemiologic study included sex, age, contact with cats, lymphadenopathy, antiretroviral treatment, and chemoprophylaxis

Address for correspondence: Magda Pape, Department of Microbiology, AHEPA University Hospital, St. Kyriakidi 1, Thessaloniki 54006, Greece. Voice: +3-23-1099-4619; fax: +3-23-1099-4621.

koumedse@med.auth.gr

Ann. N.Y. Acad. Sci. 1063: 299–301 (2005). © 2005 New York Academy of Sciences.
doi: 10.1196/annals.1355.047

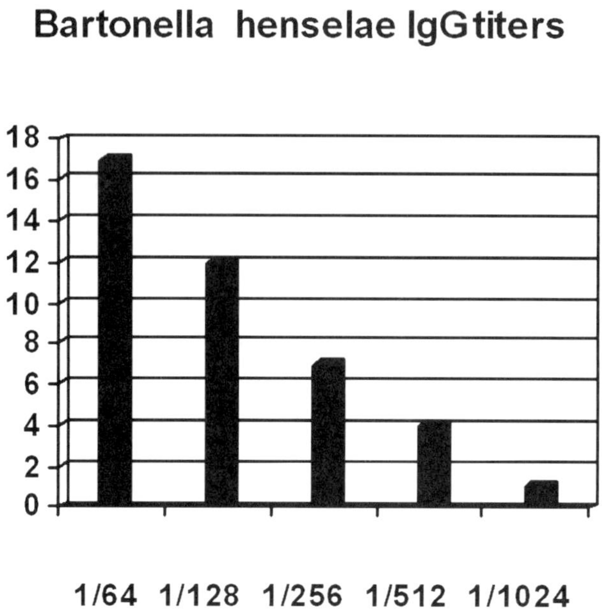

FIGURE 1. *B. henselae* IgG titers.

versus symptoms such as fever. All sera were examined using both the *B. henselae* and *B. quintana* IgG/IgM indirect immunofluorescent antibody (IFA) method (Focus, kit). The serum samples were initially diluted 1/64 and 1/20 for the detection of IgG and IgM antibodies, respectively. Titers of 1/20 for IgM and 1/64 for IgG were considered positive.

RESULTS

Of the 253 patients, 186 were men and 67 were women (mean age: 45 ± 5 years). Of these, 103 (41%) were seropositive for *B. henselae* IgG antibodies. Titers of 1/64, 1/128, 1/256, 1/512, and 1/1024 for IgG antibodies to *B. henselae* were found in 17%, 12%, 7%, 4%, and 1% of the subjects examined, respectively (FIG. 1). Fifteen (6%) subjects had IgG antibodies to both Bartonella species at a titer of 1/64. As shown in previously published data,[2] the seropositivity in the healthy population in northern Greece was statistically significantly lower at the respective levels of IgG.

Only 2 patients had IgM antibodies at a titer of 1/20 and 1/40. The IgG titers to these patients were 1/512 and 1/1024, respectively. The last one had persistent fever (temperature: 39°C) of 1-week duration without an identifiable source. During his physical examination, lymphadenopathy was observed, but no cat scratch or bite was reported.

Among the 253 patients, 4 were under chemoprophylaxis with Zithromax and none reported animal or insect exposure before the serologic tests for Bartonella species were performed. No symptoms or signs (e.g., chills, sweats, headache, weight loss, nausea, diarrhea, lymphadenopathy) were present during the study period. All patients received antiretroviral therapy (HAART).

DISCUSSION

Bartonella infections are substantially underrecognized because of the nonspecific symptomatology. Undiagnosed Bartonella infections can persist for months in immunocompromised patients and can cause chronic opportunistic infection. Our data indicate that the prevalence of Bartonella infection among HIV-infected patients is much greater than that in the healthy population of the same area and that Bartonella infection should be considered in the differential diagnosis for patients with HIV disease.[3]

REFERENCES

1. KOEHLER, J.E., M.A. SANCHEZ, S. TYE *et al.* 2003. Prevalance of Bartonella infection among human immunodeficiency virus–infected patients with fever. Clin. Infect. Dis. **37:** 559–566.
2. TEA, A., S. ALEXIOU-DANIEL, M. ARVANITIDOU *et al.* 2003. Occurrence of *Bartonella henselae* and *Bartonella quintana* in a healthy Greek population. Am. J. Trop. Med. Hyg. **68:** 554–556.
3. JACKSON, L.A., B.A. PERKINS & J.D. WENGER. 1993. Cat scratch disease in the United States: an analysis of three national databases. Am. J. Public Health **83:** 1707–1711.

Bacillary Angiomatosis Caused by *Bartonella quintana*

MONTSERRAT SALA,[a] BERNAT FONT,[a] ISABEL SANFELIU,[b] MARIELA QUESADA,[b] IMMA PONTS,[b] AND FERRAN SEGURA[a]

[a]*Infectious Diseases Program, Internal Medicine Department,*
[b]*Microbiology Laboratory, UDIAT Centre Diagnòstic, Corporació Parc Taulí, Sabadell, Barcelona, Spain*

ABSTRACT: Bacillary angiomatosis is a disorder of neovascular proliferation involving skin and lymph nodes of immunosuppressed patients. *Bartonella henselae* or *Bartonella quintana* have been inculpated as causative by direct culture or PCR amplification of DNA sequences. Here, we report the clinical evolution of a patient infected with human immunodeficiency virus (HIV) whose *B. quintana* infection was diagnosed by PCR .

KEYWORDS: bacillary angiomatosis; HIV; *Bartonella quintana*; PCR; case

An HIV-infected patient was admitted in the hospital because of fever, chills, diarrhea, and painful subcutaneous nodules in both legs, arms, and neck. Some of them were red to purple and some ulcerated (FIGS. 1 and 2). CD4 cell count was 15 cells/mm^3, and HIV RNA was >750,000 copies/mL. The biopsy of a lesion showed neovascular proliferation and foci of acute and chronic inflammation. There was vasculitis in small- and medium-sized vessels. New nodules appeared in the neck and shoulders and a new biopsy was performed. The histopathologic examination showed the characteristic changes of bacillary angiomatosis (BA), including lobular proliferation of small capillary–sized blood vessels lined with enlarged endothelial cells and mixed inflammatory infiltrate of lymphocytes and neutrophils (FIG. 3). Warthin-Starry silver staining showed numerous darkly staining organisms scattered throughout the connective tissue (FIG. 4). The culture of this biopsy was negative for *Bartonella* spp. Blood cultures were also negative. The anti-*Bartonella* IgG antibodies were positive (titer: 1/512).

For the diagnosis, we amplificated a *Bartonella*-specific sequence of the citrate synthase gene (*glt*A) by polymerase chain reaction (PCR). First, DNA was extracted from biopsy by using a QIAamp® DNA Mini Kit (QIAGEN GmbH, Germany) as recommended by the manufacturer. The oligonucleotide primers (Invitrogen™ Life Technologies) used in this PCR assay generated an amplicon of 379 bp.[1] Conditions were described previously with minor modifications.[2] A standard PCR mixture was

Address for correspondence: Montserrat Sala, Infectious Diseases Program, Internal Medicine Department, Corporació Parc Taulí, Parc Taulí s/n, E-08208 Sabadell, Barcelona, Spain. Voice: +34-93-7231010; fax: +34-93-7160646.
msala@cspt.es

**Ann. N.Y. Acad. Sci. 1063: 302–307 (2005). © 2005 New York Academy of Sciences.
doi: 10.1196/annals.1355.048**

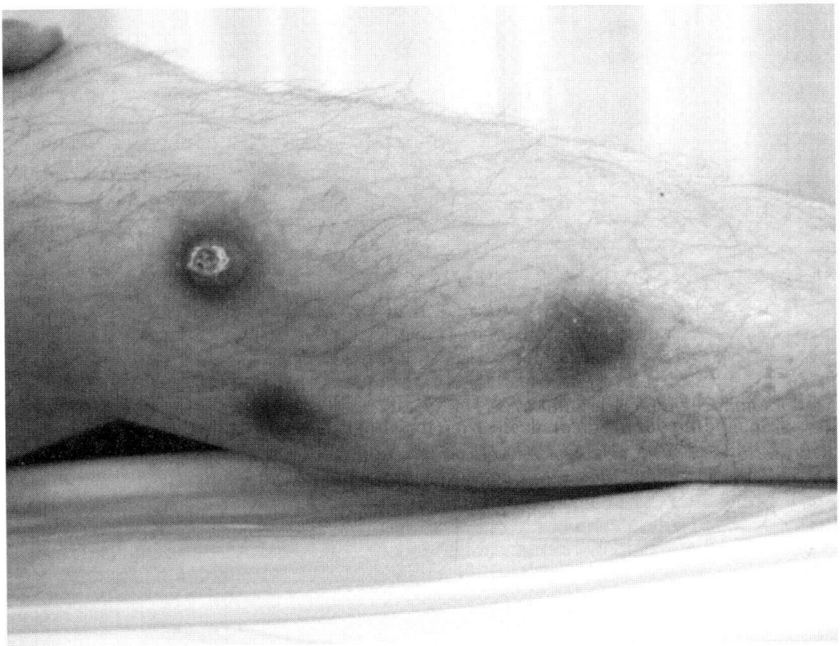

FIGURE 1. Painful subcutaneous nodules in an HIV-infected patient. Some of them were red to purple and some ulcerated.

in a final volume of 50 μL containing 0.5 μL of the appropriate DNA template, 0.5 U of Taq DNA polymerase, 5 μL of buffer (10×), 200 μM (each) deoxynucleoside triphosphate, 25 μM $MgCl_2$, and 50 pmol of each primer. As positive control, DNA of *B. henselae* H1 ATCC 49882 and *B. clarridgeiae* ATCC 51734 were used. As negative control, we used water, *Escherichia coli*, *Pseudomonas aeruginosa*, and *Staphylococcus aureus* DNA, and DNA from blood of three different newborns. PCR amplifications were carried out in a GeneAmp PCR System 9700 (PE Applied Biosystems) thermocycler, for 35 cycles with the following cycle parameters: 95°C for 20 s, 51°C for 30 s, and 72°C for 2 min. To verify the presence of amplicons of appropriate size, PCR products were electrophoresed in 1.8% agarose gels according to standard methods, and the ethidium bromide–stained amplicon bands were then visualized by using a UV transilluminator and photographed. To identify the species of *Bartonella* implicated, we amplificated the intergenic spacer region (ITS) between the 16 and the 23S rRNA genes with complementary primers, *B. henselae* [nt] 302 to 321 and *B. henselae* [nt] 473 to 454 (Invitrogen™ Life Technologies), as forward and reverse primers, respectively, as previously described by Jensen *et al.*[3] The positivity of the amplification was confirmed by electrophoresis in 1.8% and 3% agarose gels. The sizes of the ITS PCR amplification products were determined by comparison with the standard molecular weight marker VIII (Boehringer Mannheim,

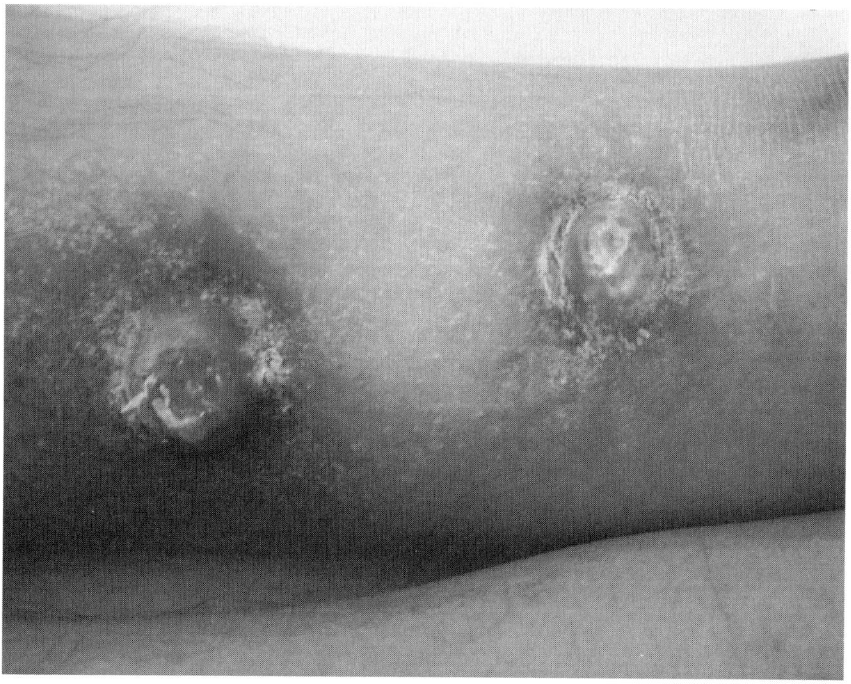

FIGURE 2. Painful subcutaneous nodules in an HIV-infected patient. Some of them were red to purple and some ulcerated.

CombA, Mannheim, Germany). PCR products were purified by using QIAquick PCR purification kit (QIAGEN) as proposed by the manufacturer and were sequenced with an automated sequencer ABI 3100 Genetic Analyzer. Their sequences were compared with the corresponding sequences for *Bartonella* species available in the DNA analysis computer program, NCBI Blast.

COMMENTS

BA is caused by *B. henselae* or *B. quintana.* Most *Bartonella* spp. are infectious agents of nonhuman mammals. Humans may be incidental hosts in most cases; in fact, animal host for *B. quintana* is not yet identified. The human body louse is its only proposed vector, although the intimacy of the relationship between bacterium and arthropod is not known.[4] Formerly named *Rickettsia quintana*, it was the etiologic agent of trench fever during World War I. Interest in it reemerged in 1983 when Stoler *et al.*[5] described the association between *R. quintana* and HIV infection. The disease was termed BA. In 1990, Perkocha *et al.*[6] described a new AIDS-related syndrome in hepatic parenchyma termed peliosis hepatis (PH), also related with

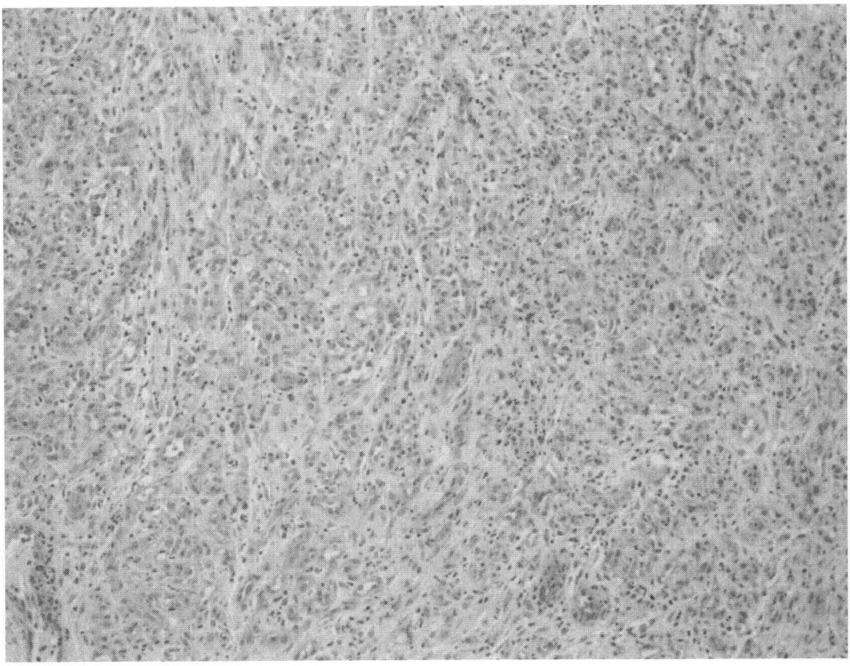

FIGURE 3. Histopathologic examination showed the characteristic changes of bacillary angiomatosis, including lobular proliferation of small capillary–sized blood vessels lined with enlarged endothelial cells and mixed inflammatory infiltrate of lymphocytes and neutrophil.

R. quintana. In 1990, Relman *et al.*[7] partially characterized the observed bacillus by PCR, and the rickettsia was cultured from skin lesions of BA patients by Koehler *et al.* in 1992.[8] *R. quintana* has been taxonomically reclassificated and is now named *Bartonella quintana*. *B. quintana* has been related with BA, PH, endocarditis, and bacteremia in homeless and chronic lymphadenopathy.[9] This infection occurs mainly in immunosuppressed patients as HIV-infected.[10] As a vascular proliferative disease, it produces lesions that are solitary or multiple, and superficial or subcutaneous. Superficial may be red, purple, or uncolored; deep are usually nodular and uncolored and either mobile or fixed. Mucosa and several organs can be involved: liver, spleen, bone marrow, lymph nodes, and cardiac valves. The diagnosis of BA is based on histopathology. Hematoxylin-eosin staining shows vascular neoproliferation and neutrophilic infiltration. Warthin-Starry silver staining is specific for detection of the bacillus seen as small dark organisms in the connective tissue. Routine blood culture methods would not allow the detection of slowly growing *Bartonella* species. The use of enriched media, prolonged incubation times, and cell lysis centrifugation are recommended. Serologic tests may not reliably distinguish between *B. quintana* and *B. henselae* antibody responses. Moreover, cross-reactivity between *Bartonella* and other organisms, including *Chlamydia*, exists.

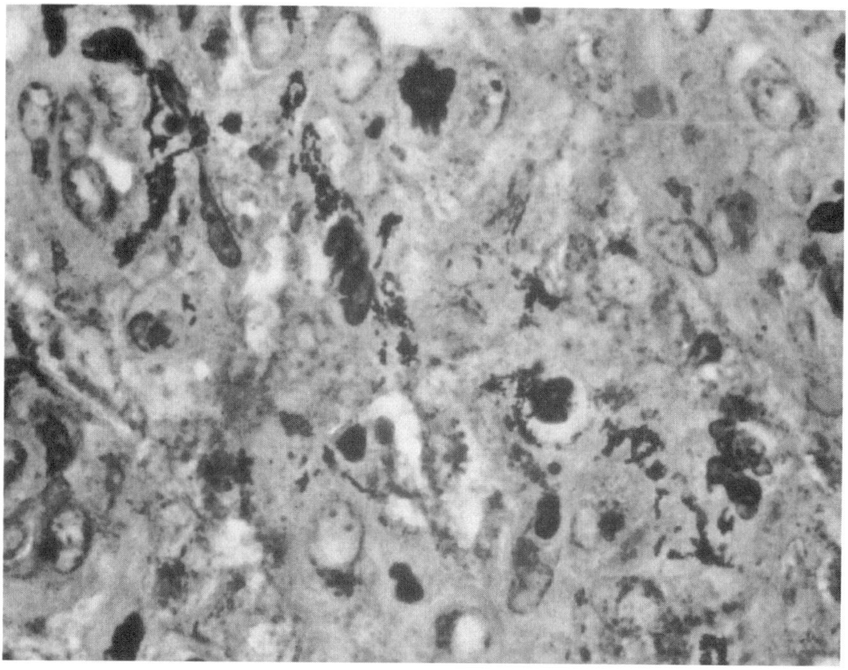

FIGURE 4. Warthin-Starry silver staining showed numerous darkly staining organisms scattered throughout the connective tissue.

PCR is the most sensitive of the existing rapid methods to detect microbial pathogens in clinical specimens. When pathogens difficult to culture *in vitro* or requiring a long cultivation period are expected to be present in specimens, the diagnostic value of PCR is known to be significant. Due to the fastidious nature of *Bartonella* species and their high degrees of antibiotic susceptibility, cultures of clinical samples most often remain sterile. We report here on the amplification and sequencing of *B. quintana* DNA from the biopsy of a patient with infective BA, which strongly implicates this bacterium as the causative agent of this disease, as has been repeatedly demonstrated in other cases. The results of the PCR assays demonstrated rapid and specific methods of detecting the organism in clinical samples.

All HIV-infected patients with *Bartonella* infection should be treated with antibiotics. Erythromycin, doxycyclin, rifampin, and gentamicin may have clinical efficacy. In patients with endocarditis, bacteremia, or PH, they should be administered intravenously. Patients should receive a minimum of four months of treatment. Patients should also be followed closely for relapse in the same or different organ. Some patients may require lifelong suppressive therapy. Our patient received three months of therapy and now is treated only with HAART. His immunological situation has improved and no new lesions of BA have appeared.

REFERENCES

1. NORMAN, A.F., R. REGNERY, P. JAMESON *et al.* 1995. Differentiation of *Bartonella*-like isolates at the species level by PCR–restriction fragment length polymorphism in the citrate synthase gene. J. Clin. Microbiol. **33:** 1797–1803.
2. AVIDOR, B., Y. KLETTER, S. ABULAFIA *et al.* 1997. Molecular diagnosis of cat scratch disease: a two-step approach. J. Clin. Microbiol. **35:** 1924–1930.
3. JENSEN, W.A., M.Z. FALL, J. ROONEY *et al.* 2000. Rapid identification and differentiation of *Bartonella* species using a single-step PCR assay. J. Clin. Microbiol. **38:** 1717–1722.
4. MAURIN, M. & D. RAOULT. 1996. *Bartonella* (*Rochalimaea*) *quintana* infections. Clin. Microbiol. Rev. **9:** 273–292.
5. STOLER, M.H., T.A. BONFIGLIO, R.T. STEIGBIGEL & M. PEREIRA. 1983. An atypical subcutaneous infection associated with acquired immunodeficiency syndrome. Am. J. Clin. Pathol. **80:** 714–718.
6. PERKOCHA, L.A., S.M. GEAGHAN, T.S. YEN *et al.* 1990. Clinical and pathological features of bacillary peliosis hepatis in association with human immunodeficiency virus infection. N. Engl. J. Med. **323:** 1581–1586.
7. RELMAN, D.A., J.S. LOUTIT, T.M. SCHMIDT *et al.* 1990. The agent of bacillary angiomatosis: an approach to the identification of uncultured pathogens. N. Engl. J. Med. **323:** 1573–1580.
8. KOEHLER, J.E., F.D. QUINN, T.G. BERGER *et al.* 1992. Isolation of *Rochalimaea* species from cutaneous and osseous lesions of bacillary angiomatosis. N. Engl. J. Med. **327:** 1625–1631
9. BROUQUI, P., B. LASCOLA, V. ROUX & D. RAOULT. 1999. Chronic *Bartonella quintana* bacteremia in homeless patients. N. Engl. J. Med. **340:** 184–189.
10. KOEHLER, J.E. 1995. *Bartonella*-associated infections in HIV-infected patients. AIDS Clin. Care **7:** 97–102.

Molecular Screening of *Bartonella* Species in Rodents from the Russian Far East

OLEG MEDIANNIKOV,[a,b,c] LEONID IVANOV,[d] NINA ZDANOVSKAYA,[d] NELYA VYSOCHINA,[d] PIERRE-EDOUARD FOURNIER,[c] IRINA TARASEVICH,[a] AND DIDIER RAOULT[a]

[a]*Laboratory of Rickettsial Ecology, Gamaleya Research Institute of Epidemiology and Microbiology, Moscow 123098, Russia*

[b]*Department of the Infectious Diseases, Far Eastern State Medical University, Khabarovsk 680000, Russia*

[c]*Unité des Rickettsies, Faculté de Médecine, CNRS UMR 6020 27, Université de la Méditerranée, 13385 Marseille, Cedex 05, France*

[d]*Khabarovsk Plague Control Station, Ministry of Health of the Russian Federation, Khabarovsk 680000, Russia*

Abstract: A potentially broad-range PCR system for *gltA* gene amplification has been designed. A nearly full (992 bp) sequence of the *gltA* gene was amplified in two steps. DNA was extracted from organs (spleen and liver) of four mostly spread species of rodents: *Apodemus agrarius* and *Apodemus peninsulae* mice; *Clethrionomys rufocanus* and *Microtus fortis* voles. All amplicons have been sequenced. The incidence of *Bartonella* species in rodents was 73%, 60%, 60%, and 83% for the above-mentioned rodents, respectively. Several genotypes have been identified, including two *gltA* genotypes close to *B. taylorii*, four *gltA* genotypes close to *B. grahamii*, and one genotype of a potentially new species. Several *Bartonella* species were found in both mice species, although each vole species harbored a single species of *Bartonella*. High incidence of *Bartonella* infection was found in all studied species of small rodents in the Russian Far East. Several amplified genotypes probably belong to local strains of *B. taylorii* and *B. grahamii*, and one genotype represents a possible new species.

Keywords: *Bartonella*; rodents; Russia; Far East

INTRODUCTION

The Russian Far East is a traditional term to name the ultimate eastern region of Russia, close to the Pacific coast. Multiple zoonoses were found in this region; nevertheless, no rodent-associated bartonellae have been described. *Bartonella* microorganisms, including *B. grahamii*[1] associated with rodents, were recently considered as possible human pathogens. Their role in human pathology is yet to be clarified,

Address for correspondence: Oleg Y. Mediannikov, Laboratory of Rickettsial Ecology, Gamaleya Institute of Epidemiology and Microbiology, ul. Gamalei 18, Moscow 123098, Russia. Voice: +7-095-193-43-10; fax: +7-095-193-61-85.
oleguss1@mail.ru; Pierre-Edouard.Fournier@medecine.univ-mrs.fr

Ann. N.Y. Acad. Sci. 1063: 308–311 (2005). © 2005 New York Academy of Sciences.
doi: 10.1196/annals.1355.049

TABLE 1. List of primers used in this study

Primer	Sequence
CS140f	TTACTTATGATCCKGGYTTTA
BhCS679f	CATGCAGATCAYGAACAAAATGC
BhCS763r	GCAGGTGTTGCITGYCTTTGGG
BhCS1133r	GAAATGTTTACTGTTCTTTTTGC

but several species are able to induce a disease in humans. In southern China,[2] a PCR-based screening study revealed a high prevalence of *Bartonella* species among small rodents. Our objectives were to describe the prevalence and genetic diversity of the *Bartonella* community found in rodents in the Khabarovsk region in the Russian Far East and to define the ecologic associations of the different *Bartonella* strains with rodent hosts.

MATERIALS AND METHODS

Fifty-one small rodents belonging to four species were captured during the late spring and summer of 2002 near Khabarovsk city. They were two species of mice (15 *Apodemus agrarius* and 15 *Apodemus peninsulae*) and two species of voles (15 *Clethrionomys rufocanus* and 6 *Microtus fortis*). These species represent the mostly common rodents in the south of the Russian Far East and were identified as reservoirs of many zoonoses, including tick-borne encephalitis, yersinioses, hemorrhagic fever with renal syndrome, leptospirosis, etc. Captured animals were anesthetized and processed according to procedures used by the Khabarovsk Plague Control Station during routine surveillance activities. DNA from the tissue samples (spleen and liver) were immediately extracted using standard Qiagen kits for DNA extraction. A potentially broad-range PCR system for *gltA* gene amplification has been designed. A nearly full (992 bp) sequence of the *gltA* gene has been amplified in two steps. In the first step, we amplified DNA with primers Cs140f[3] and BhCS1133r (TABLE 1), using annealing temperature of 46°C. The second step included amplification in the nested PCR using the products of the first step as templates for the second one at annealing temperature of 48°C. The following primer combinations were used: Cs140f + BhCS763r and BhCS679f + BhCS1133r. Finally, two amplified portions of the *gltA* gene from each positive sample were sequenced and compiled together using GENETYX-WIN software. The obtained nearly full gene sequences (992 bp) were then submitted to GenBank for assignment accession numbers (TABLE 2).

RESULTS

The prevalences of the *Bartonella* species in rodents were identified as 73%, 60%, 60%, and 83% for *A. agrarius*, *A. peninsulae*, *C. rufocanus*, and *M. fortis,* accordingly. It was found that both species of voles harbored only one (probably specific) species of *Bartonella.* It is one of two species (type I) close to *B. taylorii.* The same species also was identified in 26.7% of *A. peninsulae* mice. On the other

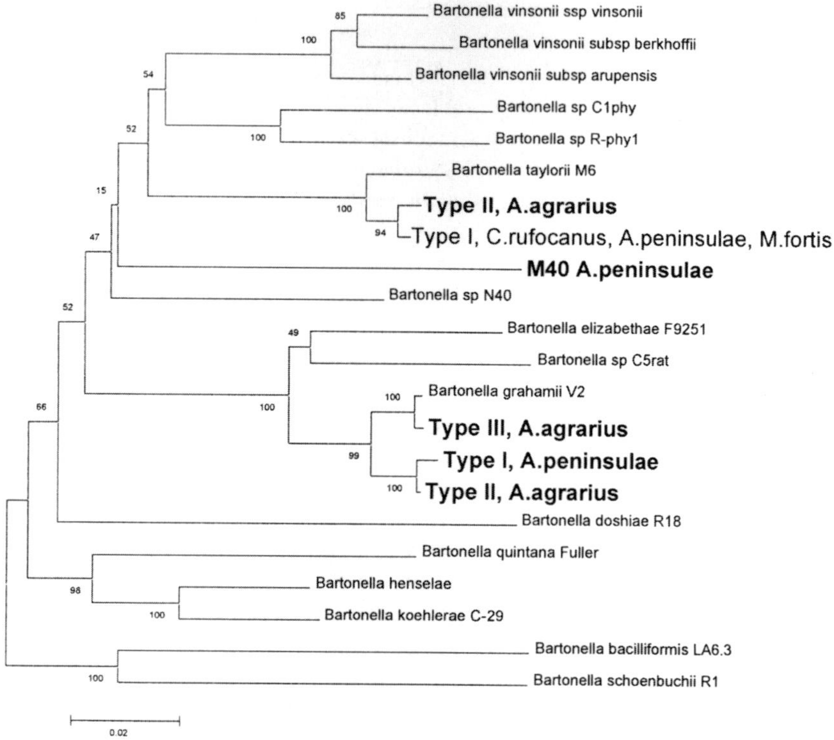

FIGURE 1. Phylogenetic tree made by MEGA 2.1 software after alignment (GENETYX-WIN 5.1) of *gltA* gene sequences obtained from GenBank and sequenced during this study. The numbers at the nodes represent the number of bootstrap replicates of 100.

TABLE 2. Genetic variants of *Bartonella* species, their host, and nucleotide accession numbers of sequences

Accession no.	Species	Type	Source
AY584859	*Bartonella* spp.	M40	*A. peninsulae, A. agrarius*
AY584854	*B. grahamii*	I	*A. peninsulae, A. agrarius*
AY584855	*B. grahamii*	II	*A. agrarius*
AY584856	*B. grahamii*	III	*A. agrarius*
AY584857	*B. grahamii*	IV	*A. agrarius*
AY584852	*B. taylorii*	I	*C. rufocanus, M. fortis, A. peninsulae*
AY584853	*B. taylorii*	II	*A. agrarius*

hand, both mice species harbored several species of *Bartonella*. *A. peninsulae* was found to be the host of three different bartonellae: one close to *B. grahamii*, one close to *B. taylorii*, and one species that significantly differs from the others. This specimen was encoded as M40. Its position on a phylogenetic tree (FIG. 1) shows that it is clustered with other rodent-associated species of *Bartonella*, but forms an independent, well-isolated clade. The common field mouse, *A. agrarius*, was found to host six different *Bartonellae*: three variants of *B. grahamii*; one variant of *B. taylorii* (type II, slightly different from the one found in voles); and possibly a new *Bartonella* species, which also was amplified in *A. peninsulae*.

CONCLUSIONS

High incidence of *Bartonella* infection was found in all studied species of small rodents in the Russian Far East. Several amplified genotypes probably belong to local strains of *B. taylorii* and *B. grahamii*, and one genotype represents a possible new species. The presence of *B. grahamii* in rodents necessitates a survey study for human bartonellosis associated with this species. The field mouse is widely spread in the Northern Hemisphere and a variety of *Bartonellae*, including multiple strains of the same species, suggest probably the beginning of evolutionary splitting of this species into several clades.

[*Competing interests statement:* The authors have reported that they have no conflicting financial interests.]

REFERENCES

1. KERKHOFF, F.T., A.M. BERGMANS, A. VAN DER ZEE & A. ROTHOVA. 1999. Demonstration of *Bartonella grahamii* DNA in ocular fluids of a patient with neuroretinitis. J. Clin. Microbiol. **37:** 4034–4038.
2. YING, B., M.Y. KOSOY, G.O. MAUPIN *et al.* 2002. Genetic and ecologic characteristics of *Bartonella* communities in rodents in southern China. Am. J. Trop. Med. Hyg. **66:** 622–627.
3. BIRTLES, R.J. & D. RAOULT. 1996. Comparison of partial citrate synthase gene (*gltA*) sequences for phylogenetic analysis of *Bartonella* species. Int. J. Syst. Bacteriol. **46:** 891–897.

Characterization of Genes Involved in Long-Term Bacteremia in Mice by *Bartonella birtlesii*

MARIA MAVRIS,[a] HENRI SAENZ,[b] MARTINE MONTEIL,[a]
HENRI-JEAN BOULOUIS,[a] CHRISTOPH DEHIO,[b] AND
MURIEL VAYSSIER-TAUSSAT[a]

[a]*UMR 956 BIPAR, Ecole Nationale Vétérinaire d'Alfort, Maisons-Alfort, France*

[b]*Division of Molecular Microbiology, Biozentrum, University of Basel, Switzerland*

KEYWORDS: signature-tagged; mutagenesis; erythrocytes infection; virulence factors

Members of the genus *Bartonella* are considered to be agents of emerging infectious diseases. They are gram-negative, arthropod-borne intracellular pathogens and are characterized by their tropism for erythrocytes.[1] Each species of *Bartonella* is adapted to one reservoir host in which infection is accompanied by a long-term bacteremia. If a member of the Bartonella sp. accidentally infects a non reservoir host, the infection can be associated with diverse pathologies. Therefore, these bacteria are considered agents of emerging infectious diseases.

The aim of our work was to characterize the molecular mechanisms of invasion of *Bartonella* in red blood cells of the reservoir host. To this end, we used *Bartonella birtlesii* for which our laboratory had already established an animal model.[2] Infection of Balb/C mice resulted in a persistent bacteremia, detectable at day 5 and lasting up to 5 to 8 weeks.

A library of mutants was constructed in *B. birtlesii* using the signature-tagged transposon mutagenesis (STM) technique (H. Saenz, manuscript in preparation). The STM technique involves constructing individual unique tags and introducing them into a plasmid containing a transposon carrying an antibiotic resistance.[3] The individual tagged plasmids are then introduced into *E. coli* and then conjugated into *B. birtlesii*. Selection of the mutants is based on a resistance to the antibiotic carried by the transposon and sensitivity to the antibiotic carried by the plasmid. For our purposes, we used 36 independent tags and isolated 96 mutants for each tag, resulting in a total of 3456 mutants. This represents more than one insertion per open reading frame if we assume a genome size of 2.2 Mb for *B. birtlesii*.

An initial screening, using 10% of the total mutant library (320 mutants), was performed by infecting Balb/C mice in duplicate. Blood samples were taken at days 7, 10, and 14 post-infection and assessed for presence of bacteria possessing individual tags. Input and output pools were analyzed by PCR amplification of individual

Address for correspondence: M. Vayssier-Taussat, Ph.D, UMR 956 BIPAR, 7 avenue du General de Gaulle, Ecole Nationale Vétérinaire d'Alfort, Maisons-Alfort, France. Voice: 33 1 4396 715; Fax: 33 1 4396 7332.
mvayssier@vet-alfort.fr

**Ann. N.Y. Acad. Sci. 1063: 312–314 (2005). © 2005 New York Academy of Sciences.
doi: 10.1196/annals.1355.050**

tags using specific oligonucleotide primers. We selected mutants unable to persist in the blood of mice, and therefore absent at all three days tested post-infection. Among the 320 mutants tested, 3 were present at days 10 and 14 but not at day 7. These mutants are likely delayed, i.e. colonize blood but with a slower growth rate. Six mutants were present at day 7 but not at day 10 and 14 and likely represent mutants with ability to invade blood but not to persist. Ten mutants were absent at all 3 days tested post-infection. These non-bacteremic mutants, representing 4% of the screened library, are the mutants of interest affected in persistence in the blood or at some earlier phase of infection.

The site of insertion of the transposon was mapped in each of the mutants. We identified insertions in genes of the Trw type IV secretion system (T4SS) known to be responsible for invasion of red blood cells.[4,5] We also identified mutations in amino acid transporter genes and other housekeeping genes. Additional insertions were identified in genes encoding adhesion proteins, proteins belonging to ABC transporters, outer membrane proteins and hypothetical proteins of unknown function. Insertions in known virulence and housekeeping genes have validated the functioning of this mutagenesis system in *B. birtlesii.* The insertions in genes of unknown function and those in genes of potential outer membrane proteins are of particular interest for further characterization.

In order to identify whether these genes may be implicated in attachment or invasion to erythrocytes, the mutants were further characterized for their ability to invade blood cells. For this purpose, an *in vitro* model has been recently established in our laboratory to examine the ability of the mutants to enter red blood cells. Briefly, mouse erythrocytes were incubated with wild type *B. birtlesii* at a multiplicity of infection varying from 0.01 to 6. *In vitro* infection of erythrocytes was observed by confocal microscopy and intracellular bacteria were quantified on the basis of protection from gentamicin (TABLE 1). We observed intracellular bacteria after 24 h of infection. At that time, 4% of erythrocytes were infected, and at 48 h and 72 h, 30% of erythrocytes were infected. Interestingly and for unknown reasons, we observed that erythrocytes incubated with *B. birtlesii* were clustered suggesting that *B. birtlesii* wild type carries molecules susceptible to linkage with erythrocytes receptor.

This *in vitro* model of murine erythrocytes invasion by *Bartonella* will be now used to study the non-bacteremic mutants that have lost the ability either to adhere or to invade or to multiply within erythrocytes. The remainder of the mutant bank could be easily screened resulting in the potential identification of other factors involved in the entry and persistence processes and will also enable us to ask other questions regarding this uncharacterized intracellular bacterium.

REFERENCES

1. SEUBERT, A., R. SCHULEIN & C. DEHIO. 2002. Bacterial persistence within erythrocytes: a unique pathogenic strategy of Bartonella spp. Int. J. Med. Microbiol. **291:** 555–560.
2. BOULOUIS, H.J., F. BARRAT, D. BERMOND, *et al.* 2002. Kinetics of *Bartonella birtlesii* infection in experimentally infected mice and pathogenic effect on reproductive functions. Infect. Immun. **69:** 5313–5317.
3. HENSEL, *et al.* 1995.

4. SCHULEIN, R. & C. DEHIO. 2002. VirB/VirD4 type IV secretion system of Bartonella is essential for establishing intraerythrocytic infection. Mol. Microbiol. **46:** 1053–1067.
5. SEUBERT, A., R. HIESTAND, F. DE LA CRUZ & C. DEHIO. 2003. A bacterial conjugation machinery recruited for pathogenesis. Mol. Microbiol. **49:** 1253–1266.

Rickettsia parkeri as a Paradigm for Multiple Causes of Tick-Borne Spotted Fever in the Western Hemisphere

CHRISTOPHER D. PADDOCK

Infectious Disease Pathology Activity, Division of Viral and Rickettsial Diseases, Centers for Disease Control and Prevention, Atlanta, Georgia 30333, USA

ABSTRACT: Among the many contributions made to rickettsiology by entomologist and rickettsiologist Ralph R. Parker was his discovery in 1937 of a novel rickettsia isolated from the Gulf Coast tick, *Amblyomma maculatum*. This bacterium was subsequently characterized as a unique rickettsial species in 1965 and named *Rickettsia parkeri* in honor of its discoverer. During the next several decades *R. parkeri* was generally considered as one of several "nonpathogenic" spotted fever group (SFG) rickettsiae that resided in ticks of the United States. The identification of novel rickettsioses on other continents during the last two decades of the twentieth century provided important evidence of the frequent coexistence of multiple and unique tick-borne SFG rickettsiae sharing common geographic regions. Surprisingly, this paradigm, which was repeatedly demonstrated in Europe, Africa, and Australia during the last 10 years, had no confirmed correlate in the United States until 2002, when *R. parkeri* was isolated from a patient from the state of Virginia. Several pieces of epidemiologic, laboratory, and clinical evidence are compelling enough to suggest that this infection has occurred in other U.S. patients who reside within the range of the Gulf Coast tick. Just as important are new data indicating relatively high infection rates of *A. maculatum* ticks with *R. parkeri*, documenting the occurrence of *R. parkeri* in *Amblyomma triste* ticks from Uruguay, and providing evidence that other *Amblyomma* species might serve as efficient vectors of *R. parkeri*. The recognition of *R. parkeri* as a cause of disease in humans will hopefully encourage a closer examination for specific etiologies of tick-borne spotted fever rickettsioses in the United States and other countries of the Western Hemisphere.

KEYWORDS: *Rickettsia parkeri*; *Rickettsia rickettsii*; *Rickettsia amblyommii*; spotted fever rickettsia; Rocky Mountain spotted fever; *Amblyomma maculatum*; Gulf Coast tick; R.R. Parker

Address for correspondence: Christopher D. Paddock, M.D., Infectious Disease Pathology Activity, Mailstop G-32, Centers for Disease Control and Prevention, 1600 Clifton Road, Atlanta, GA 30333. Voice: 404-639-1309; fax: 404-639-1377.

cdp9@cdc.gov

Disclaimer: The findings and conclusions in this article are those of the author and do not necessarily reflect the views of the Department of Health and Human Services.

Ann. N.Y. Acad. Sci. 1063: 315–326 (2005).
doi: 10.1196/annals.1355.051

RICKETTSIA PARKERI: DISCOVERY AND REDISCOVERY

> *"Circumstantial evidence suggests that this rickettsia is the causative agent of disease in some one or more of the natural hosts of* A. maculatum. *Whether or not this disease occurs in man is unknown, but if it does, the presumptive evidence from animal experimentation suggests that human infection might be confusingly similar to spotted fever."*
>
> R. R. PARKER, 1948[1]

At least 10 named spotted fever group (SFG) rickettsiae and several other non-speciated or incompletely characterized rickettsiae with distinct genotypic or serotypic characteristics have been identified in ixodid ticks in the Western Hemisphere.[2] Until 2002, all confirmed cases of tick-borne spotted fever in North, Central, and South America were attributed to one pathogen, *Rickettsia rickettsii*, the cause of Rocky Mountain spotted fever (RMSF). Paradoxically, *R. rickettsii* almost always constitutes the minority of SFG rickettsial isolates obtained from ticks, even in areas were RMSF is endemic.[3–8] Historically, tick-borne rickettsiae other than *R. rickettsii* were often described as nonpathogens.[9–11]

Entomologist and rickettsiologist Ralph Robinson Parker (FIG. 1) was among the first to document the existence of SFG rickettsiae and rickettsia-like bacteria different from *R. rickettsii* in United States ticks.[12] In 1937, he isolated a distinct rickettsial strain from Gulf Coast ticks (*Amblyomma maculatum*) collected from cattle in Liberty County, Texas.[13] Parker determined that male guinea pigs inoculated intraperitoneally with triturated pools of *A. maculatum* soon developed low-grade fever and periorchitis. The animals never died from infection with the "maculatum agent," the febrile period was generally short, and the scrotal erythema caused by this rickettsia was typically bright pink or red.[13] In contrast, male guinea pigs infected with *R. rickettsii* often died following a longer, more severe febrile period, and the scrota of these animals turned dusky purple-red and frequently became necrotic. Other animals, including monkeys, rabbits, white rats, and the Sawatch meadow mouse, showed varying severity of illness following infection with the maculatum agent, and no increase in agglutinins for *Proteus* OXK, OX2, or OX19 antigens was identified in the serum of infected rabbits.[14] Evaluations of guinea pig serum specimens for complement-fixing antibodies with heterologous SFG rickettsial antigens provided information that categorized this bacterium as an SFG rickettsia.[15] Subsequent serologic studies using murine complement-fixing antibodies characterized the maculatum agent as a unique SFG rickettsia, and in 1965, it was named *Rickettsia parkeri* in honor of R.R. Parker. The official, albeit brief, notation described *R. parkeri* as a small, rod-shaped bacterium, with an average size of 1.6×0.5 μm, found in the nucleus and cytoplasm of infected cells.[16]

R. parkeri remained a relatively obscure rickettsia for the next several decades, being mentioned occasionally as a potential cause of human illness[17,18] but more often relegated to the group of "nonpathogenic" SFG rickettsiae found in ticks in the United States. In 2002, the first confirmed infection with *R. parkeri* in a human was identified in a 40-year-old man from the Tidewater area of coastal Virginia who developed a febrile illness associated with headache, myalgias, a maculopapular rash, and multiple eschars on his lower extremities; *R. parkeri* was isolated in cell culture

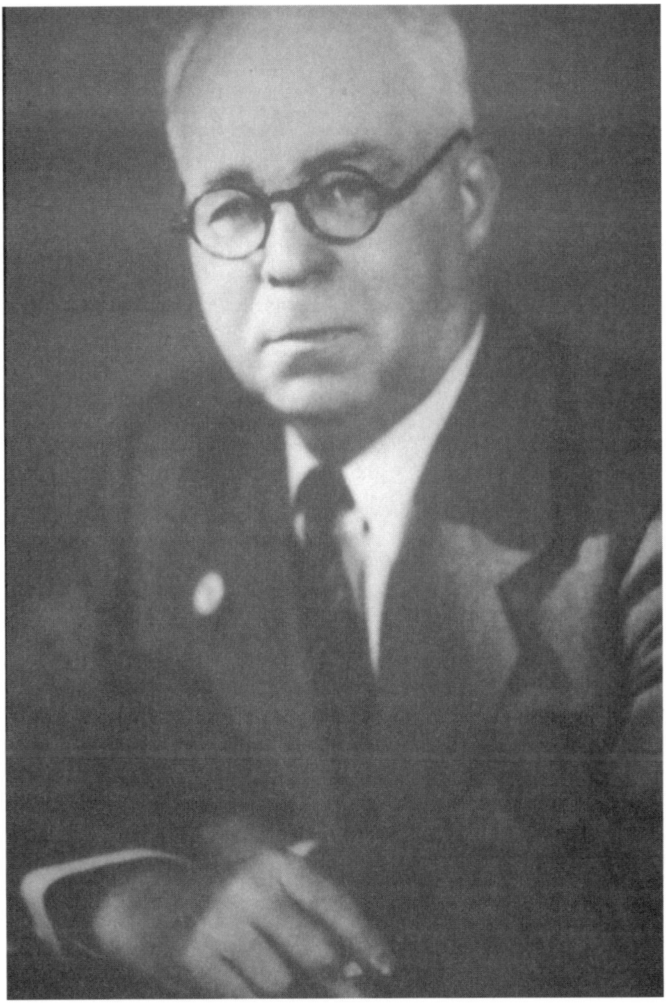

FIGURE 1. Ralph Robinson Parker, 1888–1949. Photograph provided by the Rocky Mountain Laboratories, National Institute of Allergy and Infectious Diseases, National Institutes of Health.

from one of the eschars.[19] The patient was not hospitalized and responded promptly to therapy with doxycycline.

This index patient recalled no definite tick bite; however, *A. maculatum* ticks are distributed in several southeastern states that border the Gulf and southern Atlantic coast of the United States, including the Virginia coast. Established inland populations of Gulf Coast ticks also occur in Oklahoma and Kansas.[20,21] The range of *A. maculatum* also encompasses regions of Central and South America,[22] and in this context, unrecognized cases of *R. parkeri* rickettsiosis could potentially occur across a relatively broad geographic expanse. The absence of an identifiable tick bite by the index patient, in association with the occurrence of multiple eschars, is suggestive of parasitism by infected larval stage *A. maculatum* ticks, which are <0.5 mm in greatest dimension[22] and bite sensitive mammalian hosts far more surreptitiously than do adult-stage ticks. Because *R. parkeri* can be passed from infected adult female ticks to their progeny,[23] Gulf Coast tick larvae may be capable of transmitting this agent to susceptible hosts in a manner similar to other closely related SFG rickettsiae.[24]

The actual distribution of *R. parkeri* and the frequency of its occurrence in *A. maculatum* are not well known. *R. parkeri* has been isolated from Gulf Coast ticks in Alabama, Georgia, Mississippi, and Texas.[13,14,25,26] Noncharacterized SFG rickettsiae were detected by hemolymph testing with an SFG-specific fluorescent antibody stain in 2 (3.8%) of 53 *A. maculatum* collected in South Carolina during 1974–1976,[27] and minimum infection ratios from 1.2–2.4% can be estimated by the reported success at isolating *R. parkeri* from pooled Gulf Coast ticks collected in Mississippi during the late 1940s.[25] A recent survey, using more sensitive molecular methods, of Gulf Coast ticks collected from Georgia, Florida, Kentucky, Mississippi, and Oklahoma, has shown that *R. parkeri* is associated with populations of *A. maculatum* in each of these states and that at some collection sites approximately 15% of adult-stage ticks are infected with this rickettsia (Sumner and colleagues, unpublished data).

Various investigations indicate that other *Amblyomma* ticks might also serve as potential vectors of *R. parkeri*. Microimmunofluorescence testing using mouse antiserum identified *R. parkeri* in 2 (0.5%) of 421 and 3 (0.05%) of 1,912 adult lone star ticks (*Amblyomma americanum*) collected from Mississippi and Kentucky, respectively, during 1983 and 1984,[28] and there are experimental data to suggest that *A. americanum* can transmit *R. parkeri* to guinea pigs.[23] Recent molecular studies also document the occurrence of *R. parkeri* in *Amblyomma triste* ticks in Uruguay.[29] These findings are particularly intriguing when viewed in context with earlier case reports from Uruguay of an eschar-associated SFG rickettsiosis attributed to *R. conorii* on the basis of serological test results.[30,31] Preliminary investigations suggest that *Amblyomma cajennense* (the Cayenne tick) might also support the development of *R. parkeri*.[32] There are no data available that describe the vertebrate host(s) involved as reservoirs or amplifiers in the natural transmission cycle of *R. parkeri* or that describe the life cycle of *R. parkeri* in ticks.

THE LEGACY OF R. R. PARKER: A LIFE IN RICKETTSIOLOGY

> *"Sometimes I wish (wish is not really the right word) that I were preparing to leave the Bitter Root and the tick work behind...but I fail to understand why a man should switch his work in science every few years any more than he should in other work of life."*
>
> R. R. PARKER, 1928[33]

Shortly after receiving his Ph.D. in entomology from Massachusetts Agricultural College in 1916, Parker was hired to work on the ecology of tick and reservoir species involved in the transmission and maintenance of RMSF in eastern Montana. In 1918, he was chosen to head tick eradication activities in the Bitterroot Valley by the Montana State Board of Entomology, and in 1921, was appointed Special Expert to the Public Health Service in charge of all field operations at Hamilton Station in Hamilton, Montana. In 1930, Parker became Director of Hamilton Station (which became the Rocky Mountain Laboratories [RML] in 1937) and retained that position for the subsequent 19 years.[33]

Parker's contributions to rickettsiology were as varied as they were seminal. A partial compilation of his work includes the first systematic collection, collation, and reporting of the national incidence of RMSF;[34] the description of rickettsial reactivation in tick hosts;[35] the development of a tick-derived vaccine that conferred protection against fatal infection with *R. rickettsii*;[36] the identification of multiple tick species in the United States as important potential vectors of *R. rickettsii*;[37] the isolation of the Sheila Smith strain of *R. rickettsii*;[33] and the isolation and characterization of a distinct low-virulence strain of *R. rickettsii* (Hlp) associated with the rabbit tick *Haemaphysalis leporispalustris*.[38] Parker also recruited other scientists of considerable talent and contemporary renown to work at RML, including C.B. Philip, G.E. Davis, W.L. Jellison, and H.R. Cox.[33]

Parker's scientific achievements and interests extended far beyond SFG rickettsiae. His early work so impressed Harvard pathologist and bacteriologist Simeon Burt Wolbach that he was invited by Wolbach in 1919 to participate in entomologic studies of lice with an overseas commission investigating epidemic typhus in post–World War I Poland. Parker was granted a leave of absence from his work in Montana and traveled to Boston; however, just before the group was set to disembark, Parker was hospitalized for a severe respiratory illness complicated by heart problems and missed the sailing date.[33,39] He made several important contributions to the study of tularemia, including the first work to document the role of ticks as hosts and vectors of *Francisella tularensis*.[40] During the course of their studies with this pathogen, Parker and a colleague, Dr. Roscoe R. Spencer, became ill with laboratory-acquired tularemia, and chronicled descriptions of their illnesses (patients "R.R.P" and "R.R.S.") in a subsequent report.[41]

Parker died while working at his desk at RML on September 4, 1949. At that time, Parker possessed a broader knowledge of RMSF than perhaps any other individual, and his death has been described as a turning point in the history of RML and the study of RMSF.[39] During the two decades following Parker's death, the focus of epidemiologic research on RMSF shifted from western Montana to the southeastern United States and there was a marked drop in the number of nationally reported cases of RMSF, the latter of which has been attributed in part to decreased surveillance efforts affected by his absence.[42]

Parker's scientific discoveries continue to be validated by contemporary ecologic, epidemiologic, and immunologic studies of RMSF and other SFG rickettsiae, including the recent demonstration of *Rhipicephalus sanguineus* as a vector of RMSF in the United States,[43] *R. parkeri* as a pathogen of humans,[19] and the partial cross-immunity conferred between SFG and typhus group rickettsiae.[44]

THE CASE FOR MULTIPLE CAUSES OF TICK-BORNE SPOTTED FEVER IN THE UNITED STATES

"Although boutonneuse fever has never been recorded in the western hemisphere, primary ulcers resembling the tâche noire have been reported on patients in the United States."

W. BURGDORFER, 1975[45]

"Given the early branching within the SFG of the North American, nonpathogenic species, it is somewhat surprising to find R. parkeri, *another North American species of unreported pathogenicity, clustering with the Old World pathogens* R. sibirica *and* R. conorii. *This placement suggests that* R. parkeri *may in fact be a cryptic pathogenic species, not yet identified with disease, or that this species is associated with a more mild or overlooked phenotype".*

D. R. STOTHARD AND P. A. FUERST, 1995[18]

Since 2002, no additional confirmed cases of *R. parkeri* rickettsiosis have been reported; however, several compelling lines of evidence suggest that infections with *R. parkeri*, and probably one or more other tick-borne SFG rickettsiae, are responsible for at least some of the approximately 400–1,100 cases of "RMSF" reported each year in the United States (www.cdc.gov/mmwr/summary.html). These include: (1) cases of eschar-associated spotted fevers for which species-specific confirmatory data are lacking; (2) serologic evidence of subclinical or mild infections with spotted fever group rickettsiae in tick-exposed patients; (3) evidence of mild to severe disease in various rodents inoculated with certain "nonpathogenic" SFG rickettsiae; and (4) the precedent recognition of multiple tick-borne rickettsial diseases in Europe, Africa, and Australia.[2,46]

There are rare descriptions of eschars occurring in patients diagnosed with RMSF from the United States and Brazil[47–50]; however, these infections were not confirmed by using tests specific for *R. rickettsii*, suggesting that at least some of these cases represented infections with *R. parkeri* or possibly other eschar-producing SFG rickettsiae. Interestingly, R.R. Spencer may have documented the first unrecognized human case of *R. parkeri* rickettsiosis in 1926.[51] In this brief report Spencer described a 35-year-old female patient from coastal Virginia who exhibited many clinical and epidemiologic similarities to the 2002 index patient. The patient had a moderately severe illness characterized by fever, headache, rash, inguinal adenopathy, and multiple ulcerated lesions. Each of the ulcers occurred at the bite site of an *Amblyomma*-like tick, and her systemic manifestations developed approximately 10 days after these bites. Multiple serum specimens from the patient failed to agglutinate *Proteus* OX19 antigens. When citrated whole blood from the patient was inoculated into several guinea pigs, only one animal developed fever. Spencer concluded that the patient's disease appeared to be very similar to RMSF but that the geographic location of this episode, the mild response of guinea pigs following inoculation, and absence of febrile agglutinins in the convalescing patient "make such a diagnosis very doubtful."[51]

In 1932 P. G. Shipley described similar illnesses in several children in Maryland.[52] Shipley, reporting on a condition he called "coastal tick-bite fever," indicated

TABLE 1. Selected clinical and epidemiologic characteristics of various noncharacterized, eschar-associated spotted fever rickettsioses diagnosed at the Centers for Disease Control and Prevention during 1998–2002

Year	Age (years)/ Sex	State	Tick Bite	Eschar	Rash	IFA Titer(s) to *R. rickettsii*
1998	65/M	MS	NR	+	+	128, 1,024[a]
1999	50/F	MS	+	+	+	4,096
1999	69/M	TX	+	+	+	64, 128
1999	83/M	FL	+	+	+	64, 1,024
2002	60/F	CA	NR	+	–	<16, 512

[a]An eschar biopsy specimen was also positive by immunohistochemical staining for SFG rickettsiae.
NR, none reported.

that two types of disease could be distinguished: a severe form, with an extensive rash and delirium (similar to RMSF), and a mild form, characterized by relatively low fevers and a mild rash showing only a few scattered lesions. Shipley also noted that "not infrequently the site of inoculation is marked by a small ulcer which bleeds easily on examination and there may be marked enlargement of regional lymph nodes which receive the drainage of the ulcer."[52]

During 1998–2002, at least five other cases of eschar-associated spotted fever were identified in patients from the southern and western United States during the course of routine diagnostic testing by the Viral and Rickettsial Zoonoses Branch at the Centers for Disease Control and Prevention (TABLE 1). Most of these patients recalled a tick bite at the site of the eschar, developed a maculopapular rash, and responded rapidly to doxycycline or gradually improved without specific therapy. Cases were confirmed by SFG-specific serologic or immunohistochemical assays; however, limited availability of specimens for culture or molecular-based techniques precluded agent-specific diagnoses (CDC, unpublished data).

In a recent report, an examination of 15 serum specimens from U.S. patients with reactivity to *R. rickettsii* antigens (by using an indirect immunofluorescence antibody [IFA] assay), revealed five samples with higher IFA titers when *R. parkeri* was used as antigen.[53] Four of these specimens reacted with a 120-kDa protein of *R. parkeri* by Western blot analysis, suggesting that additional cases of infection with *R. parkeri*, or possibly other SFG rickettsiae, have occurred in patients in the United States.

Contemporary serosurveys in various regions of the United States have identified remarkably high prevalences of antibodies reactive with *R. rickettsii* among persons for whom no antecedent illness of a severity comparable to microbiologically confirmed RMSF was identified. In one study, serum samples obtained from 32 (9.1%) of 352 children residing in two counties in Texas where RMSF is endemic, showed antibody titers ≥64 when tested by IFA. Eight of these children had a febrile illness associated with rash or headache in the preceding year, but none had been hospitalized or diagnosed with RMSF.[54] More recently, antibody titers ≥64 were identified in serum specimens obtained from 239 (12%) of 1999 children at medical facilities in Arkansas, Kentucky, Missouri, North Carolina, Oklahoma, and Tennessee.[55] These investigators suggested that some of these infections could represent relatively

TABLE 2. Candidate pathogens among currently recognized spotted fever rickettsiae in the United States

SFG Rickettsia (strain or species)	Tick Vector(s)	State(s) of Reported Occurrence	Evidence of Pathogenicity	Reference
Tillamook	*Ixodes pacificus*	CA, OR	Lethal to mice	58, 59
364D	*Dermacentor occidentalis*	CA	Scrotal swelling in guinea pigs; disease in humans is suggested by serologic studies	59, 60
Rickettsia rhipicephali	*Rhipicephalus sanguineus, D. occidentalis, D. andersoni, D. variabilis*	MS, NC, TX, CA, OR, MT	Scrotal swelling, splenomegaly, and death in meadow voles	6, 45, 59, 61
Nonnamed	*Amblyomma cajennense*	TX	Closely related or identical to *Rickettsia honei*	62
Rickettsia amblyommii	*Amblyomma americanum*	TN, GA, SC, NC, FL, NY, NJ, RI, IA, OK	Disease in humans suggested by serologic studies	63–66

mild infections with SFG rickettsiae other than *R. rickettsii.* Even more provocative are recent studies that documented seroconversion to *R. rickettsii* antigens in patients with recent tick bites who developed relatively mild, febrile, rash illnesses, and none of whom required hospitalization or showed severe manifestations associated with classical RMSF.[56,57]

Several candidate pathogens exist among speciated or partially characterized SFG rickettsiae endemic to the United States (TABLE 2). These represent rickettsial strains or species that are harbored by one or more human-biting tick species, some of which elicit mild to severe clinical disease when inoculated into various rodents. In the western United States, two nonspeciated SFG rickettsial strains similar to, yet distinguishable from, *R. rickettsii* are pathogenic to mice and guinea pigs. These include strain Tillamook, isolated from *Ixodes pacificus* ticks in western Oregon and California,[58,59] and strain 364D, isolated from *Dermacentor occidentalis* in California.[59] In addition, data from antibody adsorption tests of convalescent-phase serum specimens of patients in northern California with confirmed "RMSF" suggest infection with strain 364D.[60] *Rickettsia rhipicephali*, an SFG rickettsia identified in several species of U.S. ticks, causes moderately severe disease in meadow voles inoculated with this agent.[6,45,59,61] An SFG rickettsia recently identified in *A. cajennense* ticks collected from south Texas shares close genetic homology with *Rickettsia honei*, the agent of Flinders Island spotted fever in Australia, and might also elicit similar disease in tick-exposed persons in Texas.[2,62] An SFG rickettsia identified in lone star ticks,[63] *Rickettsia amblyommii*, may account for much of the serologic reactivity to SFG rickettsiae observed among tick-exposed persons residing throughout the range of *A. americanum*. In one study, the average infection prevalence of *R. amblyommii* in lone star ticks collected from multiple sites in eight states was 39% (range, 7–88%).[64] Western blot and competition enzyme-linked immunosorbent assays have also provided strong evidence that some cases of infection with this rickettsia have occurred in humans.[65,66]

The recognition of *Rickettsia africae* as a cause of disease in humans in the Caribbean[67] and the recent identification of several novel SFG rickettsiae in South America[2] also support a conclusion that additional SFG rickettsial pathogens inevitably remain to be discovered in the Americas.

Why should it be important to recognize tick-borne SFG rickettsiae other than *R. rickettsii* and the associated diseases, which even if misidentified, will uniformly respond to doxycycline? From an epidemiologic perspective alone, discrimination of cryptogenic etiologic agents and the associated infectious manifestations is crucial to define a true clinical spectrum for each particular rickettsiosis, particularly a nationally reported disease as important as RMSF. In this context, it is possible that cases of "subclinical" or "mild" RMSF occur rarely, if ever, and that geographic or temporal variations in case-fatality rates of this disease have been artefactually influenced by inclusion of inaccurately classified cases resulting from non-specific laboratory assays. The development of monoclonal immunohistochemical techniques and serologic tests with greater specificities, coupled whenever possible with traditional culture-based methods, will be necessary to dissect the collective rickettsial species that cause "RMSF," and should simultaneously enhance physician cognizance of other, less severe rickettsioses that occur in the same region.

Soon after the initial isolation of *R. parkeri*, R.R. Parker stated that "Final decision as to whether maculatum infection is or is not a new disease entity must await further research."[14] Despite a wait of nearly 65 years, the recent recognition of *R. parkeri* as a cause of disease in humans will hopefully encourage a closer examination for specific etiologies of tick-borne spotted fever in the United States and in other countries of the Western Hemisphere. After a century of a consistently monotypic diagnosis, the clinical, epidemiologic, and ecologic complexity of these infections warrants further inspection. Renewed interest, combined with contemporary and traditional laboratory techniques, will undoubtedly uncover additional cases of infection caused by *R. parkeri* and perhaps other novel rickettsial diseases.

[*Competing interests statement:* The authors of this article state that they have no competing financial interests.]

REFERENCES

1. PARKER, R.R. 1948. Symptomatology and certain other aspects of Rocky Mountain spotted fever. *In* Rickettsial Diseases of Man. F.R. Moulton, Ed.: 139–146. American Association for the Advancement of Science. Washington, D.C.
2. PAROLA, P., C.D. PADDOCK & D. RAOULT. 2005. Tick-borne rickettsioses around the world: emerging diseases challenging old concepts. Clin. Microbiol. Rev. **18:** 719–756.
3. BENACH, J.L., D.J. WHITE, W. BURGDORFER, *et al.* 1977. Changing patterns in incidence of Rocky Mountain spotted fever on Long Island (1971–1976). Am. J. Epidemiol. **106:** 380–387.
4. LINNEMANN, C.C., A.E. SCHAEFFER, W. BURGDORFER, *et al.* 1980. Rocky Mountain spotted fever in Clermont County, Ohio. II. Distribution of population and infected ticks in an endemic area. Am. J. Epidemiol. **111:** 31–36.

5. Feng, W.C., E.S. Murray, W. Burgdorfer, *et al.* 1980. Spotted fever group rickettsiae in *Dermacentor variabilis* from Cape Cod, Massachusetts. Am. J. Trop. Med. Hyg. **29:** 691–694.
6. Philip, R.N. & E.A. Casper. 1981. Serotypes of spotted fever group rickettsiae isolated from *Dermacentor andersoni* (Stiles) ticks in western Montana. Am. J. Trop. Med. Hyg. **30:** 230–238.
7. Gordon, J.C., S.W. Gordon, E. Peterson & R.N. Philip. 1984. Epidemiology of Rocky Mountain spotted fever in Ohio, 1981: serologic evaluation of canines and rickettsial isolation from ticks associated with human case exposure sites. Am. J. Trop. Med. Hyg. **33:** 1026–1031.
8. Pretzman, C., N. Daugherty, K. Poetter & D. Ralph. 1990. The distribution and dynamics of rickettsia in the tick population of Ohio. Ann. N.Y. Acad. Sci. **590:** 227–236.
9. Bell, E.J., G.M. Kohls, H.G. Stoenner & D.B. Lackman. 1963. Nonpathogenic rickettsias related to the spotted fever group isolated from ticks, *Dermacentor variabilis* and *Dermacentor andersoni* from eastern Montana. J. Immunol. **90:** 770–781.
10. Schriefer, M.E. & A.F. Azad. 1994. Changing ecology of Rocky Mountain spotted fever. *In* Ecological Dynamics of Tick-borne Zoonoses. D.E. Sonenshine & T.N. Mather, Eds.: 314–326. Oxford University Press. New York.
11. Weller, S.J., G.D. Baldridge, U.G. Munderloh, *et al.* 1998. Phylogenetic placement of rickettsiae from the ticks *Amblyomma americanum* and *Ixodes scapularis*. J. Clin. Microbiol. **36:** 1305–1317.
12. Parker, R.R. & R.R. Spencer. 1926. Rocky Mountain spotted fever. A study of the relationship between the presence of rickettsia-like organisms in tick smears and the infectiveness of the same ticks. Public Health Rep. **41:** 461–469.
13. Parker, R.R., G.M. Kohls, G.W. Cox & G.E. Davis. 1939. Observations on an infectious agent from *Amblyomma maculatum*. Public Health Rep. **54:** 1482–1484.
14. Parker, R.R. 1940. A pathogenic rickettsia from the Gulf Coast tick, *Amblyomma maculatum*. *In* Proceedings of the Third International Congress for Microbiology: 390–391. New York, NY.
15. Lackman, D.B., R.R. Parker & R.K. Gerloff. 1949. Serological characteristics of a pathogenic rickettsia occurring in *Amblyomma maculatum*. Public Health Rep. **64:** 1342–1349.
16. Lackman, D.B., E.J. Bell, H.G. Stoenner & E.G. Pickens. 1965. The Rocky Mountain spotted fever group of rickettsias. Health Lab. Sci. **2:** 135–141.
17. Walker, D.H. & D.B. Fishbein. 1991. Epidemiology of rickettsial diseases. Eur. J. Epidemiol. **7:** 237–245.
18. Stothard, D.R. & P.A. Fuerst. 1995. Evolutionary analysis of the spotted fever and typhus groups of *Rickettsia* using 16S rRNA gene sequences. Sys. Appl. Microbiol. **18:** 52–61.
19. Paddock, C.D., J.W. Sumner, J.A. Comer, *et al.* 2004. *Rickettsia parkeri*: a newly recognized cause of spotted fever rickettsiosis in the United States. Clin. Infect. Dis. **38:** 805–811.
20. Barker, R.W., A.A. Kocan, S.A. Ewing, *et al.* 2004. Occurrence of the Gulf Coast tick (Acari: Ixodidae) on wild and domestic mammals in north-central Oklahoma. J. Med. Entomol. **41:** 170–178.
21. Goddard, J. & C.D. Paddock. 2005. Observations on distribution and seasonal activity of the Gulf Coast tick in Mississippi. J. Med. Entomol. **42:** 176–179.
22. Cooley, R.A. & G.M. Kohls. 1944. The genus *Amblyomma* (Ixodidae) in the United States. J. Parasitol. **30:** 77–111.
23. Goddard, J. 2003. Experimental infection of lone star ticks, *Amblyomma americanum* (L.), with *Rickettsia parkeri* and exposure of guinea pigs to the agent. J. Med. Entomol. **40:** 686–689.
24. Kelly, P.J. & P.R. Mason. 1991. Transmission of a spotted fever group rickettsia by *Amblyomma hebraeum* (Acari: Ixodidae). J. Med. Entomol. **28:** 598–600.
25. Philip, C.B. & J.S. White. 1955. Disease agents recovered incidental to a tick survey of the Mississippi Gulf Coast. J. Econ. Entomol. **48:** 396–400.

26. PHILIP, R.N., E.A. CASPER, W. BURGDORFER, *et al.* 1978. Serologic typing of rickettsiae of the spotted fever group by microimmunofluorescence. J. Immunol. **121:** 1961–1968.
27. LOVING, S.M., A.B. SMITH, A.F. DISALVO & W. BURGDORFER. 1978. Distribution and prevalence of spotted fever group rickettsiae in ticks from South Carolina, with an epidemiological survey of persons bitten by infected ticks. Am. J. Trop. Med. Hyg. **27:** 1255–1260.
28. GODDARD, J. & B.R. NORMENT. 1986. Spotted fever group rickettsiae in the lone star tick, *Amblyomma americanum* (Acari: Ixodidae). J. Med. Entomol. **23:** 465–472.
29. VENZAL, J.M., A. PORTILLO, A. ESTRADA-PEÑA, *et al.* 2004. *Rickettsia parkeri* in *Amblyomma triste* from Uruguay. Emerg. Infect. Dis. **10:** 1493–1495.
30. CONTI-DIAZ, I.A., I. RUBIO, R.E. SOMMA MOREIRA & G. PÉREZ BÓRMIDA. 1990. Rickettsiosis cutáneo ganglionar por *Rickettsia conorii* en el Uruguay. Rev. Inst. Med. Trop. São Paulo **32:** 313–318.
31. CONTI-DÍAZ, I.A. 2003. Rickettsiosis caused by *Rickettsia conorii* in Uruguay. Ann. N.Y. Acad. Sci. **990:** 264–266.
32. SANGIONI, L.A., M.C. HORTA, M.C.B. VIANNA, *et al.* 2005. Rickettsial infection in animals and Brazilian spotted fever endemicity. Emerg. Infect. Dis. **11:** 265–270.
33. PHILIP, R.N. 2000. Rocky Mountain Spotted Fever in Western Montana. Anatomy of a Pestilence. Bitter Root Valley Historical Society. Hamilton, MT.
34. CHILDS, J.E. & C.D. PADDOCK. 2002. Passive surveillance as an instrument to identify risk factors for fatal Rocky Mountain spotted fever: is there more to learn? Am. J. Trop. Med. Hyg. **66:** 450–457.
35. SPENCER, R.R. & R.R. PARKER. 1923. Rocky Mountain spotted fever: infectivity of fasting and recently fed ticks. Public Health Rep. **38:** 333–339.
36. PARKER, R.R. 1941. Rocky Mountain spotted fever: results of fifteen years' prophylactic vaccination. Am. J. Trop. Med. **21:** 369–383.
37. PARKER, R. R., C.B. PHILIP & W.L. JELLISON. 1933. Rocky Mountain spotted fever. Potentialities of tick transmission in relation to geographical occurrence in the United States. Am. J. Trop. Med. **8:** 341-379.
38. PARKER, R.R. E.G. PICKENS, D.B. LACKMAN, *et al.* 1951. Isolation and characterization of Rocky Mountain spotted fever rickettsiae from the rabbit tick *Haemaphysalis leporis-palustris* Packard. Public Health Rep. **66:** 455–463.
39. HARDEN, V.A. 1990. Rocky Mountain Spotted Fever. History of a Twentieth-Century Disease. Johns Hopkins University Press. Baltimore, MD.
40. PARKER, R.R., R.R. SPENCER & E. FRANCIS. 1924. Tularemia infection in ticks of the species *Dermacentor andersoni* Stiles, in the Bitterroot Valley, Montana. Public Health Rep. **39:** 1057–1073.
41. PARKER, R.R. & R.R. SPENCER. 1926. Six additional cases of laboratory infection of tularemia in man. Public Health Rep. **41:** 1341.
42. BURGDORFER, W. 1975. A review of Rocky Mountain spotted fever (tick-borne typhus), its agent, and its tick vectors in the United States. J. Med. Entomol. **12:** 269–278.
43. DEMMA, L.J., M.S. TRAEGER, W.L. NICHOLSON, *et al.* 2005. Rocky Mountain spotted fever from an unexpected tick vector in Arizona. N. Engl. J. Med. **353:** 587–594.
44. VALBUENA, G., J.M. JORDAN & D.H. WALKER. 2004. T cells mediate cross-protective immunity between spotted fever group rickettsiae and typhus group rickettsiae. J. Infect. Dis. **190:** 1221–1227.
45. BURGDORFER, W., D.J. SEXTON, R.K. GERLOFF, *et al.* 1975. *Rhipicephalus sanguineus*: vector of a new spotted fever group rickettsia in the United States. Infect. Immun. **12:** 205–210.
46. RAOULT, D. 2004. A new rickettsial disease in the United States. 2004. Clin. Infect. Dis. **38:** 812–813.
47. WOLBACH, S.B. 1919. Rocky Mountain spotted fever. J. Med. Res. **41:** 2–197
48. WALKER, D.H., R.M. GAY & M. VALDES-DAPENA. 1981. The occurrence of eschars in Rocky Mountain spotted fever. J. Am. Acad. Dermatol. **4:** 571–576.
49. COX, G.M. & D.J. SEXTON. 1995. Photo quiz. Clin. Infect. Dis. **21:** 315–429.
50. PIZA, J.T. 1932. Considerações epidemiologicas e clinicas sobre typho exanthematico de S. Paulo. *In* Typho Exanthathematico de São Paulo. J.T. Piza, J.R. Meyer & L.S. Gomes, Eds.: 11–19. Sociedade Impressora Paulista. São Paulo, Brazil.

51. SPENCER, R.R. 1926. A case of typhus-like fever following tick bite. Public Health Rep. **41:** 2523–2524.
52. SHIPLEY, P.G. 1932. Tick-bite fever in children. Bull. Johns Hopkins Hosp. **51:** 83–101.
53. RAOULT, D. & C.D. PADDOCK. 2005. *Rickettsia parkeri* infection and other spotted fevers in the United States. N. Engl. J. Med. **353:** 626–627.
54. TAYLOR, J.P., W.B. TANNER, J.A. RAWLINGS, *et al.* 1985. Serological evidence of subclinical Rocky Mountain spotted fever infections in Texas. J. Infect. Dis. **151:** 367–369.
55. MARSHALL, G.S., G.G. STOUT, R.F. JACOBS, *et al.* 2003. Antibodies reactive to *Rickettsia rickettsii* among children living in the southeast and south central regions of the United States. Arch. Pediatr. Adolesc. Med. **157:** 443–448.
56. YEVICH, S.J., J.L. SANCHEZ, R.F. DEFRAITES, *et al.* 1995. Seroepidemiology of infections due to spotted fever group rickettsiae and *Ehrlichia* species in military personnel exposed in areas of the United States where such infections are endemic. J. Infect. Dis. **171:** 1266–1273.
57. MCCALL, C.L., A.T. CURNS, L.D. ROTZ, *et al.* 2001. Fort Chaffee revisited: the epidemiology of tick-borne rickettsial and ehrlichial diseases at a natural focus. Vector Borne Zoonotic Dis. **1:** 119-127.
58. HUGHES, L.E., C.M. CLIFFORD, R. GRESBRINK, *et al.* 1976. Isolation of a spotted fever group rickettsia from the Pacific Coast tick, *Ixodes pacificus*, in Oregon. Am. J. Trop. Med. Hyg. **25:** 513-516.
59. PHILIP, R.N., LANE R.S. & E.A. CASPER. 1981. Serotypes of tick-borne spotted fever group rickettsiae isolated from western California. Am. J. Trop. Med. Hyg. **30:** 722–727.
60. LANE, R.S., R.N. PHILIP & E.A. CASPER. 1981. Ecology of tick-borne agents in California. II. Further observations on rickettsiae. *In* Rickettsiae and Rickettsial Diseases. W. Burgdorfer & R.L. Anacker, Eds.: 595–602. Academic Press. New York, NY.
61. BURGDORFER, W., L.P. BRINTON, W.L. KRYNSKI & R.N. PHILIP. 1978. *Rickettsia rhipicephali*, a new spotted fever group rickettsia from the brown dog tick, *Rhipicephalus sanguineus*. *In* Rickettsiae and Rickettsial Diseases. J. Kazár, R.A. Ormsbee & I.N. Tarasevich, Eds.: 307–316, 642–646. Veda. Bratislava.
62. BILLINGS, A.N., X.J. YU, P.D. TEE & D.H. WALKER. 1998. Detection of a spotted fever group rickettsia in *Amblyomma cajennense* (Acari: Ixodidae) in south Texas. J. Med. Entomol. **35:** 474–478.
63. BURGDORFER, W., S.F. HAYES & L.A. THOMAS. 1981. A new spotted fever group rickettsia from the lone star tick, *Amblyomma americanum*. *In* Rickettsiae and Rickettsial Diseases. W. Burgdorfer & R.L. Anacker, Eds.: 595–602. Academic Press. New York, NY.
64. MIXSON, T.R, C.D. PADDOCK, J.W. SUMNER, *et al.* 2005. Prevalence of pathogenic bacteria in *Amblyomma americanum* collected throughout its range in the United States (abstract Y-009). Presented at the 105th General Meeting of The American Society of Microbiology. Atlanta, GA. May 2005.
65. DASCH, G.A., D.J. KELLY, A.L. RICHARDS, *et al.* 1993. Western blotting analysis of sera from military personnel exhibiting serological reactivity to spotted fever group rickettsiae. Am. J. Trop. Med. Hyg. **49:** 220.
66. DASCH, G.A., A. HIGHBAUGH & W.L. NICHOLSON. 2001. Direct binding and competition enzyme-linked immunosorbent assays for identifying the etiologic agents of spotted fever group (abstract 8). Presented at the American Society for Rickettsiology: Bartonella as an Emerging Pathogen Group, 2001 Joint Conference. Big Sky, Montana. August 2001.
67. PAROLA, P., G. VESTRIS, D. MARTINEZ, *et al.* 1999. Tick-borne rickettsiosis in Guadelope, the French West Indies: isolation of *Rickettsia africae* from *Amblyomma variegatum* ticks and serosurvey in humans, cattle, and goats. Am. J. Trop. Med. Hyg. **60:** 888–893.

Detection of a Typhus Group *Rickettsia* in *Amblyomma* Ticks in the State of Nuevo Leon, Mexico

AARON MEDINA-SANCHEZ,[a] DONALD H. BOUYER,[b] VIRGINIA ALCANTARA-RODRIGUEZ,[c] CLAUDIO MAFRA,[d] JORGE ZAVALA-CASTRO,[e] TED WHITWORTH,[b] VSEVOLOD L. POPOV,[b] ILDEFONSO FERNANDEZ-SALAS,[a] AND DAVID H. WALKER[b]

[a]*Laboratorio de Entomologia Medica, Facultad de Biologia, Universidad Autonoma de Nuevo Leon, Monterrey, Nuevo Leon, Mexico*

[b]*Department of Pathology, University of Texas Medical Branch, Galveston, Texas, USA*

[c]*Unidad Departamental de Vigilancia Epidemiologica, Direccion General de Servicios Medicos y Urgencias de la Secretaria de Salud del Distrito Federal, Mexico, DF, Mexico*

[d]*Departamento de Bioquimica e Biologia Molecular, Universidade Federal de Viçosa, Viçosa, MG, Brazil*

[e]*Centro de Investigaciones Regionales Dr. Hideyo Noguchi, Universidad Autonoma de Yucatan, Merida, Yucatan, Mexico*

ABSTRACT: The state of Nuevo Leon, Mexico has had outbreaks of typhus group rickettsiosis, most recently recognized in 1997. Evaluation of the sera of 345 patients with a dengue-like illness revealed that 25.5% had antibodies reactive with typhus group rickettsiae and 16% had antibodies to *Rickettsia parkeri*. Rickettsiae were detected by PCR and shell-vial isolations in the field-collected *Amblyomma* ticks. Molecular characterization by DNA sequence analysis of the *gltA*, *ompB*, and 17-kDa gene identified the organisms to be *R. prowazekii*.

KEYWORDS: typhus; rickettsiosis; *R. prowazekii*

INTRODUCTION

Typhus has been considered to be present in Mexico since the sixteenth century. Two million deaths were ascribed to typhus in the epidemic of 1576, and the illness known as *cocolixtle* and *matlazahuatl* to the indigenous peoples likely were present prior to the arrival of Europeans.[1] Public health records beginning in 1893 document numerous epidemics and a high incidence and mortality rate. During 1941, 1,166 deaths caused by epidemic typhus were reported in Mexico with Nuevo Leon among the most affected states. Previous investigations of ticks as hosts of rickettsiae in

Address for correspondence: Aaron Medina-Sanchez, Laboratorio de Entomologia Medica, Facultad de Biologia, Universidad Autonoma de Nuevo Leon, Monterrey, Mexico. medisanch@yahoo.com

Ann. N.Y. Acad. Sci. 1063: 327–332 (2005). © 2005 New York Academy of Sciences. doi: 10.1196/annals.1355.052

Mexico identified spotted fever group rickettsiae presumed to be *Rickettsia rickettsii* in *Rhipicephalus sanguineus* and *Amblyomma cajennense* ticks. More recently in the state of Nuevo Leon, outbreaks of epidemic typhus in the municipality of Galeana in 1963 and of murine typhus in Montemorelos in 1996 were diagnosed based upon serologic and clinico-epidemiologic data. This study undertook serologic investigation of patients with dengue-like illness and of ticks collected from nearby locations.

MATERIALS AND METHODS

Serology

In 2001, the public health department of Nuevo Leon, Mexico, collected sera from febrile patients in Allende and Linares who were suspected to have dengue fever. IFA for IgG antibodies against *Rickettsia prowazekii, R. typhi, and R. parkeri* was performed as previously described and a titer of 1:64 or higher was considered positive. Positive samples were titrated to a dilution of 1:1024.[2]

Western Immunoblotting

Rickettsia prowazekii, *R. typhi,* and *R. parkeri* were cultivated in Vero cells, purified by 32% Percoll density gradient centrifugation, separated by SDS-PAGE, transferred to nitrocellulose membranes by semi-dry protein blotting, reacted with a 1:100 dilution of sera in blocking buffer, and detected with affinity-purified alkaline phosphatase-labeled goat anti-human IgG diluted 1:5000 in blocking buffer prior to development with BCIP-NBT (Kirkegaard & Perry Laboratories, Gaithersburg, MD).

Tick Collection

Ticks were collected by flagging vegetation, dry ice capture, and removal from livestock. Some ticks were maintained alive and others stored at –80°C. Ticks were identified in consultation with Dr. Pete Teel, Texas A&M University, College Station, Texas. Each tick was bisected, and placed in pools of halves of five ticks or stored as individual halves.

Rickettsial Isolation

Live ticks were sterilized by immersion in 70% alcohol for 10 min followed by a bleach solution and finally washed in sterile water, and dried on sterile filter paper in a biosafety class II cabinet. The pools were homogenized in a small Petri dish using a sterile scalpel, and a 200 μL volume of tick homogenate was used for shell-vial isolation technique as described previously.[3]

Molecular Detection of Rickettsiae

DNA from the tick pools and rickettsial isolation cell cultures was extracted by using the Dneasy tissue kit (Qiagen, Chatsworth, Calif.) according to the manufacturer's protocols. DNA was subsequently extracted from individual ticks from the positive pools using alkaline hydrolysis.[4]

Approximately five microliters (60 ng) of extracted DNA from pools were used as templates for amplification of a 434 bp fragment of the rickettsial 17-kDa protein gene as previously described.[5]

Molecular Characterization of Rickettsial Isolate

The genes amplified for the phylogenetic analysis were *gltA* (citrate synthase), *ompA* and *ompB* (outer membrane proteins). PCR amplification was performed as described previously.[6] These three genes are important molecular targets for taxonomy of rickettsiae.

PCR products of the expected size were cloned using the TOPO TA Cloning Kit (Invitrogen, Carlsbad, CA) according to manufacturer's protocol. Plasmids containing the DNA inserts of the expected size were sequenced at least three times using an ABI automated sequencer with M13 forward and M13 reverse sequencing primers (Invitrogen, Carlsbad CA).

Electron Microscopy

A T75 flask with infected Vero cell monolayers was fixed in Ito's fixative, post fixed in osmium tetroxide for 1 h, and stained *en bloc* in 1% uranyl acetate–0.1 M maleate buffer (pH 5.2) as described previously.[7] Pellets were dehydrated in ethanol, embedded in epoxy resin (Poly/Bed 812), and polymerized at 60°C overnight. Ultrathin sections (thickness, 70 nm) were prepared by using a Reichert Ultracut S ultramicrotome, placed on copper grids, stained with uranyl acetate and lead citrate, and examined in a Philips CM 100 and a Philips 201 electron microscope at 60 kV.

RESULTS

Detection of Antibodies Reactive with R. prowazekii, R. typhi, *and* R. parkeri

Of the 349 sera of patients with dengue-like illness, 89 (25.5%) contained antibodies reactive with *R. prowazekii* and/or *R. typhi*, and 36 (16%) contained antibodies reactive with *R. parkeri*. Some of the sera contained antibodies reactive with OmpB of *R. prowazekii*, OmpB of *R. typhi*, or OmpA and OmpB of *R. parkeri* as detected by immunoblotting.

Detection and Identification of Rickettsiae *in Ticks*

The ticks were identified as *Amblyomma cajennense* and *Amblyomma imitator*. Of a total of 190 ticks in 38 pools of five tick halves, 19 pools contained DNA of *Rickettsia* as determined by nested PCR amplification of the 17-KDa protein gene. Extracts of another 105 ticks examined by PCR amplification of the 17-kDa protein gene revealed three that contained *Rickettsia* DNA. DNA sequence of the 17-kD protein gene amplicons from tick #70 was >99% similar to *R. prowazekii*.

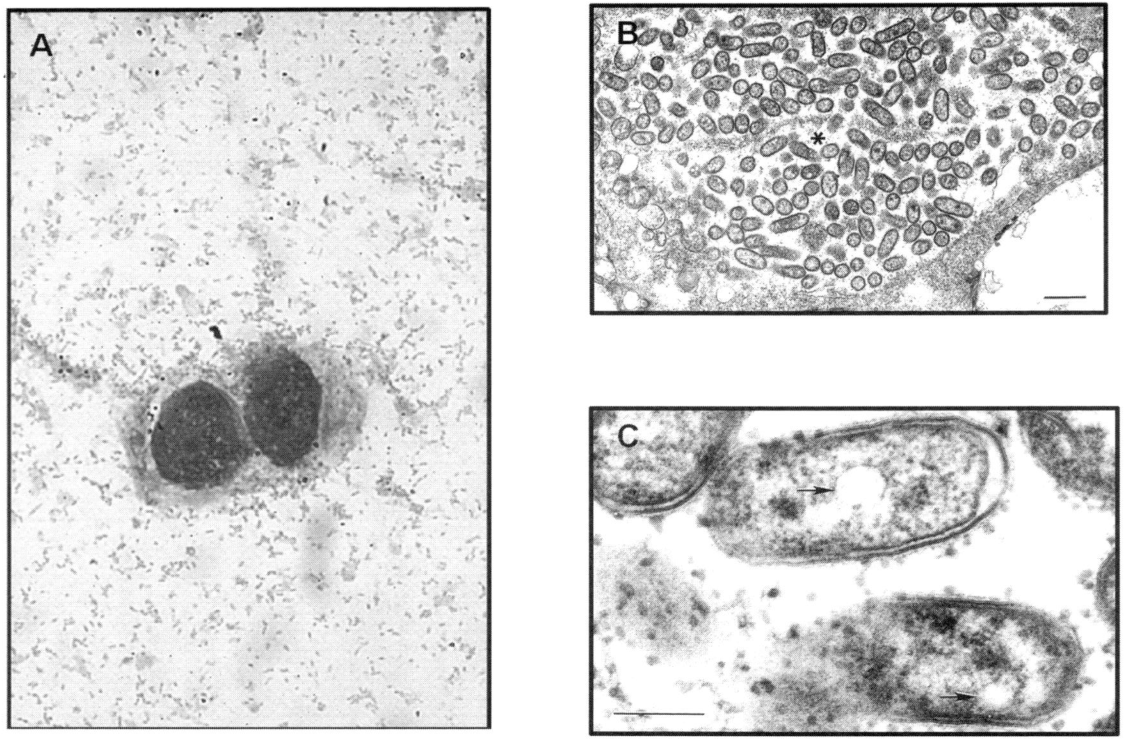

FIGURE 1. Images of *Rickettsia prowazekii* tick isolate in Vero cell culture. (**A**) Dif-Quik stain of shell-vial culture 20 days after inoculation. (**B**) Electron photomicrograph of a Vero cell heavily infected with rickettsiae (*asterisk*) isolated from ticks (*Amblyomma cajennense*) collected in the state of Nuevo Leon, Mexico. Bar: 1.0 μm. (**C**) Higher magnification of the rickettsiae reveals intracytosolic vacuoles (*arrows*), an ultrastructural hallmark of typhus group rickettsiae. Bar: 0.20 μm.

Shell vial cultures of the three pools demonstrated by PCR to contain *Rickettsia* yielded five shell vials with evidence of rickettsial growth by Dif-Quik stain. Only two remained free of contamination (FIG. 1A).

Ultrastructural examination revealed large accumulations of intracytosolic gram-negative bacteria with size, shape, and protoplasmic droplets typical of typhus group *Rickettsia* (FIG. 1B and C).

Phylogenetic analysis of alignments of a 1,211 bp fragment of *gltA* revealed >99% similarity with *R. prowazekii*; of an 838 bp fragment of *ompB*, 100% similarity with *R. prowazekii*; and of 425 bp fragment of the 17-kDa protein gene, >99% similarity with *R. prowazekii*.

DISCUSSION

Reiss-Gutfreund described isolations of *R. prowazekii* from *Amblyomma variegatum*, *Hyalomma marginatum rufipes*, and *H. truncatum* in Ethiopia in 1957, 1961, and 1966, and one of these isolates (ZRS strain) was confirmed to be *R. prowazekii* at the Rocky Mountain Laboratory.[8] Studies of ticks from Ethiopia by Burgdorfer and Philip identified a single *A. cohaerens* tick that by hemolymph test with anti–*R. prowazekii* serum was determined to contain a typhus group rickettsia that they were not able to isolate.[9]

The present study detected *R. prowazekii* in *Amblyomma* ticks in Mexico and established an isolate of *R. prowazekii* from one of the ticks. These findings again raise the question of a natural reservoir of epidemic typhus rickettsiae involving ticks and challenge our current concepts of the origin and evolution of *R. prowazekii,* which largely center on the human latent infection-reactivation-louse-human cycle or the flying squirrel-louse and/or flea-flying squirrel cycle.

The high prevalence of antibodies to typhus group rickettsiae in several populations studied recently in Mexico could reflect tick transmitted *R. prowazekii* as well as murine typhus. Further entomological, epidemiologic, clinical, and rickettsiologic studies will be required to confirm the presence of *R. prowazekii* in Mexican ticks and their public health importance.

REFERENCES

1. ALCANTARA, V.E., E.G. GALLARDO, C. HONG, *et al.* 2004. Typhus group rickettsiae antibodies in rural Mexico. Emerg. Infect. Dis. **10:** 549–550.
2. ZAVALA-VELAZQUEZ, J.E., J. RUIZ-SOSA, I. VADO-SOLIS, *et al.* 1999. Serologic study of the prevalence of rickettsiosis in Yucatan: evidence for a prevalent spotted fever group rickettsiosis. Am. J. Trop. Med. Hyg. **61:** 405–408.
3. KELLY, P.J., D. RAOULT & P.R. MASON. 1991. Isolation of spotted fever group rickettsias from triturated ticks using a modification of the centrifugation-shell vial technique. **85:** 397–398.
4. ALEKSEEV, A.N., H.V. DUBININA, I. VAN, *et al.* 2001. Identification of *Ehrlichia* spp. and *Borrelia burgdorferi* in Ixodes ticks in the Baltic regions of Russia. J. Clin. Microbiol. **39:** 2237–2242.
5. WEBB, L., M. CARL, D.C. MALLOY, *et al.* 1990. Detection of murine typhus infection in fleas by using the polymerase chain reaction. J. Clin. Microbiol. **28:** 530–534.
6. BOUYER, D.H., J. STENOS, P. CROCQUET-VALDES, *et al.* 2001. *Rickettsia felis*: molecular characterization of a new member of the spotted fever group. Int. J. Syst. Evol. Microbiol. **51:** 339–347.

7. ITO, S. & Y. RIKIHISA. 1981. Techniques for electron microscopy of rickettsiae. *In* Rickettsiae and Rickettsial Diseases. W. Burgdorfer & R.L. Anacker, Eds.: 213–227. Academic Press. New York, NY.
8. REISS-GUTFREUND, R.J. 1966. The isolation of *Rickettsia prowazekii* and *mooseri* from unusual sources. Am. J. Trop. Med. Hyg. **15:** 943–949.
9. BURGDORFER, W., R.A. ORMSBEE, M.L. SCHMIDT, *et al.* 1973. A search for the epidemic typhus agent in Ethiopian ticks. Bull. World. Health Org. **48:** 563–569.

Detection of a Non-Pathogenic Variant of *Anaplasma phagocytophilum* in *Ixodes ricinus* from La Rioja, Spain

A. PORTILLO,[a] A.S. SANTOS,[b] S. SANTIBÁÑEZ,[a] L. PÉREZ-MARTÍNEZ,[a] J.R. BLANCO,[a] V. IBARRA,[a] AND J.A. OTEO[a]

[a]*Área de Enfermedades Infecciosas, Hospitales San Millán-San Pedro-de La Rioja, Logroño, (La Rioja), Spain*

[b]*Centro de Estudos de Vectores e Doenças Infecciosas, Instituto Nacional de Saúde Dr. Ricardo Jorge, Aguas de Moura, Portugal*

ABSTRACT: Our aim was to identify variants of *Anaplasma phagocytophilum* 16S rRNA gene sequences among products amplified from *Ixodes ricinus* collected in La Rioja, Spain. *A. phagocytophilum* AP-variant 1, reported as non-pathogenic, was detected in 12 samples (two adults and ten nymphs). This finding could justify the low incidence of human anaplasmosis in our area, despite the high prevalence of *A. phagocytophilum* in ticks.

KEYWORDS: *Anaplasma phagocytophilum*; human anaplasmosis; *Ixodes ricinus*; ticks; AP-Variant 1; Spain

INTRODUCTION

Human anaplasmosis (HA), previously designated as human granulocytic ehrlichiosis or HGE,[1] is an emerging tick-borne zoonosis transmitted by *Ixodes* ticks, specifically *Ixodes ricinus* in Europe. High prevalence of *Anaplasma* (formerly, *Ehrlichia*) *phagocytophilum* infection in *I. ricinus* from the North of Spain (La Rioja and Basque Country) has been reported.[2,3] However, to date, only sporadic cases of HA in Spain have been reported.[4,5] One hypothesis is that only a subset of the *A. phagocytophilum* strains that exist in nature cause human disease.[6–8] As little information exists about the host range and pathogenicity of different strains or variants of *A. phagocytophilum* in Europe, the objective of our study was to identify possible variants of *A. phagocytophilum* in *I. ricinus* collected in La Rioja (Spain) according to the sequence of 16S rRNA gene.

Address for correspondence: José A. Oteo, Área de Enfermedades Infecciosas. Hospitales San Millán-San Pedro-de La Rioja. Avda. Viana, No. 1. 26001, Logroño (La Rioja), Spain. Voice: 34 941 297275; fax: 34 941 297267.
jaoteo@riojasalud.es

Ann. N.Y. Acad. Sci. 1063: 333–336 (2005).
doi: 10.1196/annals.1355.053

MATERIAL AND METHODS

Two hundred and forty eight *I. ricinus* were tested for the pathogen. A total of 90 specimens (84 adults and 6 nymphs) were removed from cows (*Bos taurus*) in Villoslada de Cameros, a rural mountainous area from La Rioja, during November 2003. Since the collection from bovines (or any other potential animal reservoir) would favor the identification of *A. phagocytophilum* strains to which this host were susceptible and could not be representative of tick population, samples were also collected from vegetation. For this reason, in 2004 a total of 158 questing *I. ricinus* (54 adults and 104 nymphs) collected from six different sites of our region were also analyzed.

All ticks were classified according to standard taxonomic keys. Specimens were kept in 70% ethanol solution at room temperature and individually processed. Genomic DNA extraction for PCR was performed as described before.[9,10] Ticks were taken from the 70% ethanol solution, washed with sterile water, air dried and boiled for 20 min in 100 µL of 0.7 M ammonium hydroxide to free the DNA. After cooling, the vials with the lysed material were left open in a laminar airflow cabinet for 20 min at 90°C to evaporate the ammonia. The tick lysates were either used directly for PCR or stored at –20°C until used. DNA samples were pooled for initial PCR screening of 16S rRNA gene from *A. phagocytophilum* under conditions previously reported.[11] Individual samples corresponding to vials that yielded positive PCR results were additionally tested with the same primers. In addition, another pair of primers that targets the *msp2* gene was used to confirm all individual specimens that showed positive PCR results.[12] Quality control included both positive (*A. phagocytophilum* Webster, kindly provided by Dr. Dumler, from The Johns Hopkins University School of Medicine, Baltimore, USA) and negative controls that were extracted and PCR amplified in parallel with all specimens. Negative controls consisted of sterile water instead of template DNA. Subsequent sequence analysis of both strands of each amplicon of 16S rDNA [Universidad de Alcalá de Henares (Spain)] were carried out. Homology of nucleotide sequences was determined through the BLAST National Centre for Biotechnology Information (NCBI).[13]

RESULTS

Products of the expected sizes were amplified from DNA of one of 6 nymphs removed from cows (16.6%) when tested with 16S rRNA and *msp2* primers (919 and 550 bp, respectively). *A. phagocytophilum* was not detected in adult ticks removed from cows. For ticks collected from vegetation, 9 of 104 questing nymphs (8.6%), and 2 of 54 unfed host-seeking adult ticks (3.7%) were infected with *A. phagocytophilum*. For these 11 samples, 16S rDNA and *msp2* PCR amplifications were achieved. No products were amplified from any of the negative control samples.

Sequence homology searches of 16S rRNA gene revealed that these 12 sequences analyzed were identical, and all of them differed from that of the 16S rRNA sequence of a human *A. phagocytophilum* strain (GenBank accession no. U02521) by only two nucleotides: G and A in positions 76 and 84, respectively. These changes corresponded to the AP-variant 1 strain of *A. phagocytophilum* (GenBank accession no. AY193887) previously reported as potentially non-pathogenic in USA.[6,8] These specific nucleotide substitutions were not observed in our positive control (human-infective *A. phagocytophilum*).

DISCUSSION

AP-variant 1 has been previously found in *I. scapularis* ticks and deer blood in the USA but never from a confirmed human infection.[14,15] Identical portions of 16S rRNA gene from European *A. phagocytophilum* are available in GenBank. Sequences that showed 100% of identity to AP-variant 1 were derived from *I. ricinus* ticks in Sweden and Germany, and from roe deer in Switzerland and Slovenia (GenBank accession nos. AJ242784; AF136713; AY281806; AF384212; AF481850, among others).[16–20] The impact of *A. phagocytophilum* 16S rRNA gene variants has been a matter of debate. The sequence variability in one gene is not sufficient to determine the genetic diversity of a certain strain. It is necessary to cultivate some of the *A. phagocytophilum* strains and to compare them in animal models in order to unravel the biological significance of the observed genetic differences. The latest advances in this field were presented at the Fourth International Conference on Rickettsiae and Rickettsial Diseases held in Logroño, Spain.[21,22]

In conclusion, AP-variant 1 strain of *A. phagocytophilum* in *I. ricinus* has been detected for the first time in Spain. To date, this variant has not been associated with human disease, and its presence may belie the few clinical cases of HA on the peninsula in contrast with the high prevalence of *A. phagocytophilum* infection found in *I. ricinus* in this region. To our knowledge, this is the first study in which *A. phagocytophilum* DNA sequences derived from ticks in Spain were compared. Further studies are needed to compare *A. phagocytophilum* DNA sequences derived from ticks and HA patients in our region.

ACKNOWLEDGMENTS

We thank Fátima Bacellar, Rita de Sousa, and Maria Margarida Santos Silva, from the Centro de Estudos de Vectores e Doenças Infecciosas-Instituto Nacional de Saúde (Portugal), for their help and contribution to this work.

Financial support for this research was provided in part by grants from the Fondo de Investigación Sanitaria FIS (PI021810 and G03/057) from the Ministerio de Sanidad y Consumo (Spain), and also from the Fundação para a Ciência e a Tecnologia (BD/8610/2002) from the Ministério da Educação e Ensino Superior (Portugal).

[*Competing interests statement:* The authors state that they have no competing financial interests.]

REFERENCES

1. DUMLER, J.S., A.F. BARBET, C.P.J. BEKKER, *et al.* 2001. Reorganization of genera in the families *Rickettsiaceae* and *Anaplasmataceae* in the order *Rickettsiales*: unification of some species of *Ehrlichia* with *Anaplasma*, *Cowdria* with *Ehrlichia* and *Ehrlichia*

with *Neorickettsia*, descriptions of six new species combinations and designation of *Ehrlichia equi* and "HGE agent" as subjective synonyms of *Ehrlichia phagocytophila*. Int. J. Syst. Evol. Microbiol. **51:** 2145–2165.
2. OTEO, J.A., H. GIL, M. BARRAL, *et al.* 2001. Presence of granulocytic *Ehrlichia* in ticks and serological evidence of human infection in La Rioja, Spain. Epidemiol. Infec. **127:** 353–358.
3. BARRAL, M., L. BENEDICTO, H. GIL, *et al.* 1999. Detection of *Ehrlichia phagocytophila* DNA in *Ixodes ricinus* from areas in the North of Spain. *In* Rickettsiae and Rickettsial Diseases at the Turn of the Third Millennium. D. Raoult & P. Brouqui, Eds.: 428–431. Elsevier. Paris.
4. OTEO, J.A., J.R. BLANCO, V. MARTÍNEZ DE ARTOLA, *et al.* 2000. First report of human granulocytic ehrlichiosis from Southern Europe (Spain). Emerg. Infect. Dis. **6:** 430–431.
5. GARCÍA, J.C., M.J. NÚÑEZ, B. CASTRO, *et al.* 2006. Human granulocytic anaplasmosis: the first Spanish case confirmed by PCR. Ann. N.Y. Acad. Sci. In press.
6. MASSUNG, R.F., M.J. MAUEL, J.H. OWENS, *et al.* 2002. Genetic variants of *Ehrlichia phagocytophila*, Rhode Island and Connecticut. Emerg. Infect. Dis. **8:** 467–472.
7. STUEN, S., I. VAN DE POL, K. BERGSTRÖM, *et al.* 2002. Identification of *Anaplasma phagocytophila* (formerly *Ehrlichia phagocytophila*) variants in blood from sheep in Norway. J. Clin. Microbiol. **40:** 3192–3197.
8. MASSUNG, R.F., R.A. PRIESTLEY, N.J. MILLER, *et al.* 2003. Inability of a variant strain of *Anaplasma phagocytophilum* to infect mice. J. Infect. Dis. **188:** 1757–1763.
9. GUY, E.C. & G. STANEK. 1991. Detection of *Borrelia burgdorferi* in patients with Lyme disease by the polymerase chain reaction. J. Clin. Pathol. **44:** 610–611.
10. RIJPKEMA, S., D. GOLUBIC, M. MOLKENBOER, *et al.* 1996. Identification of four genomic groups of *Borrelia burgdorferi* sensu lato in *Ixodes ricinus* ticks collected in Lyme borreliosis endemic region of northern Croatia. Exp. Appl. Acarol. **20:** 23–30.
11. CHEN, S.M., J.S. DUMLER, J.S. BAKKEN, *et al.* 1994. Identification of granulocytotropic *Ehrlichia* species as the etiologic agent of human disease. J. Clin. Microbiol. **32:** 589–595.
12. CASPERSEN, K., J.H. PARK, S. PATIL, *et al.* 2002. Genetic variability and stability of *Anaplasma phagocytophila msp2* (p44). Infect. Immun. **70:** 1230–1234.
13. http://www.ncbi.nlm.gov/BLAST/
14. BELONGIA, E.A., K.D. REED, P.D. MITCHELL, *et al.* 1997. Prevalence of granulocytic *Ehrlichia* infection among white-tailed deer in Wisconsin. J. Clin. Microbiol. **35:** 1465–1468.
15. MASSUNG, R.F., M.J. MAUEL, J.H. OWENS, *et al.* 1998. Nested PCR assay for detection of granulocytic ehrlichiae. J. Clin. Microbiol. **36:** 1090–1095.
16. VON STEDINGK, L.V., M. GURTELSCHMID, H.S. HANSON, *et al.* 1997. The human granulocytic ehrlichiosis (HGE) agent in Swedish ticks. Clin. Microbiol. Infect. **3:** 573–574.
17. BAUMGARTEN, B.U., M. ROLLINGHOFF & C. BOGDAN. 1999. Prevalence of *Borrelia burgdorferi* and granulocytic and monocytic ehrlichiae in *Ixodes ricinus* ticks from Southern Germany. J. Clin. Microbiol. **37:** 3448–3451.
18. VON LOEWENICH, F.D., B.U. BAUMGARTEN, K. SCHRÖPPEL, *et al.* 2003. High diversity of *ankA* sequences of *Anaplasma phagocytophilum* among *Ixodes ricinus* ticks in Germany. J. Clin. Microbiol. **41:** 5033–5040.
19. LIZ, J.S., J.W. SUMNER, K. PFISTER, *et al.* 2002. PCR detection and serological evidence of granulocytic ehrlichial infection in roe deer (*Capreolus capreolus*) and chamois (*Rupicapra rupicapra*). J. Clin. Microbiol. **40:** 892–897.
20. PETROVEC, M., A. BIDOVEC, J.W. SUMNER, *et al.* 2002. Infection with *Anaplasma phagocytophila* in cervids from Slovenia: evidence of two genotypic lineages. Wien. Klin. Wochenschr. **114:** 641–647.
21. MASSUNG, R.F., M.L. LEVIN, N.J. MILLER, *et al.* 2005. Reservoir competency of goats for *Anaplasma phagocytophilum*. Presented at the Fourth International Conference on Rickettsiae and Rickettsial Diseases. Logroño, Spain, June 18.
22. MASSUNG, R.F., M.L. LEVIN, U.G. MUNDERLOH, *et al.* 2005. Isolation of *Anaplasma phagocytophilum* strain AP-variant 1 in a tick-derived cell line. Presented at the Fourth International Conference on Rickettsiae and Rickettsial Diseases. Logroño, Spain, June 18.

Phylogenetic Analysis of a Novel Molecular Isolate of Spotted Fever Group Rickettsiae from Northern Peru

Candidatus Rickettsia andeanae

JU JIANG,[a,b] PATRICK J. BLAIR,[c] VIDAL FELICES,[c] CECILIA MORON,[d] MANUEL CESPEDES,[d] ELIZABETH ANAYA,[d] GEORGE B. SCHOELER,[c] JOHN W. SUMNER,[e] JAMES G. OLSON,[c] AND ALLEN L. RICHARDS[a,f]

[a]*Naval Medical Research Center Silver Spring, Maryland, 20910, USA*

[b]*Henry M. Jackson Foundation, Rockville, Maryland, 20852, USA*

[c]*Naval Medical Research Center Detachment Lima, Peru*

[d]*National Institute of Health, Ministry of Health, Lima, Peru*

[e]*Centers for Disease Control and Prevention, Atlanta, Georgia, 30033, USA*

[f]*Uniformed Services University, Bethesda, Maryland, 20814, USA*

ABSTRACT: Phylogenetic analysis of five rickettsial genes (17-kDa gene, *gltA, ompB, ompA,* and *sca4*) from two molecular isolates of *Candidatus* Rickettsia andeanae from two ticks (*Amblyomma maculatum* and *Ixodes boliviensis*) collected from two domestic horses living in two separate locations in northern Peru (Coletas and Naranjo) was conducted to more clearly characterize this recently reported novel spotted fever group (SFG) rickettsia. Following nested polymerase chain reaction (PCR) amplification of the17-kDa gene, *gltA, ompB, ompA,* and *sca4*, amplicons were purified, sequenced, and compared to those downloaded from GenBank. Phylogenetic analyses of the *Candidatus* Rickettsia andeanae sequences generated from17-kDa gene (483 bp), *gltA* (1185 bp), *ompA* (1598 bp), *ompB* (4839 bp), and *sca4* (2634 bp) demonstrated that they aligned strongly with those of SFG rickettsiae. Moreover, the sequences of these five genes most closely aligned with the following rickettsiae: *ompA*: *Rickettsia* sp RpA4 (98.03%), *R.* sp DnS28 (97.90%), and *R. rhipicephali* and *R. massiliae* (97.11%); *ompB*: *R. aeschlimannii* (97.22%), *R. rhipicephali* (97.20%), and *R.* sp Bar 29 (97.10%); and *sca4*: *R. massiliae* (97.8%), *R. rhipicephali,* and *R. slovaca* (97.7%). These results from the additional phylogenetic analyses of *Candidatus* Rickettsia andeanae confirm its inclusion within, and distance and uniqueness from, other known SFG rickettsiae.

KEYWORDS: Peru; ticks; spotted fever rickettsiae; phylogenetic analysis

Address for correspondence: Allen L. Richards, Ph.D., Director, Rickettsial Diseases Department, Naval Medical Research Center, 503 Robert Grant Avenue, Silver Spring, MD 20910-7500. Voice: (301) 319-7668; fax: (301) 319-9458.
RichardsA@nmrc.navy.mil

**Ann. N.Y. Acad. Sci. 1063: 337–342 (2005). © 2005 New York Academy of Sciences.
doi: 10.1196/annals.1355.054**

INTRODUCTION

Between May and October 2002, a number of febrile cases, including two deaths, were reported in an area around the town of Sapillica in northern Peru. A joint investigation with representatives of the Peruvian Ministry of Health and Naval Medical Research Center Detachment, Lima, documented a high prevalence of antibodies to *Rickettsia* and *Leptospira* species.[1] During the investigation nucleic acid preparations extracted from blood samples obtained from febrile humans and peri-domestic rodents, and from fleas and ticks from individual domestic and wild-trapped animals, were determined by PCR as specific for four rickettsial genes, including: the *Rickettsia* genus–specific17-kDa outer membrane antigen gene (17-kDa gene), the citrate synthase gene (*gltA*), and the outer membrane protein A (*ompA*) and B (*ompB*) genes to contain evidence for the presence of SFG rickettsiae.[2] Initially, all samples were tested for presence of the 17-kDa gene, and if detected determination of whether the amplicon was from a typhus or spotted fever group rickettsia was made. Prevalence as determined from these tests demonstrated that 24% of febrile humans (4/17), 8.3% of trapped rodents (2/24), 1.6% of flea pools (1/59), and 25% of ticks (4/16) were positive for SFG agents. Further analysis of the molecular isolates utilizing PCR specific for the *gltA*, *ompA,* and *ompB* genes and sequencing the subsequent amplicons determined the phylogenetic relationships of the molecular isolates. In addition to detecting *R. felis* in flea triturates, we identified a new SFG family member molecularly isolated from two tick samples (tick 124 and tick 163).[2] Due to the more than 3% difference in sequence identity between a 2,484 bp sequence segment of *ompB* from the novel agent and those SFG rickettsiae sequences listed in GenBank, it was proposed that the new agent be named *Rickettsia andeanae*. Herein, we describe further the characterization of *Candidatus* Rickettsia andeanae based upon phylogenetic analysis of five rickettsial genes. Four of the genes have been previously assessed (17-kDa gene 434 bp; *gltA* 381 bp; *ompA* 540 bp; and *ompB* 2,484 bp)[2] however, for this project larger amplicons from 17-kDa gene (483 bp), *gltA* (1185 bp) *ompA* (1,589 bp), and *ompB* (4,839 bp), and 2,634 bp of *sca4* (120 kDa cytoplasmic protein gene; geneD) were analyzed and the results described in this report confirmed *Candidatus* Rickettsia andeanae inclusion within, and distance and uniqueness from other known SFG rickettsiae.

MATERIALS AND METHODS

Two molecular isolates of *Candidatus* Rickettsia andeanae from two ticks (*Amblyomma maculatum* and *Ixodes boliviensis*) collected from domestic horses living in two separate locations in Northern Peru (Coletas and Naranjo)[2] were evaluated by multilocus sequence typing to determine their relationship to other rickettsiae. Following amplification by standard polymerase chain reaction (PCR) of the 17-kDa gene and nested PCR amplification of *ompB, ompA,* and *sca4*, nucleic acid–derived from the two isolates, amplicons were purified and sequenced on an automated ABI Prism 3100 gene analyzer (Applied Biosystems, Foster City, CA) similar to that described previously.[2] However, new primers were used for PCR and sequencing in this study (TABLE 1). The sequences (both forward and reverse) were assembled with

TABLE 1. Primers for PCR, nested PCR, and sequencing

Target Gene	Primer	Sequence (5′-3′)	Amplicon Size (bp)
17-kDa antigen gene	Rp17kF1[ac]	AATGAGTTTTATACTTTACAAAAT-TCTAAAAACCA	532
	Rr1175F[ac]	GCTCTTGCAACTTCTATGTT	434
	Rr2608R[ac]	CATTGTTCGTCAGGTTGGCG	
gltA	CS1dF[abc]	ATGACTAATGGCAATAATAA	1254
	CS1273R[a]	CATAACCAGTGTAAAGCTG	
	CS1234R[bc]	TCTAGGTCTGCTGATTTTTTGTTCA	
	Rp CS877F[bc]	GGG GGC CTG CTC ACG GCG G	382
	Rp CS1258R[bc]	ATTGCAAAAAGTACAGTGAACA	
ompA	190-3588F[a]	AACAGTGAATGTAGGAGCAG	1630
	190-5238R[abc]	ACTATTAAAGGCTAGGCTATT	
	RompA1F[bc]	GAATAACATTACAVGCYGGAGGAAG	
	RrA657R[c]	TATTTGCATCAATCSYATAAGWA	
	RhoA4336F[c]	AGTTCAGGAAACGACCGTA	
ompB	RompB11F[a]	ACCATAGTAGCMAGTTTTGCAG	4887
	RompB4887R[ab]	AGAGTACCTTGATGTGCRGTATAYT	
	RompB2409F[bc]	CCGTAACATTAAACAAACAAGCTG	2479
	RompB2553R[bc]	GAATTTTCAAAAGCAATYGTATCAGT	2553
	RAK1009F[bc]	ACATKGTTATACARAGTGYTAATGC	
	RAK1452R[bc]	SGTTAACTTKACCGYTTATAACTGT	
	120-2788F[c]	AAACAATAATCAAGGTACTGT	
	RompB3521F[c]	GATAATGCCAATGCAAATTTCAG	
	RompB4224F[c]	ACCAAGATTATAAGAAAGGTGATAA	
	120-4346R[c]	CGAAGAAGTAACGCTGACTT	
	RompB3637R[c]	GAAACGATTACTTCCGGTTACA	
	RompB3008R[c]	AATATCGCTGACGGTCAAGGT	
	120-607F[c]	AATATCGCTGACGGTCAAGGT	
	120-807R[c]	CCTTTTAGATTACCGCCTAA	
	RR1595F[c]	GCCGGAGTTGTCCAATTATCA	
	RompB1902R[c]	CCGTCATTTCCAATAACTAACTC	
	RompB2012F[c]	GCCGGTACAAATTTAGGTAGTG	
sca4	D1f[abc]	ATGAGTAAAGACGGTAACCT	3069
	D3069r[abc]	TCAGCGTTGTGGAGGGGAAG	
	RrD749F[abc]	TGGTAGCATTAAAAGCTGATGG	
	RrD2685R[abc]	TTCAGTAGAAGATTTAGTACCAAAT	2706
	RrD928F[bc]	ATTTATACACTTGCGGTAACAC	
	RrD1826R[bc]	TCTAAATKCTGCTGMATCAAT	
	RrD1713F[c]	CTCTGAATTAAGCAATGCGGAAA	
	T5DR1[c]	CTGATAAAGCTGTAGCTGCATTA	
	D2338f[c]	GATGCAGCGAGTGAGGCAGC	
	D928r[c]	AAGCTATTGCGTCATCTCCG	

[a]Primers used for PCR amplification; [b]Primers used for nested PCR amplification; [c]Primers used for sequencing.

TABLE 2. *Candidatus* Rickettsia andeanae sequence identity with closest neighbors

Gene	Tick Sample	Sequence Length (bp)	Length of ORF to *R. conorii*	Position to ORF	Results (percent identity with closest neighbors)	Fournier and colleagues Cutoff Values[a]
17-kDa	Tick124	422		43~464	98.49% to *R. rickettsii*; 98.28% to *R. sibirica* and *R. conorii*; 98.06% to *R. rhipicephali*; 97.84% to *R. parkeri*	[b]
	Tick163	483	480	M30~464		
gltA	Tick124	354			99.42% to *Rickettsia* sp. DnS14; 99.34% to R.sp. RpA4, *R. sibirica* and R.sp. MC16, R.sp. BJ-90; 99.26% to *R. parkeri*, *R. slovaca* 99.17% to *R. conorii*, 99.12% to *R. aeschlimannii*; 99.09% to *R. rhipicephali*	99.9%
	Tick163	1185	1308	810~1163 45~1229		
ompA	Tick124 and Tick163	1598	6066	2880~4464	98.03% to R.sp. RpA4; 97.90% to R.sp. DnS28; 97.84% to R. sp. DnS14; 97.11% to *R. rhipicephali* and *R. massiliae*	98.8%
ompB	Tick124 and Tick163	4839	4968	89~4927	97.22% *to R. aeschlimannii*; 97.20% to *R. rhipicephali*; 97.10% to R. sp. Bar 29; 97.08% to *R. massiliae*; 96.10% to *R. slovaca*	99.2%
sca4	Tick124 and Tick163	2634	3081	39~2672	97.8% to *R. massiliae*; 97.7% to *R. rhipicephali* and *R. slovaca*; 97.6% to *R. aeschlimanii*; 97.5% to *R. conorii*	99.3%

Sequencher 4.0 software (Gene Codes Corp, Ann Arbor, MI) and compared to those downloaded from GenBank. Phylogenetic analyses (Neighbor Joining Best Tree and Bootstrap methods) were performed with MacVector 7.0 software (Accelrys, Inc, San Diego, CA).

RESULTS

17-kDa Gene and gltA

Comparing sequences of the *Candidatus* Rickettsia andeanae 17-kDa gene and *gltA* fragments with GenBank sequences indicate that *Candidatus* Rickettsia andeanae belongs within the genus *Rickettsia* by showing that the 483 bp 17-kDa gene segment had >97.5% identity with five SFG rickettsiae, but with no more then 98.5% identity with any rickettsial agent (TABLE 2). Similarly, the 1,185 bp *gltA* sequence fragment of *Candidatus* Rickettsia andeanne had 99.00–99.42% identity to ten SFG rickettsiae, but no identity with any rickettsial agent >99.42% (TABLE 2). Thus, the sequencing data from the17-kDa gene and *gltA* segments indicate that *Candidatus* Rickettsia andeanae is a rickettsial agent but not identical with any agent currently listed within GenBank.

ompA

Due to presence of *ompA* among SFG rickettsiae, and the lack of a complete *ompA* among TG rickettsiae, *R. bellii* and *R. canadensis*, the production of a PCR amplicon utilizing *ompA* specific primers corroborates the *gltA* data that suggests that *Candidatus* Rickettsia andeanae is closely related to SFG rickettsiae. In addition, phylogenetic analysis of a 1598 bp segment of *ompA* indicates that *Candidatus* Rickettsia andeanae has 98.03% identity with its closest neighbor, *Rickettsia* sp. RpA4, within the SFG (TABLE 2).

ompB

Initial data from the phylogenetic analysis of *ompB* sequence (2,484 bp) from *Candidatus* Rickettsia andeanae showed that it was ≥3% divergent from other SFG rickettsiae.[2] In this investigation an *ompB* fragment almost twice as large (4,839 bp) was sequenced and evaluated for its relationship to other rickettsial (and non-rickettsial) sequences. It was determined that the larger segment also showed an approximately 3% divergence from the *ompB* sequences of the closest relations, which were determined to be SFG rickettsiae (TABLE 2). The most closely related rickettsiae based upon comparison of the 4,839 bp fragment of *ompB* were *R. aeschlimannii* (97.22% identity), *R. rhipicephali* (97.20% identity), and *R*. sp. Bar 29 (97.10% identity). The *Candidatus* Rickettsia andeanae *ompB* sequence showed only 87.7 and 87.3% identity with *R. prowazekii* and *R. typhi*, respectively.

sca4

Sequence comparisons of part or all of *sca4* have recently been described as a tool for rickettsial phylogenetic analysis because the presence of the gene among the various species of *Rickettsia* and due to its moderate sequence variability among the *Rickettsia*.[3] Blast search with the 2,634 bp *sca4* segment sequence from *Candidatus* Rickettsia andeanae, showed that it was most closely related to SFG rickettsiae *R. massiliae* (97.8%), *R. rhipicephali* and *R. slovaca* (97.7%). Similar to the sequence comparison data discerned with *ompA* and *ompB*, *Candidatus* Rickettsia andeanae *sca4* sequence shows a close relationship to SFG rickettsiae, but is divergent enough to be considered a unique rickettsial species (TABLE 2).

DISCUSSION

Multilocus sequence typing (MLST) for the characterization of pathogenic and non-pathogenic microorganisms utilizes the sequences from several gene segments to characterize the genetic makeup of an isolate.[4] The sequences are compared to those already obtained for similar and dissimilar organisms. From the comparison a determination is made as to the relationship between the new isolate and known isolates. This is very helpful in ascertaining the identity of an isolate(s) during an outbreak investigation, historical classification, or taxonomic relationships and has been used to characterize rickettsial agents.[3,5] In this investigation PCR amplified segments from five well known genes were used to validate the divergence of the novel isolate, *Candidatus* Rickettsia andeanae, from those rickettsiae previously characterized utilizing the criteria proposed by Fournier and colleagues.[3] The results presented herein confirm our earlier report[2] by extending the sequences assessed for four genes (17 kDa gene, *gltA, ompA,* ompB) and newly assessing the sequence of *sca4*. Collectively these results show the uniqueness of *Candidatus* Rickettsia andeanae, a novel agent that has been molecularly isolated from two different ticks collected from two different horses from two locations in northern Peru. However, an isolate has not been cultured in the laboratory and therefore the pathogenicity of this agent has not been ascertained. Collaborators in Peru are actively pursuing a course for cultivating this agent in their laboratory.

ACKNOWLEDGMENTS

The work reported herein was supported by the DoD GEIS program and its work unit number was 0000188M.0931.001.A0074. The opinions and assertions contained herein are the private ones of the authors and are not to be construed as official or reflecting the views of the Department of the Navy, the Department of Defense or the U.S. Government.

REFERENCES

1. BLAIR, P.J., G.B. SCHOELER, C. MORON, *et al.* 2004. Evidence of rickettsial and leptospira infections in Andean Northern Peru. Am. J. Trop. Med. Hyg. **70:** 357–363.
2. BLAIR, P.J., J. JIANG, G.B. SCHOELER, *et al.* 2004. Characterization of spotted fever group rickettsiae in flea and tick specimens from northern Peru. J. Clin. Microbiol. **42:** 4961–4967.
3. FOURNIER, P-E., J.S. DUMLER, G. GILBERT, *et al.* 2003. Gene sequence-based criteria for identification of new *Rickettsia* isolates and description of *Rickettsia heilongjiangensis* sp. nov. J. Clin. Microbiol. **41:** 5456–5465.
4. MAIDEN, M.C.J., J.A BYGRAVES, E. FEIL, *et al.* 1998. Multilocus sequence typing: a portable approach to the identification of clones within populations of pathogenic microorganisms. Proc. Natl. Acad. Sci. USA **95:** 3140–3145.
5. ISHIKURA, M., S. ANDO, Y. SHINAGAWA, *et al.* 2003. Phylogenetic analysis of spotted fever group rickettsiae based on gltA, 17-kDa, and rOmpA genes amplified by nested PCR from ticks in Japan. Microbiol. Immunol. **47:** 823–832.

Molecular and Biological Characterization of a Novel *Coxiella*-like Agent from *Carios capensis*

WILL K. REEVES,[a] AMANDA D. LOFTIS,[a] RACHAEL A. PRIESTLEY,[a] WILLIAM WILLS,[b] FELICIA SANDERS,[c] AND GREGORY A. DASCH[a]

[a]*Centers for Disease Control and Prevention, Atlanta, Georgia 30333, USA*

[b]*Clemson University, Department of Entomology, Soils, and Plant Sciences, Clemson, South Carolina, USA*

[c]*South Carolina Department of Natural Resources, Santee Coastal Reserve, McClellanville, South Carolina, USA*

ABSTRACT: The genus *Coxiella* is currently defined by a single monotypic species, *Coxiella burnetii*. Novel *Coxiella* spp. have been detected in ticks throughout the world. These bacteria have not been cultured or named, and their evolutionary relationships to *C. burnetii* are poorly known. A novel *Coxiella*-like agent was detected by PCR amplification and sequencing of DNA extracted from 64 pelican ticks, *Carios capensis*, from Devoux Bank, South Carolina, USA. PCR was used to amplify and characterize genes from the new bacterium. Sequences from some metabolic and housekeeping genes shared a 92–98% similarity to *C. burnetii*, but other genes such as the IS1111 transposon, *com*1, and 5S and 16S rRNA genes were not amplified by conventional PCR. Transovarial and transtadial transmission and environmental shedding of the agent were detected by PCR.

KEYWORDS: Argasidae; *Coxiella*; characterization; novel species

The genus *Coxiella* is currently defined by a single monotypic species, *Coxiella burnetii*. The evolutionary origin of *C. burnetii* is unknown, but novel *Coxiella* spp. and *Coxiella*-like agents have been described from species of both hard and soft ticks, including *Haemaphysalis*, *Ixodes*, *Ornithodoros,* and *Rhipicephalus.*[1–5] These bacteria have not been cultured, and their genetic diversity and biological similarity to *C. burnetii* are poorly defined. A novel genotype of *Rickettsia* was detected in a bat tick, *Carios kelleyi,*[6] so we examined *C. capensis* for a similar *Rickettsia*. *Carios capensis* bites humans and the bite can cause fever, headache, and skin irritation. These ticks are vectors of Soldado virus and their association with potential rickettsial pathogens is of concern. We discovered a novel bacterial agent in *C. capensis*

The findings and conclusions in this report are those of the authors and do not necessarily represent the views of the funding agency.

Address for correspondence: Gregory A. Dasch, Centers for Disease Control and Prevention; 1600 Clifton Rd. NE, MS G-13, Atlanta, GA 30333, USA. Voice: 404-639-4151; fax: 404-639-4436.
cui8@cdc.gov

**Ann. N.Y. Acad. Sci. 1063: 343–345 (2005). © 2005 New York Academy of Sciences.
doi: 10.1196/annals.1355.055**

and further characterized this agent by DNA sequencing using primers designed to detect *C. burnetii* genes.

All 64 *C. capensis* collected from a pelican roost at Devoux Bank, South Carolina, USA and 8 of 10 ticks from a colony maintained at Colorado State University (CSU) contained DNA most similar to that of *C. burnetii*, which was detected by PCR amplification and sequencing of the *muc*Z gene. We tested the DNA extracts with previously published primers used to amplify genes from *C. burnetii*[7–18] and designed novel primers for selected genes based on the genome sequence of *C. burnetii*. All amplicons obtained were sequenced and compared to known sequences using the BLAST 2.0 program.

Primers based on genes of *Coxiella burnetii* produced amplicons from the total DNA extracts, including the *muc*Z (DNAj-like protein) (CBU1873), *htp*B (*gro*EL) (CBU1718), *glt*A (CBU1410), *sod*B (CBU1708), 16S rDNA gene, 16S-23S internal transcribed spacer (ITS) region *rfb*I (CBU0704), export permease (CBU0461), dehydrogenase E2 component acyltransferase (CBU0638), putative dehydrogenase E1 component beta subunit (CBU0639), CTP synthase (CBU1682), ADP-heptose synthase (CBU1655), and *icd* (CBU1200) genes. Sequence similarities between these gene sequences and those of *C. burnetii* ranged from 92–98%. Previously, 16S rDNA gene sequences were the primary evidence obtained to differentiate *C. burnetii* from *Coxiella* sp. and *Coxiella*-like agents in other ticks.[1,3–5] Our success at amplifying metabolic genes such as *htp*B and *sod*B with PCR primers designed for detection of DNA of *C. burnetii* in environmental samples indicates that PCR-based diagnoses of *C. burnetii* without confirmation by DNA sequencing is unreliable.

Standard PCR assays, which failed to amplify DNA from the DNA samples, included those for the IS1111 transposon, *com*1 (CBU1910) gene, 5S and 23S rDNA genes, riboflavin synthase (CBU0646), and GDP-fucose synthase (CBU0688) genes. These genes could be lacking from this novel bacterium or could vary in sequence at the primer sites and thus be undetectable. GDP-fucose synthetase is essential in producing virenose, a polysaccharide unique to *C. burnetii*. The IS1111 transposon occurs in up to 20 copies in the *C. burnetii* genome. The apparent modification or lack of this transposable element in this *Coxiella*-like agent suggests that *C. burnetii* could have acquired this element at some later time during its evolution.

The *muc*Z PCR assay was used to amplify DNA from this novel *Coxiella*-like agent from eggs, larvae, and adult ticks, as well as the washings of tick housing chambers. Ticks that molted in the laboratory retained the DNA from this *Coxiella*-like agent and laboratory-maintained ticks from Colorado State University were infected. These data suggest that this agent is vertically maintained by the ticks both transstadially and transovarially and that the tick might shed the agent into the environment.

In conclusion, like other soft and hard ticks, *C. capensis* harbors a novel *Coxiella* sp. or *Coxiella*-like agent that appears to be maintained transovarially and transstadially. Since the prevalence of *Coxiella* spp. and *Coxiella*-like agents might vary considerably in the ticks, the near 100% carriage rate found in *C. capensis* could be typical for this species. The presence of these agents in other ticks could be underrepresented, because suitable PCR primers are not being employed. The amount of genetic and biological information on *Coxiella* spp. and *Coxiella*-like agents is limited, and they could represent one or more novel species of *Coxiella* or other microorganisms and could pose a risk to human and animal health.

[*Competing interests statement:* The authors state that they have no competing financial interests.]

REFERENCES

1. LEE, J.H., H.S. PARK, W.J. JANG, *et al.* 2004. Identification of the *Coxiella* sp. detected from *Haemaphysalis longicornis* ticks in Korea. Micro. Immun. **48:** 125–130.
2. ROSHDY, M.A. 1968. A rickettsialike (*sic*) microorganism in the tick *Ornithodoros savignyi*; observations on its structure and distribution in the tissues of the tick. J. Invert. Path. **11:** 155–169.
3. MEDIANNIKOV, O.V., L. IVANOV, M. NISKIKAWA, *et al.* 2003. Molecular evidence of Coxiella-like microorganism harbored by *Haemaphysalis concinnae* in the Russian Far East. Ann. N.Y. Acad. Sci. **990:** 226–228.
4. NODA, H., U.G. MUNDERLOH & T.J. KURTTI. 1997. Endosymbionts of ticks and their relationship to *Wolbachia* spp. and tick-borne pathogens of human and animals. Appl. Environ. Microbiol. **63:** 3926–3932.
5. BERNASCONI, M.V., S. CASATI, O. PETER & J.C. PIFFARETTI. 2002. *Rhipicephalus* ticks infected with *Rickettsia* and *Coxiella* in Southern Switzerland (Canton Ticino). Infect. Genet. Evol. **2:** 111–120.
6. LOFTIS, A.D, J.S. GILL, M.E. SCHRIFFER, *et al.* 2005. Detection of *Rickettsia*, *Borrelia*, and *Bartonella* in *Carios kelleyi* (Acari: Argasidae). J. Med. Entomol. **42:** 473–480.
7. WILLEMS, H., D. THIELE, R. FROLICH-RITTER & H. KRAUSS. 1994. Detection of *Coxiella burnetii* in cow's milk using the polymerase chain reaction (PCR). J. Vet. Med. B **41:** 580–587.
8. STEIN, A., D. KRUSZEWSKA, J. GOUVERNET & D. RAOULT. 1997. Study of the 16-23S ribosomal DNA internal spacer of *Coxiella burnetii*. Eur. J. Epidem. **13:** 471–475.
9. AFSETH, G., Y. MO & L.P. MALLAVINA. 1995. Characterization of the 23S and 5S rRNA genes of *Coxiella burnetii* and identification of an intervening sequence within the 23S rRNA gene. J. Bacteriol. **177:** 2946–2949.
10. IBRAHIM, A., L. NORLANDER, A. MACELLARO & A. SJOSTEDT. 1997. Specific detection of *Coxiella burnetii* through partial amplification of the 23S rDNA. Eur. J. Epidem. **13:** 329–334.
11. MOLLET, C., M. DRANCOURT & D. RAOULT. 1998. Determination of *Coxiella burnetii rpoB* sequence and its use for phylogenetic analysis. Gene **207:** 97–103.
12. ZHANG, G.Q., S. V. NGUYEN, H. TO, *et al.* 1998. Clinical evaluation of a new PCR assay for detection of *Coxiella burnetii* in human serum samples. J. Clin. Microbiol. **36:** 77–80.
13. SESHADRI, R. & J.E. SAMUEL. 2001. Characterization of a stress-induced alternate sigma factor, RpoS, of *Coxiella burnetii* and its expression during the development cycle. Infect. Immun. **69:** 4874–4883.
14. STEIN, A. & D. RAOULT. 1992. Detection of *Coxiella burnetii* by DNA amplification using polymerase chain reaction. J. Clin. Microbiol. **30:** 2462–2466.
15. MEDIANNIKOV, O., L. IVANOV, M. NISHIKAWA, *et al.* 2003. Molecular evidence of *Coxiella*-like microorganism harbored by *Haemaphysalis concinnae* ticks in the Russian Far East. Ann. N.Y. Acad. Sci. **990:** 226–228.
16. SEKEYOVA, Z., V. ROUX & D. RAOULT. 1999. Intraspecies diversity of *Coxiella burnetii* as revealed by *com1* and *mucZ* sequence comparison. FEMS Microbiol. Lett. **180:** 61–67.
17. LEE, J., H. PARK, W. JANG, *et al.* 2004. Identification of the *Coxiella* sp. detected from *Haemaphysalis longicornis* ticks in Korea. Microbiol. Immunol. **48:** 125–130.
18. YUASA, Y., K. YOSHIIE, T. TAKASAKI, *et al.* 1996. Retrospective survey of chronic Q fever in Japan by using PCR to detect *Coxiella burnetii* DNA in paraffin-embedded clinical samples. J. Clin. Microbiol. **34:** 824–827.

DEBONEL/TIBOLA

Is *Rickettsia slovaca* the Only Etiological Agent?

V. IBARRA,[a] A. PORTILLO,[b] S. SANTIBÁÑEZ,[a] J.R. BLANCO,[a]
L. PÉREZ-MARTÍNEZ,[a] J. MÁRQUEZ,[b] AND J.A. OTEO[a]

[a]*Área de Enfermedades Infecciosas, Hospitales San Millán-San Pedro-de La Rioja, Logroño (La Rioja), Spain*

[b]*Departamento de Biología Animal, Vegetal y Ecología, Universidad de Jaén, Spain*

KEYWORDS: **DEBONEL/TIBOLA; *Rickettsia slovaca; Rickettsia* sp.; Spain; *Dermacentor marginatus***

INTRODUCTION

A few years ago, a new disease (DEBONEL/TIBOLA) transmitted by *Dermacentor marginatus* was described.[1] The main implicated agent, *Rickettsia slovaca,* was detected in patients from France and Hungary by PCR.[2] In 2003, *R. slovaca* was isolated from a French patient's skin biopsy, which demonstrates its implication as etiological agent.[3] However, it is possible that some cases of DEBONEL/TIBOLA are caused by other related *Rickettsia* species, since other Spotted Fever Group *Rickettsia* (SFGR) have been detected in the vector.

The aim of this study was to investigate the presence of *Rickettsia* spp. in *D. marginatus* ticks attached to symptomatic and asymptomatic people.

MATERIAL AND METHODS

From January 2001 to December 2004, 14 people attended to our Hospital with a *D. marginatus* specimen attached. All ticks were removed and examined for the presence of SFGR. DNA was extracted from ticks using QIAamp Tissue Kit (QIAGEN, Hilden, Germany). PCR assays with specific primers (*ompA*, *gltA,* and 16S rRNA genes) were performed.[4–6] Sequencing reactions were carried out and results were analyzed through GenBank database.

Address for correspondence: José A. Oteo, Área de Enfermedades Infecciosas, Hospitales San Millán-San Pedro-de La Rioja, Avda. Viana, No. 1, 26001, Logroño (La Rioja), Spain. Voice: 34 941 297275; fax: 34 941 297267.
jaoteo@riojasalud.es

Ann. N.Y. Acad. Sci. 1063: 346–348 (2005). © 2005 New York Academy of Sciences.
doi: 10.1196/annals.1355.056

Human epidemiological data (age, sex, and season when disease occurred) as well as clinical features (incubation period and site of the tick attachment) were collected for each patient.

RESULTS

All ticks removed from people (*N*=14) were infected with SFGR. By sequencing procedure, eight of them (58%) were identified as *R. slovaca* (100% similarity), while the remaining six (42%) were identified as *Rickettsia* sp. strains RpA4, DnS14 and DnS28 (98% similarity). Ten patients (72%) developed symptoms and signs of DEBONEL/TIBOLA, and four of them (28%) did not develop any clinical manifestation. All patients bitten by a *D. marginatus* specimen infected with *R. slovaca* (*N*=8) developed DEBONEL/TIBOLA. Moreover, only two patients (33%) bitten by *D. marginatus* infected with *Rickettsia* sp. strains RpA4, DnS14 and DnS28 developed disease. Nevertheless, the epidemiological and clinical data were similar in both groups. Neither of the asymptomatic people was bitten by *D. marginatus* infected with *R. slovaca.*

DISCUSSION

All *D. marginatus* removed from patients with DEBONEL/TIBOLA were infected with SFGR. Eighty per cent of *Rickettsia* species detected within *D. marginatus* removed from patients were identified as *R. slovaca.* The remaining ones (20%) were similar to *Rickettsia* sp. strains RpA4, DnS14 and DnS28. These data suggest the role of *Rickettsia* sp. strains RpA4, DnS14 and DnS28 in the etiology of DEBONEL/TIBOLA. However, these *Rickettsia* strains are probably less pathogenic than *R. slovaca* since all patients bitten by *D. marginatus* infected with *R. slovaca* developed DEBONEL/TIBOLA, while only 33% patients bitten by ticks infected by *Rickettsia* sp. RpA4, DnS14, and DnS28 developed this disease.

ACKNOWLEDGMENTS

This study was supported in part by grants from the Fondo de Investigación Sanitaria (FIS PI021810 and G03/057), Ministerio de Sanidad y Consumo, Spain.

[*Competing interests statement:* The authors state that they have no conflicting financial interests.]

REFERENCES

1. Oteo, J.A., V. Ibarra, J.R. Blanco, *et al.* 2004. *Dermacentor*-borne necrosis erythema and lymphadenopathy: clinical and epidemiological features of a new tick-borne disease. Clin. Microbiol. Infect. **10:** 327–331.
2. Raoult, D., A. Lakos, F. Fenollar, *et al.* 2002. Spotless rickettsiosis caused by *Rickettsia slovaca* and associated with *Dermacentor* tick. Clin. Infect. Dis. **34:** 1331–1336.

3. CAZORLA, C., M. ENEA, F. LUCHT, *et al.* 2003. First isolation of *Rickettsia slovaca* from a patient, France. Emerg. Infect. Dis. **9:** 135.
4. REGNERY, R.L., C.L. SPRUILL & B.D. PLIKAYTIS. 1991. Genotypic identification of rickettsiae and estimation of intraspecies sequence divergence for portions of two rickettsial genes. J. Bacteriol. **173:** 1576–1589.
5. WEISBURG, W.G., M.E. DOBSON, J.E. SAMUEL, *et al.* 1989. Phylogenetic diversity of the *Rickettsiae*. J. Bacteriol. **171:** 4202–4206.
6. MÁRQUEZ, F.J., M.A. MUNIAIN, J.M. PÉREZ, *et al.* 2002. Presence of *Rickettsia felis* in the cat flea from southwestern Europe. Emerg. Infect. Dis. **8:** 89–91.

Low Risk of Developing Human *Rickettsia aeschlimannii* Infection in the North of Spain

J.A. OTEO,[a] A. PORTILLO,[a] J.R. BLANCO,[a] V. IBARRA,[a] L. PÉREZ-MARTÍNEZ,[a] C. IZCO,[a] A. PÉREZ-PALACIOS,[b] AND S. JIMÉNEZ[b]

[a]*Area de Enfermedades Infecciosas, Hospitales San Millán-San Pedro-de La Rioja, 26001 Logroño (La Rioja), Spain*

[b]*Consejería de Salud. Gobierno de La Rioja. Logroño (La Rioja), Spain*

KEYWORDS: **Human *Rickettsia aeschlimannii* infection; Spain; *Hyalomma marginatum***

INTRODUCTION

During the last twenty years, numerous *Rickettsiae* and rickettsial diseases have been described. The fact of improving culture media and the use of molecular tools such as PCR assays and sequencing, have allowed us to implicate *Rickettsia* spp. that were thought to be non-pathogenic in human infections.

Rickettsia aeschlimannii, a Spotted Fever Group *Rickettsia* (SFGR), has been recently involved as human pathogen, and at least, two cases from Africa have been published.[1,2] On the other hand, this *Rickettsia* species has been detected in Spain within the implicated vector, *Hyalomma marginatum*.[3,4] For this reason, it is possible that some Spotted Fever rickettsiosis diagnosed after tick bite are caused by this *Rickettsia* in our environment, where *H. marginatum* ticks represent 4% of human-biting ticks (data not shown). The aim of this study is to know the risk of developing human *R. aeschlimannii* infection in La Rioja (Northern Spain).

MATERIAL AND METHODS

From January 2002 to December 2004, all patients who attended to our Hospital with a *H. marginatum* specimen attached were included in the study ($N = 5$). All ticks were removed with forceps by physicians. Clinical follow-up was carried out for all cases. IgG serological tests based on indirect immunofluorescence assays (IFA) with *R. conorii* antigen (BioMerieux Laborattories, Marcy l'Etiole, France) were performed. Ticks removed from these patients were screened for the presence

Address for correspondence: José A. Oteo, Área de Enfermedades Infecciosas, Hospitales San Millán-San Pedro-de La Rioja, Avda. de Viana no. 1, 26001 Logroño (La Rioja), Spain. Voice: 34 941 297275; fax: 34 941 297267.

jaoteo@riojasalud.es

Ann. N.Y. Acad. Sci. 1063: 349–351 (2005). © 2005 New York Academy of Sciences. doi: 10.1196/annals.1355.057

of SFGR by partial amplification of the *ompA* (semi-nested PCR using primers Rr190.70p and Rr190.701n, and Rr190.70p and Rr190.602n for the primary and semi-nested amplification reactions, respectively) and *gltA* genes.[5] Questing *H. marginatum* ticks collected by blanket dragging on vegetation in La Rioja ($N = 55$; 1 adult and 54 larvae) as well as *H. marginatum* removed from cows ($N = 110$; 95 adults and 15 nymphs) were also tested with PCR using the same pairs of primers. Ticks were kept in 70% alcohol before being processed. They were rinsed in distilled water and dried on sterile filter paper. Each tick was crushed using a sterile pestle and its DNA was extracted individually using the QIAamp Tissue kit (QIAGEN, Hilden, Germany), following the manufacturer's instructions. Amplified *ompA* PCR products were purified and both strands of each product were sequenced. Nucleotide sequence homology searches were made at the network server of the National Center for Biotechnology Information (NCBI) using BLAST.

RESULTS

Patients

Neither of the patients with a *H. marginatum* specimen attached ($N = 5$) developed either clinical manifestations or IgG antibodies against SFGR. An itching papule at the site of the tick attachment was observed on two patients

Ticks from Patients

Two of 5 ticks (40%) were infected by SFGR. Comparison of the sequences to those deposited in Genbank by using BLAST service revealed that our samples were 100% identical to a portion of *ompA* gene of *R. aeschlimannii*. No other SFGR were found in the studied ticks.

Ticks from Vegetation

Neither of them was infected with SFGR.

Ticks from Cows

One adult specimen (0.9%) carried *R. aeschlimannii.*

DISCUSSION

As written above, several rickettsial diseases have been described in the last years. Some of them, such as African tick-bite fever or *R. slovaca* infection (DEBONEL-TIBOLA) seem to be very frequent in located areas, while others (i.e., *R. aeschlimannii* infection) remain to be studied. In our two cases, after being bitten by *R. aeschlimannii*–infected ticks, none was infected. Furthermore, the prevalence of infection with *R. aeschlimannii* within *H. marginatum* in our area is very low. In conclusion, the risk of human infection by *R. aeschlimannii* is very low in our region.

ACKNOWLEDGMENTS

Study partly supported by a grant from the Fondo de Investigación Sanitaria (G03/057), Ministerio de Sanidad y Consumo, Spain.

[*Competing interests statement:* The authors state that they have no conflicting financial interests.]

REFERENCES

1. Raoult, D., P.E. Fournier, P. Abboud, *et al.* 2002. First documented human *Rickettsia aeschlimannii* infection. Emerg. Infect. Dis. **8:** 748–749.
2. Pretorius, A.M. & R.J. Birtles. 2002. *Rickettsia aeschlimannii*: A new pathogenic spotted fever group rickettsia, South Africa. Emerg. Infect. Dis. **8:** 874.
3. Fernández-Soto, P., A. Encinas-Grandes & R. Pérez-Sánchez. 2003. *Rickettsia aeschlimannii* in Spain: molecular evidence in *Hyalomma marginatum* and five other tick species that feed on humans. Emerg, Infect. Dis. **9:** 889–890.
4. Oteo, J.A., A. Portillo, S. Santibáñez, *et al.* 2005. Prevalence of Spotted Fever Group *Rickettsia* (SFGR) species detected in ticks in La Rioja, Spain. Ann. N.Y. Acad. Sci. This volume.
5. Regnery, R.L., C.L. Spruill & B.D. Plikaytis. 1991. Genotypic identification of rickettsiae and estimation of intraspecies sequence divergence for portions of two rickettsial genes. J. Bacteriol. **173:** 1576–1589.

Novel Spotted Fever Group Rickettsiae (SFGR) Infecting *Amblyomma americanum* Ticks in Ohio, USA

D.J. KELLY,[a] J.R. CARMICHAEL,[b] G.C. BOOTON,[a] K.F. POETTER,[b] AND P.A. FUERST[a]

[a]*Department of Evolution, Ecology and Organismal Biology and* [b]*Department of Molecular Genetics, The Ohio State University, Columbus, Ohio 43210, USA*

KEYWORDS: ***Rickettsia*; *Amblyomma americanum; Dermacentor variabilis; Rickettsia* amblyommii sp. nov.; infection prevalence; vectors; Rocky Mountain spotted fever**

OBJECTIVES

To determine the prevalence, species composition, and genetic diversity of tick-borne rickettsiae found in *Amblyomma americanum* ticks in Ohio.

BACKGROUND

Responding to cases of tick-borne Rocky Mountain spotted fever (RMSF), the Ohio Department of Health (ODH) Vector-Borne Disease Unit (VBDU) initiated a tick testing program in 1964. Health care professionals in Ohio and other states submitted ticks collected from pets or patients. Primarily, samples of the American dog tick (*Dermacentor variabilis*), the vector of *Rickettsia rickettsii*, were tested for rickettsiae. ODH-VBDU also frequently received lone star ticks (*Amblyomma americanum*), but, as less likely vectors, these were not tested for rickettsiae until recently.

In 1974 an unknown "non-pathogenic" rickettsiae, designated WB-8-2, was isolated from an *A. americanum* tick collected in Tennessee.[1] Subsequently, in 1985, a similar form (MO-1084) was isolated from a tick collected at Fort Leonard Wood, Missouri.[2] Analyses in our laboratory of the 16S rRNA gene and the 17-kDa cell surface antigen protein gene showed that these isolates carried identical genotypes for the genes and the name "*R.* amblyommii" sp. nov. was proposed.[3] This form has so far been found in *A. americanum*, but not in ticks from the genera *Dermacentor* or *Rhipicephalus*.

Address for correspondence: D.J. Kelly, Department of Evolution, Ecology and Organismal Biology, The Ohio State University, 318 W. 12th Avenue, Columbus, OH 43210. Voice: 614-292-4570; fax: 614-292-2030.
kelly.350@osu.edu

Ann. N.Y. Acad. Sci. 1063: 352–355 (2005). © 2005 New York Academy of Sciences.
doi: 10.1196/annals.1355.058

Rickettsia bellii was isolated in 1966, and is usually associated with *Dermacentor* sp., and with some argasid ticks. To our knowledge, it has not been reported in *A. americanum*. In Ohio, *Dermacentor variabilis* is known to carry *R. rickettsii*, and *R. montanensis,* in addition to *R. bellii*. Since *D. variabilis* and *A. americanum* are likely to share mammalian hosts, *A. americanum* may serve as host for these other rickettsiae. Here, we seek to determine prevalence, species identification, and genetic diversity of nonpathogenic rickettsiae in *A. americanum* ticks collected primarily in Ohio.

MATERIALS AND METHODS

Specimens of *A. americanum* were sent directly from veterinarians, clinicians, or local health departments to ODH-VBDU from various locales as part of the tick screening program. *A. americanum* ticks, mostly attached to humans and collected primarily in Ohio in 2003 submitted to ODH-VBDU were subsequently provided to our laboratory. Frozen ticks (–20°C) were surface sterilized in 70% ethanol, washed in distilled water, and chopped in extraction buffers using a sterile needle to expose internal tissues. Genomic DNA was extracted using the PrepMan Ultra extraction solution (Applied Biosystems, Foster City, CA, USA) or a combination of the Isoquick Extraction Kit (Orca Research, Bothell, WA, USA) and DNeasy Tissue Kit (Quiagen Sciences, Valencia, CA, USA). Semi-nested PCR was done in a Whatman-Biometra thermal cycler (Biometra Biomedicine Analytik, Goettigen, Germany) with paired genus-specific oligonucleotide primers (17kD-5′ GCTTTACAAAA TTCTAAAAACCATATA; 17kD-3′ CTTGCCATTGTCCRTCAGGTTG; and 17kD-3′ nest TCACGGCAATATTGACC). These primer sequences were designed based upon work done in our laboratory.[3] Distilled water was used as a negative control for the primary PCR, a portion of which was reamplified as the semi-nested PCR negative control. Amplicons derived from semi-nested PCR were approximately 434 bp. Conditions for both primary and semi-nested PCR were as follows: 10 min at 95°C, 35 cycles of 1 min at 95°C, 1 min at 52°C, 1 min at 72°C, 15 min extension at 72°C). Direct sequencing of the PCR product was done using the Big Dye Terminator Sequencing Kit, using sequencing primer 17kD-5′seq-GGTTCTCAATTYGG and the ABI 310 system (Applied Biosystems).

RESULTS

A subset of *A. americanum* ticks obtained during the 2003 tick screening program of the ODH-VBDU were surveyed for the presence of rickettsiae using PCR and DNA sequencing. Prior to 2003, *Amblyomma* ticks were not routinely examined for the presence of tick-borne pathogens. Nine of 21 *Amblyomma* ticks examined (43%) showed evidence of carrying rickettsiae. Of the nine rickettsia-positive ticks, eight (89%) were carrying strains identified by sequence analysis as *R. amblyommii* sp. nov. A single tick was found to carry a strain identified as *R. bellii*. Geographically, the ticks that were studied in this subset of material from the ODH-VBDU tick screen represented material primarily from central and south Ohio. These are regions that have been shown to have relatively high incidence of RMSF and to have a high occurrence of *D. variabilis* ticks found to be rickettsiae-positive.

DISCUSSION

Results for the molecular survey of *A. americanum* from the 2003 ODH-VBDU tick screening program showed a high prevalence of rickettsiae-positive ticks (43%). This is much higher than seen in screens of *Dermacentor,* where rickettsiae-positive ticks, assessed by hemolymph staining and IFA screening were consistently observed in frequencies ~ 4–5% over a number of years.

Rickettsiae-positive *Amblyomma* ticks are identified in the same parts of Ohio where rickettsiae-positive *Dermacentor* ticks were observed. However, the distribution of the forms of *Rickettsia* found in *Amblyomma* compared to those found in *Dermacentor* was quite different. In *Amblyomma* from Ohio, almost all rickettsiae were identified, using molecular methods, as *R.* amblyommii sp. nov. A single tick carried a strain of *R. bellii*. In contrast, using molecular methods to identify rickettsial forms carried by *D. variabilis* ticks in Ohio from earlier years, we found that the most frequent form was *R. bellii* (82% of isolates identified using molecular screens in our laboratory). In addition, two Spotted Fever Group forms, *R. montanensis* (12.5% of isolates) and *R. rickettsii* (5.5% of isolates) are also identified in *D. variabilis*. No isolates of *R. amblyommii* sp. nov. were observed in *D. variabilis*. It appears that the two tick groups do not easily exchange rickettsiae through intermediate mammalian hosts.

A. americanum is a vector for ehrlichial pathogens. The current study has not assessed the presence of any *Ehrlichia* in these ticks. Occurrence/co-occurrence of rickettsiae and ehrlichiae within *A. americanum* should be a subject for further and future investigation.

CONCLUSIONS

We found a high rate of occurrence of *R. amblyommii* sp. nov. in *Amblyomma* ticks from Ohio. The rickettsial infection rate in *A. americanum* from Ohio is higher than in *Dermacentor.* Before 2004, ODH-VBDU did not screen *A. americanum* for rickettsiae. Now, with evidence of tick-borne rickettsial and ehrlichial pathogens in *A. americanum* in the U.S., all ticks are individually tested.

ACKNOWLEDGMENTS

We wish to thank ODH-VBDU for their cooperation in providing ticks.

[*Competing interests statement:* The authors state that they have no conflicting financial interests.]

REFERENCES

1. Burgdorfer, W., S.F. Hayes, L.A. Thomas & J.L. Lancaster, Jr. 1981. A new spotted fever group rickettsia from the Lone Star Tick, *Amblyomma americanum. In*

Rickettsiae and Rickettsial Diseases. W. Burgdorfer & R.L. Anacker, Eds: 595–602. Academic Press. New York.

2. RALPH, D., C.I. PRETZMAN, N. DAUGHERTY & K. POETTER. 1990. Genetic relationships among the members of the family Rickettsiaceae as shown by DNA restriction fragment length analysis. Ann. N.Y. Acad. Sci. **590:** 541–552.
3. STOTHARD, D. 1995. The Evolutionary History of the Genus *Rickettsia* as Inferred from 16S and 23S Ribosomal RNA Genes and the 17 Kilodalton Cell Surface Antigen Gene. Ph.D. Thesis. The Ohio State University. Columbus, OH.

Old and New Human Rickettsiosis in Minas Gerais State, Brazil

S.B. CALIC[a] C.M. BARCELLOS-ROCHA,[b] R.C. LEITE,[c] C.L. MAFRA,[d] AND M.A.M. GALVÃO[e]

[a]*Fundação Ezequiel Dias, Rua conde Pereira Carneiro, Belo Horizonte, MG, Brazil*

[b]*Universidade Federal de Lavras, MG, Brazil*

[c]*Universidade Federal de Minas Gerais, Brazil*

[d]*Universidade Federal de Viçosa, MG, Brazil*

[e]*Universidade Federal de Ouro Preto, Ouro Preto, MG, Brazil 35400-000*

ABSTRACT: The authors describe cases of Brazilian spotted fever (BSF) diagnosed in Minas Gerais state, Brazil, by the Minas Gerais Public Health Laboratory, Ezequiel Dias Foundation from 1995 to 2004. In addition they present three cases of human *Rickettsia felis* rickettsiosis from Minas Gerais diagnosed in France in 1999, and the first two suspected cases of human monocytic ehrlichiosis (HME) diagnosed in Ezequiel Dias Foundation in 2001. In both cases a differential diagnose was made with BSF.

KEYWORDS: rickettsioses; ehrlichioses; Brazilian Spotted Fever

Brazilian spotted fever (BSF) is the more common human rickettsiosis recognized in Brazil. It occurs in the states of Minas Gerais, São Paulo, Rio de Janeiro and Espírito Santo. There are also murine typhus cases reported in Minas Gerais and São Paulo.

Minas Gerais state has nearly 17 million inhabitants and 588.383 km^2 in area. It is located in the southeast area of Brazilian territory and is divided in 852 municipalities. The predominant climate is tropical with defined rainy season (summer) and dry season (winter).

From 1995 to 2004, the Minas Gerais Public Health Laboratory at the Ezequiel Dias Foundation confirmed 124 cases of BSF by IFA. Of these cases, 78% were male, and the major incidence of them was in the group of 15 years. Seventy-seven perscent of BSF cases occurred between June and November with a median of 14 cases per year.

About new rickettsiosis in Minas Gerais state we can relate three cases of human *Rickettsia felis* rickettsiosis confirmed in France in 1999,[1,2] and the first two sus-

Address for correspondence: S.B. Calic, Fundação Ezequiel Dias, Rua conde Pereira Carneiro, no. 80, 30.510.010, Belo Horizonte, MG, Brazil. Voice: 55 21 31 3371-9481; fax: 55 21 31 3371-9480.

sbcalic@funed.mg.gov.br

Ann. N.Y. Acad. Sci. 1063: 356–357 (2005). © 2005 New York Academy of Sciences. doi: 10.1196/annals.1355.059

pected cases of human monocytic ehrlichiosis (HME) diagnosed in Ezequiel Dias Foundation in 2001. In both cases a differential diagnosis was made with BSF.

Two of three confirmed cases of human *Rickettsia felis* rickettsiosis came from Coronel Fabriciano Municipality in Minas Gerais State. These cases occurred in 1999. Both were female and were 55–60 years old. These cases presented antibodies to *R. felis* by IFA with a titer of 1024 IgG and 64 IgM and 512 IgG and 64 IgM, respectively. The third case also occurred in 1999. The patient was a 36 year-old male who came from the Caeté municipality in Minas Gerais State. He had titers to *R. felis* of IgG 128 and 128 IgM as determined by IFA.

In 2003, two suspected cases of HME were detected by the epidemiologic surveillance system from Minas Gerais state as suspected cases of BSF.[3]

In both cases the serologic reactions for BSF, *A. phagocytophilum* and murine typhus by IFA, leptospirosis by macroagglutination test, and yellow fever and dengue by ELISA revealed no antibodies. The two patients were adult males. One of them recovered and the other died. The clinical and laboratory findings supported the diagnose of HME indicating for the first time the possible presence of human ehrlichioses cases in Brazil.[3] These diagnoses of HME were made based on clinical and serologic results (1/64 IgM for both;1/128 and 1/256 IgG).

Although the serologic data indicated *E. chaffeensis* as the agent involved in these episodes, the effect of crossreaction among ehrlichial species does not permit us to determine that the specific etiologic agent was *Ehrlichia chaffeensis* or another similar *Ehrlichia.* This kind of human rickettsial disease had not been described yet in Brazil, although Galvão and colleagues[4] reported for the first time the evidence of antibodies to *Ehrlichia chaffeensis* in a serologic survey of dogs from a spotted fever endemic region in Minas Gerais state.

These cases show us the necessity of studying further the epidemiology of vectors and agents involved in rickettsial diseases in Brazil and other countries of Latin America.

The implementation of molecular biology specific techniques that permit distinguishing between the different rickettsioses has been fundamental to the elicidation of infections such as ehrlichiosis and other rickettsial diseases.

[*Competing interests statement:* No competing interests statement was received.]

REFERENCES

1. Raoult, D., B. La Scola, M. Enea, *et al.* 2001. A flea-associated Rickettsia pathogenic for humans. Emerg. Infect. Dis. **7:** 73–81.
2. Galvão, M.A.M., C.L. Mafra, C.B. Chamone, *et al.* 2004. Clinical and laboratorial evidence of *Rickettsia felis* infections in Latin America. Rev. Soc. Bras. Med. Trop. **37:** 238–240.
3. Calic, S.B., M.A.M. Galvão, F. Bacellar, *et al.* 2004. Human ehrlichioses in Brazil: first suspected cases. Braz. J. Infect. Dis. **8:** 259–262.
4. Galvão, M.A.M., J.A. Lamounier, E. Bonomo, *et al.* 2002. [Emerging and reemerging rickettsiosis in an endemic area of Minas Gerais State, Brazil] Cad Saude **18:** 1593–1597.

Ehrlichia ruminantium: An Emerging Human Pathogen?

M. T. E. P. ALLSOPP,[a] M. LOUW,[b] AND E. C. MEYER[c]

[a]*Onderstepoort Veterinary Institute, Private Bag X5, Onderstepoort 0110, South Africa*

[b]*Department of Anatomical Pathology, National Health Laboratory Services, Tshwane Academic Division, PO Box 2034, Pretoria, South Africa*

[c]*Department of Family Medicine, School of Medicine, Faculty of Health Sciences, University of Pretoria, Brooklyn, Pretoria 0001, South Africa*

KEYWORDS: Encephalitis; *Ehrlichia ruminantium*; pCS20; 16S RNA gene sequences

INTRODUCTION

Ehrlichia ruminantium, transmitted by ticks of the genus *Amblyomma*, causes heartwater in ruminants in sub-Saharan Africa, Madagascar, and some Caribbean islands, but there are no authenticated reports that the organism can cause disease in nonruminants or humans. There is no reliable vaccine and infected animals frequently die before treatment with tetracyclines can be administered. Serological tests for *E. ruminantium* lack specificity, and the most reliable and sensitive test for the organism involves polymerase chain reaction (PCR) amplification and probing for a section of the organism genome referred to as the pCS20 region. We report here three fatal human cases of suspected ehrlichiosis involving unrelated individuals who were not overtly immunocompromised but for whom strong pCS20 probe positive results were obtained. The first of these, for whom few clinical details are available, died approximately three weeks after the death from "biliary fever" of her pet dog. The second, a six-year-old child, died a week after hospital admission with a clinical picture of encephalitis with complaints of severe headache, sleepiness, and unsteady gait. His condition deteriorated rapidly and a brain CT scan revealed echo dense lesions in the cerebral hemispheres. Post-mortem examination revealed severe vasculitis affecting the midbrain and pons regions, as well as prominent pulmonary edema. The third case was also a child who died after a short illness. The clinical features resembled those of the second case. Both children were accustomed to playing outdoors, one on an agricultural smallholding and the other on the borders of a game reserve, but only one child had definite evidence of tick bite. Both were seronegative

Address for correspondence: M.T.E.P. Allsopp, Onderstepoort Veterinary Institute, Private Bag X5, Onderstepoort 0110, South Africa. Voice: +27 12 529 9124; fax: +27 12 529 9417.
alsoppP@arc.agric.za

**Ann. N.Y. Acad. Sci. 1063: 358–360 (2005). © 2005 New York Academy of Sciences.
doi: 10.1196/annals.1355.060**

for rickettsial infection. Molecular evidence based on small subunit ribosomal RNA (16S) and pCS20 gene sequences indicates that *E. ruminantium* was present in DNA from all three individuals.

METHODS AND RESULTS

Aliquots (25 ng) of DNA extracted from whole blood or serum from the three patients were subjected to whole genome amplification using GenomiPhi (Amersham Biosciences, UK.) according to the manufacturer's protocol. Further PCR amplifications (50 μL) using 1μL aliquots of the GenomiPhi products were carried out using primers specific for the 16S V1 loop region of many α-proteobacteria[1] and primers specific for the pCS20 region of *Ehrlichia ruminantium*.[2]

Visible amplicons of ~320 base pairs (bp) were obtained from the V1 loop amplifications, together with faint, higher molecular weight bands at ~800 bp and 1200 bp. The V1 loop amplicons were gel-purified from 1% agarose/TBE gels using the Qiagen MinElute columns (QIAGEN, Hilden, Germany) according to the manufacturer's protocol and, after spectrophotometric quantification, were cloned into pGEM-T (Promega, Madison, USA) as recommended by the manufacturer. Bacterial colonies positive for *E. ruminantium* were identified from colony lifts on nylon filters (Magna Lift, Osmonics Inc., Minnetonka, MN, USA) by probing with a ^{32}P-labeled oligonucleotide specific for *E. ruminantium*.[1] Positive colonies were grown overnight in 3 mL aliquots of LB with tetracycline and ampicillin as recommended in the Promega protocol and plasmid preparation was carried out using the High Pure Plasmid Isolation kit (Roche Diagnostics, Mannheim, Germany).

No visible amplicons were obtained from the initial pCS20 amplifications, so nested PCR (50 μL) was carried out using 1 μL of primary amplicon and primers AB128 and AB127,[3] to give a visible 760 bp product which was gel-purified and cloned as described above. Colony lifts were probed with a ^{32}P random prime labeled fragment of the *E. ruminantium* (Welgevonden) pCS20 region[2] and plasmids extracted from probe positive colonies were digested with EcoR1 to check for the correct sized insert.

A minimum of 10 V1 loop colonies and 10 pCS20 colonies was sequenced from each of the three human samples. All V1 loop clones and pCS20 clones from the woman with suspected canine-derived ehrlichiosis had identical sequences, indicating a single *E. ruminantium* genotype. The 16S V1 loop sequence was identical to that previously identified from a dog suffering from "atypical" canine ehrlichiosis.[4] Three V1 loop sequence variants, differing from the canine derived sequence, and different pCS20 sequences, were obtained from each of the two children, indicating the presence of three different *E. ruminantium* genotypes. These observations suggest that the *E. ruminantium* present in the children came from ticks (species undetermined) which had fed on carrier domestic or wildlife animal species. Although we have no information concerning evidence of tick bites, the unique *E. ruminantium* variant detected in the woman was possibly acquired from her sick dog.

[*Competing interests statement:* The authors state that they have no conflicting financial interests.]

REFERENCES

1. ALLSOPP, M.T.E.P., E.S. VISSER, J.L. DU PLESSIS, *et al.* 1997. Different organisms associated with heartwater as shown by analysis of 16S ribosomal RNA gene sequences. Vet. Parasitol. **71:** 283–300.
2. VAN HEERDEN, H., H.C. STEYN, M.T.E.P. ALLSOPP, *et al.* 2004. Characterisation of the pCS20 region of different *Ehrlichia ruminantium* isolates. Vet. Microbiol. **101:** 279–291.
3. MAHAN, S. M., S. D. WAGHELA, T.C. MCGUIRE, *et al.* 1992. A cloned DNA probe for *Cowdria ruminantium* hybridizes with eight heartwater strains and detects infected sheep. J. Clin. Microbiol. **30:** 981–986.
4. ALLSOPP, M.T.E.P. & B.A. ALLSOPP. 2001. Novel *Ehrlichia* genotype detected in dogs in South Africa. J. Clin. Microbiol. **39:** 4204–4207.

Anaplasma and *Ehrlichia* Infection

J. STEPHEN DUMLER

Division of Medical Microbiology, Department of Pathology, The Johns Hopkins University School of Medicine, Baltimore, Maryland USA

ABSTRACT: **Human and animal infections by *Anaplasmataceae* are increasingly recognized as important and potentially fatal arthropod-transmitted diseases. Since the first recognition and implementation of diagnostic methods for human infection by *Ehrlichia chaffeensis* and *Anaplasma phagocytophilum*, the incidence of infections has linearly increased. Moreover, diagnostic and epidemiological testing indicates that "ehrlichia" infections are globally distributed and suggests that additional agents of human and veterinary "ehrlichiosis" will be identified. With increasing disease identification has come recognition that the infections can be severe, with approximately one-half of patients requiring hospitalization for complications including respiratory distress, myocarditis, neurological complications, hepatitis, a septic or toxic shock–like disease, opportunistic infections, and death in 0.5 to 3.0%. An understanding of the diseases, pathophysiology, pathogenesis, control, and management will best be developed through fundamental investigations. Advances in comprehension as to the separate contributions of bacteria and host are crucial since most data now suggest that alterations in host neutrophil function and protection from innate and adaptive immunity also contribute to disease manifestations. It is reasonable to operate from the hypothesis that these host cell functional changes ultimately benefit bacterial survival while inadvertently eliciting clinical disease in poorly adapted hosts. A firmer basis for the scientific understanding of *Anaplasmataceae* biology will allow logical and rational approaches toward infection control, prevention, and treatment.**

KEYWORDS: ***Anaplasma*; *Ehrlichia*; ehrlichiosis; pathophysiology; seroprevalence; pathogenesis**

INTRODUCTION

The terminology "ehrlichiosis" is a very non-specific descriptor used to characterize disease that occurs with infection by any of a broad range of obligate intracellular bacteria in the *Anaplasmataceae* family. The vast majority of pathogens within this family were best known as agents of veterinary disease, and only in recent years when human infections have been recognized has significant study been conducted to improve taxonomy and classification, diagnostic testing, epidemiological surveillance, and studies of pathophysiology and pathogenesis.

Address for correspondence: J. Stephen Dumler, M.D., Division of Medical Microbiology, Department of Pathology, The Johns Hopkins University School of Medicine, 720 Rutland Avenue, Ross 624, Baltimore, MD 21205. Voice: 410-955-8654; fax: 443-287-3665.
sdumler@jhmi.edu

Ann. N.Y. Acad. Sci. 1063: 361–373 (2005).
doi: 10.1196/annals.1355.069

TAXONOMY AND NOMENCLATURE

Because many of the agents of "ehrlichiosis" were discovered prior to the availability of modern tools for genetic classification, the taxonomic structure was based upon a number of relatively subjective features, including morphology, the type of cell infected, the range of animals with disease manifestations, and vague serological cross-reactivities.[1] With the introduction of molecular phylogenetic tools, it became evident that there was remarkable disarray among the organisms that comprise this group, including species in two different families, five or more genera, including multiple species names. A recent reclassification has brought more logical nomenclature,[2] including the dismantling of the tribe structure of *Rickettsiaceae*, the reassignment of *Ehrlichia*, *Neorickettsia*, and *Wolbachia* species in the tribe *Ehrlichieae* of the *Rickettsiaceae* to the family *Anaplasmataceae*, the reassignment of *Ehrlichia sennetsu* and *E. risticii* to the genus *Neorickettsia*, *Cowdria ruminantium* to the genus *Ehrlichia* under the same species name, and recognition that *Ehrlichia phagocytophila*, *Ehrlichia equi*, and the human granulocytic ehrlichiosis agent are a single species, now designated *Anaplasma phagocytophilum*, and the reassignment of *E. platys* and *E. bovis* also into the genus *Anaplasma*. While such changes are more in line with the genetic phylogeny of these organisms, the ramifications of re-naming are now being felt as clinicians cope with changes in bacterial nomenclature and disease names.[3]

HUMAN INFECTIONS BY *ANAPLASMATACEAE*

To date, at least five agents in the *Anaplasmataceae* family can infect humans, including *Ehrlichia chaffeensis*, *E. ewingii*, *E. canis*, *A phagocytophilum*, and *N. sennetsu*. Only *E. chaffeensis*, *E. ewingii,* and *A. phagocytophilum* infections have been sufficiently characterized for in depth discussion. Disease caused by *E. chaffeensis* that infects monocytes in the peripheral blood is called human monocytic or monocytotropic ehrlichiosis (HME).[4] Its close genetic relative, *E. ewingii*, shares substantial serological cross-reactivity, although it infects neutrophils,[4] a feature of the more genetically distinct *A. phagocytophilum*, etiologic agent of human granulocytic or granulocytotropic anaplasmosis (HGA).[5] To minimize confusion with prior nomenclature, it may be preferable that human infection by *E. ewingii* be referred to as human ewingii ehrlichiosis (HEE) instead of human granulocytic ehrlichiosis, the previous name for HGA. Regardless, the clinical and laboratory manifestations of these infections in humans share many features, including undifferentiated fever with thrombocytopenia, leukopenia, and/or mild elevations in serum transaminases. These features in the context of a typical exposure to ticks in endemic regions weigh heavily that HGA, HME, or HEE should be included in the differential diagnosis.

EPIDEMIOLOGY AND ECOLOGY

Since its first identification in 1986, infections by *Ehrlichia chaffeensis* have been broadly recognized across the south central, southeast, mid-Atlantic, and increasing-

TABLE 1. Meta-analysis of *Anaplasma phagocytophilum* seroprevalence among various human populations (%)

	Cumulative Analysis	Median Analysis			
	Mean (Number of Subjects)	Median	Maximum	Minimum	Number Studies
Overall					
Asia	8.9 (271)	8.9	8.9	8.9	1
Europe	7.2 (8275)	6.2	21.0	0.0	35
North America	4.5 (4070)	5.1	35.6	0.3	11
Cross-sectional[a]					
Asia	Na[4]	na	na	na	0
Europe	8.2 (4038)	5.6	15.4	0.0	19
North America	3.7 (2939)	3.0	14.9	0.3	6
At-risk[b]					
Asia	8.9 (271)	8.9	8.9	8.9	1
Europe	6.3 (3719)	9.1	21.0	0.1	15
North America	6.4 (1131)	5.3	35.6	0.4	5
Lyme disease[c]					
Asia	na	na	na	na	0
Europe	11.4 (1362)	10.8	21.0	3.8	8
North America	20.9 (230)	5.5	35.6	5.3	3

[a]Includes 6–24 year olds, blood donors, children with endocrinologic disorders, health care recipients, healthy individuals, male military personnel, non-Lyme disease patients, pre-marital individuals, and syphilis patients.

[b]Includes adult and pediatric *B. burgdorferi* seropositive patients, cat or dog-exposed individuals, farm workers, febrile patients, forestry workers, patients with fever or undetermined origin, Lyme disease patients, Lyme neuroborreliosis patients, individuals with tick bites or tick exposure.

[c]Includes adult and pediatric *B. burgdorferi* seropositive patients, Lyme disease patients, and Lyme neuroborreliosis patients.

[d]na, not available.

ly the northeast parts of the U.S.[4,6,7] Similarly, HGA is increasingly recognized in the northeast, mid-Atlantic, upper Midwest, and northern California.[5,8] The geographic regions are largely determined by the presence of known competent tick vectors and reservoir hosts, *Amblyomma americanum* (lone star tick) and *Odocoileus virginianus* (white-tailed deer) for *E. chaffeensis*, and *Ixodes scapularis* (black-legged or deer tick) and *I. pacificus* (western black-legged tick) and *O. virginianus*, *Peromyscus leucopus* (white-footed mouse), and *Neotoma fuscipes* (dusky-footed wood rat) for *A. phagocytophilum*.[4,5,9,10] Reporting of human infections was initially sporadic and incomplete after the first descriptions of these infections, but with increasing awareness, more widespread availability of improved diagnostic tests, and perhaps expansion of the infectious agent, a nearly linear increase in cases reported to the CDC has been demonstrated (FIG. 1).[8] Since 1986, at least 1,979 human

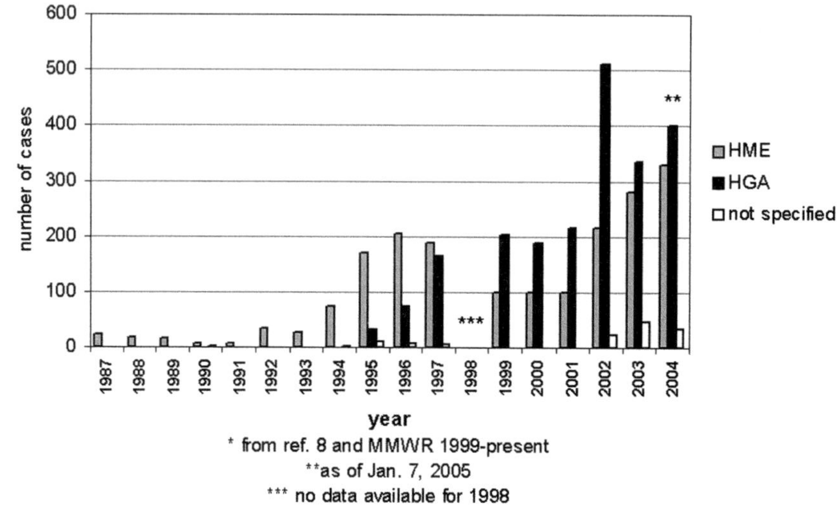

FIGURE 1. Cases of human monocytic ehrlichiosis and granulocytic anaplasmosis in the U.S. reported to the CDC, 1986–2004.

cases of HME, 2,189 cases of HGA, and 153 cases of unspecified "ehrlichiosis" have been reported to the CDC. These figures make HGA and HME the third and fourth most common tick-borne infections in the U.S. behind Lyme disease and Rocky Mountain spotted fever.

Remarkably, HGA is now reported worldwide, with recognition of clinical disease in at least 14 different European countries and perhaps in China, Siberian Russia, and Korea.[11–15] Serological evidence of *A. phagocytophilum* infection of humans is also broadly reported in North America, Europe, and in a few studies reported from Asia. A meta-analysis of seroepidemiologic studies of HGA (TABLE 1) reveals a median of 5.6% infection among 19 studies in Europe and 3.0% among 6 studies in North America, whereas the rates were substantially higher for at-risk populations (*B. burgdorferi* seropositive or Lyme disease, tick-exposed or tick-bite persons, cat- or dog-exposed, farm workers, febrile patients, forestry workers) in Europe (median 9.1% in 15 studies), in North America (5.3% in 5 studies), and in Asia (8.9% in 1 study). Likewise, seroepidemiologic evidence of infection among patients with Lyme disease (*Ixodes* spp. tick bites) is even higher at 5.5% in North America (3 studies) and 10.8% in Europe (8 studies). While the vast majority of these studies were conducted in regions known to be endemic for tick-borne infections, even these rates are startling high given the perception that HGA is a rare disease.

CLINICAL AND LABORATORY FINDINGS

Although different bacteria cause HME and HGA, the clinical and laboratory manifestations are similarly dominated by fever, headache, myalgia, and malaise

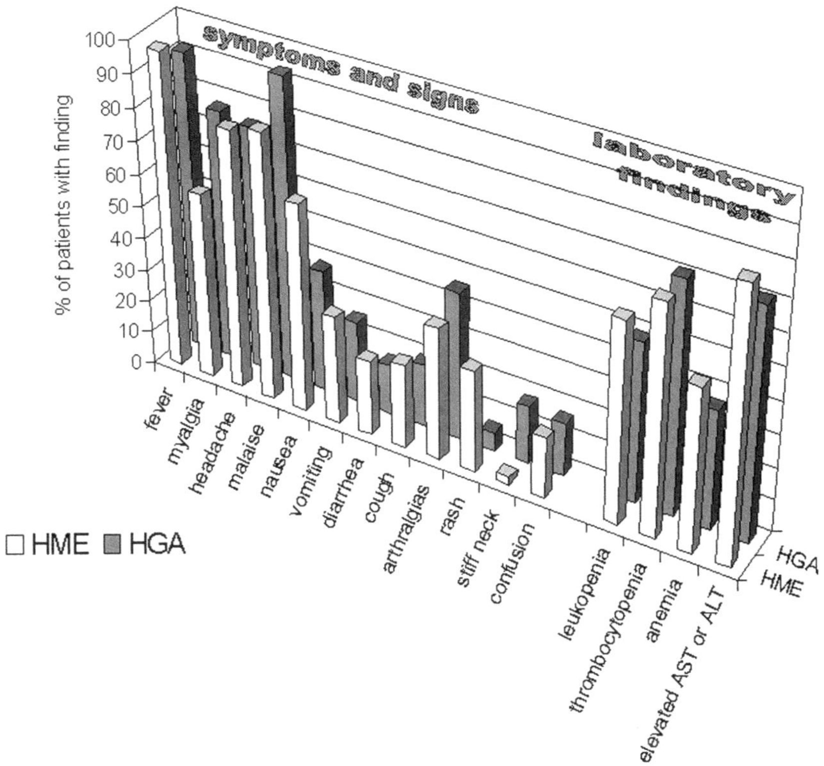

FIGURE 2. Meta-analysis of HME and HGA clinical and laboratory findings (HME N = 143–633, HGA N = 22–685).

(FIG. 2).[7,11,16–28] In addition, the gastrointestinal and respiratory systems are frequently affected, although skin rash is generally infrequent with HME and rare with HGA. Central nervous system infection is present in about 20% of patients with HME but is exceedingly rare with HGA, probably owing to the effects of the infection on the host cell. Laboratory findings can be very helpful in patients with suggestive epidemiological histories that include tick exposure or bites and an appropriate clinical presentation. These include thrombocytopenia, leukopenia, anemia, and increased serum transaminase activities suggesting mild to moderate liver injury.

After identification of infection, approximately 50% of patients with either HME or HGA require hospitalization, and approximately 7% of HGA patients require admission to an intensive care unit.[5,7] However, most patients respond within 24 to 48 hours to treatment with doxycycline, although some with advanced infections may take longer to resolve or may have persistent residual symptoms and signs reflecting slow resolution of inflammation or accumulated tissue injury. Complications of

TABLE 2. Clinical complications with human monocytic ehrlichiosis and human granulocytic anaplasmosis

HME *Ehrlichia chaffeensis*	HGA *Anaplasma phagocytophilum*
50% hospitalized	56% hospitalized (7% ICU)
Hypotension	Septic or toxic shock-like syndrome
Respiratory failure	Acute respiratory distress syndrome (ARDS)
interstitial pneumonitis	atypical pneumonitis
noncardiogenic pulmonary edema	
Acute abdominal syndrome	Acute abdominal syndrome
Acute renal failure	Acute renal failure
Coagulopathy	Coagulopathy
Opportunistic infections	Opportunistic infections
Hemorrhage	Hemorrhage
Cardiac failure	Myocarditis
	Rhabdomyolysis
	Demyelinating polyneuropathy
	Brachial plexopathy
Hepatitis and cholestasis	Hepatitis
Cranial nerve palsies	Cranial nerve palsies
Meningoencephalitis	
Photophobia	
Stupor	
Hallucinations	
Seizures	
Coma	
CSF pleocytosis (23% neutrophil dominated)	
Death	Death
3% case fatality rate	0.5% case fatality rate

HME and HGA vary and can involve many organ systems (TABLE 2), and include toxic and septic shock–like syndromes, coagulopathy, hemorrhage, respiratory distress syndrome, acute abdominal syndromes, acute renal failure, heart failure and myocarditis, opportunistic infections, and cranial nerve neuropathies.[4,5,24] In addition, meningitis and meningoencephalitis occur in approximately 20% of patients with HME, but rarely with HGA. Other neuropathies such as brachial plexopathy and demyelinating polyneuropathy are reported with HGA, but not HME. Fulminant *E. chaffeensis* infection can occur in immunocompromised hosts, including those with HIV infection, high dose corticosteroid therapy, organ transplantation, and monoclonal gammopathy.[29] The case fatality rate for HME is approximately 3%, whereas that of HGA is 0.5%. Only a limited number of patients with ewingii ehrlichiosis have been reported, many with HIV infection or organ transplantation, and the rate of complications appears to be low with no deaths reported.[30]

Whether asymptomatic infection occurs with E. *chaffeensis* and *A. phagocytophilum* infection is controversial. The sheer number of infections documented in seroprevalence studies compared to reported symptomatic infections implies that most are subclinical or mild. However, the seroprevalence rates of HME in highly endemic areas such as Tennessee (3.3 to 12.5%) or Arkansas (1.3%) approximate those identified among symptomatic patients in Tennessee and nearby southeastern Missouri (330 to 414 cases/100,000 [0.3 to 0.4%]).[27,28,31] A similar situation exists for HGA where active surveillance in northwest Wisconsin (26 to 58 cases/100,000 [0.03 to 0.06%]) and Connecticut (24 to 51 cases/100,000 [0.02 to 0.05%]) comes within tenfold less than the seroprevalence rates in these regions (0.6 to 14.9%).[16,32,33] Using these figures, the estimated comparative rates of disease vs. subclinical infection are 0.3–3:100 for HME and 0.4–6:100 for HGA. In Europe, approximately 65 cases of HGA have been described, whereas the seroprevalence rate (8.2% overall) appears to exceed this by a very large margin implying a much higher frequency of subclinical infection.[12]

PATHOLOGY AND PATHOPHYSIOLOGY

Diagnostic tissue examinations or autopsies have only been examined to a limited extent with HME and HGA. Most evaluations now illustrate that tissues have inflammatory changes especially enriched for macrophages and histiocytes, including noncaseating granulomas with HME.[34–37] The presence of hemophagocytosis in bone marrow and lymph node tissues suggests widespread macrophage activation. The bone marrow is almost always normocellular to hypercellular with all hematopoietic elements present in normal numbers.[35,36] Coupled with the evidence of peripheral consumption of marrow elements, this finding strongly suggests that pancytopenia results mostly from peripheral destruction or sequestration of leukocytes, platelets, and erythrocytes, and not from hypoplasia or myelosuppressive events, although a contribution toward suppression cannot be totally excluded.[38] Similarly, changes in the liver vary from focal apoptotic hepatocytes with or without scattered inflammatory cells, to lobular hepatitis and lobular necrosis.[34,37] The lungs are also variably involved in both HME and HGA.[36,39] Most often, the appearance is mild interstitial pneumonitis, with occasional cases demonstrating focal or diffuse alveolar injury, and in severe cases, macrophage-dominated intra-alveolar infiltrates that significantly compromise airways and respiratory function.[34] These findings are pathologic correlates of acute lung injury and acute respiratory distress syndrome, a frequent component of severe and fatal HME, and perhaps with HGA as well.[40]

The underlying mechanisms of tissue injury and disease are not well understood for either HME or HGA. The initial observation of leukopenia in patients with intracellular infections of leukocytes misleads one to conclude that disease simply results from bacterial killing of host cells and subsequent inflammation. However, there is a marked discrepancy between the quantity of bacteria in the blood or tissues, the degree of pancytopenia, and the degree of histopathologic injury.[34,36] Kinetic studies of the distribution of *A. phagocytophilum*–infected neutrophils and inflammatory injury in mouse models suggest a triggering function for the infected cells, related to the induction of proinflammatory cytokines such as interferon (IFN) γ.[41] The discrepancy between bacterial load and inflammatory tissue injury is dramatically illustrated with infection of IFNγ knockout mice that despite bacterial loads exceeding six- to sevenfold higher than wild-type controls, do not develop any histopathologic lesions in liver or other tissues.[42] In contrast when mice devoid of IL-10, the main repressor of IFNγ, are infected, the bacterial load is identical to that of wild-type mice but the degree of inflammatory histopathologic liver injury and apoptosis is substantially greater. It is no surprise that disease and histopathologic evidence of tissue injury are linked to inflammatory reactions, since many investigators have demonstrated the production of inflammatory cytokines and chemokines or other biologically active products with *E. chaffeensis* and *A. phagocytophilum* infections *in vitro* and *in vivo*.[43–50]

Thus, an important unresolved question is to what degree is disease and histopathologic injury in HME and HGA governed by the bacterium or the host? In HME, the mean leukocyte count is 2,100 cells/μL, or an average reduction of 5,600 cells/μL below normal concentrations.[7,27] However, the mean absolute infected cell count is only 3 cells/μL,[28] indicating that 1,900 times more cells are lost in HME than can be accounted for by direct bacterial infection and leukocyte lysis or loss. Although the figure is lower for HGA where 15-fold more cells are lost than can be accounted for by direct bacterial infection,[51] the data strongly imply a role for host-mediated processes in pancytopenia and by extension, injury to other tissues such as liver or lung.

In contrast, clinical evaluations clearly indicate that both HME and HGA severity are linked to the interval of time before diagnosis and therapy, and both infections respond rapidly to doxycycline treatment.[5,7] Additionally, severity in HGA is related to the proportion of infected neutrophils observed in blood during the active infection.[52] One hypothesis that would encompass all of these observations is the induction of a poorly regulated, cytokine-mediated inflammatory process—such as a macrophage activation or hemophagocytic syndrome—both supported by histopathologic analyses of infected humans, naturally infected animals, experimentally infected animals, and by the demonstration of high levels of the macrophage activating cytokine IFNγ in the blood of human patients, mice, cats, and non-human primates with HGA.[5,34,36,41,43,53–55] In contrast, immunocompetent mice are not generally susceptible to *E. chaffeensis* infection,[56] yet SCID mice rapidly die after infection associated with unrestricted bacterial growth, suggesting that intact immunologic mechanisms are protective rather than detrimental.[57] Another animal model that closely mimics HME uses the related *Ixodes ovatus* ehrlichia, and fatal infection in this system is associated with high serum TNFα, low serum IL-12, TNFα-producing CD8 cells, and low levels of IFNγ-producing CD4 cells.[47] Although the specific immunologic mechanisms have yet to be discerned, it is clear that there is an inter-relationship between the bacterial trigger and subsequent immunologically mediated tissue and organ injury.[42,47,58]

Cytokine dysregulation and hyperproduction syndromes, including toxic and septic shock, hemophagocytosis, and macrophage activation syndrome often present with similar clinical manifestations dominated by fever, pancytopenia, alterations in vascular permeability, hypotension, and end-organ injury.[59,60] Septic shock is driven by high bacterial loads that deliver unrestricted stimulation by pathogen-associated molecular patterns (such as lipopolysaccharide, peptidoglycan, or glycolipids).[59,61] Macrophage activation and hemophagocytic syndromes are generally associated with low to moderate pathogen loads and dysfunctional macrophage activation.[61,62] While many cases of macrophage activation and hemophagocytic syndrome are associated with infection, there are genetically determined conditions for which this phenotype is also observed, including familial hemophagocytic lymphohistiocytosis (PRF1 [perforin] mutations), Griscelli syndrome (RAB27A mutations [secretory vesicle trafficking]), Chediak-Higashi syndrome (LYST mutations [lysosomal trafficking regulator]), and X-linked lymphoproliferative syndrome (SH2D1A mutations involved in NKT cell development).[62,63] Similarly, herpesvirus-associated hemophagocytic syndromes are characterized by non-functional NK cells that lack or are deficient in the cytolytic secretory product, perforin.[59,62,63] The recurring theme among these processes, whether infection-associated or genetically defined, is interference with vesicular trafficking that could confound function of critical innate or adaptive immune effector cells, such as NK, NKT, or CD8 T cells, that are in part responsible for direct cytotoxicity and regulation of cytokine networks.

Based upon these data and the recognized alterations in cell function with infection by *E. chaffeensis* and *A. phagocytophilum*, a model for the pathophysiology of HME and HGA could start with infection of the host leukocyte that gains access to the bloodstream, circulating systemically (FIG. 3). Owing to the intrinsic intracellular location and direct downregulatory effects on host cell protective mechanisms such as scavenging of reactive oxygen species or downregulating phagocyte oxidase components, or downregulation of IL12, IL15, or IL18 gene expression,[48,64–66] infected cells resist mechanisms of innate immune response. Not withstanding this intrinsic resistance, *A. phagocytophilum*–infected cells are dichotomously activated[67] whereas uninfected immune cells could respond to free bacterial components leading to cellular activation, generation of proinflammatory response, including effectors of tissue injury. The effects of poorly regulated inflammatory and immune response, including hypercytokinemia, could result in increased vascular permeability, persisting inflammation, and further exacerbation of tissue injury.[43]

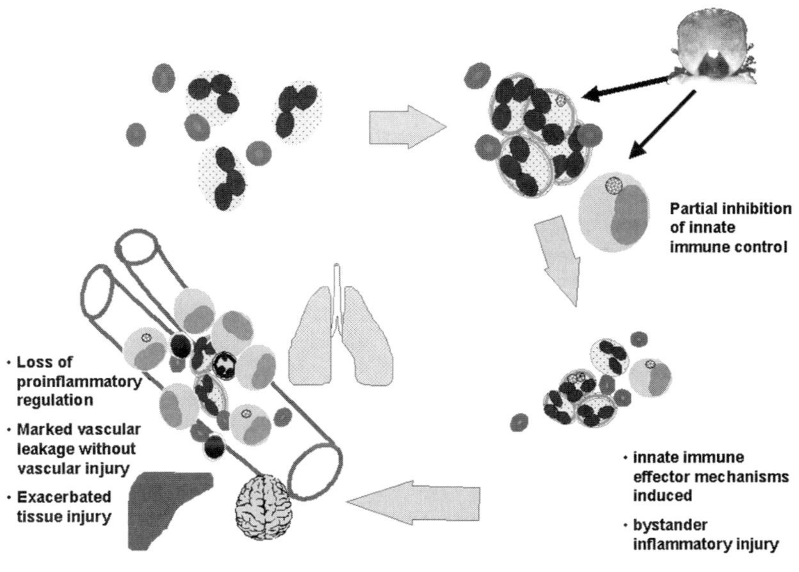

FIGURE 3.

What are the potential advantages of an infection that incites proinflammatory tissue injury rather than suppressing the innate and adaptive immune responses? Akkoyunlu showed improved propagation of A. *phagocytophilum* that results from its intrinsic activation of chemokine secretion among infected neutrophils.[68] A side effect of chemokine production by infected neutrophils is the amplification of inflammation, also facilitated by protracted degranulation,[67] inhibited apoptosis,[69] and downregulation of phagocyte oxidase[66] that dampens inflammation by metabolizing proinflammatory mediators.[70] It is likely that the continued inflammatory response contributes to the recruitment of potential host cells and their persistence in the blood providing more ready access to feeding ticks. Whether such consequences also benefit *E. chaffeensis* survival, or whether there are different fitness mechanisms involved will require much more study. This situation is an interesting contrast to those recently observed for many other bacterial infections that manipulate the host's responses by depressing proinflammatory and innate immunity signaling in order to promote bacterial survival.[71–73] Thus, inciting inflammatory disease is a survival adaptation of *A. phagocytophilum* and possibly *E. chaffeensis* that permits mammalian propagation and intracellular survival and assures sufficient bacteremia for transmission to ticks. Given the availability of suitable animal models, tick transmission models, effective cell culture models, and all the tools of cell biology and the molecular era, these hypotheses can and should be tested. Unraveling the mysteries of survival and propagation of *Anaplasmataceae* may be critical to advance the understanding of the pathogenesis of infections by these agents.

[*Competing interests statement:* The authors state that they have no conflicting financial interests.]

REFERENCES

1. RIKIHISA, Y. 1991. The tribe *Ehrlichieae* and ehrlichial diseases. Clin. Microbiol. Rev. **4:** 286–308.
2. DUMLER, J.S., A.F. BARBET, C.P. BEKKER, *et al.* 2001. Reorganization of genera in the families *Rickettsiaceae* and *Anaplasmataceae* in the order *Rickettsiales*: unification of some species of *Ehrlichia* with *Anaplasma*, *Cowdria* with *Ehrlichia* and *Ehrlichia* with *Neorickettsia*, descriptions of six new species combinations and designation of *Ehrlichia equi* and "HGE agent" as subjective synonyms of *Ehrlichia phagocytophila*. Int. J. Syst. Evol. Microbiol. **51:** 2145–2165.
3. UILENBERG, G., F. THIAUCOURT & F. JONGEJAN. 2004. On molecular taxonomy: what is in a name? Exp. Appl. Acarol. **32:** 301–312.
4. PADDOCK, C.D. & J.E. CHILDS. 2003. *Ehrlichia chaffeensis*: a prototypical emerging pathogen. Clin. Microbiol. Rev. **16:** 37–64.
5. BAKKEN, J.S. & J.S. DUMLER. 2000. Human granulocytic ehrlichiosis. Clin. Infect. Dis. **31:** 554–560.
6. MAEDA, K., N. MARKOWITZ, R.C. HAWLEY, *et al.* 1987. Human infection with *Ehrlichia canis*, a leukocytic rickettsia. N. Engl. J. Med. **316:** 853–856.
7. FISHBEIN, D.B., J.E. DAWSON & L.E. ROBINSON. 1994. Human ehrlichiosis in the United States, 1985 to 1990. Ann. Intern. Med. **120:** 736–743.
8. MCQUISTON, J.H., C.D. PADDOCK, R.C. HOLMAN, *et al.* 1999. The human ehrlichioses in the United States. Emerg. Infect. Dis. **5:** 635–642.
9. CHILDS, J.E. & C.D. PADDOCK. 2003. The ascendancy of *Amblyomma americanum* as a vector of pathogens affecting humans in the United States. Annu. Rev. Entomol. **48:** 307–337.

10. BELONGIA, E.A., K.D. REED, P.D. MITCHELL, *et al.* 1997. Prevalence of granulocytic *Ehrlichia* infection among white-tailed deer in Wisconsin. J. Clin. Microbiol. **35:** 1465–1468.
11. BLANCO, J.R. & J.A. OTEO. 2002. Human granulocytic ehrlichiosis in Europe. Clin Microbiol. Infect. **8:** 763–772.
12. STRLE, F. 2004. Human granulocytic ehrlichiosis in Europe. Int. J. Med. Microbiol. **293:** 27–35.
13. ZHAO, Q., W. CAO, J. LI, *et al.* 2002. [Detection and sequential analysis of Granulocytic ehrlichia 444-Epank gene]. Zhonghua. Liu. Xing. Bing. Xue. Za. Zhi. **23:** 286–288.
14. SIDEL'NIKOV, I.N., O. MEDIANNIKOV, L.I. IVANOV, *et al.* 2003. [The first case of granulocytic ehrlichiosis in the Far East of the Russian Federation]. Klin. Med. (Mosk.). **81:** 67–68.
15. HEO, E.J., J.H. PARK, J.R. KOO, *et al.* 2002. Serologic and molecular detection of *Ehrlichia chaffeensis* and *Anaplasma phagocytophila* (human granulocytic ehrlichiosis agent) in Korean patients. J. Clin. Microbiol. **40:** 3082–3085.
16. BAKKEN, J.S., J. KRUETH, C. WILSON-NORDSKOG, *et al.* 1996. Clinical and laboratory characteristics of human granulocytic ehrlichiosis. J. Am. Med. Assoc. **275:** 199–205.
17. AGUERO-ROSENFELD, M.E., H.W. HOROWITZ, G.P. WORMSER, *et al.* 1996. Human granulocytic ehrlichiosis: a case series from a medical center in New York State. Ann. Intern. Med. **125:** 904–908.
18. ARNEZ, M., T. LUZNIK-BUFON, T. AVSIC-ZUPANC, *et al.* 2003. Etiology of tick-borne febrile illnesses in Slovenian children. Ann. N.Y. Acad. Sci. **990:** 353–354.
19. BJOERSDORFF, A., B. WITTESJO, J. BERGLUN, *et al.* 2002. Human granulocytic ehrlichiosis as a common cause of tick-associated fever in Southeast Sweden: report from a prospective clinical study. Scand. J. Infect. Dis. **34:** 187–191.
20. BELONGIA, E.A., K.D. REED, P.D. MITCHELL, *et al.* 2001. Tickborne infections as a cause of nonspecific febrile illness in Wisconsin. Clin. Infect. Dis. **32:** 1434–1439.
21. BELONGIA, E.A., K.D. REED, P.D. MITCHELL, *et al.* 1999. Clinical and epidemiological features of early Lyme disease and human granulocytic ehrlichiosis in Wisconsin. Clin. Infect. Dis. **29:** 1472–1477.
22. WALLACE, B.J., G. BRADY, D.M. ACKMAN, *et al.* 1998. Human granulocytic ehrlichiosis in New York. Arch. Intern. Med. **158:** 769–773.
23. LOTRIC-FURLAN, S., M. PETROVEC, T. AVSIC-ZUPANC, *et al.* 2004. Comparison of patients fulfilling criteria for confirmed and probable human granulocytic ehrlichiosis. Scand. J. Infect. Dis. **36:** 817–822.
24. BAKKEN, J.S. & J.S. DUMLER. 2005. Clinical diagnosis and treatment of human granulocytotropic anaplasmosis. Ann. N.Y. Acad. Sci. This volume.
25. ENG, T.R., J.R. HARKESS, D.B. FISHBEIN, *et al.* 1990. Epidemiologic, clinical, and laboratory findings of human ehrlichiosis in the United States, 1988. J. Am. Med. Assoc. **264:** 2251–2258.
26. OLANO, J.P., W. HOGREFE, B. SEATON, *et al.* 2003. Clinical manifestations, epidemiology, and laboratory diagnosis of human monocytotropic ehrlichiosis in a commercial laboratory setting. Clin. Diagn. Lab. Immunol. **10:** 891–896.
27. OLANO, J.P., E. MASTERS, W. HOGREFE, *et al.* 2003. Human monocytotropic ehrlichiosis, Missouri. Emerg. Infect. Dis. **9:** 1579–1586.
28. STANDAERT, S.M., T. YU, M.A. SCOTT, *et al.* 2000. Primary isolation of *Ehrlichia chaffeensis* from patients with febrile illnesses: clinical and molecular characteristics. J. Infect. Dis. **181:** 1082–1088.
29. SAFDAR, N., R.B. LOVE & D.G. MAKI. 2002. Severe *Ehrlichia chaffeensis* infection in a lung transplant recipient: a review of ehrlichiosis in the immunocompromised patient. Emerg. Infect. Dis. **8:** 320–323.
30. PADDOCK, C.D., S.M. FOLK, G.M. SHORE, *et al.* 2001. Infections with *Ehrlichia chaffeensis* and *Ehrlichia ewingii* in persons coinfected with human immunodeficiency virus. Clin. Infect. Dis. **33:** 1586–1594.
31. STANDAERT, S.M., J.E. DAWSON, W. SCHAFFNER, *et al.* 1995. Ehrlichiosis in a golf-oriented retirement community. N. Engl. J. Med. **333:** 420–425.

32. IJDO, J.W., J.I. MEEK, M.L. CARTER, *et al.* 2000. The emergence of another tickborne infection in the 12-town area around Lyme, Connecticut: human granulocytic ehrlichiosis. J. Infect. Dis. **181:** 1388–1393.
33. LEIBY, D.A., A.P. CHUNG, R.G. CABLE, *et al.* 2002. Relationship between tick bites and the seroprevalence of *Babesia microti* and *Anaplasma phagocytophila* (previously *Ehrlichia* sp.) in blood donors. Transfusion **42:** 1585–1591.
34. WALKER, D.H. & J.S. DUMLER. 1997. Human monocytic and granulocytic ehrlichioses. Discovery and diagnosis of emerging tick-borne infections and the critical role of the pathologist. Arch. Pathol. Lab. Med. **121:** 785–791.
35. DUMLER, J.S., J.E. DAWSON & D.H. WALKER. 1993. Human ehrlichiosis: hematopathology and immunohistologic detection of *Ehrlichia chaffeensis*. Hum. Pathol. **24:** 391–396.
36. LEPIDI, H., J.E. BUNNELL, M.E. MARTIN, *et al.* 2000. Comparative pathology, and immunohistology associated with clinical illness after *Ehrlichia phagocytophila*-group infections. Am. J. Trop. Med. Hyg. **62:** 29–37.
37. SEHDEV, A.E. & J.S. DUMLER. 2003. Hepatic pathology in human monocytic ehrlichiosis. *Ehrlichia chaffeensis* infection. Am. J. Clin. Pathol. **119:** 859–865.
38. PEARCE, C.J., M.E. CONRAD, P.E. NOLAN, *et al.* 1988. Ehrlichiosis: a cause of bone marrow hypoplasia in humans. Am. J. Hematol. **28:** 53–55.
39. MARTY, A.M., J.S. DUMLER, G. IMES, *et al.* 1995. Ehrlichiosis mimicking thrombotic thrombocytopenic purpura. Case report and pathological correlation. Hum. Pathol. **26:** 920–925.
40. WONG, S. & L.J. GRADY. 1996. *Ehrlichia* infection as a cause of severe respiratory distress. N. Engl. J. Med. **334:** 273.
41. MARTIN, M.E., J.E. BUNNELL & J.S. DUMLER. 2000. Pathology, immunohistology, and cytokine responses in early phases of human granulocytic ehrlichiosis in a murine model. J. Infect. Dis. **181:** 374–378.
42. MARTIN, M.E., K. CASPERSEN & J.S. DUMLER. 2001. Immunopathology and ehrlichial propagation are regulated by interferon-gamma and interleukin-10 in a murine model of human granulocytic ehrlichiosis. Am. J. Pathol. **158:** 1881–1888.
43. DUMLER, J.S., E.R. TRIGIANI, J.S. BAKKEN, *et al.* 2000. Serum cytokine responses during acute human granulocytic ehrlichiosis. Clin. Diagn. Lab. Immunol. **7:** 6–8.
44. LEE, E.H. & Y. RIKIHISA. 1996. Absence of tumor necrosis factor alpha, interleukin-6 (IL-6), and granulocyte-macrophage colony-stimulating factor expression but presence of IL-1beta, IL-8, and IL-10 expression in human monocytes exposed to viable or killed *Ehrlichia chaffeensis*. Infect. Immun. **64:** 4211–4219.
45. LEE, E.H. & Y. RIKIHISA. 1997. Anti-*Ehrlichia chaffeensis* antibody complexed with *E. chaffeensis* induces potent proinflammatory cytokine mRNA expression in human monocytes through sustained reduction of IκB-alpha and activation of NF-κB. Infect. Immun. **65:** 2890–2897.
46. KIM, H.Y. & Y. RIKIHISA. 2000. Expression of interleukin-1β, tumor necrosis factorα, and interleukin-6 in human peripheral blood leukocytes exposed to human granulocytic ehrlichiosis agent or recombinant major surface protein P44. Infect. Immun. **68:** 3394–3402.
47. ISMAIL, N., L. SOONG, J.W. MCBRIDE, *et al.* 2004. Overproduction of TNF-α by CD8+ type 1 cells and down-regulation of IFN-γ production by CD4+ Th1 cells contribute to toxic shock-like syndrome in an animal model of fatal monocytotropic ehrlichiosis. J. Immunol. **172:** 1786–1800.
48. ZHANG, J.Z., M. SINHA, B.A. LUXON, *et al.* 2004. Survival strategy of obligately intracellular *Ehrlichia chaffeensis*: novel modulation of immune response and host cell cycles. Infect. Immun. **72:** 498–507.
49. KLEIN, M.B., S. HU, C.C. CHAO, *et al.* 2000. The agent of human granulocytic ehrlichiosis induces the production of myelosuppressing chemokines without induction of proinflammatory cytokines. J. Infect. Dis. **182:** 200–205.
50. BORJESSON, D.L., S.D. KOBAYASHI, A.R. WHITNEY, *et al.* 2005. Insights into pathogen immune evasion mechanisms: *Anaplasma phagocytophilum* fails to induce an apoptosis differentiation program in human neutrophils. J. Immunol. **174:** 6364–6372.

51. BAKKEN, J.S., M.E. AGUERO-ROSENFELD, R.L. TILDEN, *et al.* 2001. Serial measurements of hematologic counts during the active phase of human granulocytic ehrlichiosis. Clin. Infect. Dis. **32:** 862–870.
52. BAKKEN, J.S., J.S. DUMLER, S.M. CHEN, *et al.* 1994. Human granulocytic ehrlichiosis in the upper Midwest United States. A new species emerging? J. Am. Med. Assoc. **272:** 212–218.
53. OLANO, J.P. & D.H. WALKER. 2002. Human ehrlichioses. Med. Clin. North. Am. **86:** 375–392.
54. FOLEY, J.E., N.W. LERCHE, J.S. DUMLER, *et al.* 1999. A simian model of human granulocytic ehrlichiosis. Am. J. Trop. Med. Hyg. **60:** 987–993.
55. FOLEY, J.E., C.M. LEUTENEGGER, J.S. DUMLER, *et al.* 2003. Evidence for modulated immune response to *Anaplasma phagocytophila* sensu lato in cats with FIV-induced immunosuppression. Comp. Immunol. Microbiol. Infect. Dis. **26:** 103–113.
56. SOTOMAYOR, E.A., V.L. POPOV, H.M. FENG, *et al.* 2001. Animal model of fatal human monocytotropic ehrlichiosis. Am. J. Pathol. **158:** 757–769.
57. WINSLOW, G.M., E. YAGER, K. SHILO, *et al.* 1998. Infection of the laboratory mouse with the intracellular pathogen *Ehrlichia chaffeensis*. Infect. Immun. **66:** 3892–3899.
58. MATTNER, J., K.L. DEBORD, N. ISMAIL, *et al.* 2005. Exogenous and endogenous glycolipid antigens activate NKT cells during microbial infections. Nature **434:** 525–529.
59. FISMAN, D.N. 2000. Hemophagocytic syndromes and infection. Emerg. Infect. Dis. **6:** 601–608.
60. DINARELLO, C.A. 1997. Proinflammatory and anti-inflammatory cytokines as mediators in the pathogenesis of septic shock. Chest. **112:** 321S–329S.
61. MOSSER, D.M. 2003. The many faces of macrophage activation. J. Leukoc. Biol. **73:** 209–212.
62. LARROCHE, C. & L. MOUTHON. 2004. Pathogenesis of hemophagocytic syndrome (HPS). Autoimmun, Rev. **3:** 69–75.
63. Grom, A.A. 2004. Natural killer cell dysfunction: A common pathway in systemic-onset juvenile rheumatoid arthritis, macrophage activation syndrome, and hemophagocytic lymphohistiocytosis? Arthritis Rheum. **50:** 689–698.
64. CARLYON, J.A., D. ABDEL-LATIF, M. PYPAERT, *et al.* 2004. *Anaplasma phagocytophilum* utilizes multiple host evasion mechanisms to thwart NADPH oxidase-mediated killing during neutrophil infection. Infect. Immun. **72:** 4772–4783.
65. IJDO, J.W. & A.C. MUELLER. 2004. Neutrophil NADPH oxidase is reduced at the *Anaplasma phagocytophilum* phagosome. Infect. Immun. **72:** 5392–5401.
66. BANERJEE, R., J. ANGUITA, D. ROOS, *et al.* 2000. Cutting edge: infection by the agent of human granulocytic ehrlichiosis prevents the respiratory burst by down-regulating $gp91^{phox}$. J. Immunol. **164:** 3946–3949.
67. CHOI, K.S., D.J. GRAB & J.S. DUMLER. 2004. *Anaplasma phagocytophilum* infection induces protracted neutrophil degranulation. Infect. Immun. **72:** 3680–3683.
68. AKKOYUNLU, M., S.E. MALAWISTA, J. ANGUITA, *et al.* 2001. Exploitation of interleukin-8-induced neutrophil chemotaxis by the agent of human granulocytic ehrlichiosis. Infect. Immun. **69:** 5577–5588.
69. YOSHIIE, K., H.Y. KIM, J. MOTT, *et al.* 2000. Intracellular infection by the human granulocytic ehrlichiosis agent inhibits human neutrophil apoptosis. Infect. Immun. **68:** 1125–1133.
70. SEGAL, B.H., D.B. KUHNS, L. DING, *et al.* 2002. Thioglycollate peritonitis in mice lacking C5, 5-lipoxygenase, or p47phox: complement, leukotrienes, and reactive oxidants in acute inflammation. J. Leukoc. Biol. **71:** 410–416.
71. PUJOL, C. & J.B. BLISKA. 2005. Turning *Yersinia* pathogenesis outside in: subversion of macrophage function by intracellular yersiniae. Clin. Immunol. **114:** 216–226.
72. CORNELIS, G.R. 2002. *Yersinia* type III secretion: send in the effectors. J. Cell. Biol. **158:** 401–408.
73. OHL, M.E. & S.I. MILLER. 2001. *Salmonella*: a model for bacterial pathogenesis. Annu. Rev. Med. **52:** 259–574.

The Interactions of *Anaplasma phagocytophilum*, Endothelial Cells, and Human Neutrophils

MICHAEL J. HERRON,[a] MARNA E. ERICSON,[b] TIMOTHY J. KURTTI,[a] AND ULRIKE G. MUNDERLOH[a]

[a]*Department of Entomology, University of Minnesota, St. Paul, Minnesota 55108*

[b]*Department of Dermatology, University of Minnesota ,Minneapolis, Minnesota 55455*

ABSTRACT: *Ixodes scapularis* ticks transmit *Anaplasma phagocytophilum* (Ap), agent of human granulocytic anaplasmosis (HGA). Invasion of neutrophil granulocytes (PMN) by Ap is the hallmark of the disease, but these short-lived phagocytes are not likely the sole cell type required for productive infection. We analyzed infection of microvascular endothelial cells during pathogenesis of anaplasmosis *in vivo* and *in vitro*. Organs from Ap-infected mice were processed for confocal microscopy 41 days p.i. Fluorescent labeling of heart and liver sections using anti-factor VIII and anti-MSP2 antibodies allowed colocalization of Ap and vascular endothelium, indicating infection. Ap rapidly invaded and grew within HMEC-1 human microvascular endothelial cells and readily transferred to PMN. Over 50% of PMN became infected within two hours of coincubation with HMEC-1. PMN adhered to, polarized, and migrated upon infected endothelial monolayers. The Ap receptor on human PMN is PSGL-1, and infected endothelial cells upregulate ICAM-1 (CD54), but the mechanisms of transfer of Ap remain unknown. To elucidate the cellular determinants involved, we tested relevant antibodies and lectins. Anti-PSGL-1 reduced infection of PMN, but did not inhibit adherence of PMN to Ap infected HMEC-1 cells while anti-CD18 did. Sialidase pretreatment increased, and EDTA and fucoidan decreased binding of Ap to HMEC-1, whereas several other lectins had no effect. An endothelial reservoir of Ap offers opportunities for ongoing, direct cell-to-cell infection of PMN, avoidance of host immune effectors, and completion of the Ap life cycle by infection of circulating leukocytes available for transfer to blood-feeding ticks.

KEYWORDS: human anaplasmosis; tick-borne pathogen; pathogenesis; microvascular endothelium; confocal microscopy; immunofluorescence; neutrophil granulocyte; CD54, ß2-integrin

Address for correspondence: Ulrike G. Munderloh, Department of Entomology, University of Minnesota, 219 Hodson Hall, 1980 Folwell Avenue, St. Paul, Minnesota, 55108. Voice: 612-624-4740; fax: 612-625-5299.
munde001@umn.edu

**Ann. N.Y. Acad. Sci. 1063: 374–382 (2005). © 2005 New York Academy of Sciences.
doi: 10.1196/annals.1355.090**

INTRODUCTION

Ticks are capable of transmitting a wide range of pathogens, including viruses, rickettsial agents, other bacteria, and protozoa. Unlike mosquitoes, ticks do not pierce a blood vessel directly, but lodge their mouthparts in the dermis and subcuticular tissue where they create a feeding lesion aided by salivary secretions and infiltrating neutrophil granulocytes (PMN) that degranulate, releasing collagenase and other substances.[1] This causes local blood vessel walls to erode during the last days of feeding, when ticks undergo rapid engorgement and ingest 80–90% of their blood meal.[2] The human granulocytic anaplasmosis (HGA) agent, *Anaplasma phagocytophilum* (Ap), is an obligate intracellular bacterium transmitted via the bite of an infected *Ixodes scapularis* tick during the first 1–2 days following attachment.[3] Therefore, it is unlikely that the cells involved in early pathogenesis are extravasated PMN which, once they have left the blood stream, are not known to return. Instead, PMN degranulate and/or phagocytize the intruding agent and die. Moreover, PMN are very short-lived cells, surviving for only hours after their release into the blood from bone marrow. Although infection with Ap inhibits normal apoptosis in PMN,[4–6] the extension of PMN survival is not sufficient to account for the duration of the disease, namely a few weeks in human patients to months in animals.[7,8] This suggested the involvement of one or more other cell types at the tick bite site that could be involved both during the early period after infection as well as long-term persistence. The endothelial lining of the microvasculature represents cells that are abundant in the skin and other organs. They interact with PMN during many inflammatory and infectious processes, thereby providing for the possibility of Ap transfer to PMN, as well as acting as a reservoir for ongoing infection. We have previously shown that human primary cells and cell lines derived from primate and bovine microvascular endothelium are susceptible to infection with Ap.[9] In the present publication, we examined the interaction between these bacteria, microvascular endothelial cells, and PMN *in vitro*. Further, we demonstrate vascular endothelial infection in the liver and heart of SCID mice.

MATERIALS AND METHODS

Animals

Female C3H/HeJ SCID (severe combined immuno-deficiency) mice, 8 weeks of age, were purchased from Jackson Laboratories (Bar Harbor, ME), and maintained according to guidelines issued by the National Institutes of Health (NIH) and the United States Department of Agriculture (USDA). Mice were inoculated intraperitoneally (i.p.) with 10^7 Ap strain HGE1-infected human PMN, and monitored by examination of tail blood (Giemsa-stained thin blood smears and PCR[10]) one, two and six weeks p.i., as well as on day 41 when they were sacrificed. Liver and heart tissue were fixed in Zamboni's fixative, and 200 μm sections reacted with rabbit antibody to von Willebrand factor VIII (endothelial marker; Zymed, San Francisco, CA) and a monoclonal antibody to MSP2 of Ap (R5E4[11]). Bound antibody was detected using TRITC-labeled anti-rabbit IgG, and FITC-labeled anti-mouse IgG, by imaging sections with a BioRad MRC1024 confocal system.

Materials

Antibodies to CD18 and CD54 (ICAM-1) were purchased from Ancell (Bayport, MN). Monoclonal antibody KPl-1 to P-selectin glycoprotein ligand 1 (PSGL-1, CD162) was a generous gift from Dr. Karen Snapp.[12] Lectin (fucoidan) and sialidase were from Sigma (Sigma, St. Louis. MO). Antibodies were diluted to 10 μg/mL in cell culture medium, and added to confluent cell layers in 96-well culture plates for 30 min before addition of Ap. Lectins were diluted in phosphate buffered saline (PBS), and added to wells at a concentration of 1 mg/ml for 1 hour at 37°C. Vybrant Green CFDA vital cell stain was obtained from Molecular Probes (Eugene, OR) and used at a concentration of 2 μM to visualize live *Anaplasma* inside host cells. To examine upregulation of CD54 (ICAM-1), infected HMEC-1[13] were washed once with culture medium, fixed with 1% *p*-formaldehyde in PBS, and incubated for 1 h at 37°C with rabbit anti-CD54 antibody diluted 1:50 in phosphate-buffered saline (PBS) with 3% bovine serum albumin (BSA). After 3 washes in PBS, cells were reacted with anti-rabbit IgG labeled with TRITC, and visualized using a Nikon Diaphot fitted for epifluorescence.

Cell Lines and Bacteria

The human promyelocytic leukemia cell line HL-60 (ATCC CCL-240) was used to propagate Ap.[10] HL-60 cells were grown in RPMI1640 (Bio-Whittaker, Walkersville, MD, USA) supplemented with 10% FBS (fetal bovine serum; Harlan, Indianapolis, IN) and 25 mM HEPES (4-(2-hydroxyethyl)piperazine-1-ethanesulfonic acid). The human microvascular endothelial line HMEC-1[13] was grown in MCDB131 (Mediatech, Herndon, VA, USA) supplemented with 10% FBS and 0.5 μg/mL cortisone and propagated on gelatin-coated tissue culture ware in 5% CO_2 in humidified air at 37°C. For functional assays HMEC-1 were seeded in 100 μL of MCDB 131 supplemented with 10% FBS and 0.5 μg/mL cortisone and propagated on gelatin-coated 96-well plates (Nalge Nunc Int. Rochester, NY) one day prior to infection with Ap.

The HGE2 isolate of Ap was propagated in HL-60 cells,[10] and used throughout for *in vitro* studies. The HGE1 isolate was grown the same way and used to infect mice.

Infection of Endothelial Cells with A. phagocytophilum

Initially, 0.2 mL of an Ap culture in which 80% or more of the HL-60 cells were infected with the HGE2 isolate[10] was added to a each well of a 96-well plate containing a confluent cell layer of HMEC-1 cells. Control wells received a similar number of uninfected HL-60 cells. Plates were incubated for 24 h at 37°C in a humid atmosphere of 5% CO_2 in air, and then infected and uninfected HL-60 were removed by gentle rinsing with two changes of RPMI1640 supplemented with 10% FBS and 25 mM HEPES.

To determine the effect of lectins on subsequent binding of Ap to HMEC-1 cells, 1 mg/mL of Fucoidan was added to cultures in microtiter wells and incubated for 1 h at 37°C before addition of Vybrant Green Ap. After 1 h at 37°C, wells were washed twice with PBS, and then fixed in 1% *p*-formaldehyde for 15 minutes. Cells were photographed at 40 × magnification under UV epifluorescence and analyzed using

ImageJ (W. Rasband, National Institutes of Health and available on the Internet at <http://rsb.info.nih.gov/ij/>) to count bacteria in 3 areas/well. Experiments were repeated 3 times. For experiments using sialidase, established monolayers of HMEC-1 were pretreated with 1 U/mL of Cp neuraminidase (=sialidase, from *Clostridium perfringens*) at *p*H6 for 2 h, and Vybrant Green–labeled Ap were then added. Binding of Ap was determined the same way as outlined for lectin experiments.

Isolation and Infection of PMN

peripheral blood was obtained from healthy volunteers by venipuncture using EDTA (ethylenediaminetetraacetic acid) as an anticoagulant. Neutrophil granulocytes (PMN) were isolated by density gradient centrifugation as described.[14] The PMN layer was collected and washed twice in Dulbecco's phosphate buffered saline, and resuspended in RPMI1640 with 10% FBS.

Twenty five thousand freshly isolated human PMN were added to microtiter wells containing infected HMEC-1 monolayers[9] and incubated for the times shown in HEPES buffered RPMI1640 with 10% FBS in a 5% CO_2 atmosphere. At the specified intervals the medium containing PMN was removed by pipetting and cytospin slides of these cells were prepared and Giemsa stained. The percentage of infected PMN was determined microscopically.

PMN Adhesion

Freshly isolated human PMN were incubated for 15 minutes in 2 μM Vybrant Green CFDA in Dulbecco's PBS, centrifuged at 400 × *g* for 5 min, resuspended in HEPES buffered RPMI1640 with 10% FBS and incubated for 15 min at 37°C. Cells were again centrifuged at 400 × *g* for 5 min and resuspended in HEPES buffered RPMI1640 with 10% FBS. Vybrant Green–labeled human PMN, 10^5, were added to microtiter wells containing infected HMEC-1 monolayers[9] and incubated in HEPES buffered RPMI1640 with 10% FBS in a 5% CO_2 atmosphere. At the specified intervals non-adherent PMN were removed by washing with two changes of HEPES buffered RPMI1640 with 10% FBS. Adherent cells were imaged with a Nikon DXM1200 digital camera and a 4 × objective on a Nikon Diaphot, using epifluorescence illumination. Adherent PMN were counted automatically with ImageJ.

PMN Migration and Polarization

Twenty five thousand freshly isolated human PMN were added to microtiter wells containing infected HMEC-1 monolayers[9] and incubated for 30 min in HEPES buffered RPMI1640 with 10% FBS in a 5% CO_2 atmosphere. The plates were imaged every 15 sec with a Nikon DXM1200 digital camera and a 40× objective on a Nikon Diaphot, using phase contrast optics. Images were assembled in ImageJ and the paths of migrating PMN were traced manually using this software.

Light Microscopy

Live endothelial cultures were monitored daily by phase contrast microscopy, and HL-60 cultures containing Ap were monitored every second day with Giemsa-staining. Cells were spun onto microscope slides using a Cytospin (Shandon Southern Instruments, Sewickley, PA, USA) centrifuge at 100 × *g* for 2 min. Slides were fixed in methanol for 5 min, air-dried briefly, and immersed in a buffered (pH 6.8) solution of 4% Giemsa's stain (Karyomax, Gibco, Grand Island, NY, USA) for 30 min at 37°C.

Slides were viewed and photographed under oil immersion at 100 × magnification using a Nikon Eclipse E400 microscope, fitted for epifluorescence and equipped with a Nikon DXM1200 digital camera.

RESULTS AND DISCUSSION

Several lines of evidence led us to consider involvement of microvascular endothelium during pathogenesis of granulocytic anaplasmosis. These included the development of the tick feeding lesion, the dynamics of transmission of Ap by ticks which occurs within 24 h post tick attachment[3] when blood vessels at the bite site remain intact, and the fact that PMN won't return to the blood stream once they have emigrated into tissue. Moreover, we found it intriguing that Ap adhere to PMN via P-selectin glycoprotein ligand 1 (PSGL-1), which PMN use to engage P-selectin displayed on inflamed endothelium during rolling adhesion.[15] We had previously shown that Ap productively infects microvascular endothelial cells *in vitro*.[9] Here, we dem-

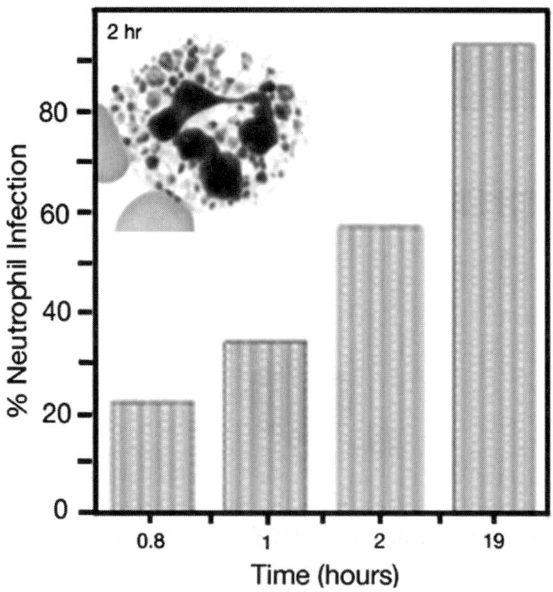

FIGURE 1. Rapid rate of transfer of *Anaplasma phagocytophilum* isolate HGE2 from infected HMEC-1 monolayers to human neutrophil granulocytes (PMN). Human PMN cocultured with HMEC-1 endothelial cells in microtiter plate wells were sampled at the times indicated, stained with Giemsa's stain, and the percent infected cells determined microscopically. Inset: Infected PMN after 2 h of coculture.

onstrated infection of vascular endothelium of heart and liver in SCID mice infected for seven weeks. We chose SCID mice to optimize our chances of finding infected endothelial cells in animals that had a truly chronic infection, unlike non-SCID mice which clear the microbes in 2–3 weeks. Using antibodies to von Willebrand factor VIII (red signal) and a mAb, R5E4 (green signal), to an immune-dominant major surface protein, MSP2, produced a yellow signal indicative of endothelial infection with Ap in merged overlapping areas (not shown).

In vitro, transfer of Ap to PMN was highly efficient: within 30 min, 20% of PMN were infected, increasing to 35% by 1 h, and over 50% by 2 h (FIG. 1). At this time point, spread of Ap between PMN is unlikely, whereas after 19 h, when nearly all PMN contained bacteria, infection could have resulted both from contact with endothelial cells and release of Ap from other PMN. The infection of PMN was possibly mediated by their enhanced adhesion to infected HMEC-1 cells. Infected HMEC-1 displayed upregulation of CD54 (ICAM-1) and the number of adherent PMN was about 15- to 20-fold higher than in controls (FIG. 2). Neutrophils coincubated with infected HMEC-1 monolayers were observed to change shape, i.e., to become polarized, and to migrate upon the endothelial cell layer in a directional pattern, suggesting involvement of integrins in the adhesion process.[15] As expected, pre-incubation of HMEC-1 with antibodies to CD18 (the β2-integrin arm of the heterodimer which

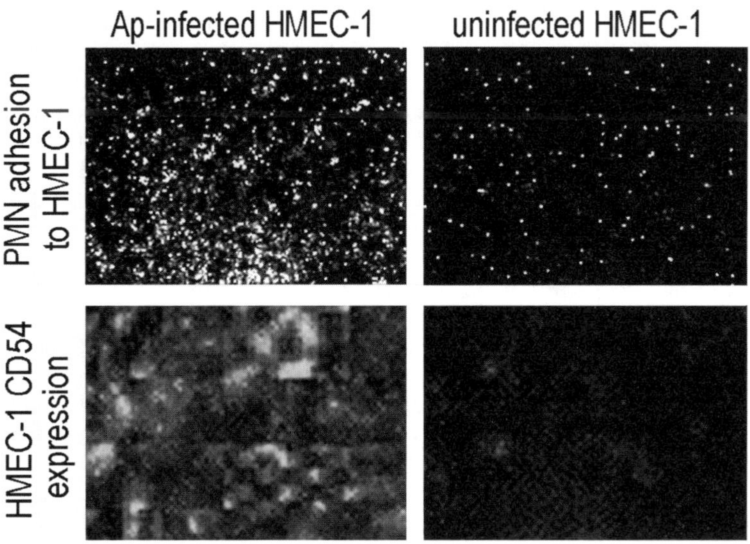

FIGURE 2. Adhesion of human neutrophil granulocytes (PMN) to infected (*upper left panel*) and uninfected (*upper right panel*) human microvascular endothelial cells, line HMEC-1. Enhanced adherence of PMN to infected HMEC-1 cells correlates with increased expression of CD54 (ICAM-1) by infected HMEC-1 (*lower left panel*) as compared to uninfected HMEC-1 (*lower right panel*). PMN were labeled with the vital dye Vybrant Green CDFA, and CD54 was detected using anti-CD54 and a TRITC-labeled second antibody visualized under UV epifluorescence.

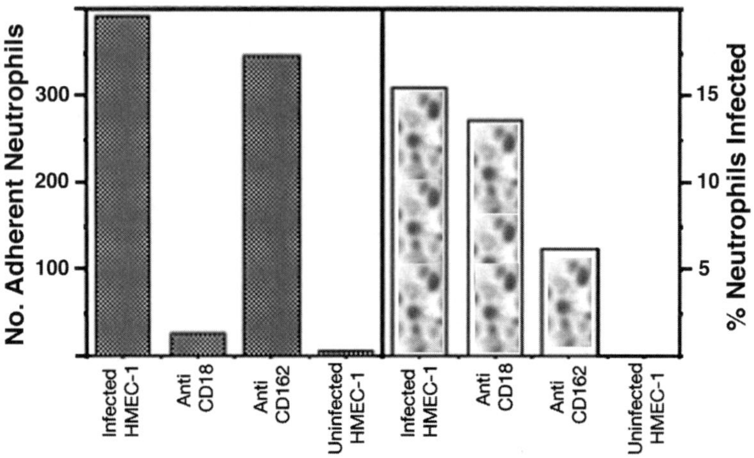

FIGURE 3. Effect of antibodies to PSGL-1 (CD162) and CD18 (β2 integrin) on binding to endothelial cells and infection of PMN. While anti-CD18 reduced PMN-binding to nearly the level of the negative control, it had little effect on infection. Anti-CD162, on the other hand, did not affect adherence of PMN to HMEC-1, but significantly reduced infection.

constitutes the leukocyte integrin CD11b/CD18, or Mac-1) greatly reduced PMN adherence to HMEC-1 (FIG. 3, left panel), but, unexpectedly, had little effect on transfer of Ap to PMN (FIG. 3, right panel). We expect that results will be different under flow conditions. Mac-1 plays an important role in adhesion of PMN to endothelium and extravasation into inflammatory foci,[15] and we hypothesize that its function may be modulated in infected neutrophils. On the other hand, antibodies to PSGL-1 minimally affected PMN adhesion to infected HMEC-1 (FIG. 3, left panel), but significantly reduced PMN infection (to about 30% of untreated controls; FIG. 3, right panel), confirming the role of CD162 in invasion of PMN by Ap.[16]

Lectins are involved in many microbe-host cell interactions. Of several lectins tested, only fucoidan, a sulfated polysaccharide that is known to inhibit leukocyte rolling on inflamed endothelium,[15] interfered with Ap binding to HMEC-1 cells. At a concentration of 4 mM EDTA similarly reduced adherence of Ap to HMEC-1 (Fig. 4), likely reflecting a requirement of divalent cations, especially calcium, in the adhesion process. Like fucoidan, EDTA is a known inhibitor of leukocyte rolling on endothelium.[15]

Intracellular pathogens commonly engage sialylated mammalian cell surface receptors, and Ap specifically uses the neutrophil PSGL-1 decorated with sialyl-Lewis^{x}[16] for invasion of PMN. We were, therefore, surprised to find that pretreatment of HMEC-1 layers with sialidase increased binding of Ap to the cells, instead of decreasing it (FIG. 5).

In conclusion, we have uncovered an additional step in the pathogenesis of human granulocytic anaplasmosis, involving infection of microvascular endothelium. Our finding of endothelial infection in deep organs of mice infected for nearly seven weeks supports the notion that this may serve as a mechanism to maintain long-term

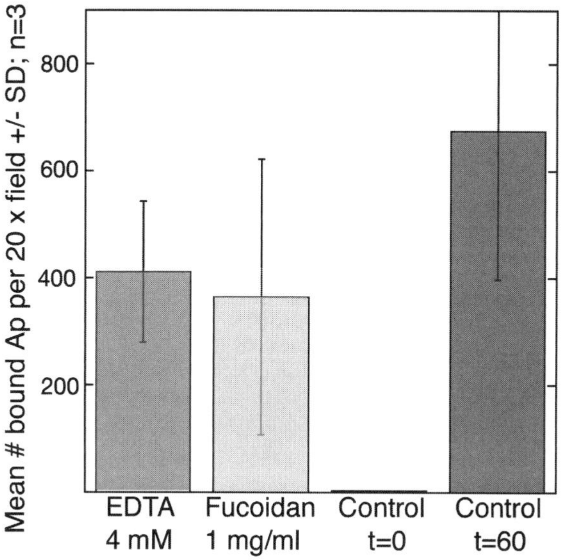

FIGURE 4. Effects of EDTA and Fucoidan on adhesion of *Anaplasma* to HMEC-1 endothelial cells *in vitro*. Both compounds similarly reduced binding of bacteria to the cells after 1 h of coincubation.

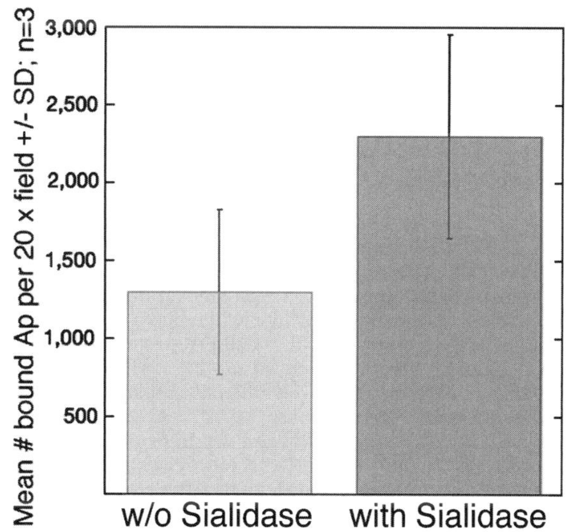

FIGURE 5. Effect of sialidase treatment of HMEC-1 endothelial cell layers on subsequent binding of *Anaplasma*. Bacterial adhesion increased after sialidase treatment, suggesting that the bacteria do not bind to sialylated cell surface moieties.

infection. More research is needed to unravel the interactions between Ap and endothelium at the cellular level, but our results suggest that these bacteria utilize different ligands and receptors for invasion of the various tissues they infect in the mammalian host.

[*Competing interests statement:* The authors state that they have no competing financial interests.]

REFERENCES

1. TATCHELL R.J. & D.E. MOORHOUSE. 1970. Neutrophils: their role in the formation of a tick feeding lesion. Science **167:** 1002–1003.
2. FIELDEN, L.J, R.M. JONES, M. GOLDBERG & Y. RECHAV. 1999. Feeding and respiratory gas exchange in the American dog tick, *Dermacentor variabilis*. J. Insect Physiol. **45:** 297–304.
3. KATAVOLOS P., P.M. ARMSTRONG, J.E. DAWSON & S.R. TELFORD 3rd. 1998. Duration of tick attachment required for transmission of granulocytic ehrlichiosis. J. Infect. Dis. **77:** 1422–1425.
4. SCAIFE H., Z. WOLDEHIWET, C.A. HART & S.W. EDWARDS. 2003. *Anaplasma phagocytophilum* reduces neutrophil apoptosis in vivo. Infect. Immun. **71:** 1995–2001.
5. BORJESSON D.L, S.D. KOBAYASHI, A.R. WHITNEY, *et al.* 2005. Insights into pathogen immune evasion mechanisms: *Anaplasma phagocytophilum* fails to induce an apoptosis differentiation program in human neutrophils. J. Immunol. **174:** 6364–6372.
6. GE Y., K. YOSHIIE, F. KURIBAYASHI, *et al.* 2005. *Anaplasma phagocytophilum* inhibits human neutrophil apoptosis via upregulation of bfl-1, maintenance of mitochondrial membrane potential and prevention of caspase 3 activation. Cell Microbiol. **7:** 29–38.
7. DUMLER J.S. & J.S. BAKKEN. 1996. Human granulocytic ehrlichiosis in Wisconsin and Minnesota: a frequent infection with the potential for persistence. J. Infect. Dis. **173:** 1027–1030.
8. FOLEY J.E., V. KRAMER & D. WEBER. 2002. Experimental infection of dusky-footed wood rats (*Neotoma fuscipes*) with *Ehrlichia phagocytophila* sensu lato. J. Wildl. Dis. **38:** 194–198.
9. Munderloh, U.G., M.J. Lynch, M.J. Herron, *et al.* 2004. Infection of endothelial cells with *Anaplasma marginale* and *A. phagocytophilum*. Vet. Microbiol. **101:** 53–64.
10. GOODMAN J.L., C. NELSON, B. VITALE, *et al.* 1996. Direct cultivation of the causative agent of human granulocytic ehrlichiosis. N. Engl. J. Med. **334:** 209–215. Erratum in: N. Engl. J. Med. 1996. **335**: 361.
11. RAVYN, M.D., L.J. LAMB, R. JEMMERSON, *et al.* 1999. Characterization of monoclonal antibodies to an immunodominant protein of the etiologic agent of human granulocytic ehrlichiosis. Am. J. Trop. Med. H yg. **61:** 171–176.
12. SNAPP, K.R., H. DING, K. ATKINS, *et al.* 1998. A novel P-selectin glycoprotein ligand-1 monoclonal antibody recognizes an epitope within the tyrosine sulfate motif of human PSGL-1 and blocks recognition of both P- and L-selectin. Blood **91:** 154–164.
13. ADES, E.W., F.J. CANDAL, R.A. SWERLICK, *et al.* 1992. HMEC-1: establishment of an immortalized human microvascular endothelial cell line. J. Invest. Dermatol. **99:** 683–690.
14. FERRANTE, A. & Y. H. THONG 1980. Optimal conditions for simultaneous purification of mononuclear and polymorphonuclear leucocytes from human blood by the Hypaque-Ficoll method. J. Immunol. Methods **36:** 109–117.
15. SIMON S.I., & C.E. GREEN. 2005. Molecular mechanics and dynamics of leukocyte recruitment during inflammation. Annu. Rev. Biomed. Eng. **7:** 151–185.
16. HERRON M.J. C.M. NELSON, J. LARSON, *et al.* 2000. Intracellular parasitism by the human granulocytic ehrlichiosis bacterium through the P-selectin ligand, PSGL-1. Science **288:** 1653–1656.

Balancing Protective Immunity and Immunopathology

A Unifying Model of Monocytotropic Ehrlichiosis

NAHED ISMAIL AND DAVID H. WALKER

Department of Pathology, Department of Microbiology and Immunology, Sealy Center for Vaccine Development, and Center for Biodefense and Emerging Infectious Diseases, University of Texas Medical Branch, Galveston, Texas 77555-0609, USA

ABSTRACT: Interactions among pathogens, antigen-presenting cells (APCs) and lymphocytes are critical in maintaining balance in the daily challenges to the immune system. Monocytotropic ehrlichiosis, caused by *Ehrlichia chaffeensis*, is a multisystem inflammatory ailment. A complex interaction between *Ehrlichia* and the immune systems of a number of mammalian hosts, in human disease and animal models, has been described. The presence of an overwhelming ehrlichial infection in immunocompromised individuals suggests that severe tissue damage is most likely due to direct bacterial effect. However, clinical and experimental observations indicate that this is an oversimplified concept. First, immunocompetent patients with severe ehrlichiosis have a low bacterial burden. Second, severe and fatal murine ehrlichiosis in immunocompetent animals, which mimics human disease, is associated with a low bacterial burden in different organs and late systemic and local overproduction of TNF-α by T cells. In order to counterbalance overshooting immune responses, T cells and APCs secrete anti-inflammatory cytokines that are key for maintaining a healthy balance between protection and immunopathology. CD4+ T cell–mediated immunity and antibody responses of a Th1 phenotype play critical roles in protection against *Ehrlichia*. Of particular importance for the generation of protective immunity is the induction of activation programs in APCs directly by pathogens or by T cell–derived factors. In this study, we consider the roles of innate and adaptive immune responses in terms of protection from severe ehrlichiosis and their potential roles in immunopathology.

KEYWORDS: **Th1/Th2 cells; cytokines; TNF-α; bacteria; inflammation**

INTRODUCTION

Human monocytotropic ehrlichiosis (HME) is an emerging, tick-borne, zoonotic disease caused by infection of monocytes by the obligate intracellular bacterium, *Ehrlichia chaffeensis*.[1] Infection of humans with *E. chaffeensis* results in a spectrum of clinical manifestations, ranging from fatal to self-limited disease. In immunocom-

Address for correspondence: Nahed Ismail, M.D., Ph.D., Assistant Professor and Associate Director, Department of Pathology, Associate Director, Clinical Microbiology Division, Member of Center for Biodefense and Emerging Infectious Diseases, 301 University Blvd., Galveston, Texas, 77555-0609. Voice: (409) 772-3111; fax: (409) 772-3568.
naismail@utmb.edu

Ann. N.Y. Acad. Sci. 1063: 383–394 (2005).
doi: 10.1196/annals.1355.070

promised individuals, such as those infected with HIV[2] or treated with immunosuppressive drugs, *E. chaffeensis* infection can result in a severe, life-threatening disease. Immunocompetent individuals who do not receive doxycycline treatment until ≥8 days after the onset of symptoms are also at increased risk of developing fatal HME. Severe cases of HME are often comparable in severity to Rocky Mountain spotted fever or toxic shock syndrome.[3]

Current animal models of monocytotropic ehrlichiosis that employ infection of immunocompetent or mice lacking CD4+ T cells with *Ehrlichia chaffeensis* have demonstrated that cell-mediated immunity in particular CD4+ T cells is essential for complete clearance of organisms. SCID mice are highly susceptible to infection with *E. chaffeensis*, while MHC class II knockout mice develop persistent infection. Intracellular killing of *E. chaffeensis* requires CD4+ T cell–dependent cellular effector mechanisms, including NO production by IFN-γ–activated macrophages, and granulomatous inflammation.[4,5] The role of the humoral response in the host defense against *Ehrlichia* is supported by the observations showing that transfer of immune serum obtained from immunocompetent C57BL/6 mice as well as antibodies specific to the 28-kDa major outer membrane proteins of *E. chaffeensis* to C57BL/6 SCID mice provides significant, but transient, protection from disease.[6] Since infection of immunocompetent mice with *E. chaffeensis* does not result in severe disease, and infection of SCID mice results in fatal disease that does not mimic the histopathological findings in HME, we examined the immunopathological mechanisms of resistance and susceptibility to monocytotropic ehrlichiosis in immunocompetent mice employing other ehrlichial species that are phylogenetically related to *E. chaffeensis.* The first is a highly virulent ehrlichial strain isolated from *Ixodes ovatus* ticks (IOE) native to Japan[7] that causes fatal disease in immunocompetent mice.[8]

The second agent is a mildly virulent organism (*Ehrlichia muris*) that causes mild and self-limited disease in immunocompetent mice.[9] Phylogenetic analysis supports the close relationships among monocytotropic *Ehrlichia* spp., including *E. chaffeensis*, *E. muris*, and IOE.[10,11] Additionally, serological cross-reactions occur among closely related monocytotropic *Ehrlichia* species, attributed mainly to molecularly characterized major outer membrane proteins (p28s) of *Ehrlichia* and major antigenic protein 2, the P28 orthologue identified in *E. ruminantium.*[12,13]

In this study we assessed the course of infection and immune responses in C57BL/6 mice susceptible to fatal infection with IOE, but resistant to severe disease caused by *E. muris* infection. Furthermore, we examined whether imbalance between the level of pro-inflammatory and anti-inflammatory cytokines played a critical role in the pathogenesis of severe ehrlichiosis.

MATERIALS AND METHODS

Mice

Sex-matched C57BL/6, C3H/HeJ, and C3H/HeN mice were obtained from The Jackson Laboratory (Bar Harbor, ME) and were used at 6–8 weeks of age in all experiments. Mice were injected intraperitoneally with 1 mL of fresh inoculum at the following doses: 10^{-2} or 10^{-4} dilution of IOE stock or 10^{-1}, 10^{-2}, or 10^{-3} dilution of *E. muris* stock. Quantitative real-time PCR determined that the 10^{-2} dilution of IOE stock (high dose IOE) contained 4×10^6 bacterial genomes, whereas the 10^{-1} dilution of *E. muris* stock (high dose *E. muris*) contained 6 × 10^8 bacterial genomes. Control mice were given 1 mL of a 10^{-1} or 10^{-2} dilution of a spleen homogenate from naive C57BL/6 mice. On the indicated days of infection, mice were sacrificed, and immune responses were assessed. Selected organs were harvested for histology, immunohistochemistry, and determination of bacterial load by real-time PCR as described previously.[14]

Preparation of Host Cell-Free Ehrlichia

IOE and *E. muris* antigens were prepared from either IOE-infected spleens and livers harvested from day 7–infected mice or *E. muris*–infected P388D1 cells as described before.[14] A mixture of spleen and liver from naive mice (mock Ag) was used as a negative control in all experiments using cell-free IOE Ags, while uninfected cell culture lysate (mock Ag) was used as a negative control in all experiments using *E. muris* Ags.

ELISPOT Assays for Antigen-Specific Th1 or Th2 Cytokine-Producing T Cells

Single-cell suspensions were obtained from the spleens of control and infected mice. CD4+ and CD8+ T cells were isolated by negative selection using mouse CD4 or CD8 subset enrichment columns (R&D Systems), and the purity ranged from 80–90% as determined by flow cytometric analysis. Splenocytes and purified T cell subsets were assessed via ELISPOT for cytokine production, as described previously.[14,15]

Lymphocyte Culture and Cytokine Detection

For *in vitro* cytokine measurements, splenocytes were plated in 24-well tissue culture plates at a final concentration of 3 × 10^6 cells/mL in complete RPMI medium. Cells were stimulated with Con A (5 μg/mL), relevant cell-free *E. muris* or IOE antigens, or medium alone, and supernatant fluids were harvested at 72 h. TNF-α and IL-10 levels were measured by specific capture ELISA kits supplied by R&D Systems following the manufacturer's instructions. The detection limits were 150 pg/mL and 5 pg/mL for IL-10 and TNF-α, respectively.

Statistics

Values for secreted Ag-specific cytokine proteins, quantitative real-time PCR, and serum cytokine levels were compared using Student's two-tailed *t* test; $P<0.05$ was regarded as significant.

RESULTS

Course of Infection and Bacterial Burden in Animal Models Of Mild and Fatal Human Monocytotropic Ehrlichiosis

We compared the course of disease in mice infected with different doses of highly virulent IOE or mildly virulent *E. muris*. C57BL/6 mice given a high dose (10^{-2} dilution) of IOE developed progressive disease with weight loss and severe hypogly-

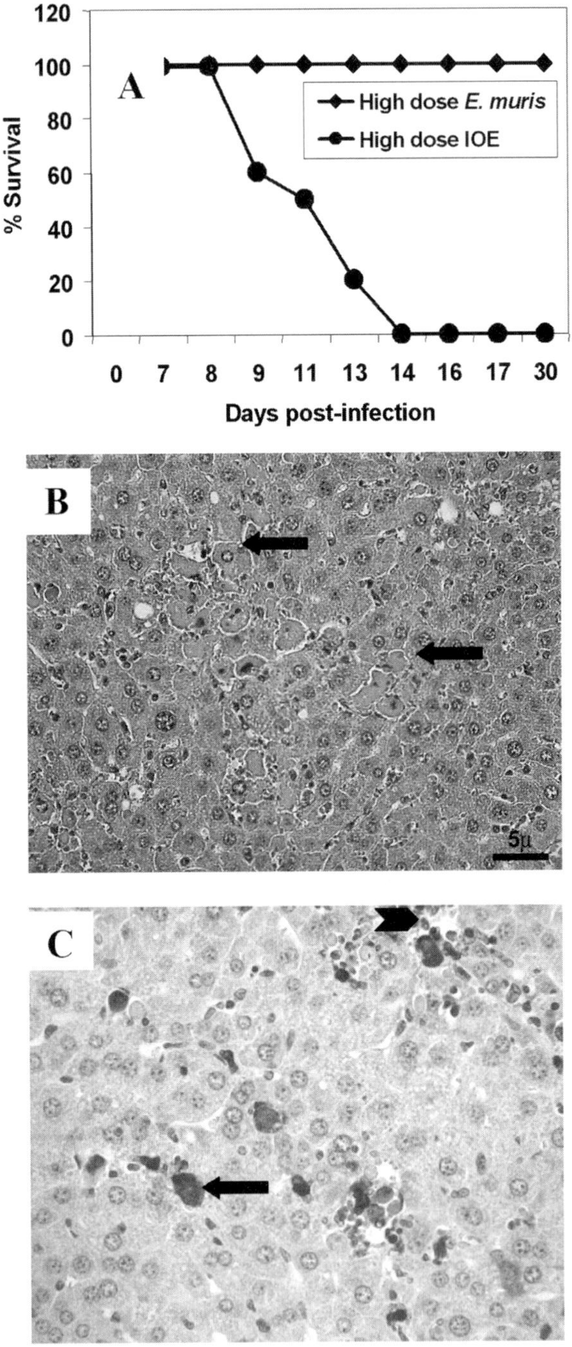

FIGURE 1. *See following page for legend.*

cemia (data not shown), and all died between days 8 and 10 as a result of toxic shock-like syndrome as has been described before (FIG. 1A).[14] These two models were used to evaluate the host immune response associated with fatal ehrlichiosis caused by the highly virulent ehrlichial strain.

Histopathological examination of the liver on day 7 postinfection of mice with high dose IOE revealed abundant, partially confluent foci of cell death of contiguous hepatocytes with regions of cellular infiltration (FIG. 1B). Apoptotic cells were observed diffusely throughout the liver, which is consistent with the presence of a large number of TUNEL-positive cells (FIG. 1C). In contrast, histopathological examination of the liver in mice infected with a high dose of *E. muris* showed moderate focal accumulation of lymphocytes in the perisinusoidal and perivascular areas. The hepatocytes manifested no evidence of injury and were similar to hepatocytes in control animals.

Analysis of the bacterial burden in different organs on day 7 postinfection using quantitative real-time PCR showed that both IOE and *E. muris* organisms were equally capable of dissemination *in vivo*, with marked tropism to the spleen, liver, and lung (FIG. 2A). However, mice infected with high dose IOE had two- to threefold more ehrlichiae in the lung and liver than *E. muris*–infected mice. In contrast, the concentrations of IOE and *E. muris* were comparable in the spleen of infected mice. These data suggest that mortality of IOE-infected mice and severe ehrlichiosis are not due to an overwhelming infection but rather due to an immune-mediated mechanism. A similar observation has been also found in immunocompetent patients infected with *E. chaffeensis*, suggesting that mice infected with a high dose of IOE clinically and pathologically mimic HME.

Roles of TNF-α in IOE-Induced Toxic Shock-Like Syndrome

The systemic pathology during lethal IOE infection suggested that tissue damage might be a consequence of overinduction of proinflammatory cytokines.[16] Therefore, serum levels of TNF-α were determined at different time points during acute infection. An extremely high serum level (~900 pg/mL) of TNF-α was detected on day 7 postinfection in mice infected with high dose IOE (FIG. 2B). In contrast, serum levels of TNF-α in naive mice infected with *E. muris* were not significantly different from those in uninfected mice.

Late IL-10 Overproduction in Wild Type Mice following Lethal IOE Infection

The production of pro-inflammatory TNF-α is regulated by the anti-inflammatory effect of IL-10.[17] We hypothesized that overproduction of TNF-α following lethal

FIGURE 1. Infection with a high dose of IOE causes severe and fatal ehrlichiosis associated with extensive focal hepatic apoptosis. (**A**) Survival/mortality of C57BL/6 mice following intraperitoneal injection with a high (4×10^6) dose of high virulence IOE strain (●), a high dose (6×10^8) of low virulence *E. muris* strain (◆). (**B**) Hepatic histopathology. Mice infected with high dose IOE developed extensive hepatic necrosis and apoptosis (*arrows*) on day 7 postinfection. (**C**) TUNEL staining of liver section from mice infected with a high dose of IOE, day 7 postinfection. The liver section shows apoptotic hepatocytes (*arrows*) and an apoptotic cell lining a hepatic sinusoid (*arrowhead*). Original magnification, ×400. (Reprinted by permission from the American Association of Immunologists, Inc. J. Immunol. **172:** 1786–1800. Copyright 2004.)

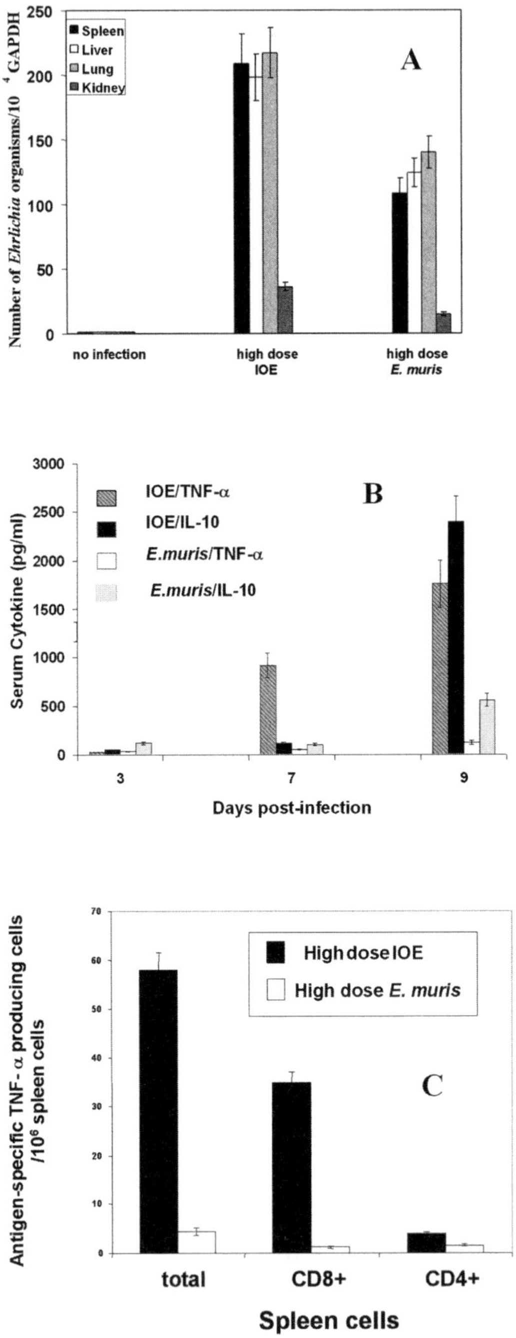

FIGURE 2. *See following page for legend.*

IOE infection is due to defective production of anti-inflammatory IL-10. To test this hypothesis, the levels of serum and splenic IL-10 were measured in wild type mice infected with high doses of either *E. muris* or IOE. At early time points postinfection, lethal infection with high dose IOE induced IL-10 to an extent not significantly different from that induced by *E. muris* infection (FIG. 2B). In contrast, at later time points, a very high level of serum IL-10 was detected in IOE-infected, but not in *E. muris*–infected, mice with a peak at 1–2 days before death (FIG. 2B). These data suggest that late IL-10 overproduction plays a detrimental role in the pathogenesis of severe and fatal ehrlichiosis.

Ehrlichia-Specific CD8+ T Cells Are the Major Source of TNF-α in Severe and Fatal Ehrlichiosis

To determine the source of TNF-α overproduction in mice infected with high dose of IOE, the number of TNF-α producing total splenocytes, and purified splenic CD4+ and CD8+ T cells were enumerated by ELISPOT assay. IOE infection resulted in generation of a substantially higher number of IOE-specific, TNF-α–producing cells in the spleen of IOE-infected mice than *E. muris*–specific cells in mice infected with *E. muris* ($P < 0.01$) (FIG. 2C). Unstimulated spleen cells did not produce TNF-α. More intriguing, IOE-specific CD8+ T cells comprised ~60% of the TNF-α–producing cells, whereas little TNF-α was produced by IOE-specific CD4+ T cells (FIG. 2C).

Downregulation of the Type 1 Response Is Associated with Susceptibility to IOE Infection

To determine whether the Th1/Th2 cytokine profile predicts the resistance or susceptibility of a host to infection with monocytotropic ehrlichiae, we quantified the number of *Ehrlichia*-specific, IFN-γ– and IL-4–producing cells in the spleen of different mice groups using ELISPOT assays. On day 7, splenocytes from mice resistant to infection with high dose *E. muris* contained substantially higher numbers of *Ehrlichia*-specific, IFN-γ–producing cells than mice susceptible to infection with a high dose of IOE (FIG. 3). A substantial number of IFN-γ–producing spleen cells was detected when splenocytes from all mouse groups, including IOE-infected mice, were stimulated with Con A in the ELISPOT assay (not shown). All groups contained negligible numbers of *Ehrlichia*-specific, IL-4–producing cells by ELISPOT

FIGURE 2. Severe and fatal ehrlichiosis following lethal IOE infection is associated with overproduction of TNF-α and IL-10 in the absence of an overwhelming infection. **(A)** Quantitative real-time PCR and relative bacterial load on day 7 postinfection with IOE or *E. muris*. **(B)** Serum IL-10 and TNF-α levels following infection with lethal IOE and nonlethal *E. muris*. High levels of serum TNF-α and IL-10 were detected in mice primarily infected with a high dose of IOE on days 7 and 9 postinfection, respectively. *E. muris*–infected mice had a low level of serum TNF-α and IL-10 at all time points. **(C)** ELISPOT analysis of the number of TNF-α–producing total splenocytes, and purified CD4+ and CD8+ T cells from IOE- and *E. muris*–infected mice. Lethal IOE infection resulted in generation of high number of IOE-specific-TNF-α–producing CD8+ T cells on day 7 postinfection. Data represent the average and SD of triplicate amplifications with three mice per group. Similar results were observed in three independent experiments. (Reprinted by permission from the American Association of Immunologists, Inc. J. Immunol. **172:** 1786–1800. Copyright 2004.)

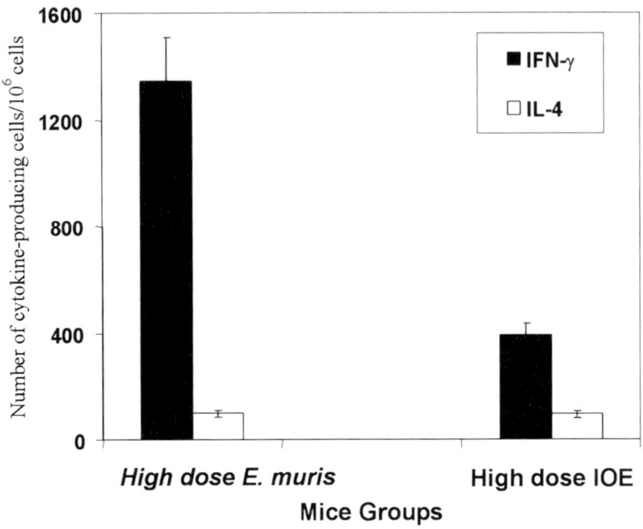

FIGURE 3. Downregulation of type-1 response characterized by IFN-γ production is associated with susceptibility to IOE infection. ELISPOT assay showing the frequency of Ag-specific IFN-γ– or IL-4–producing cells in mice injected intraperitoneally with a high dose of *E. muris* or IOE, on day 7 postinfection. Data represent the average and SD of four mice per group. Similar results were observed in three independent experiments (N = 12/group).

assay (FIG. 3), and we did not detect significant IL-4 production in the culture supernatant of splenocytes from any infected group by ELISA (data not shown).

Host Response and Control of Mildly or Highly Virulent Ehrlichia Is Independent of TLR4

TLR4 interacts with various bacterial products and thereby functions as an important component of the innate immune response against bacterial pathogens.[18,19] We therefore tested whether pathogen recognition via TLR4 that signals through the major adaptor protein of the TLR, MyD88, is involved in control of *Ehrlichia*. C3H/HeJ mice that are deficient in MyD88-dependent TLR4 signaling[18,19] were infected with a high dose of IOE or *E. muris*, and the course of infection and bacterial burden were compared to that encountered in *E. muris*– and IOE-infected C3H/HeN wild-type mice, in which the TLR4 as well as other TLR signaling is intact. Both C3H/HeJ TLR4$^{-/-}$ and C3H/HeN mice were able to control *E. muris* infection. However, both strains succumbed to lethal intraperitoneal infection with IOE on days 8–10, similar to wild type C57BL/6 mice (FIG. 4A).

TNF-α Overproduction and Suppressed CD4+ Th1 Response after Lethal Intraperitoneal Infection with IOE Are Independent of TLR4

In mice, TLR4 is expressed in antigen presenting cells, such as myeloid DCs, and is pivotal in the initiation of adaptive immunity.[18] To test the requirement for TLR4

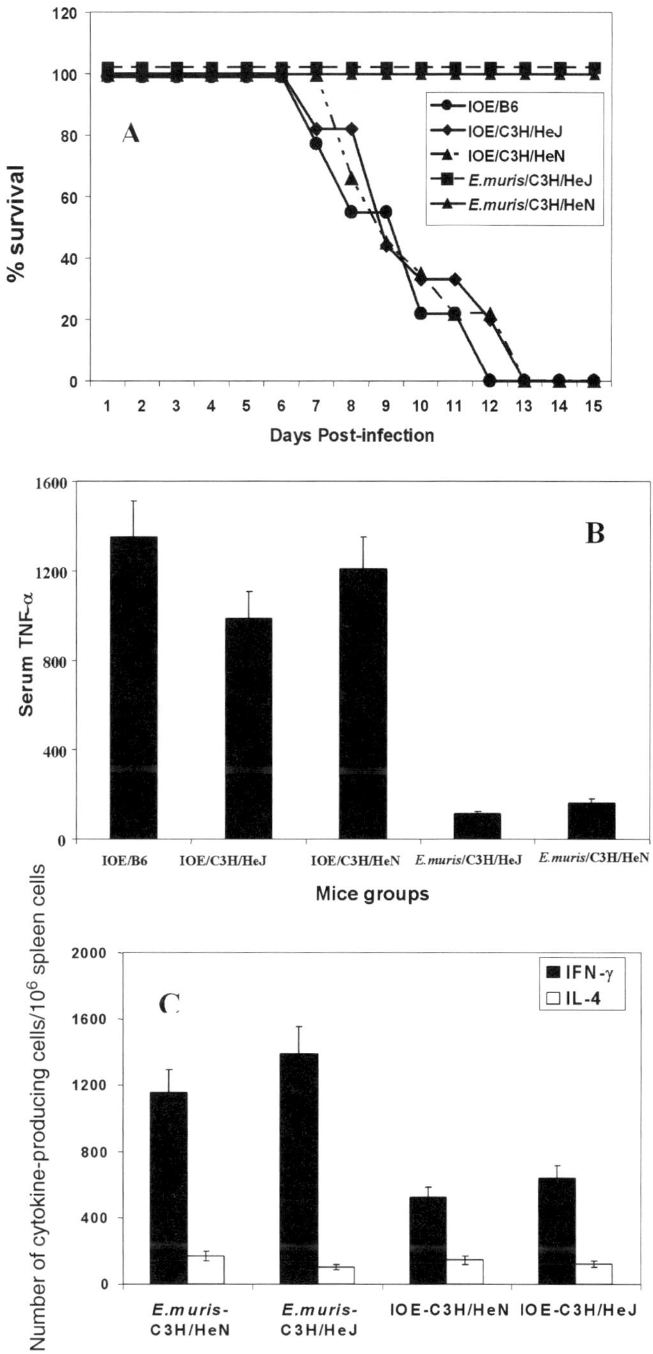

FIGURE 4. *See following page for legend.*

stimulation in the induction of acquired immune response following lethal and non-lethal infection with IOE or *E. muris,* respectively, we examined TNF-α production in the serum and spleen as well as the Th1/Th2 response in the spleen of $TLR4^{-/-}$ C3H/HeJ and $TLR4^{+}$C3H/HeN mice on day 7 postinfection with a high dose of either IOE or *E. muris*. Similar to C3H/HeN mice, lethal IOE infection in $TLR4^{-/-}$ C3H/HeJ mice resulted in a high level of TNF-α in the serum (FIG. 4B) and spleen, which was associated with the generation of a weak Th1 response (FIG. 4C). On the

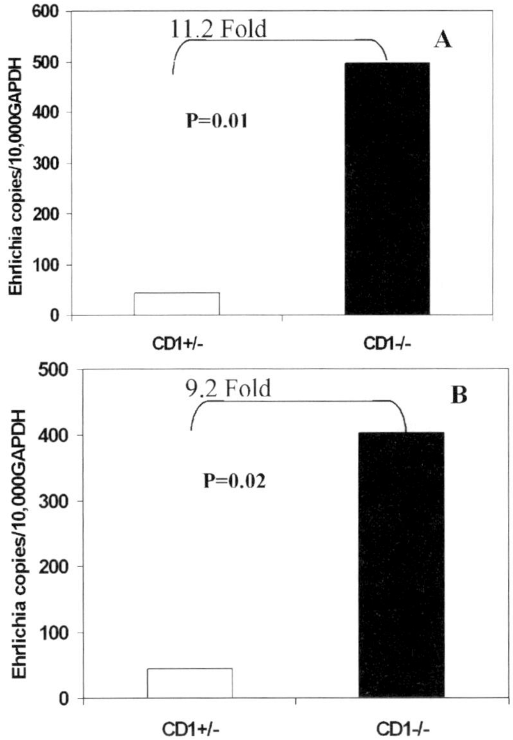

FIGURE 5. *In vivo* role of NKT cells during ehrlichial infection. *Ehrlichia* PCR counts in spleens of $CD1d^{+/-}$ and $CD1d^{-/-}$ mice at 2 days (**A**) and 7 days (**B**) postinfection. Data represent mean ± SD from three mice; one experiment representative of two is shown. Fold increase and *P* values are indicated. (Reprinted by permission from Macmillan Publisher, Ltd. Nature **434:** 525–529. Copyright 2005.)

FIGURE 4. Host defense and immune response against *Ehrlichia* is TLR4 independent. Infected $TLR4^{-/-}$ deficient mice (C3H/HeJ) display comparable survival rate (**A**), serum level of TNF-α (**B**), and type-1 (IFN-γ)/type-2 (IL-4) response (**C**) relative to both TLR-competent C3H/HeN and C57BL/6 wild type mice. Survival of C3H/HeJ $TLR4^{-/-}$, C3H/HeN $TLR4^{+/+}$, and WT C57BL/6 mice (N = 10–15/group) was monitored following intraperitonal injection with a high dose of IOE or *E. muris*. Data are pooled results from two separate experiments that gave nearly identical results.

other hand, non-lethal *E. muris* infection resulted in low level of serum and splenic TNF-α, but a substantial Th1 response, similar to C3H/HeN mice (FIG. 4B and C). These results suggest that TNF-α and IFN-γ secretion is completely independent of TLR4 after lethal or non-lethal ehrlichial infections.

Control of Ehrlichial Replication Is Dependent on CD1-Restricted NKT Cells

CD1d-restricted natural killer T (NKT) cells are innate-like lymphocytes that express a conserved T-cell receptor and contribute to host defense against various microbial pathogens.[20] To test the central role that NKT cells might play *in vivo* against LPS-lacking *Ehrlichia*, $CD1^{-/-}$ mice deficient in NKT cells and wild type C57BL/6 mice were infected intravenously with a high dose of *E. muris*, and bacterial burdens were determined in different organs on day 7 postinfection. $CD1d^{-/-}$ mice had higher ehrlichial burden and delayed bacterial clearance in the spleens on days 2 and 7 postinfection (FIG. 5 A and B, respectively) compared with heterozygous littermate controls. This demonstrates the antimicrobial function of NKT cells in host defense against ehrlichia. Further studies by Mattner and colleagues[20] have demonstrated that the splenic IFN-γ response to LPS-negative *Ehrlichia* and another LPS-negative organism, *Sphingomonas,* is largely independent of MyD88. $CD1d^{-/-}$ spleen cells lacking NKT cells failed to respond to *Ehrlichia* and *Sphingomonas*, whereas the response to LPS-containing *Salmonella* was only marginally reduced. Similarly, wild-type NKT cells co-cultured with MyD88-deficient DCs responded to *Sphingomonas* and *Ehrlichia* but not *Salmonella.*[20] Taken together, these results suggest that IFN-γ stimulation by *Ehrlichia* and *Sphingomonas* is primarily dependent on NKT cells and CD1d, with minimal contribution from TLRs.[20]

[Competing interests statement: The authors report that they have no conflicts of interest.]

REFERENCES

1. OLANO, J.P. & D.H. WALKER. 2002. Human ehrlichioses. Med. Clin. North Am. **86:** 375.
2. PADDOCK, C. D., D.P. SUCHARD, K.L. GRUMBACH, *et al.* 1993. Brief report: fatal seronegative ehrlichiosis in a patient with HIV infection. N. Engl. J. Med. **329:** 1164.
3. FICHTENBAUM, C.J., L.R. PETERSON & G.J. WEIL. 1993. Ehrlichiosis presenting as a life-threatening illness with features of the toxic shock syndrome. Am. J. Med. **95:** 351.
4. WINSLOW, G.M., E. YAGER, K. SHILO, *et al.* 1998. Infection of the laboratory mouse with the intracellular pathogen *Ehrlichia chaffeensis*. Infect. Immun. **66:** 3892.
5. GANTA, R.R., M.J. WILKERSON, C. CHENG, *et al.* 2002. Persistent *Ehrlichia chaffeensis* infection occurs in the absence of functional major histocompatibility complex class II genes. Infect. Immun. **70:** 380.
6. LI, J. S., F. CHU, A. REILLY, *et al.* 2002. Antibodies highly effective in SCID mice during infection by the intracellular bacterium *Ehrlichia chaffeensis* are of picomolar affinity and exhibit preferential epitope and isotype utilization. J. Immunol. **169:** 1419.
7. SHIBATA, S., M. KAWAHARA, Y. RIKIHISA, *et al.* 2000. New *Ehrlichia* species closely related to *Ehrlichia chaffeensis* isolated from *Ixodes ovatus* ticks in Japan. J. Clin. Microbiol. **38:** 1331.
8. SOTOMAYOR, E.A., V.L. POPOV, H-M. FENG, *et al.* 2001. Animal model of fatal human monocytotropic ehrlichiosis. Am. J. Pathol. **158:** 757.

9. KAWAHARA, M., T. ITO, C. SUTO, *et al.* 1999. Comparison of *Ehrlichia muris* strains isolated from wild mice and ticks and serologic survey of humans and animals with *E. muris* as antigen. J. Clin. Microbiol. **37:** 1123.
10. SUMNER, J.W., G.A. STORCH, R.S. BULLER, *et al.* 2000. PCR amplification and phylogenetic analysis of *groESL* operon sequences from *Ehrlichia ewingii* and *Ehrlichia muris*. J. Clin. Microbiol. **38:** 2746.
11. SHIBATA, S., M. KAWAHARA, Y. RIKIHISA, *et al.* 2000. New *Ehrlichia* species closely related to *Ehrlichia chaffeensis* isolated from *Ixodes ovatus* ticks in Japan. J. Clin. Microbiol. **38:** 1331.
12. ALLEMAN, A.R., A.F. BARBET, M.V. BOWIE, *et al.* 2000. Expression of a gene encoding the major antigenic protein 2 homolog of *Ehrlichia chaffeensis* and potential application for serodiagnosis. J. Clin. Microbiol. **38:** 3705
13. ALLEMAN, A.R., L.J. MCSHERRY, A.F. BARBET, *et al.* Recombinant major antigenic protein 2 of *Ehrlichia canis*: a potential diagnostic tool. J. Clin. Microbiol. **39:** 2494.
14. ISMAIL N., L. SOONG, J.W. MCBRIDE, *et al.* 2004. Overproduction of TNF-alpha by CD8+ type 1 cells and down-regulation of IFN-gamma production by CD4+ Th1 cells contribute to toxic shock-like syndrome in an animal model of fatal monocytotropic ehrlichiosis. J. Immunol. **172:** 1786.
15. POWER, C.A., C.L. GRAND, N. ISMAIL, *et al.* 1999. A valid ELISPOT assay for enumeration of ex vivo, antigen-specific, IFN-γ-producing T cells. J. Immunol. Methods **227:** 99.
16. HACK, C.E., L.A. AARDEN & L.G. THIJS. 1997. Role of cytokine in sepsis. Adv. Immunol. **66:** 101.
17. SCHOPF, L.R., K.F. HOFFMANN, A.W. CHEEVER, *et al.* 2002. IL-10 is critical for host resistance and survival during gastrointestinal helminth infection. J. Immunol. **168:** 2383.
18. GOLDSTEIN, D.R. 2004. Toll-like receptors and other links between innate and acquired alloimmunity. Curr. Opin. Immunol. **16:** 538.
19. FENG, C.G., C.A. SCANGA & C.M. COLLAZO-CUSTODIO. Mice lacking myeloid differentiation factor 88 display profound defects in host resistance and immune responses to *Mycobacterium avium* infection not exhibited by Toll-like receptor 2 (TLR2)- and TLR4-deficient animals. J. Immunol. **171:** 4758.
20. MATTNER, J., K.L. DEBORD, N. ISMAIL, *et al.* 2005. Exogenous and endogenous glycolipid antigens activate NKT cells during microbial infections. Nature **434:** 525.

Susceptibility and Resistance to Monocytic Ehrlichiosis in the Mouse

GARY M. WINSLOW,[a] CONSTANTINE BITSAKTSIS,[a] AND ERIC YAGER[b]

[a]*Wadsworth Center, New York State Department of Health, Albany, New York 12201-2002, USA*

[b]*The Department of Biomedical Sciences, School of Public Health, University at Albany, Albany, New York 12201-0509, USA*

ABSTRACT: To address the role of cellular immunity during ehrlichia infection, we have utilized a model of monocytic ehrlichiosis that results from infection of mice by *Ixodes ovatus* ehrlichia (IOE). Although ehrlichiosis in humans is largely a disease of immunocompromised individuals, the use of the IOE model has allowed us to identify factors required for host defense in normal mice. Using a low-dose infection C57BL/6 mouse model, we have demonstrated that host defense requires immune mechanisms involving CD4 T cell-mediated, TNF-α-, IL-12-, and IFN-γ–dependent, macrophage activation. We have also provided formal evidence that IFN-γ produced by CD4 Th1 cells is sufficient for protective immunity. Our recent studies have demonstrated, in addition, an essential role for IL-10, which is probably important in inhibiting immunopathological responses, and for inducible nitric oxide synthase. The latter observation establishes an important role for reactive nitrogen intermediates in bacterial elimination *in vivo*. In contrast, evaluation of mice carrying wild-type and mutant alleles of *Nramp1* revealed at most a modest role for this gene in resistance to fatal IOE infection. Other studies in low-dose infected mice have indicated that the generation of immunological memory may be impaired during low-dose IOE infection, possibly due to bacterial immune subversion. These studies highlight the utility of the IOE mouse model in identifying important parameters of the immune response during ehrlichiosis.

KEYWORDS: ehrlichia; cellular immunity; intracellular bacteria; CD4 T cell; CD8 T cell

INTRODUCTION

The ehrlichiae are obligate intracellular rickettsiae that cause a range of diseases in humans in humans and animals.[1–3] The understanding of host defense during ehrlichiosis is relatively undeveloped, however, so our laboratory has been employing a number of approaches to investigate host immunity and susceptibility in mouse models. The mouse is an ideal animal model for investigation, because many, al-

Address for correspondence: Gary Winslow, Wadsworth Center, 120 New Scotland Avenue, Albany, NY 12208. Voice: 518-473-2795; fax 518-486-9858.
gary.winslow@wadsworth.org.

**Ann. N.Y. Acad. Sci. 1063: 395–402 (2005). © 2005 New York Academy of Sciences.
doi: 10.1196/annals.1355.071**

though not all, ehrlichiae infect mice as part of their natural life cycle, and also because a wide range of immunological tools are available for experimental studies. Our previous studies investigated humoral immunity in a model of monocytic ehrlichiosis in SCID mice. A particularly novel aspect of that work was that antibodies were found to be highly effective in controlling *Ehrlichia chaffeensis* infection, even when administered well after infection had become established. As antibodies are generally considered to be of little value during most intracellular bacterial infections, an implication is that mechanisms of host defense used against the ehrlichiae differ from those used during other intracellular bacterial infections.

Although the SCID mouse provided an excellent model in which to examine the role of exogenous antibodies in host defense in the absence of adaptive cellular immunity, an obvious limitation of the model was that humoral and/or cellular immunity could not be studied in the context of a normal host response. *E. chaffeensis* infects immunocompetent mice, but infection is largely self-limiting; a feature that has made it more difficult, although not impossible,[4,5] to identify correlates of immune protection. For example, in our unpublished studies, we failed to identify any gene-targeted mouse strains (including IFN-γ–deficient, and several other immunodeficient strains) that were susceptible to acute fatal *E. chaffeensis* infection.

Recent studies have described the development of a mouse model of fatal monocytic ehrlichiosis infection[6] that results from infection with *Ixodes ovatus* ehrlichia (IOE[7,8]). Subsequent studies using this model led to a study of immunity during high-dose fatal infection.[9] This work revealed that fatal infection was associated with cytokine dysregulation by both CD4 and CD8 T cells.[9] We have modified this experimental model to examine resistance and susceptibility following sublethal, low-dose IOE infection. Here we will describe some of our recent studies that have utilized this model to identify factors affecting host susceptibility and resistance to ehrlichia infection.

MATERIALS AND METHODS

Mice

All mice were obtained from the Jackson Laboratories, including mice deficient for IL-10 (B6.129P2-IL10^{tn1Cgn}/J), inducible nitric oxide synthase (B6.129P2-Nos2^{tm1iLau}), and the IFN-γ receptor (B6.129S7-Ifngr). Although some of the gene-targeted mutations were available only on a B6.129 genetic background, infection studies of B6.129 mice have not revealed any differences in susceptibility to IOE infection, as compared to C57BL/6 mice. For the *Nramp1* studies, *Nramp1*$^{+/+}$ (129x1/SvJ) and C57BL/6 mice (*Nramp1*$^{asp169/asp169}$) were used. The studies were performed in accordance with institutional guidelines for animal welfare.

Methods

All methods, including IOE infection and quantitation, and T cell purification and adoptive transfer, have been described previously.[10]

RESULTS AND DISCUSSION

Investigation of Immunity to Ehrlichiosis in Gene-Targeted and Inbred Mice

Using a low-dose infection model, we have demonstrated that C57BL/6 and BALB/c mice are susceptible to surprisingly low numbers of IOE administered intraperitoneally. As it is not yet possible to culture or to quantify viable IOE, IOE-infected splenocytes were used as an inoculum, and the infectious dose was quantified by determining the copy number of the IOE 16S rDNA gene (a single-copy gene) using quantitative PCR. In this way, the LD_{50} in C57BL/6 and BALB/c mice was determined to be 500–1000 bacteria.[10] C57BL/6 and BALB/c mice inoculated with lower numbers of bacteria (100–200 bacteria) were resistant to fatal infection. In contrast, C57BL/6-*scid* mice, which lack adaptive immunity required for host resistance, did not survive infection with inocula estimated to contain as few as a single bacterium. These data indicated that our infectious inoculum contained a high percentage of viable bacteria, and that the model can be used to study infection with relatively low numbers of ehrlichiae (100–200 bacteria); plausibly, these numbers are comparable to those that might be expected to be transmitted by a feeding tick. On the basis of the studies in SCID mice, we have made the simplifying assumption that copy number and viable bacteria were essentially equivalent in our experimental model.

Because immunocompetent mice survived low-dose infection, and whereas SCID mice did not, we used the model to identify and characterize cells and factors involved in host defense. Available strains of gene-targeted mice, deficient for a number of important immune cell subsets and factors, were examined for resistance and susceptibility to IOE infection. In striking contrast to their response to *E. chaffeensis* infection, many of the gene-targeted strains examined were susceptible to a low-dose IOE inoculum that was sublethal for immunocompetent mice. Mice infected with an inoculum of approximately 100 IOE were shown to require CD4 T cells, IFN-γ, TNF-α, IL-12p40, the IFN-γ receptor, and TNF receptors I and II, in order to mount a protective response to fatal infection.[10] Only two gene-targeted strains examined were resistant to infection, the IL-4– and CD8-deficient mice. Association of resistance with these phenotypes suggested that CD4 Th1 cells are essential for host defense, and that CD8 T cells are dispensable for resistance to low-dose IOE infection.

More recent studies have revealed that both IL-10, and inducible nitric oxide synthase (iNOS), in addition to the above described factors, are essential for IOE host defense (FIG. 1). The requirement for the former finding likely indicates that IL-10 is required to suppress excessive inflammatory cytokine responses during infection, as has been observed in studies of other intracellular pathogens.[11] The requirement for iNOS was not unexpected, given that a major function for iNOS is in IFN-γ–induced killing of intracellular pathogens.[12–14] A role for iNOS has also been suggested from studies of the related rickettsia, *Anaplasma phagocytophila*.[15] Nevertheless, our studies provide definitive evidence that reactive-nitrogen intermediates are utilized for bacterial elimination *in vivo* during ehrlichia infection.

Although the gene-targeted mouse strains provide a powerful approach for identifying pathways of host defense, some caution is warranted regarding the interpretation of findings that rely solely on the use of such mice. Many of the mutations can cause pleiotropic defects in a number of other pathways and cell types, sometimes

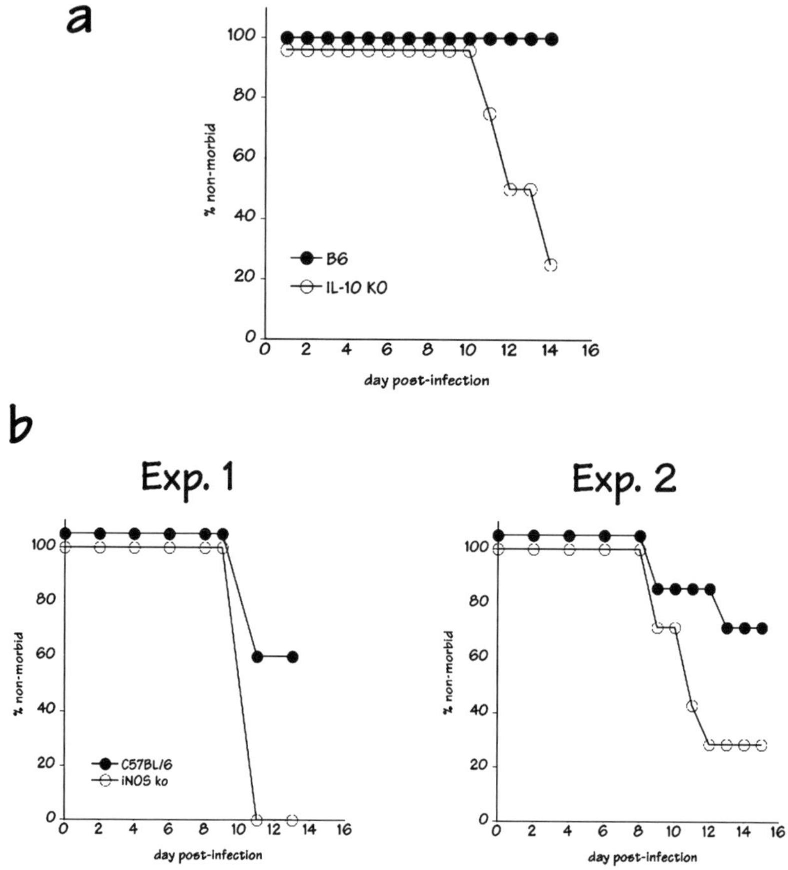

FIGURE 1. IOE infection in selected gene-targeted mouse strains. (**a**) C57BL/6 (B6) and IL-10–deficient mice were infected with a low-dose inoculum of IOE (approximately 100 bacteria) and were monitored for morbidity (as evidenced by symptoms such as immobility, hunched posture, and wasting) on the days indicated. (**b**) In similar experiments C57BL/6 mice, or mice deficient in iNOS, were infected with a low-dose inoculum of IOE. In the two experiments shown, 5 of 5 and 5 of 7 iNOS-deficient mice succumbed to low-dose infection, while only 2 of 5 and 2 of 7 control C57BL/6 mice died, respectively. In our model, C57BL/6 mice on occasion die of fatal low-dose IOE infection.

in quite unexpected ways. For example, deficiencies in particular cell subsets (e.g., CD4 T cells) may affect the maturation of other lymphocytes.[16,17] Alterations of cell frequencies in gene-targeted mice may result from changes that occur during lymphocyte development, or from changes in immune regulation that occur during lymphocyte differentiation. Thus, although findings in gene-targeted mouse models may suggest a requirement for a particular cell type or factor, definitive evidence for the involvement of a particular component in host defense requires additional confirmation.

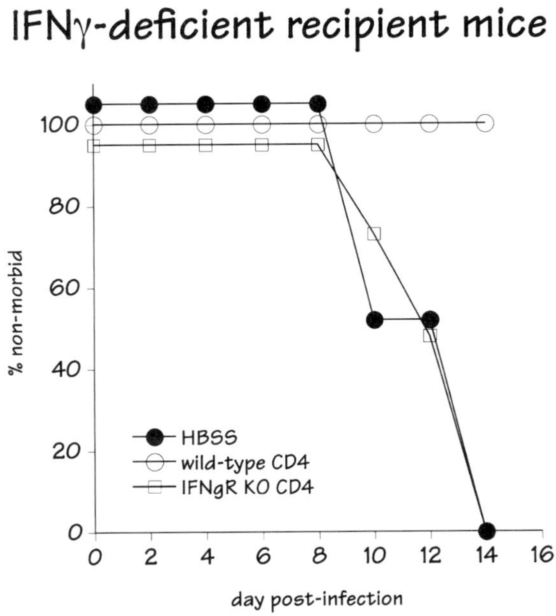

FIGURE 2. IFN-γ production by CD4 T cells was sufficient to rescue IFN-γ–deficient mice from fatal low-dose IOE infection. IFN-γ–deficient recipient mice were administered buffer (HBSS), purified wild-type CD4 T cells, or IFN-γ receptor–deficient CD4 T cells (IFNγR–KO) ($2{\times}10^6$) 1 day prior to low-dose IOE challenge. Each group contained three mice.

One strategy in our laboratory has been to utilize adoptive transfer approaches to evaluate the role of specific cells more precisely. For example, although our gene-targeted mouse data indicated that both the CD4 receptor and IFN-γ are required for IOE host defense, it was unclear whether CD4 T cells are themselves required (CD4 is also expressed on a subset of dendritic cells[18]), or whether the requirement for IFN-γ indicated that IFN-γ production by CD4 T cells was essential (IFN-γ is produced by other cells, including NK cells). To test the latter hypothesis, we addressed whether wild-type CD4 T cells could complement the IFN-γ deficiency, by transferring wild-type CD4 T cells into in susceptible IFN-γ–deficient mice one day prior to low-dose IOE infection. For these studies the CD4 T cells were obtained from IOE-infected mice four weeks following infection, purified by magnetic bead negative selection, and administered ($2{\times}10^6$ cells) intravenously. Wild-type CD4 T cells fully protected the IFN-γ–deficient mice from otherwise fatal infection (FIG. 2). In other studies, antibody-mediated IFN-γ ablation was used to confirm that the protection afforded by the donor CD4 T cells is IFN-γ–dependent,[10] rather than due to some other function of the transferred CD4 T cells. In similar transfer studies, we demonstrated that the IFN-γ receptor (IFN-γR) is required on the donor CD4 T cells; this requirement likely indicates a requirement for the IFN-γR for the generation of fully functional CD4 effector T cells (FIG. 2). These studies provided direct evidence for the importance of both IFN-γ and CD4 T cells in protection, and they indicated that

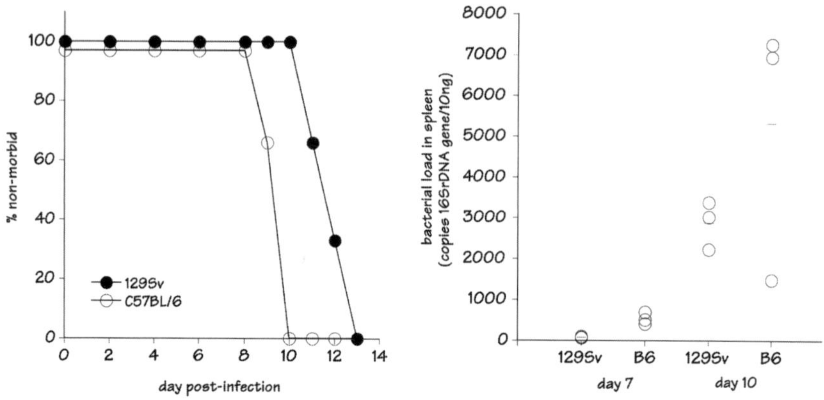

FIGURE 3. Nramp1 plays at most a modest role in host resistance to IOE infection. Mice carrying wild-type (129Sv) or mutant alleles of *Nramp1* (C57BL/6) were infected with a high-dose IOE challenge (approximately 2000 organisms). Morbidity (*left panel*) and bacterial colonization in spleen tissue (*right panel*) were monitored on the indicated days postinfection. In the *right panel* each *circle* represents a single mouse, and the mean value for each group is indicated by a *dash*. A trend is seen toward higher bacterial loads in the *Nramp1*-deficient (B6) mice, although the differences were statistically significant ($P < 0.5$) only on day 7, as determined using Fisher's exact test (95% confidence level).

IFN-γ production by the CD4 T cells was sufficient—and likely necessary—for immunity. The studies, however, do not rule out important roles for other IFN-γ–producing cells during infection. Thus, although the gene-targeted mice are very powerful tools to investigate host defense, additional experimental approaches are necessary to confirm the involvement of cell subsets and factors during host defense.

The use of the IOE model has also allowed us to examine host resistance and susceptibility in conventional inbred mouse strains. In particular, we have examined the possible involvement of Nramp1, a factor involved in divalent-metal influx at the phagosomal membrane and known to play a role in host immunity to several pathogenic intracellular bacteria.[19–21] Nramp1 is non-functional in many inbred mouse strains, including C57BL/6, but it is fully functional in 129x1/SvJ (129Sv) mice (both strains are H-2^b). Because common inbred strains are resistant to low-dose IOE infection, we compared susceptibility to a high-dose IOE infection (2× LD_{50}; approximately 2000 bacteria) in 129Sv and C57BL/6 mice. The *Nramp1*-positive strain 129Sv exhibited a 2–3 day increase in the time to morbidity after high-dose IOE challenge, suggesting a partial role for Nramp1 in host defense (FIG. 3a). Analysis of bacterial colonization of spleen tissue revealed a similar trend toward increased resistance, as the *Nramp1*-positive 129Sv mice exhibited lower bacterial loads on days 7 and 10 postinfection (FIG. 3b). These data reveal that although Nramp1 appears to play a role in host resistance to IOE infection, its contribution is at best modest under the conditions of high-dose IOE infection used in our studies. Thus, although Nramp1 does not play a major role in host resistance to IOE infection, it may nevertheless contribute to host defense, and may play a greater role under different infection conditions, such as persistent infection.[21]

MEMORY T CELL RESPONSES DURING IOE

The study of immunological memory in ehrlichiosis is largely undeveloped. Such studies are clearly needed for vaccine development, especially for vaccines designed to elicit protective cellular immunity. Indeed, many vaccines have been tested with little knowledge of the development of immunological memory. Although empirical approaches have been successful on occasion, it is likely that optimal vaccine design will require detailed knowledge of immunological memory. Whereas in most experimental models prior infection generates protective immunity to a higher challenge infection (a hallmark of immunological memory), we have observed that a prior low-dose IOE or *E. chaffeensis* infection does not protect against subsequent high-dose IOE challenge (unpublished data).[10] This failure of protective recall responses was not due to the inability to generate protective memory responses against IOE, because prior *E. muris* infection induces highly protective memory responses (unpublished data).[9]

Our efforts to boost immunity to high-dose IOE infection by repeated immunizations with low-dose IOE led to the surprising finding that a second low-dose infection resulted in fatal recall responses (unpublished data). Thus, immunological memory is impaired in IOE-infected mice, perhaps as a result of immune subversion. In subsequent studies we have shown that the fatal recall responses were entirely dependent on CD8 T cells, as CD8-deficient mice were unaffected by secondary low-dose challenge (unpublished data). These findings contrast with our published findings that CD8 T cells are not necessary for immunity to a primary low-dose IOE infection.[10] Thus, paradoxically, CD8 T cells, although unnecessary during primary infection, nevertheless develop into memory T cells that, upon re-challenge, can generate fully functional but deleterious secondary responses. These data may bear some relation to observations made by Ismail and colleagues, who provided evidence that CD8 T cells are a possible source of high levels of TNF-α during fatal high-dose IOE infection.[9] Indeed, our preliminary data have suggested an involvement of TNF-α in the deleterious CD8 memory T cells responses that we have observed (unpublished data). Thus, CD8 T cells may play a key role in immunopathological responses elicited during IOE challenge infection in mice. Hence, the study of immunological memory during ehrlichia infection may not only provide information necessary for vaccine development, but may also broaden our understanding of how immunological memory can be subverted, to allow persistent and/or repeated infections to occur in both natural and accidental hosts, including humans.

ACKNOWLEDGMENTS

This work was supported by U.S. Public Health Service grant R01-AI47963-01.

[*Competing interest statement:* The authors declare that they have no competing interests.]

REFERENCES

1. Paddock, C.D. & J.E. Childs. 2003. *Ehrlichia chaffeensis*: A prototypical emerging Pathogen. Clin. Microbiol. Rev. **16:** 37–64.

2. WINSLOW, G. & B. BITSAKTSIS. 2005. Immunity to the ehrlichiae: New tools and recent developments. Curr. Op. Inf. Dis. **18:** 217–221.
3. DUMLER, J.S. & D.H. WALKER. 2001. Tick-borne ehrlichioses. Lancet Infect. Dis. (April 2001): 21–28.
4. GANTA, R.R. *et al.* 2002. Persistent *Ehrlichia chaffeensis* infection occurs in the absence of functional major histocompatibility complex class II genes. Inf. Immun. **70:** 380–388.
5. GANTA, R.R. *et al.* 2004. Delayed clearance of *Ehrlichia chaffeensis* infection in CD4+ T-cell knockout mice. Infect. Immun. **72:** 159–167.
6. SOTOMAYOR, E.A. *et al.* 2001. Animal model of fatal human monocytotropic ehrlichiosis. Am. J. Pathol. **158:** 757–769.
7. SHIBATA, S. *et al.* 2000. New Ehrlichia species closely related to *Ehrlichia chaffeensis* isolated from *Ixodes ovatus* ticks in Japan. J. Clin. Microbiol. **38:** 1331–1338.
8. OKADA, H. *et al.* 2003. Distribution of Ehrlichiae in tissues as determined by in-situ hybridization. J. Comp. Pathol. **128:** 182–187.
9. ISMAIL, N. *et al.* 2004. Overproduction of TNF-alpha by CD8+ type 1 cells and down-regulation of IFN-gamma production by CD4+ Th1 cells contribute to toxic shock-like syndrome in an animal model of fatal monocytotropic ehrlichiosis. J. Immunol. **172:** 1786–1800.
10. BITSAKTSIS, C. *et al.* 2004. Production of Interferon-γ by CD4 T cells is essential for resolving ehrlichia infection. J. Immunol. **172:** 6894–6901.
11. REDPATH, S. *et al.* 2001. Hijacking and exploitation of IL-10 by intracellular pathogens. Trends Microbiol. **9:** 86–92.
12. VAZQUEZ-TORRES, A. *et al.* 2000. Antimicrobial actions of the NADPH phagocyte oxidase and inducible nitric oxide synthase in experimental salmonellosis. I. Effects on microbial killing by activated peritoneal macrophages in vitro. J. Exp. Med. **192:** 227–236.
13. MACMICKING, J.D. *et al.* 1997. Identification of nitric oxide synthase as a protective locus against tuberculosis. Proc. Natl. Acad. Sci. USA **94:** 5243–5248.
14. WEI, X.Q. *et al.* 1995. Altered immune responses in mice lacking inducible nitric oxide synthase. Nature **375:** 408–411.
15. BANERJEE, R. *et al.* 2000. Granulocytic ehrlichiosis in mice deficient in phagocyte oxidase or inducible nitric oxide synthase. Infect. Immun. **68:** 4361–4362.
16. KHANOLKAR, A. *et al.* 2004. CD4 T cell-dependent CD8 T cell maturation. J. Immunol. **172:** 2834–2844.
17. LIU, H. *et al.* 2002. Reduced functional capacity of CD8+ T cells expanded by post-exposure vaccination of gamma-herpesvirus-infected CD4-deficient mice. J. Immunol. **168:** 3477–3483.
18. SHORTMAN, K. & Y.J. LIU. 2002. Mouse and human dendritic cell subtypes. Nat. Rev. Immunol. **2:** 151–161.
19. BELLAMY, R. 1999. The natural resistance-associated macrophage protein and susceptibility to intracellular pathogens. Microbes. Inf. **1:** 23–27.
20. FORBES, J.R. & P. GROS. 2001. Divalent-metal transport by NRAMP proteins at the interface of host-pathogen interactions. Trends Microbiol. **9:** 397–403.
21. MONACK, D.M. *et al.* 2004. *Salmonella typhimurium* persists within macrophages in the mesenteric lymph nodes of chronically infected Nramp1+/+ mice and can be reactivated by IFN{gamma} neutralization. J. Exp. Med. **199:** 231–241.

Overcoming Barriers to the Transformation of the Genus *Ehrlichia*

S. WESLEY LONG, TED J. WHITWORTH, DAVID H. WALKER, AND XUE-JIE YU

Department of Pathology, University of Texas Medical Branch, Galveston, Texas 77555-0609, USA

ABSTRACT: While bacterial transformation has evolved since the early 20th century to allow for the genetic manipulation of a variety of microbial agents, rickettsial organisms have proved resistant to such advances until only recently. The *Ehrlichia* are small, gram-negative, obligately intracellular bacterial parasites, which belong to the family Anaplasmataceae and cause a variety of infections in human and animal hosts. *E. chaffeensis* is the causative agent of human monocytotropic ehrlichiosis and is transmitted by *Amblyomma americanum*, the Lone Star tick. In this work, we describe the first report of successful transformation of a closely related ehrlichial species, the murine monocytotropic species *E. muris*. Application of these techniques should allow for a wide variety of molecular studies to be performed that were previously impossible. This heralds the beginning of a new era in ehrlichial research.

KEYWORDS: *Ehrlichia*; *E. chaffeensis*; *E. muris*; transformation; PCR; chloramphenicol

INTRODUCTION

Ehrlichia are small, gram-negative obligately intracellular parasites, which belong to the family Anaplasmataceae and cause a variety of infections in human and animal hosts. *E. chaffeensis* is the causative agent of human monocytotropic ehrlichiosis and is transmitted by *Amblyomma americanum*, the Lone Star tick.[1] Thus far, *Ehrlichia* have proven resistant to attempts at genetic transformation and lack naturally occurring plasmids or phage. This situation has posed a significant obstacle to progress in the field, preventing genetic manipulations routinely available in most fields of bacteriology.

The transformation of *Rickettsia prowazekii* was first reported by Rachek *et al.* in 1998.[2] The barriers to the transformation of *Ehrlichia* were many. First, only one antibiotic family has been shown to have reliable clinical utility against *E. chaffeensis*, the tetracyclines. Doxycycline is the gold standard drug for treatment of ehrlichial infections and, therefore, it would be unwise to create tetracycline-resistant *E. chaffeensis*. Chloramphenicol would be a possible choice for antibiotic selection, based upon retrospective data from one clinical series; however, previous work had shown

Address for correspondence: S. Wesley Long, Department of Pathology, University of Texas Medical Branch, 301 University Boulevard, Route 0609, Galveston, TX 77555-0609. Voice: 409-772-4813; fax: 409-747-2415.
swlong@utmb.edu

**Ann. N.Y. Acad. Sci. 1063: 403–410 (2005). © 2005 New York Academy of Sciences.
doi: 10.1196/annals.1355.072**

E. chaffeensis to be resistant to chloramphenicol treatment *in vitro*.[3] Because of these issues surrounding *E. chaffeensis*, it was decided to use the murine ehrlichial species *E. muris*. Testing of *E. muris* showed it to be susceptible to chloramphenicol *in vitro*.

A plasmid containing the chloramphenicol resistance gene, chloramphenicol acetyltransferase (CAT), under the control of an ehrlichial promoter cloned from *E. chaffeensis*, was chosen for transforming *E. muris*. *E. muris*, purified from host cells, was transformed by electroporation based upon a protocol modified from that of Rachek *et al.* for transformation of rickettsiae.

MATERIALS AND METHODS

The Organism and Cell Culture

An isolate of *E. muris* (originally obtained from Y. Rikihisa) was cultured in the DH82 canine monocyte cell line. The wild-type cells were cultured in high glucose Dulbecco's Modified Eagle Medium (Gibco) in 5% fetal bovine serum (FBS) (Gibco) and 1 mM 4-(2-hydroxyethyl)-1-piperazine ethanesulfonic acid (HEPES) (Mediatech, Herndon, VA), at 37°C with 5% CO_2. Transformed *E. muris* were maintained in the same medium, with a reduced amount of serum (2.5% FBS).

Polymerase Chain Reaction (PCR)

PCR was used to verify the presence of *E. muris* DNA in wild-type and transformant cell cultures. For increased sensitivity, a nested PCR of the 16S rRNA gene was used. The first-round PCR used the primers ECC and ECB, while the nested PCR used primers ECC and HE3.[4] The PCRs were carried out using 2.5× HotMasterMix (Eppendorf, New York, NY) and PCR-grade water. All primers and probes were obtained from Sigma Genosys.

Transformation of Ehrlichia

Infected 150-cm^2 cell culture flasks (Corning, Corning, NY) with nearly 100% of cells infected with wild-type *E. muris* were harvested by scraping. The cells were centrifuged in a Hettich Universal 32 R centrifuge (Hettich, Tuttlingen, Germany) at 240*g*, at 4°C, for 5 min. The supernatant was removed with a vacuum aspirator, and the cell pellets resuspended in 5 mL of sterile 10% glycerol in double-distilled water. Approximately 5 g of sterile glass beads were added to the 50-mL tube, and the cells were lysed by vortexing for 3 min. The resulting suspension was removed from the beads by pipetting to a new 50-mL Falcon tube. The lysed cell suspension was centrifuged at 240*g*, at 4°C, for 3 min. The supernatant was removed by aspiration and placed into a sterile Oakridge centrifuge tube, and the cell debris pellet discarded. The supernatant was then centrifuged in a Beckman centrifuge, J20 rotor, at 17,640*g* for 20 min. The supernatant was removed by aspiration, and the ehrlichial cell pellet then resuspended in 1 mL of sterile 10% glycerol prepared as described above; 100 μL of this suspension was placed into a 1-mm-gap GenePulser electroporation cuvette (Biorad, Hercules, CA). One μg of plasmid DNA was then added into the cuvette, along with 1 μL of TypeOne restriction inhibitor (Epicentre, Madison, WI).

The samples were then electroporated at 2.5 kV, 200 ohms, and 25 μF. For recovery, 1 mL of fresh Minimum Essential Medium Eagle (MEM) was then added into the cuvette, and the cells were allowed to recover at 37°C for 30 min to 1 h. The entire contents of the cuvette were then added to a 25-cm^2 cell culture flask (Corning) containing a monolayer of DH82 cells in fresh DMEM with 2.5% FBS and 1 mM HEPES. Approximately 24 h later, chloramphenicol was added at a concentration of 16 μg/mL (Sigma). Fresh antibiotic was added during medium changes, which occurred approximately every 3 days, typically for 2 weeks to a month. Appearance of wild-type ehrlichiae after withdrawal of antibiotics after at least 2 weeks of treatment has not been observed.

Confocal Microscopy

DH82 cells infected with wild-type or transformed *E. muris* were centrifuged using a cytospin apparatus onto glass slides and fixed in cold acetone/methanol (1:1) at –20°C for 10 min. The slides were then washed in PBS three times, 5 min per wash. After the wash, the slides were placed in a blocking solution containing 1% normal goat serum, 5% BSA (fraction V), and 0.3% Triton X-100 at room temperature for 30 min. Mouse anti–*E. chaffeensis* 1A9 monoclonal antibody (1:500 dilution) was used as the primary antibody to stain ehrlichiae, and sheep anti-CAT digoxigenin-labeled antibody (1:1000) was used as the primary antibody to stain the CAT protein. The primary antibodies were diluted in 1% BSA in PBS, centrifuged at 13,400*g* for 5 min, and then added to each slide. The slides were washed in PBS three times for 20 min each. Rhodamine-labeled sheep anti-DIG Fab fragments (1:100 dilution) and FITC-labeled anti-mouse IgG (1:100 dilution) were used as secondary antibodies and diluted in PBS containing 1% BSA, as described above. Slides were incubated with the secondary antibodies for 2 h in the dark and then washed with PBS at room temperature three times for 10 min each wash. Fluorescent mounting medium was added, the coverslip was affixed, and the slides then placed into a dark slide box and stored at 4°C until examined by confocal microscopy.

Electron Microscopy

Monolayers infected with either wild-type or transformed *E. muris* were fixed in a mixture of 0.5% glutaraldehyde, 2.5% formaldehyde, 0.03% trinitrophenol, and 0.03% $CaCl_2$ in 0.05 M cacodylate buffer at a pH of 7.3.[5] The cells were scraped from the flasks and pelleted. For immunogold electron microscopy, the cell pellets were stained en bloc with 1% uranyl acetate in 0.1 M cacodylate at a pH of 5.2. The pellets were then embedded in LR White resin. For ultrastructural examination in plastic, the cell pellets were stained in 1% OsO_4 in 0.1 M cacodylate buffer after primary fixation. The cell pellets were then stained with 1% uranyl acetate in 0.1 M cacodylate, dehydrated in a series of ethanol dilutions, and embedded in Poly/Bed 812. Ultrathin sections were cut using a Sorvall MT-6000 ultramicrotome and examined in a Philips CM 100 electron microscope at 60 kV.

Immunogold Staining

LR White sections on nickel Formvar-coated grids were stained with a mixture of a mouse anti-p28 monoclonal antibody (1A9)[5] at a dilution of 1:10 and a rabbit anti-CAT monoclonal antibody (Roche) at a dilution of 1:10. The diluent was 1% BSA in TBS. The sections were incubated with the primary antibodies for 1 h at room temperature and then overnight at 4°C. The secondary antibodies used to stain the LR White sections were a mixture of goat anti-mouse IgG + IgM (H + L) labeled with 5-nm gold particles (AuroProbe RPN430) and goat anti-rabbit IgG (H + L) labeled with 15-nm gold particles (AuroProbe RPN422), both at a dilution of 1:20 in 1% BSA in TBS. The sections were incubated with the secondary antibodies for 1 h at room temperature. The sections were then washed, fixed with 2% aqueous glutaraldehyde, and stained with 2% aqueous uranyl acetate (5 min) and lead citrate (30 s). The grids were then examined in a Philips CM 100 electron microscope at 60 kV.

Statistical Analyses

The transformed and nontransformed *E. muris* from both the plastic-embedded cells and the LR White-embedded cells were measured (at least 15 bacteria were measured from each group) and the average sizes determined. The average sizes from each group were statistically compared by the chi-square (χ^2) method and were considered statistically significant if $P < 0.05$.

RESULTS

PCR amplification of the *cat* gene was used to detect the presence and prolonged maintenance of the resistance gene in the transformants. PCR products were cloned, and sequencing verified that the amplicons contained the *cat* gene. Southern blots also verified the identity of the *cat* gene PCR amplicons. The expression of the *cat* resistance gene was verified by detection of the presence of the CAT protein in infected host cell lysates.

Confocal microscopy demonstrated the expression of the *cat* gene in transformed ehrlichiae by dual-labeling and colocalization of ehrlichial cells and the CAT protein (FIG. 1). Confocal microscopy demonstrated a higher degree of infection than visualized by light microscopy and DifQuik staining. The transformant-containing morulae appeared to be smaller than the wild-type morulae, which may partially account for the difficulty in visualization by DifQuik staining. Southern blots and dot blots using a *cat* gene-specific oligonucleotide probe (5′-ACGGGGGCGAA-GAAGTTGTCCATA-3′) confirmed the presence of the *cat* gene in samples of transformed *E. muris* and the absence of *cat* gene staining in wild-type controls.

Ultrastructurally, wild-type *E. muris* possessed typical gram-negative morphology with an outer membrane separated from the inner membrane by an electron lucent periplasmic space. Ehrlichiae were identified as possessing either dense cored cell morphology or reticulate cell morphology. The nontransformed *E. muris* were typically coccoid, although a few coccobacilli were also identified. They ranged in size from 320 nm to 917 nm in diameter, with an average size of 565 nm. In contrast, the transformed *E. muris* existed as protoplasts completely lacking outer membranes. They were small, with a range of sizes from 93 nm to 470 nm and an average size of 230 nm. The transformants were identified as possessing either a small electron dense morphology or a slightly larger electron lucent morphology, and both forms

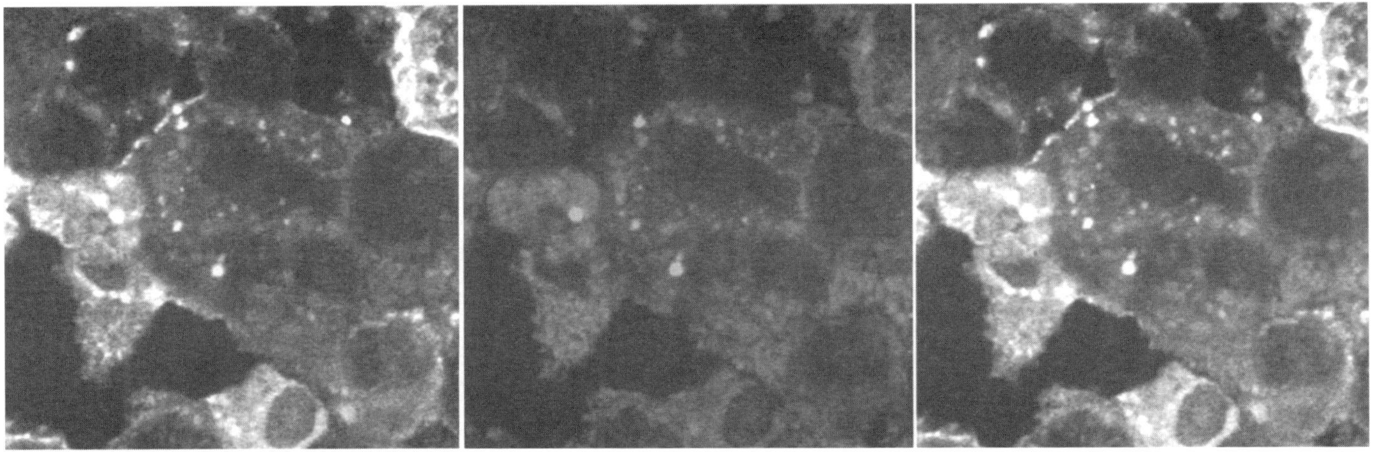

FIGURE 1. Confocal microscopy of the same field of DH82 cells infected with transformed *E. muris*. Mouse anti–*E. chaffeensis* 1A9 monoclonal antibody (1:500 dilution) was used as the primary antibody to stain ehrlichia (*left*), and sheep anti-CAT digoxigenin-labeled antibody (1:1000) was used as the primary antibody to stain the CAT protein (*middle*). Rhodamine-labeled anti-DIG antibody (1:100 dilution) and FITC-labeled anti-mouse IgG (1:100 dilution) were used as secondary antibodies. The merged image of the same field (*right*) demonstrates the colocalization of ehrlichiae and CAT protein within the morulae. This figure appears in color at Annals Online.

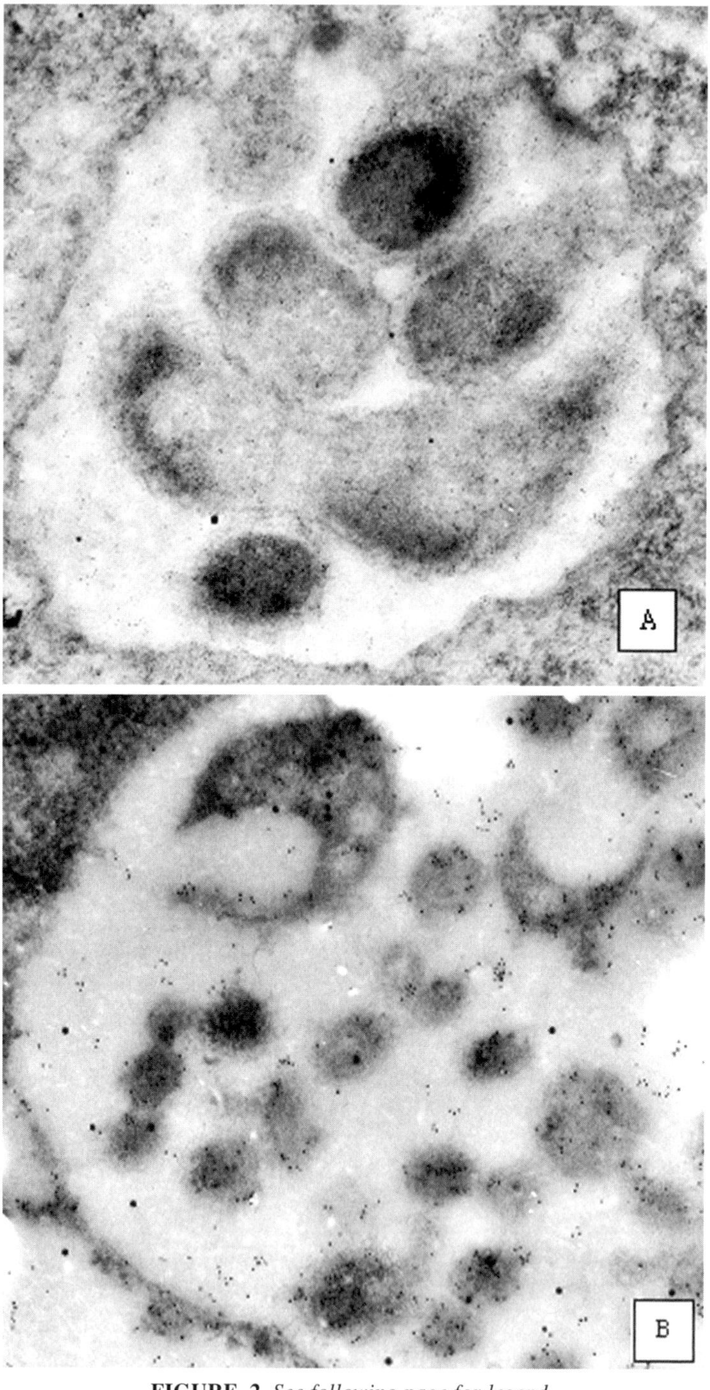

FIGURE 2. *See following page for legend.*

were often pleomorphic. Several transformants were observed to possess voluminous invaginations of the cytoplasmic membrane up to 325 nm deep.

The transformed *E. muris* were significantly smaller than the wild-type *E. muris* ($P < 0.001$). Immunogold staining with anti-p28 antibody confirmed that the transformants did indeed exist as smaller particles without outer cell membranes (FIG. 2). Dual immunogold staining with anti-p28 antibody (5-nm particles) and anti-CAT antibody (15-nm particles) confirmed the presence of CAT in the transformants and its absence in the wild-type *E. muris* (FIG. 2). These transformed *E. muris* have a morphological appearance similar to cell wall–deficient bacteria or L-forms described for other gram-negative bacteria.

DISCUSSION

The field of rickettsial disease research had been held back for many years due to the lack of suitable transformation systems, and only recently have experimental options begun to be elucidated. These systems have not yet been replicated in the *Ehrlichia*, and certain technical modifications were required to develop a system that was suitable for use with these related rickettsial pathogens.

Transformed *E. muris* exhibited ultrastructural changes typical of cell wall–deficient forms, which are observed as a minority population of wild-type ehrlichial cultures.[6] It was originally postulated that *Ehrlichia* formed these cell wall–deficient forms in response to harsh environmental conditions as a means of survival, similar to the L-transformation observed in other gram-negative bacteria in response to antibiotics or nutrient restriction.[6]

The appearance of the transformants as L-forms may be indicative of a decreased fitness for replication within the environment of the monocyte. In some cases, the appearance of L-forms in other gram-negative bacteria was attributed to decreased production of structurally important membrane proteins due to interference of antibiotics in protein expression.

It is important to note that exposure to chloramphenicol alone has been shown to induce L-transformation of *Staphylococcus aureus* in the presence of serum at the concentrations of chloramphenicol used in our transformation experiments.[7] In order to eliminate this as a possible explanation for the morphologic variation observed in our transformants, wild-type *E. muris*–infected DH82 cells were briefly exposed to chloramphenicol (32 μg/mL) for 2 and 4 days and then allowed to recover in normal medium. These infected cultures were examined by electron microscopy for morphologic variation. The *E. muris* after chloramphenicol exposure were found to be morphologically consistent in both size and overall appearance with wild-type *E. muris*.

FIGURE 2. Ultrastructural comparison of DH82 cells infected with wild-type *E. muris* (**A**) or transformed *E. muris* (**B**) stained for CAT protein and p28 antigen using immunogold. The characteristic morphologic changes in the transformants (L-transformation) can be appreciated along with their diminished size compared to the wild type. The CAT protein (15-nm gold particles) was present in the transformed *E. muris* (**A**), but not the untransformed *E. muris* (**B**), which are identified by their expression of p28 (5-nm gold particles).

[*Conflict of interest statement:* The authors of this research declare that they have no conflict of interest.]

REFERENCES

1. CHILDS, J.E. & C.D. PADDOCK. 2003. The ascendancy of *Amblyomma americanum* as a vector of pathogens affecting humans in the United States. Annu. Rev. Entomol. **48:** 307–337.
2. RACHEK, L.I., A.M. TUCKER, H.H. WINKLER & D.O. WOOD. 1998. Transformation of *Rickettsia prowazekii* to rifampin resistance. J. Bacteriol. **180:** 2118–2124.
3. BROUQUI, P. & D. RAOULT. 1992. *In vitro* antibiotic susceptibility of the newly recognized agent of ehrlichiosis in humans, *Ehrlichia chaffeensis*. Antimicrob. Agents Chemother. **36:** 2799–2803.
4. ANDERSON, B.E., J.W. SUMNER, J.E. DAWSON *et al.* 1992. Detection of the etiologic agent of human ehrlichiosis by polymerase chain reaction. J. Clin. Microbiol. **30:** 775–780.
5. POPOV, V.L., X-J. YU & D.H. WALKER. 2000. The 120 kDa outer membrane protein of *Ehrlichia chaffeensis*: preferential expression on dense-core cells and gene expression in *Escherichia coli* associated with attachment and entry. Microb. Pathog. **28:** 71–80.
6. POPOV, V., V.C. HAN, S-M. CHEN *et al.* 1998. Ultrastructural differentiation of the genogroups in the genus *Ehrlichia*. J. Med. Microbiol. **47:** 235–251.
7. GODZESKI, C.W., G. BRIER & D.E. PAVEY. 1962. L-phase growth induction as a general characteristic of antibiotic-bacterial interaction in the presence of serum. Antimicrob. Agents Chemother. **11:** 843–853.

Mechanisms of Immunological Control of *Anaplasma phagocytophilum* in Mice

CHRISTINA RINKLER, YVONNE KERN, CHRISTIAN BOGDAN, AND FRIEDERIKE D. VON LOEWENICH

Institute of Medical Microbiology and Hygiene, University of Freiburg, D-79104 Freiburg, Germany

KEYWORDS: ***Anaplasma phagocytophilum*; mouse model**

Anaplasma phagocytophilum is a Gram-negative, obligate intracellular bacterium.[1] It is transmitted by ticks and elicits febrile diseases in animals and humans. *A. phagocytophilum* is unique in that it replicates within the hostile environment of its host cell, the neutrophil. The laboratory mouse is a suitable model to study *A. phagocytophilum* infection *in vivo*.[2] In order to investigate by which defense mechanism *A. phagocytophilum* is controlled in the mouse system, we studied the course of infection in various transgenic mouse strains with defects of the immune system.

Mice were i.p. injected with *A. phagocytohilum*–infected SCID mouse blood. DNA was prepared from groups of three mice sacrificed at each time point and each experiment was repeated twice. The bacterial load was measured in the blood and various organs by a quantitative PCR technique as described.[3]

We previously showed that T- and/or B-cells are required for the control of *A. phagocytophilum in vivo*, because C.B17 SCID mice were persistently infected and developed a 60-fold higher bacterial load in the blood compared to wild-type mice. In contrast to wild-type mice which controlled the pathogen, SCID mice succumbed to infection.[3] To define whether T- and or B-cells are critical to overcoming the infection we used T-cell deficient BALB/c nude mice and BALB Ig$\alpha^{-/-}$ mice which lack mature B-cells. BALB/c nude mice developed a 120-fold (P = 0.00021) and 107-fold (P = 0.0055) higher bacterial load in the blood compared to wild-type mice at day 14 and day 21, respectively. However, C57BL/6 MHC class I-or II deficient mice were able to control *A. phagocytophilum*.

With respect to the mechanisms of pathogen recognition and killing, we found that mice deficient for Toll-like receptor (TLR) 2 and 4, MyD88, tumor necrosis factor, inducible nitric oxide synthase (iNOS), or phagocyte NADPH oxidase (gp91$^{phox-/-}$) were fully able to overcome a systemic infection with *A. phagocytophilum*.[3]

From our study, we conclude that effector mechanisms which are crucial in the defense against numerous other intracellular pathogens are dispensable for control

Address for correspondence: Dr. Friederike von Loewenich, Institut für Medizinische Mikrobiologie und Hygiene, Hermann-Herder-Str. 11, D-79104 Freiburg, Germany. Voice: +49-761-203-5359; fax: +49-761-203-6651.
friederike.loewenich@uniklinik-freiburg.de

Ann. N.Y. Acad. Sci. 1063: 411–412 (2005). © 2005 New York Academy of Sciences.
doi: 10.1196/annals.1355.073

of *A. phagocytophilum,* whereas innate and/or adaptive T cell the immune responses are critical.

[*Competing interests statement:* The authors declare that they have co conflicting financial interests.]

REFERENCES

1. DUMLER, J.S. *et al.* 2001. Reorganization of genera in the families *Rickettsiaceae* and *Anaplasmataceae* in the order *Rickettsiales:* unification of some species of *Ehrlichia* with *Anaplasma, Cowdria* with *Ehrlichia* and *Ehrlichia* with *Neorickettsia,* descriptions of six new species combinations and designation of *Ehrlichia equi* and "HGE agent" as subjective synonyms of *Ehrlichia phagocytophila.* Int. J. Syst. Evol. Microbiol. **51:** 2145–2165.
2. BORJESSON, D.L. & S.W. BARTHOLD. 2002. The mouse as a model for investigation of human granulocytic ehrlichiosis: current knowledge and future directions. Comp. Med. **52:** 403–413.
3. VON LOEWENICH, F.D. *et al.* 2004. Control of *Anaplasma phagocytophilum*, an obligate intracellular pathogen in the absence of inducible nitric oxide synthase, phagocyte NADPH oxidase, tumor necrosis factor, Toll-like receptor (TLR) 2 and 4, or the TLR adaptor molecule MyD88. Eur. J. Immunol. **34:** 1789–1797.

Platelet Dysfunction after Association with *Anaplasma phagocytophilum in Vitro*

DORI L. BORJESSON, JENNIFER L. BRAZZELL, AND REGINA FEFERMAN

Department of Veterinary Population Medicine, College of Veterinary Medicine, University of Minnesota, St. Paul, Minnesota 55108, USA

ABSTRACT: Granulocytic anaplasmosis is a tick-borne, zoonotic disease caused by an obligate intracellular granulocytotropic bacterium, *Anaplasma phagocytophilum*. *A. phagocytophilum* and other *Anaplasma* and *Ehrlichia* spp. have been variably implicated with an associated hematologic alteration, platelet dysfunction, that can result in potentially serious clinical sequelae including hemorrhage. The objective of this work was to define an *in vitro* model to assess alterations in platelet function associated with *A. phagocytophilum*.

KEYWORDS: *A. phagocytophilum*; platelet dysfunction; platelet; pathogen

Granulocytic anaplasmosis is a tick-borne, zoonotic disease caused by an obligate intracellular granulocytotropic bacterium, *Anaplasma phagocytophilum*.[1,2] Regardless of host species, infection with *A. phagocytophilum* typically results in characteristic hematologic abnormalities, including a moderate to marked thrombocytopenia, leukopenia, and frequently anemia.[3,4] *A. phagocytophilum* and other *Anaplasma* and *Ehrlichia* spp. have also been variably implicated with an associated hematologic alteration, platelet dysfunction, that can result in potentially serious clinical sequelae including hemorrhage, bleeding diatheses, toxic shock–like syndrome, and death.[5–7]

Platelet dysfunction associated with viral and bacterial infections is a well-described phenomenon.[8–10] Some alterations in platelet function can be attributed to direct platelet-pathogen interaction, with resultant platelet invasion or induction of aggregation.[11–13] Other alterations in platelet function are indirect, including platelet interaction with inflammatory cells, inflammatory mediators, coagulation by-products, or bacterial products (e.g., exotoxins or LPS).[14,15] Platelet dysfunction secondary to infectious diseases can be manifested either as platelet activation and potentiation of coagulation leading to a prothrombotic state[8,14] or as a decrease in function leading to bleeding diatheses/hemorrhage.[10,15] The thrombocytopenia noted during *A. phagocytophilum* infection is moderate and would not, in and of itself, result in bleeding. However, experimental evidence with closely related organisms, *E. canis* and *A. platys*, and anecdotal evidence in human case reports of anaplasmosis

Address for correspondence: Dr. Dori L. Borjesson, Department of Veterinary Population Medicine, College of Veterinary Medicine, University of Minnesota, 1333 Gortner Avenue, St. Paul, MN 55108. Voice: 612-624-7400; fax: 612-624-8707.
borje002@umn.edu

Ann. N.Y. Acad. Sci. 1063: 413–415 (2005).
doi: 10.1196/annals.1355.074

suggest that platelet dysfunction and bleeding may be significant components of the disease process.[5–7,16] Platelet function associated with *A. phagocytophilum* infection has not been evaluated. The objective of this work was to define an *in vitro* model to assess alterations in platelet function associated with *A. phagocytophilum*. Although platelets are likely not infected by the pathogen, we hypothesized that platelet dysfunction is a feature of *A. phagocytophilum* infection.

Human platelets were incubated with cell-free *A. phagocytophilum* in a platelet aggregometer. Platelet response to agonists was examined utilizing a wide range of pathogen dose, multiple pathogen isolates, and various incubation periods. Flow cytometric detection of the active conformation of $GPII_bIII_a$ (fibrinogen receptor) was also assessed. Electron microscopy was employed to directly visualize platelet-pathogen interactions. Electron microscopy did not demonstrate a direct association between *A. phagocytophilum* and platelets. Platelet uptake or direct platelet interaction with *A. phagocytophilum* does not occur, occurs rarely, or is rapid and transient. *A. phagocytophilum* failed to directly stimulate platelet aggregation, unlike other extracellular bacteria examined (positive control: *Streptococcus sanguis*). Incubation of human platelets with *A. phagocytophilum* resulted in platelet hypofunction as shown by a decreased response to collagen, adenosine diphosphate, and epinephrine. Alterations in platelet function were dependent on *A. phagocytophilum* dose, with higher pathogen concentration associated with more significant alterations in function. Functional alterations were mostly independent of viable pathogen. Platelet dysfunction was induced by multiple pathogen isolates. Flow cytometric detection of fibrinogen binding suggested that altered function may be associated with altered fibrinogen binding to $GPII_bIII_a$. This *in vitro* model will be utilized to assess platelet-pathogen interaction and will complement *in vivo* animal model studies.

[*Competing interests statement:* The authors of this research declare that they have no conflicts of interest.]

REFERENCES

1. CHEN, S.M. *et al.* 1994. Identification of a granulocytotropic *Ehrlichia* species as the etiologic agent of human disease. J. Clin. Microbiol. **32:** 589–595.
2. DUMLER, J.S. *et al.* 2001. Reorganization of genera in the families Rickettsiaceae and Anaplasmataceae in the order Rickettsiales: unification of some species of Ehrlichia with Anaplasma, Cowdria with Ehrlichia, and Ehrlichia with Neorickettsia, descriptions of six new species combinations, and designation of *Ehrlichia equi* and "HGE agent" as subjective synonyms of *Ehrlichia phagocytophila*. Int. J. Syst. Evol. Microbiol. **51:** 2145–2165.
3. BAKKEN, J.S. *et al.* 1996. Clinical and laboratory characteristics of human granulocytic ehrlichiosis. J. Am. Med. Assoc. **275:** 199–205.
4. BORJESSON, D.L. *et al.* 2001. Thrombocytopenia in a mouse model of human granulocytic ehrlichiosis. J. Infect. Dis. **184:** 1475–1479.
5. FICHTENBAUM, C.J., L.R. PETERSON & G.J. WEIL. 1993. Ehrlichiosis presenting as a life-threatening illness with features of the toxic shock syndrome. Am. J. Med. **95:** 351–357.
6. HARRUS, S. *et al.* 1996. Platelet dysfunction associated with experimental acute canine ehrlichiosis. Vet. Rec. **139:** 290–293.
7. VARELA, F. *et al.* 1997. Thrombocytopathia and light-chain proteinuria in a dog naturally infected with *Ehrlichia canis*. J. Vet. Intern. Med. **11:** 309–311.

8. Boudreaux, M.K. *et al.* 1990. Potentiation of platelet responses *in vitro* by feline infectious peritonitis virus. Vet. Pathol. **27:** 261–268.
9. Herzberg, M.C. 1996. Platelet-streptococcal interactions in endocarditis. Crit. Rev. Oral Biol. Med. **7:** 222–236.
10. Russell, K.E. *et al.* 1999. Platelets from thrombocytopenic ponies acutely infected with equine infectious anemia virus are activated *in vivo* and hypofunctional. Virology **259:** 7–19.
11. Chia, J.S. *et al.* 2004. Platelet aggregation induced by serotype polysaccharides from *Streptococcus mutans*. Infect. Immun. **72:** 2605–2617.
12. Coburn, J., J.M. Leong & J.K. Erban. 1993. Integrin alpha IIb beta 3 mediates binding of the Lyme disease agent *Borrelia burgdorferi* to human platelets. Proc. Natl. Acad. Sci. USA **90:** 7059–7063.
13. Heilmann, C. *et al.* 2004. *Staphylococcus aureus* fibronectin-binding protein (FnBP)–mediated adherence to platelets, and aggregation of platelets induced by FnBPA but not by FnBPB. J. Infect. Dis. **190:** 321–329.
14. Elizalde, J. *et al.* 1997. Platelet activation in mice and human *Helicobacter pylori* infection. J. Clin. Invest. **100:** 996–1005.
15. Sheu, J.R. *et al.* 1998. Mechanisms involved in the antiplatelet activity of *Escherichia coli* lipopolysaccharide in human platelets. Br. J. Haematol. **103:** 29–38.
16. Gaunt, S.D., D.C. Baker & S.S. Babin. 1990. Platelet aggregation studies in dogs with acute *Ehrlichia platys* infection. Am. J. Vet. Res. **51:** 290–293.

Anaplasma phagocytophilum Infection Reduces Expression of Phagocytosis-Related Receptors on Neutrophils

JUSTIN W. A. GARYU AND J. STEPHEN DUMLER

Division of Medical Microbiology, Department of Pathology, Johns Hopkins University School of Medicine, Baltimore, Maryland 21205, USA

ABSTRACT: *Anaplasma phagocytophilum* is a tick-transmitted obligate intracellular bacterium of neutrophils that causes human granulocytic anaplasmosis. Previous data confirm that *in vitro* infection by *A. phagocytophilum* modifies neutrophil functions, including a 50% or greater reduction in phagocytosis and shedding of neutrophil cell surface adhesion molecule receptors. If these receptors are downregulated or shed from the surface of neutrophils with *A. phagocytophilum* infection, it may prevent neutrophils from effective phagocytosis. We hypothesized that diminished phagocytosis in neutrophils is partly associated with the loss of surface phagocytic receptors. To address this, we assayed the expression of these receptors after 24 h of *A. phagocytophilum* infection in human neutrophils.

KEYWORDS: *Anaplasma phagocytophilum*; neutrophils; phagocytosis; Fc receptors; complement receptors; opsonophagocytic receptors

Anaplasma phagocytophilum is a tick-transmitted obligate intracellular bacterium of neutrophils that causes human granulocytic anaplasmosis (HGA). Previous data confirm that *in vitro* infection by *A. phagocytophilum* modifies neutrophil functions, including a 50% or greater reduction in phagocytosis and shedding of neutrophil cell surface adhesion molecule receptors.[1,2] Opsonophagocytic receptors on neutrophil surfaces include FcγRI, FcγRII, FcγRIII, FcεRII, FcαR, CR1, and C1qRp, each binding to an opsonizing ligand such as IgG, IgA, IgE, or various complement components. If these receptors are downregulated or shed from the surface of neutrophils with *A. phagocytophilum* infection, it may prevent neutrophils from effective phagocytosis. We hypothesized that diminished phagocytosis in neutrophils is partly associated with the loss of surface phagocytic receptors. To address this, we assayed the expression of these receptors after 24 h of *A. phagocytophilum* infection in human neutrophils.

A. phagocytophilum were propagated in HL-60 cells grown in RPMI 1640 medium with 1% fetal bovine serum (FBS) and 2 mM L-glutamine until at least 90% were infected. Cell-free *A. phagocytophilum* were prepared from sonicated infected HL-

Address for correspondence: J. Stephen Dumler, M.D., Division of Medical Microbiology, Department of Pathology, Johns Hopkins University School of Medicine, 720 Rutland Avenue, Ross 624, Baltimore, MD 21205. Voice: 410-955-8654; fax: 443-287-3665.
sdumler@jhmi.edu

**Ann. N.Y. Acad. Sci. 1063: 416–419 (2005). © 2005 New York Academy of Sciences.
doi: 10.1196/annals.1355.075**

60 cells from which intact cells, nuclei, and cell debris were removed by centrifugation (750*g* for 10 min). Cell-free bacteria suspended in 6 mL of RPMI 1640 with 10% FBS were then used to infect neutrophils at a ratio that provided an approximate MOI of 100:1.

Human neutrophils were obtained from EDTA-anticoagulated peripheral blood under a protocol approved by the JHMI IRB. Dextran-sedimented, leukocyte-rich plasma was centrifuged through Ficoll-Paque density gradients, mononuclear cells were discarded, and residual erythrocytes were lysed in hypotonic buffer to obtain purified neutrophils (>95% pure, 95% viable). These cells were cultivated for 24 h with or without cell-free *A. phagocytophilum.* Medium only was used as mock-infection for controls

Infected and mock-infected neutrophils were stained with fluorescein- or phycoerythrin-conjugated antibodies to FcγRI, FcγRII, FcγRIII, FcεRII, FcαR, CR1, and C1qRp, paired with appropriate fluorescently labeled isotype-matched control antibodies (all from BD-Pharmingen) and analyzed by flow cytometry. Gates were based on forward and side scatter morphology, and a fluorescent threshold was established above the value at which 95% of cells stained with the appropriate isotype control antibody. A threshold was established separately for mock-infected and infected neutrophils for each antibody pair. An adjusted geometric mean fluorescent value (GMFV) was calculated by subtracting the geometric mean of the isotype-matched control from that of the cells stained with the receptor antibody. GMFVs for cell populations were compared using two-tailed, unpaired Student's *t* tests if values exceeded threshold; P values of <.05 were considered significant.

A. phagocytophilum–infected neutrophils had significantly reduced levels of surface-exposed receptors C1qRp, FcαR, FcγRII, and FcγRIII at 24 h after infection ($P < .05$; FIG. 1). The expression of CR1 was slightly reduced ($P = .076$), but was very low or absent for FcεRII and FcγRI in all cells.

A. phagocytophilum infection alters neutrophils in many ways. We recently provided controlled *in vitro* evidence of defective phagocytosis among infected neutrophils.[1] The mechanism by which *A. phagocytophilum* alters neutrophil phagocytic capacity is poorly understood. Choi *et al.* demonstrated that neutrophil infection leads to protracted degranulation, including a variety of metalloproteases.[2,3] This ultimately results in surface shedding of adhesion molecules such as platelet selectin glycoprotein ligand-1 (PSGL1) and neutrophils unable to bind to endothelium. Additionally, Carlyon *et al.* showed that *A. phagocytophilum*–infected HL-60 cells have completely inhibited *RAC2* expression,[4] a critical signaling molecule in mobilizing the actin-based machinery for phagocytosis and vesicular trafficking.

One potential mechanism by which *A. phagocytophilum* alters neutrophil phagocytosis could be through loss of surface opsonophagocytic receptors, via shedding as with PSGL1, with LPS-induced loss of FcγRIII, or by decreased receptor expression as with the loss of *RAC2*.[2,4,5] These data provide new information supporting the concept of reduced expression or loss of surface molecules with *A. phagocytophilum* infection as a mechanism for reduced phagocytosis. Whether phagocytosis is also impacted by loss of signaling owing to *RAC2* downregulation or by the reduction of triggering[6] with diminished surface receptor density still needs to be determined. Elucidation of mechanisms leading to perturbation of neutrophil phagocytosis could define the spectrum of abnormalities and could assist in identification of host cell targets important in *A. phagocytophilum* pathogenesis.

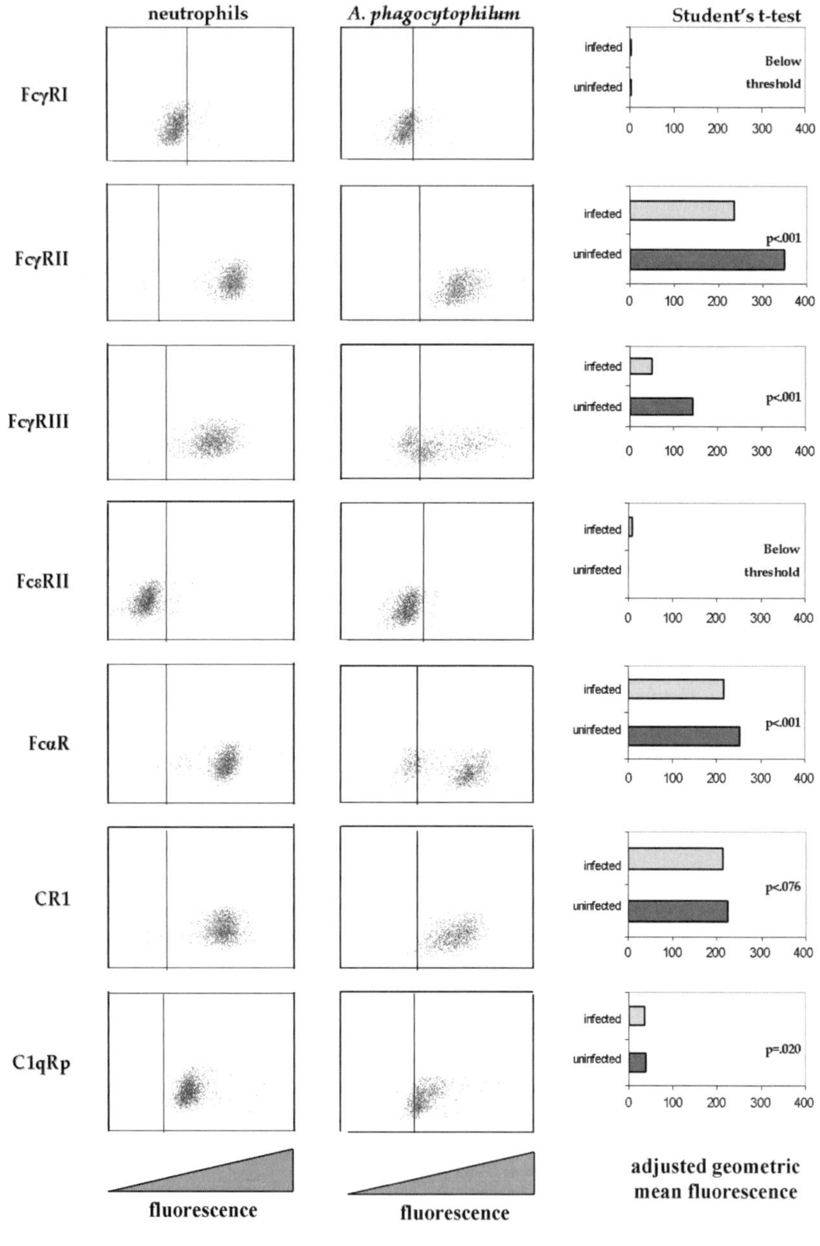

FIGURE 1. *See following page for legend.*

[*Competing interests statement:* The authors of this research declare that they have no conflict of interest.]

REFERENCES

1. GARYU, J.W., K.S. CHOI, D.J. GRAB *et al.* 2005. Defective phagocytosis in *Anaplasma phagocytophilum*–infected neutrophils. Infect. Immun. **73:** 1187–1190.
2. CHOI, K.S., J. GARYU, J. PARK *et al.* 2003. Diminished adhesion of *Anaplasma phagocytophilum*–infected neutrophils to endothelial cells is associated with reduced expression of leukocyte surface selectin. Infect. Immun. **71:** 4586–4594.
3. CHOI, K.S., D.J. GRAB & J.S. DUMLER. 2004. *Anaplasma phagocytophilum* infection induces protracted neutrophil degranulation. Infect. Immun. **72:** 3680–3683.
4. CARLYON, J.A., W.T. CHAN, J. GALAN *et al.* 2002. Repression of *rac2* mRNA expression by *Anaplasma phagocytophila* is essential to the inhibition of superoxide production and bacterial proliferation. J. Immunol. **169:** 7009–7018.
5. WAGNER, C., R. DEPPISCH, B. DENEFLEH *et al.* 2003. Expression patterns of the lipopolysaccharide receptor CD14, and the Fcγ receptors CD16 and CD64 on polymorphonuclear neutrophils: data from patients with severe bacterial infections and lipopolysaccharide-exposed cells. Shock **19:** 5–12.
6. SALMON, J.E., N.L. BROGLE, J.C. EDBERG *et al.* 1991. Fcγ receptor III induces actin polymerization in human neutrophils and primes phagocytosis mediated by Fcγ receptor II. J. Immunol. **146:** 997–1004.

FIGURE 1. Flow cytometry of opsonophagocytic receptors on *A. phagocytophilum*– and mock-infected human neutrophils after 24 h of culture. Dot plots (left and middle columns) demonstrate the relative distribution of fluorescence on the x-axis (and side light scatter on the y-axis). The quantified fluorescence data and *P* values for comparison of infected and mock-infected cells are shown in the right-hand column. Below threshold: insufficient fluorescence above background to enable statistical assessment.

Analysis of Ehrlichial p28 Gene Expression in a Murine Model of Persistent Infection

PATRICIA A. CROCQUET-VALDES, JERE W. McBRIDE, HUI-MIN FENG, NAHED ISMAIL, MELISSA A. SMALL, XUE-JIE YU, AND DAVID H. WALKER

Department of Pathology, Sealy Center for Vaccine Development, and WHO Collaborating Center for Tropical Diseases, University of Texas Medical Branch, Galveston, Texas 77555-0609, USA

ABSTRACT: Historically, ehrlichioses were tick-borne diseases of veterinary medical importance and are now important emerging infectious diseases in humans. p28s are encoded by multigene families with ORFs tandemly arranged with intergenic spaces of variable lengths. We reported initial sequencing of the *Ehrlichia muris p28* locus. A model of persistent infection was described and provided tools for study of persistent ehrlichial infection. We completed the sequence of the *E. muris p28* locus and examined mRNA expression.

KEYWORDS: Ehrlichia; multigene family; outer membrane proteins; RT-PCR

INTRODUCTION

Historically, ehrlichioses were tick-borne diseases of veterinary medical importance and are now important emerging infectious diseases in humans. *Ehrlichia muris* is a member of the genus *Ehrlichia* based on morphological, antigenic, and genetic criteria.[1,2] The first isolate was obtained in 1983 from a wild mouse and subsequently from *Haemaphysalis flava* ticks in Japan and by polymerase chain reaction (PCR) in *Ixodes persulcatus* ticks in Russia.[3]

p28's are encoded by multigene families with ORFs tandemly arranged with intergenic spaces of variable lengths. We reported initial sequencing of the *E. muris p28* locus.[4] Recently, a model of persistent infection was described[5] and provided tools for study of persistent ehrlichial infection. We completed the sequence of the *E. muris p28* locus and examined mRNA expression.

MATERIALS AND METHODS

PCR Amplification of the E. muris p28 *Multigene Locus*

Amplification of the *p28* gene locus of *E. muris* genomic DNA was initially performed by PCR using primers IOEnc3 (TCACAGATATTTTTCGTAA) and

Address for correspondence: Patricia Crocquet-Valdes, University of Texas Medical Branch, 301 University Boulevard, Galveston, TX 77555-0609. Voice: 409-772-4813; fax: 409-747-2455. pavaldes@utmb.edu

Ann. N.Y. Acad. Sci. 1063: 420–424 (2005). © 2005 New York Academy of Sciences. doi: 10.1196/annals.1355.076

Ecasec3R (CTTCCCCTGTCTTCATTTC) to produce amplicon EM28-2, and primers IOEnc3 and Echafsec5R (TTCCATTTTTGAGTTCTTCTTTGA) specific for conserved regions of *secA* and an intergenic region of the *Ixodes ovatus Ehrlichia* (IOE) *p28* sequence (unpublished data, McBride 2001) to produce amplicon EM30-2. Reactions contained 50 pmoles of each primer and 90 ng of *E. muris* (strain AS145) genomic DNA and 2× PCR Master (Roche Applied Science, Indianapolis, IN). The thermal cycling protocol consisted of 94°C for 5 min followed by 30 cycles of 94°C for 1 min, 50°C for 1 min, and 72°C for 4 min; and a final extension at 72°C for 7 min. Amplicons were analyzed on a 1% agarose gel and visualized by ethidium bromide staining. Unknown sequences adjacent to our amplified product were determined using a genome walking technique as previously described[6] and by long-range PCR using EXL™ DNA polymerase (Stratagene, La Jolla, CA).

DNA Sequencing

The amplicons were gel-purified using a QIAquick Gel Extraction Kit (Qiagen, Santa Clarita, CA) and cloned into pCR®4-TOPO or pCR®-XL-TOPO (Invitrogen, Carlsbad, CA) for sequencing. Sequences were determined at the Protein Chemistry Laboratory at the University of Texas Medical Branch using an ABI Prism 377 DNA Sequencer (Perkin-Elmer Applied Biosystems, Foster City, CA).

Gene Analysis

DNA sequences were analyzed using Lasergene software (DNAstar, Madison, WI) and Web interface software Seqweb version 2.1 for GCG® Wisconsin Package™ (Accelrys, San Diego, CA). Amino acid alignments were performed using Clustal W.

RT-PCR of **E. muris p28**

Primers for gene-specific RT-PCR amplification of *E. muris p28* mRNA were designed. RNA (0.125 μg) isolated using RNAqueous® (Ambion, Austin, TX) from mice spleens harvested at days 9, 60, and 90 postinoculation with *E. muris* was amplified using Invitrogen's SuperScript™ III RT-PCR Kit (Invitrogen, Carlsbad, CA). Primer pairs (0.2 μM) were used to amplify each *p28* gene in a one-step RT-PCR reaction. A negative control that included all reagents and inactivated the reverse transcriptase with a 5-min incubation at 95°C was included to confirm that genomic DNA was not present in the RNA preparation. PCR products were submitted for sequencing to verify the identity of specific *p28* amplicons.

RESULTS

Sequence Analysis of the **E. muris p28** *Locus*

Primers designed from IOE *p28* sequence were used to amplify two amplicons, EM28-2 and EM30-2, from *E. muris* genomic DNA. Sequence analysis of these two amplicons showed significant similarity to the 3′ end of the *E. chaffeensis p28* locus (FIG. 1). From these two clones, primers were designed for genome walking, and 13

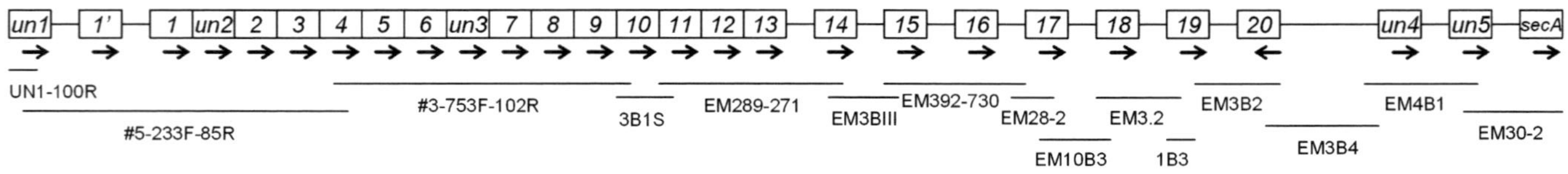

FIGURE 1. Schematic representation of the *E. muris p28* locus described in this report. Open boxes represent open reading frames (ORFs). Thick black lines below the locus represent clone fragments used in sequencing. Arrows indicate direction of transcription for each *p28*.

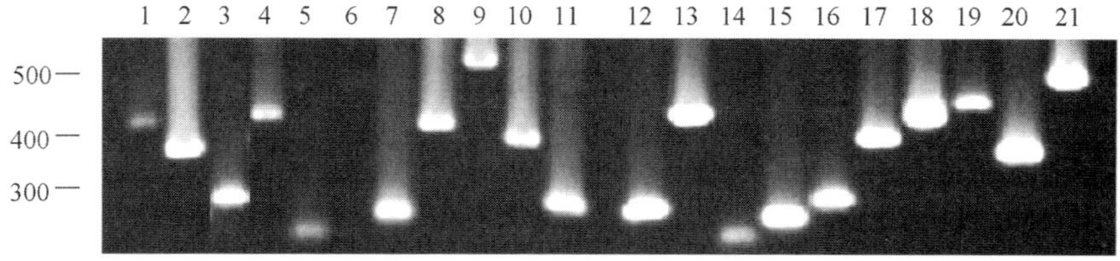

FIGURE 2. RT-PCR of *E. muris p28* genes from *E. muris*–infected mouse spleen at 9 days postinoculation. Lanes 1–21 represent *p28* genes 1′–20, respectively. Markers (in base pairs) are represented at left.

more amplicons were obtained to complete the locus for a total length of 26.86 kb (GenBank accession no. DQ335244).

Twenty-one *p28* tandemly arranged paralogs were identified (*p28-1′–p28-20*), along with *un1*, a hypothetical transcription regulator at the 5′ end, and an ORF with high similarity to *secA*, part of an enzyme involved in protein translocation, at the 3′ end. Four ORFs, *un2–un5*, did not show any homology to any known protein in a database search. The *E. muris p28*'s were more closely related to the *E. chaffeensis p28*'s than to the *E. canis* orthologs (data not shown). The same could be said for *secA* and *un1–un5* ORFs (data not shown). However, at the 3′ end of the locus, no ortholog to *p28-21* was present in *E. muris* when compared to *E. chaffeensis*. The amino acid sequence identities among the p28 paralogs in *E. muris* were 20.9% to 82.8%. The most similar p28's of *E. muris* were p28-17 and p28-19, and the least similar were p28-3 and p28-5.

The most significant differences between the *E. muris* locus and *p28* loci in other *Ehrlichia* species were found in the intergenic sequences, where many deletions and substitutions were present (data not shown).

RT-PCR of E. muris p28

RT-PCR analysis of the 21 *p28* genes of *E. muris* demonstrated that they were all transcriptionally active on day 9 (FIG. 2) in an *in vivo* mouse model of persistent infection. However, by 60 days postinoculation, few organisms were present in the spleen, and expression of only *p28-1′*, *p28-2*, and *p28-19* was barely detectable (data not shown). By 90 days postinoculation, no *p28* expression was detected (data not shown).

CONCLUSIONS

Phylogenetically, *E. muris* is most closely related to IOE. However, because of the absence of sufficient IOE *p28* data, *E. muris p28*'s share greatest similarity to *E. chaffeensis p28*'s. *p28* loci gene organization is well conserved among ehrlichial species. The majority of the differences between *p28* paralogs and orthologs were found in the hypervariable regions. Identifying the *E. muris p28*'s allows us to study their role in the mouse model of persistent infection.

Our RT-PCR results indicate that all *p28* genes of *E. muris* are transcribed. These results differ from RT-PCR analysis of *E. chaffeensis* reported by Long *et al.*,[7] where detection of transcription of only 16 of the 22 genes was observed. For *E. canis*, Ohashi *et al.*[8] reported all *p28*'s to be expressed. Data from Cheng *et al.*[9] indicated that only some *p28*'s are expressed in *E. canis*.

ACKNOWLEDGMENTS

This work was supported by National Institutes of Health Grant No. RO1 AI 31431. The technical support of Colette Keng and Mengyi Ye is gratefully acknowledged.

[*Competing interests statement:* The authors declare that they have no competing interests.]

REFERENCES

1. KAWAHARA, M., C. SUTO, Y. RIKIHISA *et al.* 1993. Characterization of ehrlichial organisms isolated from a wild mouse. J. Clin. Microbiol. **31:** 89–96.
2. WEN, B., Y. RIKIHISA, J. MOTT *et al.* 1995. *Ehrlichia muris* sp. nov., identified on the basis of 16S rRNA base sequences and serological, morphological, and biological characteristics. Int. J. Syst. Bacteriol. **45:** 250–254.
3. ALEKSEEV, A., H. DUBININA, I. VAN DE POL & L. SCHOULS. 2001. Identification of *Ehrlichia* spp. and *Borrelia burgdorferi* in *Ixodes* ticks in the Baltic region of Russia. J. Clin. Microbiol. **39:** 2237–2242.
4. CROCQUET-VALDES, P.A., J.W. MCBRIDE, X-J. YU & D.H. WALKER. 2003. Molecular characterization of the 28 kDa multigene locus of *Ehrlichia muris*. Ann. N.Y. Acad. Sci. **990:** 714–716.
5. OLANO, J.P., G. WEN, H-M. FENG *et al.* 2004. Histologic, serologic, and molecular analysis of persistent ehrlichiosis in a murine model. Am. J. Pathol. **165:** 997–1006.
6. YU, X-J., J.W. MCBRIDE, X. ZHANG & D.H. WALKER. 2000. Characterization of the complete transcriptionally active *Ehrlichia chaffeensis* 28 kDa outer membrane protein multigene family. Gene **248:** 59–68.
7. LONG, S.W., X-F. ZHANG, H. QI *et al.* 2002. Antigenic variation of *Ehrlichia chaffeensis* resulting from differential expression of the 28-kilodalton protein gene family. Infect. Immun. **70:** 1824–1831.
8. OHASHI, N., Y. RIKIHISA & A. UNVER. 2001. Analysis of transcriptionally active gene clusters of major outer membrane protein multigene family in *Ehrlichia canis* and *E. chaffeensis*. Infect. Immun. **69:** 2083–2091.
9. CHENG, C., C.D. PADDOCK & R.R. GANTA. 2003. Molecular heterogeneity of *Ehrlichia chaffeensis* isolates determined by sequence analysis of the 28-kilodalton outer membrane protein genes and other regions of the genome. Infect. Immun. **71:** 187–195.

Innate Immune Tissue Injury and Murine HGA

Tissue Injury in the Murine Model of Granulocytic Anaplasmosis Relates to Host Innate Immune Response and Not Pathogen Load

DIANA G. SCORPIO,[a] FRIEDERIKE D. VON LOEWENICH,[b] CHRISTIAN BOGDAN,[b] AND J. STEPHEN DUMLER[c]

[a]*Department of Comparative Medicine, Johns Hopkins University School of Medicine, Baltimore, Maryland 21205, USA*

[b]*Institute of Medical Microbiology and Hygiene, University of Freiburg, Freiburg, Germany*

[c]*Department of Pathology, Johns Hopkins University School of Medicine, Baltimore, Maryland 21205, USA*

ABSTRACT: *Anaplasma phagocytophilum* is an obligate intracellular tick-borne bacterium that propagates within neutrophils and causes human and animal granulocytic anaplasmosis (HGA). In the murine model of HGA, host immune response plays a more important role in histopathologic lesions than does pathogen load. We examined the role of CYBB, NOS2, and TNFα as effectors of innate immune–related injury. Our hypothesis is that the innate immune response to *A. phagocytophilum* results in inflammatory histopathology, but does not control the pathogen.

KEYWORDS: *Anaplasma phagocytophilum*; TNF; NOS2; phagocyte oxidase; innate immunity; mouse model

Anaplasma phagocytophilum is an obligate intracellular tick-borne bacterium that propagates within neutrophils and causes human and animal granulocytic anaplasmosis (HGA). In the murine model of HGA, host immune response plays a more important role in histopathologic lesions than does pathogen load.[1,2] Previous investigations of host innate immune response on pathogen propagation revealed no differences in *A. phagocytophilum* blood or tissue loads between wild type and mice deficient in TNFα, gp91^{phox} (CYBB), NOS2, TLR2, TLR4, or MyD88.[3] However, previous studies showed that blood and tissue bacterial burdens do not correlate with histopathology.[1,2] We examined the role of CYBB, NOS2, and TNFα as effectors of

Address for correspondence: Diana G. Scorpio, DVM, MPH, DACLAM, Department of Comparative Medicine, Johns Hopkins University School of Medicine, 720 Rutland Avenue, Ross 459, Baltimore, MD 21205. Voice: 410-955-3273; fax: 410-502-5068.
dscorpio@jhmi.edu

Ann. N.Y. Acad. Sci. 1063: 425–428 (2005). © 2005 New York Academy of Sciences.
doi: 10.1196/annals.1355.077

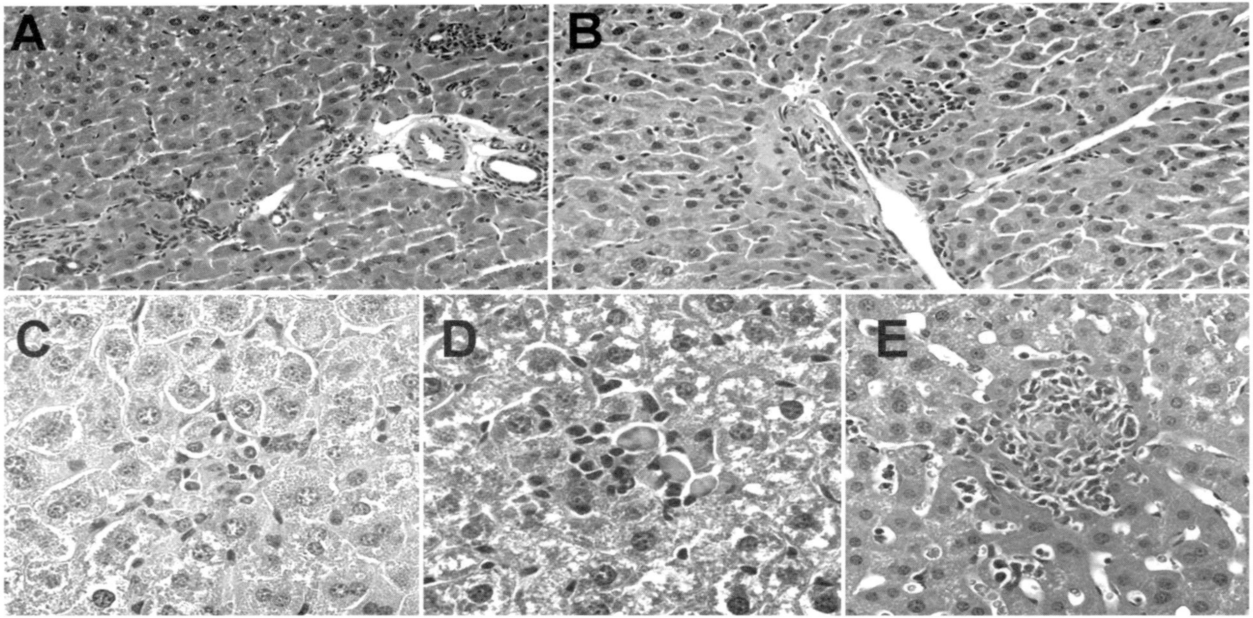

FIGURE 1. Examples of hepatic histopathology among mice infected with *A. phagocytophilum*. Wild-type and knockout mice had widely distributed inflammatory lesions throughout the hepatic parenchyma and perivascular regions. Characteristics of lesions included mild to moderate lobular hepatitis (**A**); perivenular and periportal infiltrates (**B**); focal lobular lesions with mixed inflammatory infiltrates (**C**); apoptotic hepatocytes with associated inflammatory infiltrate (**D**); and in some cases (*CYBB–/–* mice), small- to medium-sized hepatic granulomas and granulomatous inflammatory cell infiltrates (**E**).

innate immune–related injury. Our hypothesis is that the innate immune response to *A. phagocytophilum* results in inflammatory histopathology, but does not control the pathogen.

A. phagocytophilum (MRK strain)–infected SCID mouse blood was used as inoculum. *TNF*- ($n = 6$), *CYBB*- (gp91^{phox}) ($n = 9$), and *NOS2*-knockout mice ($n = 9$) and the same number of wild-type B6 mice were inoculated intraperitoneally with 10^4–10^6 genome equivalents of *A. phagocytophilum.* For the *CYBB* and *NOS2* experiments, the same numbers of mice were inoculated with blood from uninfected SCID mice; for the *TNF* experiment, 2 uninfected B6 animals served as controls. *CYBB–/–*, *NOS2–/–*, and B6 controls were examined at day 7, 21, and 42, whereas *TNF–/–* and B6 controls were tested at day 3 and 7 postinfection. Histopathology was assessed for inflammatory lesions by severity ranking after normalizing for uninfected controls. Differences in medians were assessed by one-sided nonparametric Mann-Whitney tests (Cuzick's trend test for small sample sizes); P values of $<.05$ were considered significant.

Wild-type B6 and knockout mice had inflammatory lesions distributed throughout the hepatic parenchyma and perivascular regions (FIG. 1). Characteristics included mild to moderate lobular hepatitis; perivenular and periportal infiltrates; focal lobular lesions with mixed inflammatory infiltrates; apoptotic hepatocytes with associated inflammatory infiltrate; and in day 42 *CYBB–/–* mice, focal and multifocal small- to medium-sized hepatic granulomas and granulomatous inflammatory cell infiltrates.

At the earliest time point (day 3), wild-type B6 mice had significantly more severe hepatic histopathology ($P < 0.05$) than did matched *TNF–/–* mice, a trend also noted for the day 7 time point ($P < 0.10$). Likewise, B6 mice had significantly higher hepatic severity ranks than did matched *NOS2–/–* mice, but only on day 7 ($P < 0.05$). Compared to infected *CYBB–/–* mice, significantly more hepatic inflammation was noted for infected B6 mice on day 7 ($P < 0.05$). One *CYBB–/–* mouse necropsied on day 7 had a purulent skin infection and was excluded from the analyses. On day 42, hepatic lesions in *CYBB–/–* mice included small to medium granulomatous infiltrates in all mice, and severity exceeded those in matched B6 mice, although this was not statistically significant ($P = 0.10$).

It was previously shown that innate immunity is not essential to control *A. phagocytophilum* infection since infected wild-type and knockout mice have similar bacterial loads.[3] However, the pathogen still induces an innate immune response leading to tissue injury even before adaptive immunity is initiated. The innate immune response that dominates at days 3 to 7 elicits inflammatory tissue lesions related to the generation of both reactive oxygen and nitrogen species, supported by the observation that significantly less histopathology was observed in mice deficient in TNFα, phagocyte oxidase, and nitric oxide synthase. Inflammatory lesions resolved with time and, in *CYBB–/–* mice, a trend toward more severe histopathology was noted at day 42, characterized by the presence of noncaseating granulomas and granulomatous inflammatory infiltrates, similar to those observed with chronic granulomatous disease. The prolonged inflammation observed in *CYBB–/–* mice in the absence of any bacteria suggests, as previously noted, that phagocyte oxidase is important for dampening and downregulating the inflammatory response.[4,5] Since *A. phagocytophilum* is known to downregulate expression of phagocyte oxidase, it could contribute locally to poor resolution of inflammation or could promote persistent inflammation. An advantage of persistent inflammation with *A. phagocytophilum* is the continued recruitment of new potential host cells to expand bacterial populations.[2,6] Whether *A. phagocytophilum*–induced downregulation of phagocyte oxidase also contributes to disease and the pathogenesis of HGA by locally impairing resolution of inflammation should be further investigated.

[*Competing interests statement:* The authors declare that they have no conflicting interests.]

REFERENCES

1. MARTIN, M.E., K. CASPERSEN & J.S. DUMLER. 2001. Immunopathology and ehrlichial propagation are regulated by interferon-gamma and interleukin-10 in a murine model of human granulocytic ehrlichiosis. Am. J. Pathol. **158:** 1881–1888.
2. SCORPIO, D.G., M. AKKOYUNLU, E. FIKRIG & J.S. DUMLER. 2004. CXCR2 blockade influences *Anaplasma phagocytophilum* propagation but not histopathology in the mouse model of human granulocytic anaplasmosis. Clin. Diagn. Lab. Immunol. **11:** 963–968.
3. VON LOEWENICH, F.D., D.G. SCORPIO, U. REISCHL *et al.* 2004. Frontline: control of *Anaplasma phagocytophilum*, an obligate intracellular pathogen, in the absence of inducible nitric oxide synthase, phagocyte NADPH oxidase, tumor necrosis factor, Toll-like receptor (TLR) 2 and TLR4, or the TLR adaptor molecule MyD88. Eur. J. Immunol. **34:** 1789–1797.
4. CARLYON, J.A., D. ABDEL-LATIF, M. PYPAERT *et al.* 2004. *Anaplasma phagocytophilum* utilizes multiple host evasion mechanisms to thwart NADPH oxidase–mediated killing during neutrophil infection. Infect. Immun. **72:** 4772–4783.
5. SEGAL, B.H., D.B. KUHNS, L. DING *et al.* 2002. Thioglycollate peritonitis in mice lacking C5, 5-lipoxygenase, or $p47^{phox}$: complement, leukotrienes, and reactive oxidants in acute inflammation. J. Leukocyte Biol. **71:** 410–416.
6. AKKOYUNLU, M., S.E. MALAWISTA, J. ANGUITA & E. FIKRIG. 2001. Exploitation of interleukin-8-induced neutrophil chemotaxis by the agent of human granulocytic ehrlichiosis. Infect. Immun. **69:** 5577–5588.

Cytokine Responses in Dogs Infected with *Ehrlichia canis* Oklahoma Strain

TOMOKO TAJIMA[a,b] AND YASUKO RIKIHISA[b]

[a]*Laboratory of Veterinary Microbiology, Graduate School of Life and Environmental Science, Osaka Prefecture University, Osaka 599-8531, Japan*

[b]*Department of Veterinary Biosciences, School of Veterinary Medicine, The Ohio State University, Columbus, Ohio 43210-1093, USA*

ABSTRACT: *Ehrlichia canis* causes persistent infection of monocytes/macrophages and causes canine monocytic ehrlichiosis. Other than antibody development, very little is known how the dog immune system responds to this pathogen. In the present study, we examined the temporal expression of cytokine mRNA in peripheral blood mononuclear cells (PBMCs) from dogs inoculated with *E. canis* Oklahoma strain. We also examined production of interferon-gamma (IFN-γ) by canine PBMCs infected with *E. canis in vitro*.

KEYWORDS: *Ehrlichia canis*; dog; interferon-gamma (IFN-γ)

Ehrlichia canis causes persistent infection of monocytes/macrophages and causes canine monocytic ehrlichiosis.[1] Other than antibody development, very little is known how the dog immune system responds to this pathogen. In the present study, we examined the temporal expression of cytokine mRNA in peripheral blood mononuclear cells (PBMCs) from dogs inoculated with *E. canis* Oklahoma strain. We also examined production of interferon-gamma (IFN-γ) by canine PBMCs infected with *E. canis in vitro*.

Four 1- to 2-year-old specific pathogen-free female Hound-mixed breed dogs were intravenously inoculated with *E. canis* Oklahoma strain cultured in DH82 cells and the blood specimens were collected following the time course of infection. As negative controls, two dogs were inoculated with uninfected DH82 cells. PBMCs were isolated from peripheral blood buffy coat by using Histopaque-1077 (Sigma, MO). Expression of tumor necrosis factor alpha (TNF-α), interleukin-1β (IL-1β), IL-2, IL-4, IFN-γ, and IL-6 mRNA were examined by reverse transcription (RT)–PCR.[2] To examine *in vitro* production of IFN-γ, PBMCs from uninfected dogs were infected with *E. canis* and cultured for 5 days. IFN-γ in the culture supernatant was assayed by using Quantikine Canine IFN-γ Immunoassay Kit (R & D Systems). Antibodies against *E. canis* were examined by enzyme-linked immunosorbent assay (ELISA) using purified *E. canis* Oklahoma as antigen. Horseradish peroxidase–conjugated

Address for correspondence: Tomoko Tajima, Laboratory of Veterinary Microbiology, Graduate School of Life and Environmental Science, Osaka Prefecture University, 1-1 Gakuen-cho, Sakai, Osaka 599-8531, Japan. Voice: +81-72-254-9484; fax: +81-72-254-9918.
tajima@vet.osakafu-u.ac.jp

Ann. N.Y. Acad. Sci. 1063: 429–432 (2005). © 2005 New York Academy of Sciences.
doi: 10.1196/annals.1355.078

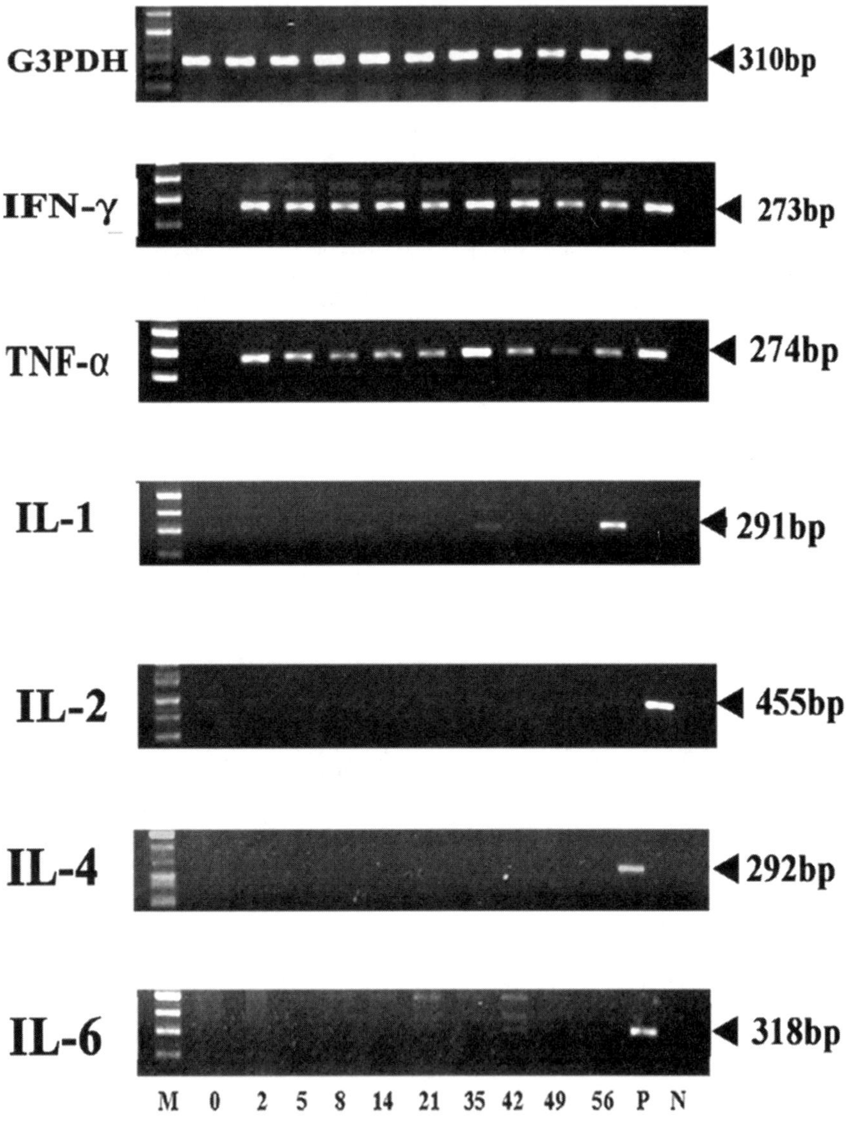

FIGURE 1. Time course of cytokine mRNA expression by PBMCs of dog no. 1 infected with *E. canis* as detected by RT-PCR. Similar results were obtained from three other dogs. Numbers indicate days postinoculation. M: molecular size marker (100-bp ladder). P: positive control, pokeweed mitogen–stimulated dog PBMC. N: negative control, no template.

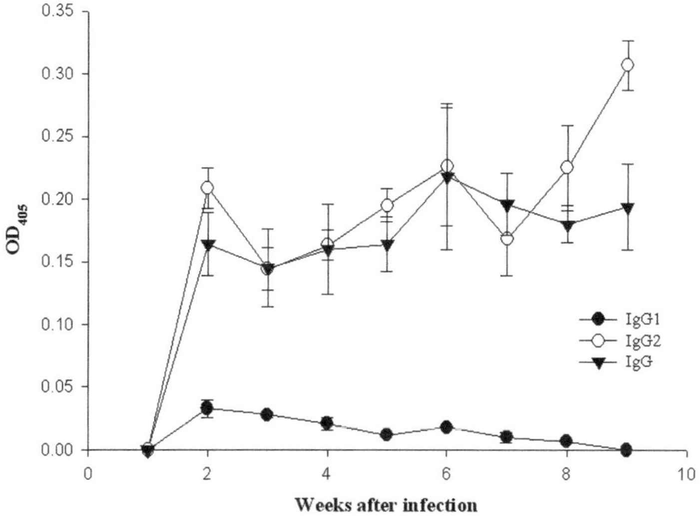

FIGURE 2. Development of antibody against *E. canis* antigen in dog no. 1 infected with *E. canis*. Similar results were obtained from three other dogs.

goat anti-dog IgG, IgG1, and sheep anti-dog IgG2 (Bethel Lab Inc., TX) were used as secondary antibodies, and colorimetric reaction was done with ABTS.

Clinical signs of the dogs were slight with transient fever (40°C for 2 days) and decrease in platelet counts. Infection of *E. canis* was confirmed by PCR in all dogs. There was persistent expression of IFN-γ and TNF-α mRNA starting on day 2 or 8 and continuing to day 56 postinoculation in all four dogs. Every dog shows very low to undetectable levels of IL-1β, IL-2, IL-4, and IL-6 mRNA expression (FIG. 1). Expression of these cytokine mRNAs was not detected in two dogs inoculated with uninfected DH82 cells. IFN-γ was detected at concentrations of 435 and 1029 pg/mL in culture supernatant of canine PBMCs at 2 and 3 days, respectively, after being infected with *E. canis*. The concentration of IFN-γ reached 2734 pg/mL on 5 days after infection. By ELISA, IgG and IgG2 specific to *E. canis* were detected, whereas IgG1 antibody was at low level (FIG. 2).

In vivo expression of IFN-γ mRNA, *in vitro* production of IFN-γ, and production of IgG2 antibody suggest that Th1 type immune response is dominant in dogs with canine mild ehrlichiosis caused by infection with Oklahoma strain. In contrast to present results, persistent upregulation of IL-1β and IL-8 and relatively low levels of IFN-γ and TNF-α mRNA expression were observed in dogs with acute severe ehrlichiosis caused by infection with New Mexico strain.[3] This suggests *E. canis* strain–dependent pathogenicity and association of Th1 type immune response with mild canine ehrlichiosis. In support for this observation, IFN-γ generated by CD4 T cells was reported to be essential in resolution of ehrlichia infection in mice.[4] However, Ismail *et al.* reported that production of high levels of TNF-α in mice contributes to toxic shock–like syndrome in fatal monocytotropic ehrlichiosis.[5] The present study and the study using highly pathogenic *E. canis* strain[3] suggest that expression of TNF-α mRNA is involved in milder disease in canine ehrlichiosis in natural hosts. The role of TNF-α on *E. canis* infection and pathogenesis in dogs remains to be elucidated.

ACKNOWLEDGMENTS

This work was supported by the Ohio State University Canine Research Fund and Grant-in-Aids for Scientific Research from the Japan Society for the Promotion of Science.

[Competing interests statement: The authors declare no conflicts of interest.]

REFERENCES

1. HARRUS, S., T. WANER, D. STRAUSS-AYALI *et al.* 1999. Recent advances in determining the pathogenesis of canine monocytic ehrlichiosis. J. Clin. Microbiol. **37:** 2745–2749.
2. GRÖNE, A., A.L. FRISK & W. BAUMGÄRTNER. 1998. Cytokine mRNA expression in whole blood samples from dogs with natural canine distemper virus infection. Vet. Immunol. Immunopathol. **65:** 11–27.
3. UNVER, A., H. HUANG & Y. RIKIHISA. 2006. Cytokine gene expression by peripheral blood leukocytes in dogs experimentally infected with a new virulent strain of *Ehrlichia canis*. Ann. N.Y. Acad. Sci. In press.
4. BITSAKTSIS, C., J. HUNTINGTON & G. WINSLOW. 2004. Production of IFN-γ by CD4 T cells is essential for resolving ehrlichia infection. J. Immunol. **172:** 6894–6901.
5. ISMAIL, N., L. SOONG, J.W. MCBRIDE *et al.* 2004. Overproduction of TNF-α by CD8+ type 1 cells and down-regulation of IFN-γ production by CD4+ Th1 cells contribute to toxic shock–like syndrome in an animal model of fatal monocytotropic ehrlichiosis. J. Immunol. **172:** 1786–1800.

Molecular Characterization of *E. canis* gp36 and *E. chaffeensis* gp47 Tandem Repeats among Isolates from Different Geographic Locations

C. KUYLER DOYLE,[a] ANA MARIA CARDENAS,[a] DANIEL M. AGUIAR,[b] MARCELO B. LABRUNA,[b] LUCY M. NDIP,[c] XUE-JIE YU,[a] AND JERE W. McBRIDE[a]

[a]*Department of Pathology, University of Texas Medical Branch, Galveston, Texas 77555-0609, USA*

[b]*Departamento de Medicina Veterinaria Preventiva, Universidade de Sao Paulo, Sao Paulo, Brazil*

[c]*Department of Life Sciences, University of Buea, Buea, South West Province, Cameroon*

KEYWORDS: glycoprotein; tandem repeats; *Ehlrichia chaffeensis*; *Ehrlichia canis*; gp36; gp47

We recently discovered and characterized major immunoreactive orthologous glycoproteins of *Ehrlichia canis* and *E. chaffeensis*, gp36 and gp47.[1] The genes encoding these proteins contain tandem repeats near the carboxyl-terminus that are sites of O-linked glycosylation. Single repeat units from both gp36 and gp47 contain epitopes that are recognized by dog antisera but are not cross-reactive. Comparative analyses in limited numbers of North American *E. canis* and *E. chaffeensis* determined that the tandem repeats varied in number and sequence among the isolates. To gain further understanding of the global conservation or heterogeneity of these proteins, particularly with respect to the tandem repeat regions, the gp36 and gp47 genes were amplified and compared in several continentally separated strains of *E. canis* and numerous geographically dispersed North American *E. chaffeensis* isolates.

Primers were designed to intergenic regions upstream and downstream of the *E. canis* and *E. chaffeensis* gp36 and gp47 coding regions (*E. canis* gp36 forward 5′-AAT CAA TGT AGT ATG TTT CTT TTA and reverse 5′- ATT TTA CAG GTT ATA TTT CAG TTA; *E. chaffeensis* gp47 forward 5′- TTG TGC AGG GAA AGT TG and reverse 5′- AAT GAA AGT AAA TAA GAA AGT GTA), and amplification was carried out as previously described.[1] The *E. canis gp36* gene sequences from the Louisiana (DQ146151), Florida (DQ146152), DJ (North Carolina)(DQ146153), Sao Paulo (DQ146154), and Cameroon 71 (DQ146155) isolates and *E. chaffeensis gp47*

Address for correspondence: Jere W. McBride, Department of Pathology, University of Texas Medical Branch, Galveston, Texas 77555-0609. Voice: 409-747-2498, fax: 409-747-2455. jemcbrid@utmb.edu

Ann. N.Y. Acad. Sci. 1063: 433–435 (2005).
doi: 10.1196/annals.1355.079

TABLE 1. Tandem repeats of gp36 and gp47 in different *E. canis* and *E. chaffeensis* strains

Tandem repeat	Strain	Repeat number	Percent homology
***E. canis* gp36**	Jake	12.2	100
	Oklahoma	5.2	100
TEDSVSAPA (9 amino acids)	Demon	16.2	99
	Louisiana	5.2	99
	Florida	4.2	100
	DJ	18.2	100
	Sao Paulo	18.2	100
	Cameroon 71	16.2	100
***E. chaffeensis* gp47**			
ASVSEGDAVVNAVSQETPA (19 amino acids)	Arkansas	7.0	99
EGNASEPVVSQEAAPVSE	Jax	4.5	98
SGDAANPVSSSENAS (33 amino acids)	St. Vincent	3.4	98
	Sapulpa	4.5	99
	V3	4.5	97
	V8	4.5	98

gene sequences from the Jax (DQ146156), St. Vincent (DQ146157), V3 (Vanderbilt) (DQ146158) and V8 (DQ146159) isolates were deposited into GenBank for this manuscript. The *E. canis gp36* gene sequences from the Jake (DQ085427), Oklahoma (DQ085428), and Demon (DQ085429) isolates and *E. chaffeensis gp47* gene sequences from the Arkansas (DQ085430) and Sapulpa (DQ085431) isolates were previously deposited. Sequence analysis was performed as previously described.[1]

The tandem repeat sequence from North American, Brazilian, and Cameroonian *E. canis* isolates was completely conserved, consisting of nine amino acids (TEDSVSAPA). However, the number of repeats varied between 4 and 18 copies of the repeat (see TABLE 1). The N-terminal pre-repeat region (143 amino acids) was highly conserved among all isolates, with the Jake, Oklahoma, Demon, and Louisiana strains containing complete homology. The Brazil and Cameroon isolates contained the most divergent sequences (four differences in amino acids), but these still retained 97.2% amino acid homology with the consensus.

Similarly, the *E. chaffeensis* isolates tested demonstrated limited diversity of gp47 tandem repeats. The Arkansas strain exhibited a unique 19 amino acid repeat unit compared to all of the other isolates sequenced. Seven repeats of the 19 amino acid sequence were identified in the Arkansas strain *gp47* gene. Five additional *E. chaffeensis* isolates from geographically dispersed locations had a conserved 33 amino acid repeat unit that exhibited minor variability in repeat sequence (see TABLE 1). The number of copies among this repeat was identical among three of four isolates (4.5 repeats), with the St. Vincent containing one fewer repeat (see TABLE 1). The N-terminal repeat pre-repeat regions (154 amino acids) were completely conserved between the Sapulpa, St. Vincent, V3, and V8 strains. This sequence contained 99.4% amino acid (one alteration) conservation with the pre-repeat region of the Arkansas strain. More divergence was found in the Jax strain, with 91.6% amino acid homology (13 substitutions) in the pre-repeat region compared with the rest of the strains.

Although these proteins are highly immunoreactive and tandem repeat units of gp36 and gp47 contain the B cell epitopes,[1] interestingly, the lack of sequence divergence suggests that there is little immune selective pressure on these proteins to alter their sequence or they must be conserved to retain function. Similarly, comparative sequence analysis failed to detect significant similarity between the repeat units, demonstrating the tandem repeats are not derived from common sequence that went through multiple mutations to gain diversity. The distinct tandem repeats of gp47 will further assist in differentiating variant strains into clades, and may provide insight into pathogenic differences among the strains.

As these orthologous glycoproteins are highly immunogenic,[1] the complete conservation of tandem repeats between strains of *E. canis* around the world and limited divergence between *E. chaffeensis* could have positive implications for future use of these proteins. With the tandem repeat units containing epitopes, a sensitive immunodiagnostic assay for *E. canis* could be developed using a recombinant protein with these tandem repeats.

ACKNOWLEDGMENTS

This work was supported by the Clayton Foundation for Research, the John Sealy Memorial Foundation, and the Sealy Center for Vaccine Development.

[*Competing interests statement:* The authors declare that they have no competing interests.]

REFERENCE

1. DOYLE, C.K., V.L. POPOV & J.W. MCBRIDE. 2006. Differentially expressed and secreted major immunoreactive protein orthologs of *Ehrlichia canis* and *E. chaffeensis* elicit early antibody responses to epitopes on glycosylated tandem repeats. Infect. Immun. **74**. In press.

Prophylactic Use of Sustained-Release Doxycycline Blocks Tick-Transmitted Infection by *Anaplasma phagocytophilum* in a Murine Model

ROBERT F. MASSUNG,[a] NORDIN S. ZEIDNER,[b] MARC C. DOLAN,[b] DAWN ROELLIG,[a] ELIZABETH GABITZSCH,[b] DANIELLE R. TROUGHTON,[a] AND MICHAEL L. LEVIN[a]

[a]*Division of Viral and Rickettsial Diseases, Centers for Disease Control and Prevention, Atlanta, Georgia 30333, USA*

[b]*Division of Vector-Borne Infectious Diseases, Centers for Disease Control and Prevention, Ft. Collins, Colorado, USA*

ABSTRACT: A sustained-release formulation of doxycycline hyclate was tested for its ability to block *Anaplasma phagocytophilum* infection in mice. Mice treated with sustained-release doxycycline showed no splenomegaly and their blood samples were negative by PCR on days 7, 14, and 21. Control mice treated with either oral doxycycline or water had significant splenomegaly and were PCR positive at multiple time points. The sustained-release doxycycline formulation was shown to be efficacious for preventing tick-transmitted *A. phagocytophilum* infection in a mouse model.

KEYWORDS: *Anaplasma phagocytophilum*; *Ixodes scapularis*; doxycycline; human granulocytic anaplasmosis; treatment

Anaplasma phagocytophilum is the etiologic agent of human granulocytic anaplasmosis (HGA), an acute febrile illness with > 500 confirmed cases in the United States in the year 2002.[1] *Ixodes scapularis* ticks are the primary vector involved in maintenance of the agent in natural reservoirs and in its transmission to humans.[2,3] Doxycycline is very effective for the treatment of acute HGA infections with defervescence generally within 24 hours after the initiation of treatment.[4] However, prophylactic treatment of individuals bitten by infected *I. scapuraris* ticks has not been evaluated. The goal of this study was to determine whether a sustained-release formulation of doxycycline hyclate (Atridox™) will prevent productive infection by *A. phagocytophilum* in a mouse model.

Groups of five nymphal *I. scapularis* ticks that had fed as larvae upon *A. phagocytophilum*-infected mice were fed on each of 15 naive mice. Ticks were removed after 72 hours and sets of 5 mice were treated with either oral doxycycline (OD; 2 mg

Address for correspondence: Robert F. Massung, Centers for Disease Control and Prevention, 1600 Clifton Rd., MS G-13, Atlanta, GA 30333. Voice: 404-639-1082; fax: 404-639-4436. rfm2@cdc.gov

Ann. N.Y. Acad. Sci. 1063: 436–438 (2005). © 2005 New York Academy of Sciences. doi: 10.1196/annals.1355.080

in water), sustained-release doxycycline hyclate (AD; 4.2 mg subcutaneous), or a control (either H_2O or copolymer minus doxycycline). EDTA-treated blood samples were drawn at 7, 14, and 21 days post treatment and spleens harvested on day 21. DNA was extracted from each sample using the Qiagen DNeasy Tissue Kit (Qiagen, Valencia, CA, USA) and tested using a quantitative PCR assay that amplified the spacer between the 23S and 5S rRNA genes as previously described.[5] The viability of organisms detected by PCR in murine spleens was evaluated by inoculating homogenized spleen samples on human promyelocytic (HL-60) cells (100 μL spleen homogenate per 10^6 cells) and into naive mice (200–300 μL spleen homogenate per mouse). Growth in HL60 cells was monitored by light microscopy of cytocentrifuge-prepared cells fixed in methanol and stained using Diff-Quik (Dade Behring, Newark, DE, USA). Replication in mice was monitored by PCR testing of DNA extracted from murine blood samples drawn on days 7, 14 and 21 post injection.

Previous studies have shown that the spleen is a site of bacterial replication and accumulation in mice infected with *A. phagocytophilum* and that splenomegaly is an excellent indicator of infection.[5] Splenomegaly was significant for each mouse treated with OD or controls (range 105–182 mg), but not found in mice treated with AD (57.0 mg +/– 4.0 mg) as shown in FIGURE 1. *A. phagocytophilum* DNA was not detected in the blood of mice treated with AD on days 7, 14, or 21 but was detected in the spleens with an average copy number of 21.6 per 2 mg. Mice treated with OD had *A. phagocytophilum* DNA in blood on days 7 (416 copies), 14 (4257 copies), and 21 (148 copies) and in spleens (18962 copies/2 mg). Mice treated with H_2O were PCR positive on days 7 (1059 copies), 14 (1125 copies), and 21 (73 copies), and in spleens (708 copies/2 mg). Viability testing for *A. phagocytophilum* in day 21 spleen samples revealed that spleens from mice treated with either OD or controls were infectious while those treated with AD were not infectious. The lack of splenomegaly

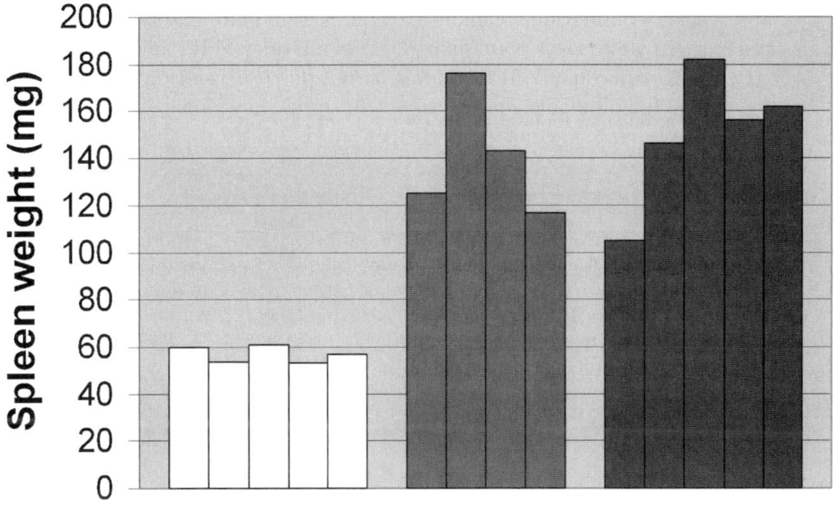

FIGURE 1. Splenomegaly in mice on day 21 after treatment with Atridox™, oral doxycycline, or control.

in AD-treated mice and our results demonstrating that the spleens from AD-treated mice did not contain infectious organisms suggest that *A. phagocytophilum* did not replicate in the spleens of these mice. Rather, the low levels of DNA detected in the spleens of AD-treated mice likely represent the clearance of non-infectious materials derived either from the initial tick feeding or from limited replication in granulocytes in the peripheral blood.

In summary, a novel prophylactic treatment using a sustained-release doxycycline formulation was shown to be efficacious for preventing tick-transmitted *A. phagocytophilum* infection in a mouse model. Additional studies in humans will be needed to determine if the prophylactic treatment of humans following tick bites will be helpful for the control and prevention of HGA and other tick-borne infections.

[*Competing interests statement:* The authors declare that they have no competing interests.]

REFERENCES

1. Groseclose, S.L., W.S. Brathwaite, P.A. Hall, *et al.* 2004. Summary of notifiable diseases—United States, 2002. Morb. Mortal. Wkly. Rep **51:** 1–84.
2. Pancholi, P., C.P. Kolbert, P.D. Mitchell, *et al.* 1995. *Ixodes dammini* as a potential vector of human granulocytic ehrlichiosis J. Infect. Dis. **172:** 1007–1012.
3. Telford, S.R., III, J.E. Dawson, P. Katavolos, *et al.* 1996. Perpetuation of the agent of human granulocytic ehrlichiosis in a deer tick-rodent cycle Proc. Natl. Acad. Sci. USA **93:** 6209–6214.
4. Dumler, J.S. & J.S. Bakken. 1995. Ehrlichial diseases of humans: emerging tick-borne infections Clin. Infect. Dis. **20:** 1102–1110.
5. Massung, R.F., R.A. Priestley & M.L. Levin. 2004. Transmission route efficacy and kinetics of Anaplasma phagocytophilum infection in white-footed mouse, *Peromyscus leucopus.* Vector Borne Zoonotic Dis. **4:** 310–318.

Concentration of Procalcitonin and C-Reactive Protein in Patients with Human Granulocytic Anaplasmosis and the Initial Phase of Tick-Borne Encephalitis

STANKA LOTRIC-FURLAN, TEREZA ROJKO, AND FRANC STRLE

Department of Infectious Diseases, University Medical Center Ljubljana, 1525 Ljubljana, Slovenia

ABSTRACT: The aim of this prospective study was to assess the value of procalcitonin (PCT) level and serum concentration of C-reactive protein (CRP) in differentiating viral from bacterial infection in selected groups of patients, including those with acute human granulocytic anaplasmosis (HGA), which is caused by an intracellular bacteria *Anaplasma phagocytophilum*, and patients with the initial phase of tick-borne encephalitis (TBE), which is a viral disease caused by an RNA virus belonging to the *Flavivirus* genus of the family Flaviviridae.

KEYWORDS: human granulocytic anaplasmosis; initial phase of tick-borne encephalitis; procalcitonin; C-reactive protein

Slovenia is a small central European country known to be endemic for tick-borne encephalitis (TBE) for more than 50 years, whereas the presence of human granulocytic anaplasmosis (HGA) has been established only recently. Several hundred patients with TBE and a few patients with proven acute HGA are registered each year in Slovenia. In at least two-thirds of patients who develop central nervous system involvement due to TBE virus infection, it is well known that the disease has a characteristic biphasic course. The initial phase of TBE has a clinical and laboratory presentation remarkably similar to acute HGA. It is characterized by fever, headache, malaise, and normal cerebrospinal fluid findings. In addition, TBE as well as acute HGA are usually associated with laboratory abnormalities, including leukopenia and thrombocytopenia, and in several patients also by elevated values of liver function test results.[1]

Prompt diagnosis of acute HGA and TBE virus infection is difficult to achieve, especially early in the course of the illness when antibodies are still absent as a rule. It is important to differentiate acute HGA and the initial phase of TBE at the time of their clinical presentation because therapeutic approaches differ considerably. Thus,

Address for correspondence: Stanka Lotric-Furlan, Department of Infectious Diseases, University Medical Center Ljubljana, Japljeva 2, 1525 Ljubljana, Slovenia. Voice: +386-1-522-21-10; fax: +386-1-522-24-56.
stanka.lotric-furlan@mf.uni-lj.si

**Ann. N.Y. Acad. Sci. 1063: 439–441 (2005). © 2005 New York Academy of Sciences.
doi: 10.1196/annals.1355.081**

it would be of practical importance for clinicians to obtain some simple laboratory indicators that could distinguish the initial phase of TBE from acute HGA.

Among several markers of inflammation, concentration of C-reactive protein (CRP) and more recently procalcitonin (PCT) level have been most often studied for their suitability for the diagnosis of bacterial infections. The reported accuracy of PCT and CRP has been rather variable. In general, elevated PCT levels were found to quite reliably support the diagnosis of disseminated bacterial infection and to be a useful parameter enabling distinction between viral and bacterial diseases.[2]

The aim of this prospective study was to assess the value of PCT level and serum concentration of CRP in differentiating viral from bacterial infection in selected groups of patients, including those with acute HGA, which is caused by an intracellular bacteria *Anaplasma phagocytophilum*, and patients with the initial phase of TBE, which is a viral disease caused by an RNA virus belonging to the *Flavivirus* genus of the family Flaviviridae.

Eleven adult patients with proven HGA and 17 patients with the initial phase of TBE were diagnosed at the Department of Infectious Diseases, University Medical Center Ljubljana, Ljubljana, Slovenia, in the period from January 2002 to December 2004, during a prospective study on the etiology of febrile illness occurring within 6 weeks after a tick bite. The patients were older than 18 years and had no known chronic underlying diseases or clinical indications of other bacterial or viral infection.

Criteria for the initial phase of TBE were fulfilled in patients with a febrile illness occurring 6 weeks after a tick bite, who had serologically proven recent TBE virus infection and normal cerebrospinal fluid examination result. The presence of IgM and IgG antibodies to TBE virus was assessed in acute and convalescent serum by enzyme-linked immunosorbent assay (ELISA) (Dade Behring Marburg GmbH, Marburg, Germany) according to the manufacturer's instructions. Demonstration of specific serum IgM antibodies to TBE virus or seroconversion in acute and convalescent sera was interpreted as an indicator of a recent infection.

A case of proven acute HGA was established by the following findings: febrile illness and seroconversion (or at least fourfold change in serum antibody titers) to *A. phagocytophilum* and/or a positive polymerase chain reaction result with subsequent sequencing of the amplicons that demonstrated specific ehrlichial DNA.

To determine serum PCT level and concentration of CRP, blood specimens were obtained on the initial examination prior to the institution of antimicrobial therapy. The concentration of CRP was determined by enhanced immunoassay nephelometry. Concentration of CRP < 5 mg/L was interpreted as a normal value. Serum PCT level was determined by LUMI®PCT (supplied by BRAMHS Diagnostica, Berlin, Germany). This is an immunoluminometric assay used to measure the concentration of PCT in human serum using two antigen-specific monoclonal antibodies that bind PCT at two different sites (the calcitonin and katacalcin segments) added in excess. The detection limit of the assay is 0.1 μg/mL. With this assay, serum levels of PCT in healthy adults are usually <0.5 μg/mL, and values of >0.5 μg/mL are considered to be elevated. Differences in the quantitative data between the two groups were determined by a Kruskal-Wallis test, with use of Epi Info software, version 6.04 (Centers for Disease Control and Prevention, Atlanta, GA). *P* values below 0.05 were considered statistically significant.

The concentration of CRP was elevated in all patients with proven HGA (100%), but in only 3 patients with the initial phase of TBE (17.6%). Elevated serum PCT level was found in 10 (90.9%) out of 11 patients with proven HGA, while in no patients with the initial phase of TBE. The concentrations of CRP for patients with proven HGA and for patients with the initial phase of TBE were 121 (15–314) mg/L and 5 (3–16) mg/L, respectively ($P < 0.001$), while corresponding values of serum PCT levels were 2.5 (0.289–7.200) μg/L and 0.121 (0.021–0.465) μg/L, respectively ($P < 0.001$). Positive predictive values of serum PCT and CRP were 100% and 79%, respectively, while the corresponding negative predictive values were 94% and 100%, respectively.

In conclusion, the results of this study show that, in a patient with a febrile illness occurring after a tick bite, elevated concentration of CRP and elevated serum PCT level point toward the diagnosis of acute HGA and against the initial phase of TBE.

[*Competing interests statement:* The authors declare that they have no competing interests.]

REFERENCES

1. LOTRIC-FURLAN, S., M. PETROVEC, T. AVSIC-ZUPANC *et al.* 2002. Epidemiological, clinical, and laboratory distinction between human granulocytic ehrlichiosis and the initial phase of tick-borne encephalitis. Wien. Klin. Wochenschr. **114:** 636–640.
2. SIMON, L., F. GAUVIN, D.K. AMRE *et al.* 2004. Serum procalcitonin and C-reactive protein levels as markers of bacterial infection: a systematic review and meta-analysis. Clin. Infect. Dis. **39:** 206–217.

Genome Analysis of *Coxiella burnetii* Species

Insights into Pathogenesis and Evolution and Implications for Biodefense

REKHA SESHADRI[a] AND JAMES SAMUEL[b]

[a]*The Institute for Genomic Research, Rockville, Maryland 20850, USA*

[b]*Department of Medical Microbiology and Immunology, Texas A&M University System Health Science Center, 407 Reynolds Bldg.,College Station, Texas 77843-1114, USA*

ABSTRACT: *Coxiella burnetii*, the etiological agent of Q fever, is a class B biodefense agent. We are continuing the momentum of discovery generated by the first *Coxiella* genome sequences by extending the breadth of genomics to include four additional heterogeneous *C. burnetii* strains. We are also sequencing the genome of *Rickettsiella grylli*, an intracellular parasite of grasshoppers and the closest known phylogenetic relative to the *Coxiella* group. These data will enable the investigation of fundamental questions about *Coxiella* pathogenicity and virulence as well as broader evolutionary questions about the transition to obligate intracellular life. Specifically, sequence comparisons will permit examination of genetic differences, allowing us to address key questions: What core genes are necessary for an obligate intracellular lifestyle and developmental cycle of the genus? What specific genetic determinants can be linked to virulence properties such as host preference, disease severity, and pathology (i.e., acute vs. chronic disease)? What are the frequencies of mutation and intragenomic recombination, and levels of genome reduction? What specific factors are relevant to colonization and virulence in human hosts (based on comparisons with *R. grylli*)? From a public health and biodefense perspective, exposure to different strains, either natural or due to illegitimate release, may have different outcomes. With extensive genomic-level information from diverse strains, investigators can determine effective drug and vaccine targets and design methods to accurately type *Coxiella* based on a subset of genes, opening the way for cost-effective targeted PCR- or antibody-based tests.

KEYWORDS: ***Coxiella burnetii*; genomics; biodefense**

INTRODUCTION

C. burnetii is the causative agent of Q fever, and as a highly virulent zoonotic pathogen and category B bioterror agent, it is a serious public health concern for civilians and military personnel.[1] It is an obligate intracellular acidophile that is highly adapted for life within the eukaryotic phagolysosome. *C. burnetii* can overcome phagocytic cells and has a novel, nonsporulating strategy to survive in the environ-

Address for correspondence: Rekha Seshadri, The Institute for Genomic Research, 9712 Medical Center Drive, Rockville, MD 20850. Voice: 301-795-7858; fax: 301-838-0208. rekha@tigr.org

Ann. N.Y. Acad. Sci. 1063: 442–450 (2005). © 2005 New York Academy of Sciences. doi: 10.1196/annals.1355.063

ment for extensive periods.[2–4] The agent was weaponized independently under various biological warfare programs initiated by the U.S. and U.S.S.R.,[5] and epidemics of Q fever were reported amongst troops during World Wars I and II. Multiple reports of outbreaks demonstrate that Q fever is undoubtedly a disease of military significance with an estimated 23–77% loss of manpower and acute impairment of operational efficiencies in a severe epidemic.[6]

BIOLOGY OF *C. BURNETII*

A hallmark property of *C. burnetii* is its ability to remain infectious after extended exposure to extreme environmental circumstances (e.g., high temperature, desiccation, osmotic shock, ultraviolet light, and chemical disinfectants).[2] This ability to survive a harsh intra- and extracellular environment may rely, in part, on a developmental life cycle with various forms specialized for propagation, surviving intracellular stress and persisting in the extracellular environment (in a non-replicating state) for long periods between hosts.[2,7] *In vitro*, *C. burnetii* passively enters and replicates within a variety of epithelial, fibroblast, and macrophage-like cell lines.[8] Internalization into host cells occurs by a microfilament-dependent parasite-directed endocytic process.[9] The nascent bacteria-containing phagosomes mature through the endocytic pathway acquiring the properties of secondary lysosomes. *C. burnetii* has an absolute requirement for an acidic pH to activate metabolism, fulfilled by living in this phagolysosomal compartment.[3,4,10] The organism replicates to high numbers, albeit at a slow replication rate (~12 h doubling time) within this vacuole, despite the presence of toxic host factors, such as acid hydrolase, oxygen and nitrogen radicals, and defensins, which are normally considered bactericidal.[8]

C. burnetii is generally maintained in nature by cycles involving many species of vertebrate animals, as well as arthropods which become infected by taking a blood meal.[11,12] Domestic animals are involved in the cycle of infection (cattle, sheep, and goats are the primary reservoirs) and humans become infected via aerosols that originate from contaminated animal products.[13] These infectious cycles might select for highly virulent genetic variants. Isolates obtained from a variety of vertebrates and arthropods have been classified into genomic groups by various methods, and while these groups do not correlate with host, geographical location, or date of isolation, the type of human disease caused by isolates in each group is similar, implying that specific isolate groups have a particular virulence potential in humans, determined by specific factors and molecular mechanisms encoded by each.

BIOMEDICAL ASPECTS

C. burnetii causes a wide spectrum of human disease. The disease manifestations of *C. burnetii* infection in humans can be separated into acute and chronic illnesses. Acute disease commonly presents as a flu-like illness with hallmark cyclic fever and periorbital headache.[14] Pneumonitis and hepatitis are regular complications but acute disease is commonly self-limiting. Various antibiotics, including tetracyclines, are effective for overcoming acute disease.[15] Until recently, clinically, the illness fell within the group of FUO (fever of unknown origin) syndromes and was not com-

TABLE 1. ***C. burnetii*** **isolates selected for sequencing**

Group	Plasmid	Isolate	Original Source	Disease
VI	QpDG	Dugway 7E22-57	Utah, rodents, 1958	–
II	QpH1	RSA331	Italy, human blood, 1945	Acute
IV	QpRS	MSU Goat Q177	Montana, goat cotyledon, 1980	Abortion
I	QpH1	African RSA334(>)	Central Africa, human blood, 1949	Acute, Congolese Red Fever
IV	QpRS	K Q154	Oregon, human heart valve, 1976	Endocarditis
V	NP	G Q212	Nova Scotia, human heart valve, 1981	Endocarditis

NP, no extrachromosomal plasmid.

monly recognized or diagnosed. In many areas of the world, a high percentage of the population (10–20%) has serological evidence of previous infection.[16] In contrast, chronic infection is much less common and manifests as endocarditis.[17,18] Chronic infections have not responded well to a variety of antibiotic regimens, with patients receiving a combination of doxycycline plus chloroquine, administered over 1–2 years, showing the best outcome.[19] From a public health and biodefense perspective, exposure to different strains, either natural, or due to illegitimate release, may have quite different outcomes. Exposure to acute disease isolates would likely result in predominantly flu-like illness with the potential for long term cardiovascular disease risk. Exposure of a population to chronic disease isolates would probably not result in significant immediate disease cases, but may result in chronic illnesses developing months or years from initial exposure.

C. burnetii was previously classified in the family Rickettsiaceae, based solely on their close association with arthropods and intravacuolar location, however they have been subsequently placed within the gamma subclass of phylum Proteobacteria. Phylogenetic analysis of 16S rRNA gene sequences and a variety of individual housekeeping gene sequences reveals it is most closely related to the pathogens *Rickettsiella* and *Legionella* (FIG. 1).[20–22] Similarities in intracellular replication in membrane-bound vacuoles and other virulence mechanisms have underscored the relationships with these other two pathogens, particularly the *Rickettsiella* spp.

BIOLOGY OF *RICKETTSIELLA GRYLLI*

Rickettsiella grylli is an obligate intracellular parasite of *Gryllus bimaculatus,* and related species of crickets. Members of the genus *Rickettsiella* are intracellular pathogens of invertebrates, including insects, crustaceans, and arachnids.[23,24] Studies of virulence in hosts other than the host of isolation have shown that *R. grylli* can multiply in the mouse when large doses are inoculated by the intraperitoneal route or by inhalation, but the mouse overcomes infection and organisms are cleared in about 2 weeks. Since studies of host specificity, cultivation, or antigenic analyses are not extensive, most of the knowledge is based on light and electron microscopic observations. The infectious forms are gram-negative rod-shaped organisms that develop intracellularly into larger vegetative forms, similar to the developmental cycle observed for *Chlamydia* spp. and *Coxiella*. Bacterial replication takes place in cell vacuoles in the fat body, the hepatopancreas, and other organs of invertebrate hosts. Growth in cell-free media has not been demonstrated. They are pathogenic for their larval hosts and young and mature stages of invertebrate hosts, but display little virulence for vertebrates. They are maintained in the soil for years, and infection arises from contaminated soil rather than transovarian passage.

RESULTS FROM THE FIRST *C. BURNETII* GENOME SEQUENCE

To date, only one genome sequence for *C. burnetii* has been published.[25] The Nine Mile Phase I strain RSA493, a highly virulent tick isolate, was chosen because of its known virulence and potential for subsequent comparison with other isolate groups. The elucidation of the genome analysis was an important milestone in *Coxiella* research, contributing significantly to our understanding of the physiology and pathogenesis of this organism. Novel genes implicated in adhesion, invasion, intracellular trafficking, host modulation, and detoxification were identified. The genome sequence has advanced investigations on the molecular mechanisms of virulence and the development of genetic tools for functional analysis of virulence genes. *C. burnetii* possesses a small reduced genome apparently resulting from strong selection for conservation of genes necessary for maintaining a complex developmental cycle and highly evolved pathogenesis mechanisms. The presence of numerous dispersed insertion sequence (IS) elements and palindromic repeats indicated great genome plasticity and a previously unappreciated degree of genomic flux in the *Coxiella*. Numerous pseudogenes attested to an ongoing process of reductive evolution; genes that once had an important function accumulate mutations and eventually disappear either because they are no longer under strong selective pressures (e.g., if the organism's niche has changed) or because of population level phenomena that lead to an inability to maintain genes under weak selection. Thus the single existing genome sequence hints at potentially great genome diversity resulting from point mutations, frameshifts, and potential intragenomic recombination mediated by IS transposases, extragenic palindromic repeats, and other elements.

STRAIN DIVERSITY AND SELECTION OF ADDITIONAL CANDIDATES FOR SEQUENCING

We proposed to study *C. burnetii* isolates using comparative genome analyses of heterogeneous strains to identify key factors critical for virulence and host interactions. Our central hypothesis was that changes in gene repertoire underpin differences in host interactions and disease pathology, and the evolution of infective and virulence mechanisms. Just as sequencing of individual genomes has invigorated molecular pathogenesis studies in bacteria, knowledge of the genomic content of multiple strains will help answer questions about the nature of *Coxiella* pathogenesis.

Isolates from mammalian and arthropod hosts have been differentiated based on genetic and phenotypic differences into at least six different genomic groups.[26–29] Members of the groups have significant differences with respect to disease association (acute or chronic disease), virulence, and antigenicity. While these groups do not correlate with host, geographical location, or date of isolation, the type of human disease caused by isolates in each group is similar. For example, group I contains acute disease isolates only while two groups of chronic disease isolates are distinguished (groups IV and V), each having unique restriction patterns, and also unique plasmid type, and no acute disease isolates—implying that specific isolate groups have a particular virulence potential in humans. Most isolates maintain a large, low-copy plasmid (e.g., QpH1, 36 kb in Nine Mile isolate). One isolate group has lost this endogenous plasmid but maintained a significant portion of the DNA by insertion into the chromosome. Plasmid functions remain cryptic, and a correlation with virulence phenotypes is not evident. The potential difference between isolates was underscored by a report that the genome size between isolates might vary by nearly 1 Mb (ranging from 1.5–2.4 Mb). DNA-DNA hybridization on selected isolates has also been used to quantify relatedness (90–95%) between several groups supporting the classification of the isolates into distinct groups.[30] Recently, a high-density oligonucleotide Affymetrix array (RMLchip) containing oligonucleotide probe sets corresponding to all open reading frames of the index strain RSA493 Nine Mile Phase I (NMI) of *C. burnetii* was interrogated with 12 *C. burnetii* strains.[30] The genomic diversity of environmental and human acute or chronic disease isolates was ascertained by deletion polymorphism analysis through hybridization of genomic DNA to the RMLchip. In this preliminary study, four strains (group I acute isolates) were identical to NMI whereas the remaining strains contained significant chromosomal deletions. The number of polymorphisms ranged from 1 to 22, with the size of each deletion ranging from 1 to 20 gene(s). Based on these differences, specific genomic groups containing similar chromosomal deletions could be defined and corresponded with previous RFLP-based genomic grouping.

We proposed to have a representative strain from each genomic group sequenced. The strains selected constituted a selection based on the virulence potential, disease phenotypes, host organism, geographical distribution, and gross genomic distinctions with the goal of maximizing known biology with genomic data.

C. burnetii *Dugway*

This strain was isolated from rodents in Utah and belongs to genomic group VI. It has a distinct, previously unsequenced plasmid designated QpDG. In recent guinea pig aerosol-challenge experiments with this strain, no fever was detected in experimental animals.[31] No human infection was reported from Camp Detrick studies.[32] Comparison of IS1111A insert pattern identified as few as 11 copies compared with 20–22 copies for other isolate groups, suggesting either major chromosomal deletions or an alternate evolutionary divergence mechanism.

C. burnetii *RSA331*

We propose to sequence Henzerling strain RSA331 that was isolated from blood of an infected patient in Italy in 1945. This strain belongs in genomic group II, possesses a previously sequenced plasmid (QpH1), and is primarily associated with acute Q fever. Preliminary analysis of nine variable-number tandem repeat (VNTR) loci and 18 single nucleotide polymorphism (SNP) loci suggest this strain is a suitably divergent candidate for sequencing to closure.[33] This strain is commonly used for vaccine preparation. Higher infectivity, distinct structural properties of LPS, and other biological distinctions have been demonstrated.

C. burnetii *MSU Goat Q177*

This strain isolated from goat cotyledons belongs to genomic group IV, contains a distinct plasmid type, QpRS, and was associated with goat abortions in Montana in 1980. Virulence studies in a guinea pig model suggest an intermediate phenotype for this strain, including low fever and no death in an aerosol-challenge experiment compared to highly virulent acute isolate groups.[31] Virulence studies in a SCID immunocompromised mouse model noted an inability to induce cachexic death.[34] An intermediate-length lipopolysaccharide is described for this strain.[35] Growth studies in tissue culture suggest defects in replication rates in macrophages.[36]

C. burnetii *RSA 334*

This strain is comparable to Nine Mile phase I (RSA 493) in virulence in animal models of infection and growth *in vitro*. It was isolated in Africa in 1949 from a patient with "Congolese red fever" and represents the potential diversity within the acute isolate group (I) of *C. burnetii*. Comparison of this genome with Nine Mile would allow prediction of the rate of evolutionary divergence for a species that replicates in a niche relatively protected from exogenous DNA for recombination.

Two additional human endocarditis isolates (Q154 and Q212) are being sequenced by Robert Heinzen's group at Rocky Mountain laboratories in Hamilton, Montana.

SUMMARY

Genome sequencing has dramatically changed the landscape of microbiology research over the past ten years. Advances in sequencing technologies and bioinformatics have made genome sequencing a routine practice. A genomic approach is particularly critical when studying an organism like *Coxiella* that has fastidious requirements for growth inside living host cells and has been refractory to conventional molecular-genetic methods. Additionally *Coxiella* are suitable subjects for sequencing due to their small size and relatively non-repetitive genomes. Analysis of the first genome of *C. burnetii* Nine Mile RSA493 provided substantial insights into the physiology, genetics, and the process of reductive evolution in this species. The availability of the genome has also helped facilitate various global gene expression (microarray) and proteomic approaches towards examining *Coxiella* diversity, molecular mechanisms of pathogenesis, host interaction, and other aspects of its biology.

The availability of genome sequences for individual as well as multiple strains of a given species is central in fostering biopreparedness efforts as exemplified by the multi-strain sequencing effort with *Bacillus anthracis* strains for development of forensic methods for attribution purposes when illegitimate use is suspected. The long-term outcomes projected for this study include development of novel diagnostic markers, sampling diversity, and epidemiological information for *C. burnetii*, increased knowledge of variation in this lineage, etc. Specifically, the genome sequences will provide key resources for addressing major biodefense needs.

Vaccine and Drug Targets

The utility of genome sequence in novel vaccine development has already been demonstrated with great success in the case of *Neisseria meningitidis* serogroup B strains.[37] The approach involved identifying 570 candidate surface-exposed or exported antigens from the genome sequence, expressing these genes (350 ORFs were successfully expressed) in *E. coli*, and development of immune-sera against purified protein. These were further tested for suitability in conferring protection against heterologous Meningococcus B strains by using ELISA and FACS techniques. Several vaccine candidates were identified from the genome using this method, which are currently undergoing clinical trials.

Since a vaccine must induce protection against an array of strains, this study will help characterize the genetic heterogeneity among geographically and biologically diverse isolates of *C. burnetii*. With extensive genomic-level information from diverse strains, investigators can build alignments of proteins under consideration as drug or vaccine targets to find regions conserved across the group. Understanding mechanisms used for replication and pathogenesis may be helpful in identifying targets for drug development.

Diagnostic Assays for Specific Subtypes

Genome sequences may enhance methods to accurately type *Coxiella* based on a subset of genes opening the way for cost-effective targeted PCR- or antibody-based tests for clinical settings. A successful response to threat also requires accurate and rapid means for detection. Inherent to this is the use of molecular epidemiological methods to understand baseline diversity and persistence in the environment. There is currently little information on baseline genomic diversity, and what genetic changes are occurring within groups from different animal and human sources and geographic locales. A knowledge of microbial diversity and forces effecting diversity and evolution of a species may be exploited to select valid signature sets and typing systems for attribution purposes in a forensic investigation by law enforcement or national security agencies.

Previous studies have underscored the advantages of having additional individual genome sequences and increasing the value of existing genomes through the power of comparative genomics, yielding useful information regarding physiological and other phenotypic differences. Examining variance in gene content will help us to understand the subtle nuances of bacterial adaptation in response to specific hosts and other conditions, as well as other aspects of species divergence.

[*Competing interests statement:* The authors declare that they have no competing interests.]

REFERENCES

1. ANONYMOUS. 2003. NIAID Biodefense Research Agenda for Category B and C Priority Pathogens. Vol. No. 03-5315. NIH Publication.
2. HEINZEN, R.A., T. HACKSTADT & J.E. SAMUEL. 1999. Developmental biology of *Coxiella burnettii.* Trends Microbiol. **7:**149–154.
3. AKPORIAYE, E.T. *et al.* 1983. Lysosomal response of a murine macrophage-like cell line persistently infected with *Coxiella burnetii.* Infect. Immun. **40:** 1155–1162.
4. HACKSTADT, T. & J.C. WILLIAMS. 1981. Biochemical stratagem for obligate parasitism of eukaryotic cells by *Coxiella burnetii.* Proc. Natl. Acad. Sci. USA **78:** 240–3244.
5. REGIS, E. 1999. The Biology of Doom: The History Of America's Secret Germ Warfare Project. Henry Holt and Associates. New York.
6. SPICER, A.J. *et al.* 1977. Q fever and animal abortion in Cyprus. Trans. R. Soc. Trop. Med. Hyg. **71:** 16–20.
7. MCCAUL, T.F., N. BANERJEE-BHATNAGAR & J.C. WILLIAMS. 1991. Antigenic differences between *Coxiella burnetii* cells revealed by postembedding immunoelectron microscopy and immunoblotting. Infect. Immun. **59:** 3243–3253.
8. BACA, O.G. & D. PARETSKY. 1983. Q fever and *Coxiella burnetii:* a model for host-parasite interactions. Microbiol. Rev. **47:** 127–149.
9. BACA, O.G., D.A. KLASSEN & A.S. ARAGON. 1993. Entry of *Coxiella burnetii* into host cells. Acta Virol. **37:** 143–155.
10. HEINZEN, R.A. *et al.* 1996. Differential interaction with endocytic and exocytic pathways distinguish parasitophorous vacuoles of *Coxiella burnetii* and *Chlamydia trachomatis.* Infect. Immun. **64:** 796–809.
11. MARRIE, T.J. 1990. Epidemiology of Q fever. *In* Q Fever, The Disease. T.J. Marrie, Ed.: 49–70. CRC Press. Boca Raton, FL.
12. KAPLAN, M.M. & P. BERTAGNA. 1955. The geographical distribution of Q fever. Bull. World Health Org. **13:** 829–860.
13. BABUDIERI, C. 1959. Q fever: a zoonosis. Adv. Vet. Sci. **5:** 81–84.
14. RAOULT, D. & T. MARRIE. 1995. Q fever. Clin. Infect. Dis. **20:** 489–495; quiz 496.
15. RAOULT, D. 1993. Treatment of Q fever. Antimicrob. Agents Chemother. **37:** 1733–1736.
16. HTWE, K.K. *et al.* 1993. Prevalence of antibodies to *Coxiella burnetii* in Japan. J. Clin. Microbiol. **31:** 722–723.
17. SIDWELL, R.W., B.D. THORPE & L.P. GEBHARDT. 1964. Studies of latent Q fever infections. II. Effects of multiple cortisone injections. Am. J. Hyg. **79:** 320–327.
18. BROUQUI, P. *et al.* 1993. Chronic Q fever. Ninety-two cases from France, including 27 cases without endocarditis. Arch. Intern. Med. **153:** 642–648.
19. JABARIT-ALDIGHIERI, N., H. TORRES & D. RAOULT. 1992. Susceptibility of *Rickettsia conorii, R. rickettsii,* and *Coxiella burnetii* to PD 127,391, PD 131,628, pefloxacin, ofloxacin, and ciprofloxacin. Antimicrob. Agents Chemother. **36:** 2529–2532.
20. ROUX, V. *et al.* 1997. Reassessment of the taxonomic position of *Rickettsiella grylli.* Int. J. Syst. Bacteriol. **47:** 1255–1257.
21. RELMAN, D.A. *et al.* 1992. Phylogenetic relationships among the agent of bacillary angiomatosis, *Bartonella bacilliformis,* and other alpha-proteobacteria. Mol. Microbiol. **6:** 1801–1807.
22. WEISBURG, W.G. *et al.* 1989. Phylogenetic diversity of the Rickettsiae. J. Bacteriol. **171:** 4202–4206.
23. WEISS, E., G.A. DASCH & K. CHANG. 1984. Rickettsiella. *In* Bergey's Manual of Systematic Bacteriology. N.R. Krieg, Ed.: 713–717. Williams and Wilkins. Baltimore, MD.
24. VAGO, C. & R. MARTOJA. 1963. [Rickettsiosis in the *Gryllidae* (*Orthoptera*)]. C. R. Hebd. Seances Acad. Sci. **256:** 1045–1047.
25. SESHADRI, R. *et al.* 2003. Complete genome sequence of the Q-fever pathogen *Coxiella burnetii.* Proc. Natl. Acad. Sci. USA **100:** 5455–5460.
26. HEINZEN, R. *et al.* 1990. Use of pulsed field gel electrophoresis to differentiate *Coxiella burnetii* strains. Ann. N.Y. Acad. Sci. **590:** 504–513.

27. Vodkin, M.H., J.C. Williams & E.H. Stephenson. 1986. Genetic heterogeneity among isolates of *Coxiella burnetii.* J. Gen. Microbiol. **132:** 455–463.
28. Hendrix, L.R., J.E. Samuel & L.P. Mallavia. 1991. Differentiation of *Coxiella burnetii* isolates by analysis of restriction-endonuclease-digested DNA separated by SDS-PAGE. J. Gen. Microbiol. **137:** 269–276.
29. Jager, C. *et al.* 1998. Molecular characterization of *Coxiella burnetii* isolates. Epidemiol. Infect. **120:** 157–164.
30. Beare, P.A. *et al.* 2004. Genome and Transcriptional Analysis of *Coxiella burnetii* using a Custom Multi-Pathogen Affymetrix GeneChip. *In* ASM Conference on Functional Genomics and Bioinformatics Approaches to Infectious Disease Research. Portland, OR.
31. Russell-Lodrique, K.E. *et al.* 2005. *C. burnetii* virulence is isolate-group specific in guinea pig aerosol-challenge model. *In* 4th International Conference on Rickettsiae and Rickettsial Diseases. Logrono, Spain. Trama Impresores S.A.L.
32. Stoenner, H.G. & D.B. Lackman. 1960. The biologic properties of *Coxiella burnetii* isolated from rodents collected in Utah. Am. J. Hyg. **71:** 45–51.
33. Keim, P. 2004. Personal Communication.
34. Andoh, M. *et al.* 2003. SCID mouse model for lethal Q fever. Infect. Immun. **71:** 4717–4723.
35. Lukacova, M. *et al.* 1993. Phase variation of lipopolysaccharide of *Coxiella burnetii,* strain Priscilla during chick embryo yolk sac passaging. FEMS Microbiol. Lett. **113:** 285–289.
36. Roman, M.J. *et al.* 1991. Analysis of *Coxiella burnetii* isolates in cell culture and the expression of parasite-specific antigens on the host membrane surface. Acta Virol. **35:** 503–510.
37. Tettelin, H. *et al.* 2000. Complete genome sequence of *Neisseria meningitidis* serogroup B strain MC58. Science **287:** 1809–1815.

Attack Scenarios with Rickettsial Species

Implications for Response and Management

G. PAPPAS, N. AKRITIDIS,[a] AND E.V. TSIANOS

First Department of Internal Medicine, University Hospital of Ioannina, Ionnina, Greece

[a]*General Hospital "G. Hatzikosta" of Ioannina Ioannina, Greece*

KEYWORDS: **Coxiella burnetii; Q fever; biological agent; scenario**

Rickettsial species have been significant pathogens for military medicine in the past, mainly through epidemic typhus and Q fever outbreaks in military expeditions of the twentieth century.[1] *Coxiella burnetii*, the etiological agent of Q fever, has been invariably acknowledged as a potential biological agent, while certain Rickettsial species possess some of the characteristics of a potential biological weapon. However, excluding *Rickettsia prowazekii,* this potential is not universally accepted and is subject to limitations. Currently, only these two agents are listed, in Category B, by the Centers for Disease Control and Prevention (CDC) as potential bioterrorism agents.

WHO AND WHY *COXIELLA BURNETII*?

Potential occasions for the use of *Coxiella burnetii* as a biological weapon are abundant in present times—especially since the events of Autumn 2001 drastically altered our perception of the impossible. In an era characterized by the presence of multiple religious, ethnic, and political extremist movements, focusing both on domestic and international issues, a specialized threat such as biowarfare might cause not only significant morbidity and mortality, but would disrupt the society's perception of normal life through the sheer public shock produced. For reasons of political correctness we will presume in this paper that the person responsible for the attack is a mad scientist out to hold the world at ransom, in the vein of various films that have long shaped public perception.[2]

Why would this mad scientist use *Coxiella burnetii*? The pathogen is cheap and easy to find, easy to aerosolize, and extremely stable in various environmental circumstances.[3] Its use, as outlined in this paper, would result in massive morbidity with limited mortality, kind of a "dress rehearsal" for the use of more grave pathogens.

Address for correspondence: Dr. Georgios Pappas, Internal Medicine Department, University Hospital, 45110, Ioannina, Greece. Voice: 30 26510 49453; fax: 30 26510 49045.
gpele@otenet.gr

Ann. N.Y. Acad. Sci. 1063: 451–458 (2005). © 2005 New York Academy of Sciences.
doi: 10.1196/annals.1355.065

FACTORS AFFECTING THE OUTCOME

The idea of simulating a biowarfare attack in order to outline the optimal response is not new,[4,5] although few scenarios have actually focused on the impact of a number of factors related to the pathogen and the time and space of the attack.[6] These factors will be analyzed through a hypothetical scenario and their influence on its outcome.

AN ATTACK SCENARIO

The aforementioned mad scientist decides to use *Coxiella burnetii* in a small city of an unnamed Southern European country belonging to the European Union, with a population of 100,000. The city is located in a rural province with a low per capita income, adjacent to a small mountain, and is rather isolated from the rest of the country due to geographical reasons (two planes arrive daily from the capital, there is no train connection, and the national road network leading to the city is not modern). The weather in the summer is mildly hot, but windy conditions commonly occur during this season. The city has two hospitals that are on call every other day, with a total 1,300-bed capacity and intensive care units (ICUs) that can handle 30 patients in total. The hospitals serve as referral hospitals for the neighboring regions that have total population of 250,000. The hospitals are usually overcrowded. The microbiology laboratories are adequately developed. A 30-bed infectious diseases unit with adequate isolation capacity exists in the larger of the hospitals. Zoonotic infectious diseases are commonly diagnosed in these hospitals, and an average of 10 cases of Q fever are hospitalized annually. There exists no special bioterrorism preparedness plan, apart from published guidelines from the National Authorities for Infectious Diseases.

One summer afternoon (day 0), the mad scientist releases a significant amount of aerosolized *Coxiella burnetii* from the nearby hill. The breeze carries the mixture towards the city, but none of the citizens notices or complains about anything. Nothing happens for the next 10 days.

On the morning of day 11, doctors at the emergency department notice a higher than usual number of patients complaining of fever with flu-like symptoms. Two of these patients are admitted to the Infectious Diseases Department and one more patient is admitted to the Department of Respiratory Medicine. The on-call doctors discuss with each other the unusually high number of patients, finding it strange, especially for this season, but no alerts, epidemiological investigations, or specialized serologic tests for the persons admitted are ordered.

On day 12, the situation gets worse in the second hospital, which is now on call. More than 100 patients complain of similar symptoms, and 15 of them are hospitalized. A neutropenic patient with cancer and a pregnant woman who have similar complaints are admitted to the departments of Oncology and Obstetrics, respectively. The doctors of the second hospital seem worried about the situation, and a brief epidemiologic surveillance among patients admitted yields no common characteristics. The second hospital ends its day on call overcrowded.

On the morning of day 13, a casual communication of one of the doctors of the second hospital with a general practitioner reveals that the latter has consulted an unusually high number of patients with similar symptoms during the previous day. There are 400 patients with fever present that day at the first hospital, 60 of them admitted, three of them at the ICU.

By the afternoon of day 13, the doctors of the first hospital have been persuaded that there is an ongoing epidemic, presumably by an unidentified viral pathogen. At emergency meeting of the heads of various departments of the first hospital the situation is discussed, all doctors are asked to be on call, and the second hospital goes on call too in order to handle the huge burden of patients. Local media are advised to avoid creating panic, doctors of the emergency department are asked to draw samples from every patient with related symptoms, the microbiology laboratory is asked to actively pursue a diagnosis through cultures and serology, and samples are sent to the Reference Microbiology Laboratory of the country's capital. It is decided that all admitted patients should be further hospitalized in the Infectious Diseases Department under the best isolation procedures possible. The National Authorities for Infectious Diseases (NAID) are informed about the outbreak of an unidentified infectious disease. Regional hospitals are contacted, to determine if similar cases exist and to determine their ability to handle the heavy patient burden. The mayor of the city and the district chairman are contacted and a meeting is arranged later that day. Local press is advised to avoid creating panic until after the meeting. The possibility of a bioterrorist attack is not considered at all, as being simply impossible. The Minister of Health is informed, and a specialist from NAID catches the next flight to the city. Regional doctors consider contacting the CDC and the European CDC (ECDC) but are advised by NAID not to, until NAID specialists know the whole picture. The Minister of Health contacts authorities of the European Union and the World Health Organization (WHO) and asks for further assistance in the form of Infectious Diseases experts. The local meeting is held without the mayor and two of the senior doctors who are also experiencing symptoms and are admitted to the hospital. There is a constant dispute during the meeting about who is in charge: the district health director, the district chairman, the NAID representative, the Infectious Diseases and Respiratory Medicine specialists, the Hospitals' chairmen, and the Head of the Epidemiology Department all consider that they should be in charge.

By midnight of day 13, they produce a public announcement that states that the public should stay at home, avoid direct contact with patients with symptoms, and avoid visiting the hospital if they are asymptomatic. General practitioners are advised to evaluate every patient possible and avoid referring to the hospitals patients with mild or moderate symptoms. No specific advice regarding antibiotic use is issued. The public is informed that a specific diagnosis will be achieved in less than 24 hours, and that no deaths have been reported yet. A national and international warning for persons who have been visiting the city during the previous three weeks is also issued. On reviewing the epidemiological, clinical, and laboratory data of the first 500 patients, it is concluded that the disease is an atypical pneumonia-like infection, with no obvious epidemiological source. Fear of an emerging SARS-like epidemic is eminent. Samples from all kinds of regional animals are drawn in order to investigate a possible animal origin of the infection. Medical specialists conclude that antibiotic use should not be deferred for hospitalized patients, and suggest the combined use of ceftriaxone and a macrolide. No decision is made regarding suggested treatment of outpatients, although some suggest the empirical use of doxycycline or moxifloxacin.

During the night of day 13, more than 500 patients visit the emergency department, while a significant number of medical and paramedical staff are also sick, further compromising the hospital response. Medical specialists have already concluded that all cases arise from a 20 kilometer–diameter circle around the city. The possibility of an airborne-spread pathogen is seriously entertained, and national and international organizations are informed. Tularemia and Q fever are high on the list of the differential diagnosis, but a viral pathogen is not excluded yet.

On the eve of day 14, an unidentified specialist from the country capital is interviewed by a national television program and speaks of bioterrorism, naming the all the potential pathogens and their consequences, and accusing the local and state authorities of inadequacy. All sorts of "experts" turn up at other national programs, while the Ministry of Health responds, "all possible scenarios are under investigation and all proper preventive measures are actively evolving."

Later that night one of the first patients admitted to the ICU dies. The news creates even more unrest, both at local and national levels. More than 1,000 people visit local pharmacies and buy, at any cost, various antibiotics: by dawn, all stocks of ciprofloxacin tablets are exhausted. About 1,000 people flee the city.

In the morning of day 14, the situation seems out of control: by noon, more than 8,000 people experience symptoms, the majority of whom are seeking hospital advice. More than another 1,000 people abandon the city by noon, some of them moving to the city capital, seeking medical advice there. The majority of the pharmacies are closed, finding it difficult to refuse to sell a variety of antibiotics to anxious customers. More than 200 people require hospitalization by noon, while a significant percentage of medics and paramedics are also sidelined by illness. Medical students are recruited to compensate for the shortage of medical personnel. A minority of paramedics refuses to participate in patient admission and care, proclaiming possible personal health harm. By noon, the government has arranged for a significant number of specialists to arrive at the city, and certain schools and hotels are selected to act as temporary hospital wards.

At noon, a North Atlantic Treaty Organization (NATO) special team arrives at the city and sets up an epidemiologic and diagnostic investigation. Army units from other country areas arrive and set up temporary hospital wards. Local army units are largely sidelined though, due to illness. Experts from ECDC and CDC are also expected by the end of day 14. Self-proclaimed "experts" continue to rant on national channels, despite a strict government suggestion to keep down the tone.

During the following two hours, the local microbiology laboratory, the national reference laboratory, and international reference laboratories will confirm that the pathogen is *Coxiella burnetii*. An urgent meeting is arranged both in the city capital and the targeted city in order for a plan to be arranged. There is once more significant dispute over who is in charge. This controversy ends when the prime minister decides to move to the targeted city to coordinate action. World experts are contacted and asked for advice. There are two main disputes: Should it be confirmed that the outbreak was most probably the result of deliberate spread? Should all the inhabitants of the targeted area receive antibiotic prophylaxis?

In the afternoon of day 14, the prime minister arrives at the city. At the same time, it is officially announced by the Ministry of Health that the pathogen is *Coxiella burnetii*. A special leaflet with information for the public developed by NAID is presented. Isolation procedures are recalled. The NAID guidelines are distributed in the targeted area, and all patients with symptoms are put on doxycycline or other drastic antibiotics. Transportation of stocks of doxycycline from all over the country and abroad is arranged. Initially the public is advised to use doxycycline only when symptomatic, and hospital emergency departments are confirmed as distribution points. Prophylaxis is advocated for medical and paramedical staff, immunosuppressed patients, and patients with valvular heart disease. The situation with pregnant women though remains obscure, some experts advocating the use of prophylactic rifampin regimens, while other suggest that only symptomatic women should receive antibiotics. The first opinion finally prevails. The minimal mortality of the disease is overemphasized, but soon further dispute grows, when certain infectious diseases specialists interviewed on television support the prophylactic use of doxycycline for all city inhabitants.

During the following two days, the two hospitals and a large hotel serving as hospital are flooded with patients, and by the end of day 16 more than 15,000 patients have experienced symptoms, more than 1,000 patients are hospitalized, and 5 people have died due to Q fever. More than 50,000 citizens end up using antibiotics, sometimes delivered through illegal sales at extreme prices. Control of the outbreak is not evolving though without further problems: as soon as the increased risk of special populations is announced, practically every such patient rushes to the hospital demanding prophylactic hospitalization. More than 5,000 patients are referring during days 15 and 16 to cardiologists worrying about possibly undiagnosed valvular heart disease. Dispute over the use of alternative antibiotic regimens such as quinolones, trimethoprim-sulfamethoxazole, and rifampin continues, and although the rates of infection in the pediatric population are relatively low, rare voices advocating the use of prophylactic antibiotic administration for children also emerge, further adding to panic. A report from the literature on direct transmission of Q fever[7] emerges on a television network, and certain patients complain about the absence of isolation procedures. One patient with no symptoms at day 14 develops symptoms at day 16 and rapidly dies, further fuelling the discussion of the prophylactic antibiotic administration for all the population. A self-proclaimed expert interviewed in a television news program accuses the government of not informing the public about the use of a vaccine in Australia, and it takes many hours for the authorities, busy with facing the outbreak, to respond appropriately. After a comment from the authorities that *Coxiella burnetii* is not an unknown pathogen for the area, many patients with pre-existing valvular heart disease are suing their cardiologists on the grounds of not being informed in the past of the dangers related to certain everyday practices. Misdiagnoses of other infections of the respiratory tract do occur, but doxycycline proves effective for these patients too. Of the more than 50,000 citizens receiving antibiotics, 40 experience serious adverse reactions requiring hospitalization, but no deaths are noted. Minor attacks from extremist groups against religious and ethnic minorities are noted in the city capital. The effect of the outbreak is obvious also in the animal population of the area, with a significant percentage of miscarriages and deterioration of meat consumption, resulting in significant economic loss. Environmental pollution with a highly resistant pathogen is also raised as an issue by the NATO special unit, and a projection of multiple localized outbreaks in the future further raises worries about the safety of living in that area on the future.

By day 19, no new cases occur. The scientists are now concerned about the cases of chronic Q fever that will emerge, and initially all high-risk patients are advised to continue treatment indefinitely. An initial estimate of 1,500 cases of chronic disease is added to an estimate of at least 2000 cases with chronic subjective symptoms, being in the form of chronic fatigue syndrome or purely depressive. TABLE 1 summarizes the outcome of this attack and compares this outcome to a hypothetical non-intervention scenario.

FACTORS THAT INFLUENCE THE OUTCOME

An important number of factors, related both to the pathogen and the place and time of the attack, could significantly influence the outcome of the attack. A lower bacterial inoculum or less optimal climate parameters would result in a significantly lower percentage of exposed population.

Although Q fever is traditionally considered as potentially caused by a single pathogen, there is ample evidence of the relationship between the inoculum and the severity of the disease induced.[9] The use of a class A pathogen would on the other hand result in a significantly higher number of deaths, thus possibly further influencing the social disruption and the public terror caused. The use of a pathogen transmitted from person to person would undoubtedly cause a global epidemic.[10]

On the other hand, *Coxiella burnetii* has a potential for chronicity[11] and for chronic environmental pollution, thus extending the local medical and social effect of such an attack. Furthermore, it is a zoonotic disease, affecting animal productivity, with serious financial implications for the targeted area.

The method of transmission also affects the outcome: using *Rickettsia prowazekii* as a weapon, one would presume that the attack would use animal and insect vectors of the pathogen: the presence of huge numbers of rats or lice would rapidly alert authorities, and the possibility of epidemic typhus would be soon entertained: prophylactic measures would be initiated immediately, and few cases of epidemic typhus would be recorded (yet, the overall death toll might finally be the same).

The inoculation period of Q fever also affects the weapon potential. The disease induced is also important, since the ease of diagnosis and the ease of differential diagnosis directly influence the initiation of response: in this attack scenario, the nonspecific symptoms caused significant delay in the recognition of the outbreak and furthermore initially guided the differential diagnosis towards other possibilities. The existence of specific treatment and prophylactic regimens is also paramount in determining the outcome, in terms of both death toll and social disruption. An attack with *Ebola* virus, still theoretically possible, would have grave consequences. The ability of rapid microbiological diagnosis is also paramount, but is related not only to the pathogen, but also to the local microbiology department's ability to proceed with the diagnosis. Facilities for diagnosing *Coxiella burnetii* through serology would be expected by an adequate microbiological laboratory: the evolution of this serology though, relating to the inoculation period, might further delay a definite diagnosis.

Factors related to the time and place of the attack are also crucial: obviously, a higher number of citizens would be exposed in summer days, relating to outdoor activities of the majority of the population. Climate parameters, such as a windy weather,[12] would also directly influence the percentage of the population exposed and the extent of the targeted area. A bigger targeted city might be related to an increased

TABLE 1. Outcome of a potential bioterrorist attack with *Coxiella burnetii*[a]

No Intervention	Moderately Rapid Response
Population exposed: 100,000	Population exposed: 100,000
Symptomatic patients: 40,000	Symptomatic patients: 15,000
In need of admission: 2,000	In need of admission: 1,000
Deaths: 20	Deaths: 5
Chronic cases/endocarditis: 1000–2000	Chronic cases/endocarditis: 600–900
Chronic cases/other: 600	Chronic cases/other: 400

[a]Data for an attack on a city with a population of 100,000, under optimal dispersion circumstances. Projections are based on large series and the clinical manifestations of the disease, as summarized by Raoult and colleagues.[8]

number of citizens exposed, although in cities expanding over great areas, only a fraction of the population might be exposed.

The importance of a prompt response cannot be overemphasized, and this response is multifactorial. TABLE 1 readily outlines the effect of a median response on the outcome, and especially on its medical aspects. A faster response, for example the initiation of specific action 12 hours earlier, would result in a further decrease of the patient burden and the social disruption inflicted. Preparedness is multifactorial: awareness of local medical authorities of the pathogen and bioterrorism in general should be emphasized. An attack with *Coxiella burnetii* in Marseille, France, would result in an almost immediate identification of the pathogen; an attack with *Brucella* in Ioannina, Greece would similarly be rapidly identified. Preparedness can vary among personnel of the same healthcare organization: a physician with an interest in infectious diseases would recognize the evolution of an outbreak more rapidly than a physician with other interests. Furthermore, the recognition of this evolving trend is definitely related to the awareness of the non-specialized medical and paramedical staff of the pathogen and of bioterrorism in general, a high level of educationally induced awareness would result in a coordinated response with minimal delays and shortcomings.

The most obvious aspect of preparedness though is the existence of a specific plan that should evolve as soon as an outbreak is suspected. Admittedly, such plans may initially lead to a great number of "false alarms."[13] Our scenario definitely outlines that conflict over hierarchy can influence the time needed for implementation of an adequate response.

The chosen targeted city and its characteristics would further influence the outcome: in a smaller city, physicians of the single non-tertiary hospital would face a continuously increasing burden of patients and might recognize the evolving epidemic faster, on the other hand though the inadequacies of a non-reference microbiological laboratory would delay diagnosis, the absence of an infectious diseases specialist would complicate the differential diagnosis, and the sheer burden for the hospital would result in a premature disruption of a proper local response, further enhancing the panic inflicted. On the other hand, if such an attack targeted a country's capital, where multiple hospitals are daily on call, the recognition of the evolving outbreak might be delayed if an infectious diseases alert network did not exist, and thus the response would be delayed, although reference laboratories might offer a prompt diagnosis. The existence of ample stock of treatment options would further affect the overall preparedness.

Finally the effect the mass media will have on the public perception cannot be underestimated. Although control of news content cannot be considered ethical when implemented by the authorities, the responsibility of the media should be expected to prevail over their quest for ratings: this though cannot be ascertained at times of emergency, and such a media response should be implemented when developing a plan of action.

REFERENCES

1. Kelly, D.J., A.L. Richards, J. Temenak, *et al.* 2002. The past and present threat of rickettsial diseases to military medicine and international public health. Clin. Infect. Dis. **34:** S145–169.
2. Pappas, G., S. Seitaridis, N. Akritidis, *et al.* 2003. Infectious diseases in cinema: virus hunters and killer microbes. Clin. Infect. Dis. **37:** 939–942.
3. Madariaga, M.G., K. Rezai, G.M. Trenhole, *et al.* 2003. Q fever: a biological weapon in your backyard. Lancet Infect. Dis. **3:** 709–721.
4. O'Toole, T. 1999. Smallpox: An attack scenario. Emerg. Infect. Dis. **5:** 540–546.
5. Bardi, J. 1999. Aftermath of a hypothetical smallpox disaster. Emerg. Infect. Dis. **5:** 547–551.
6. Inglesby, T.V., R. Grossman & T. O'Toole. 2001. A plague on your city: observations from TOPOFF. Clin. Infect. Dis. **32:** 436–445.
7. Mann, J.S., J.G. Douglas, J.M. Inglis, *et al.* 1986. Q fever: person to person transmission within a family. Thorax **41:** 974–975.
8. Raoult, D., T. Marrie & J. Mege. 2005. Natural history and pathophysiology of Q fever. Lancet Infect. Dis. **5:** 219–226
9. Vorobeychikov, E.V., G.M. Kurtzer, A.Z. Vasilenko, *et al.* 2003. Probabilistic evaluation of aspirating doses of a Q fever pathogen. Ann. N.Y. Acad. Sci. **990:** 743–750.
10. Casadevall, A. & L.A. Pirofski. 2004. The weapon potential of a microbe. Trends Microbiol. **12:** 259–263.
11. Maurin, M. & D. Raoult. 1999. Q fever. Clin. Microbiol. Rev. **12:** 518–553.
12. Tissot-Dupont, H., M.A. Amadei, M. Nezri, *et al.* 2004. Wind in November, Q fever in December. Emerg. Infect. Dis. **10:** 1264–1269.
13. Seward, J.F., K. Galil, I. Damon, *et al.* 2004. Development and experience with an algorithm to evaluate suspected smallpox cases in the United States, 2002–2004. Clin. Infect. Dis. **39:** 1477–1483.

The Pathogen Resource Integration Center

Implications for *Rickettsial* Research

MARK E. HANCE,[a] MICHAEL J. CZAR,[a] ABDU AZAD,[b] ANJAN PURKAYASTHA,[a] ERIC E. SNYDER,[a] OSWALD R. CRASTA,[a] JOAO C. SETUBAL,[a] AND BRUNO W. SOBRAL[a]

[a]*Virginia Bioinformatics Institute, Virginia Polytechnic Institute and State University, Washington Street, Blacksburg, Virginia 24061-0477, USA*

[b]*University of Maryland School of Medicine, Baltimore, Maryland 20742, USA*

KEYWORDS: **Pathogen Resource Integration Center; bioinformatics**

INTRODUCTION

The PathoSystems Resource Integration Center (PATRIC) was established in July, 2004, at the Virginia Bioinformatics Institute (VBI), to serve as a bioinformatics resource center (BRC) for scientists engaged in the development of vaccines, diagnostics, and therapeutics for three bacteria (*Rickettsiae, Coxiellae,* and *Brucellae*) and five classes of viruses (calici, corona, hepatitis A, hepatitis E, and rabies). PATRIC is one of eight such Bioinformatics Resource Centers for Biodefense and Emerging or Re-Emerging Infectious Diseases (BRCs) funded for five years by the National Institute of Allergy and Infectious Diseases (NIAID). The objective of the BRCs is to create a comprehensive database of information on selected CDC category A, B, and C pathogens and other organisms causing emerging and re-emerging human diseases. PATRIC will integrate and disseminate a variety of diverse data types, such as genome sequence, comparative genomics, genome polymorphisms, gene expression, proteomics, pathways, and host/pathogen interactions. This information will be stored in a relational database and made available to the scientific community through a user-friendly web interface. Herein, we will describe our mission goals as a participating BRC, detail the PATRIC infrastructure and our approach to biological data annotation/curation, and present our strategy for developing resources for the *Rickettsial* scientific community as well as the other scientific communities served by PATRIC.

NIAID's goal is to better understand, treat, and ultimately prevent infectious, immunologic, and allergic diseases (http://www3.niaid.nih.gov/about/overview/). Within the past several years, NIAID has funded a number of initiatives to provide comprehensive genomics resources to the scientific community.

Address for correspondence: Mark E. Hance, Virginia Bioinformatics Institute, Virginia Polytechnic Institute and State University, Washington Street, Blacksburg, VA 24061-0477. Voice: 540-231-2100; fax: 540-231-2606.

Ann. N.Y. Acad. Sci. 1063: 459–465 (2005). © 2005 New York Academy of Sciences.
doi: 10.1196/annals.1355.066

NIAID has been investing in genomic sequencing of invertebrate disease vectors and pathogenic microorganisms including both those of primary medical significance as well as those considered to be relevant to biodefense. The sequence data from these organisms coupled with other experimentally and computer-generated information are expediting the development of diagnostic and epidemiological markers, drug targets, and vaccines.

Since the early 1980s molecular sequence data has undergone exponential growth, attributable largely to the availability of DNA sequencing methods. High throughput sequencing has become commonplace; high throughput gene expression data and proteomics data are rapidly following suit. Microbial genomes can now be almost completely sequenced within a few days (Sobral and colleagues, unpublished data). NIAID recognized a need with respect to the integration and analysis of this data and established eight BRCs. Each center is assigned the task of constructing cyberinfrastructures to integrate genomic, proteomic, biochemical, and literature information (http://www.niaid.nih.gov/dmid/genomes/brc/default.htm). This integration should provide the scientific community with a valuable research resource, including access to genomic and related data pertaining to the organisms under each BRC's purview as well as bioinformatic tools to aid the researcher in the interpretation of the data. These resources will be freely available for public use. Specific objectives set forth by NIAID for the BRC initiative are: (1) to provide the scientific community with a point of entry into a comprehensive database with access to genomic and related data designed to maximize ease of use; (2) to have each center focus on the organisms listed in the NIAID Category A–C priority list of pathogens causing emerging or re-emerging diseases relevant to biodefense; and (3) ultimately to aid in the discovery of therapeutic targets, vaccines, diagnostics, and epidemiological markers.

Making sense of this abundance of data requires a new paradigm—a bioinformatic cyberinfrastructure (http://www.communitytechnology.org/nsf_ci_report/). The goal of this new environment is the integration of multiple data types using distributive database, computer, information, and communication technology. Ultimately, through this new paradigm, complete computer-generated representations of living cells and organisms will be made available and from this, powerful new investigative strategies will emerge to benefit the biomedical research community. The high rate of data generation in the life sciences, and its expected increases, poses a challenge for scientists who hope to capitalize on the value that the databases hold. Implementation of a cyberinfrastructure and the requisite bioinformatic tools for the exploration of these data by the scientific community is crucial and should enhance the research on the discovery of therapeutic targets, vaccines, and diagnostic markers.

THE PATHOSYSTEMS RESOURCE INTEGRATION CENTER (PATRIC)

The Pathosystems Resource Integration Center (PATRIC) was established at the Virginia Bioinformatics Institute (VBI) at Virginia Polytechnic Institute and State University, or Virginia Tech.(http://patric.vbi.vt.edu/). For each of the above organisms listed we will annotate and curate biological information from a number of species/strains. Specifically for *Rickettsia*, we expect to work with at least 10 genomic sequences (TABLE 1).

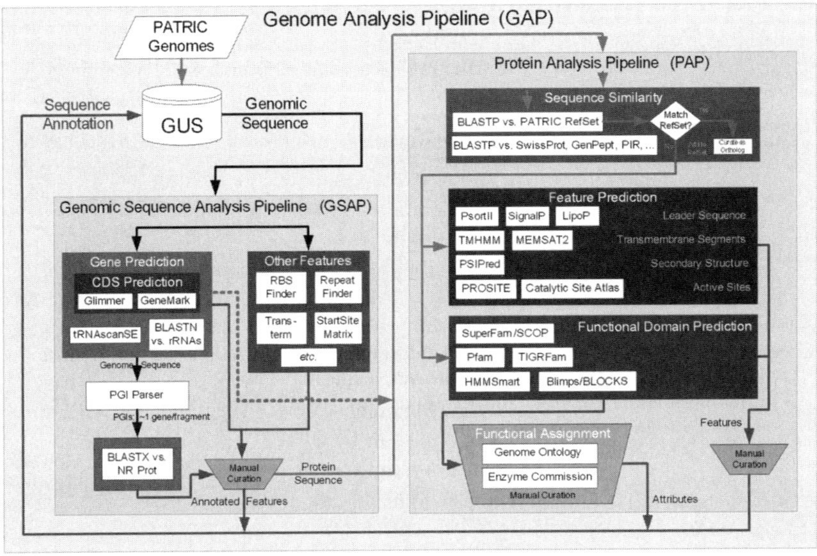

FIGURE 1. The PATRIC Genome Sequence Analysis Pipeline and Protein Analysis Pipelines. Gene prediction and protein functional prediction and assignment will be performed through automated analysis pipelines, the Genomic Sequence Analysis Pipeline (*left*) and the Protein Analysis Pipeline (*right*). Individual tools are listed within the flow diagrams for each of the pipelines.

TABLE 1. ***Rickettsia*** **genomes available or in progress as of July 2005. The** ***Rickettsia*** **genomes listed are publicly available or are currently being sequenced**

Pathogen	Accession Number(s)	Replicon Size (bp)
Rickettsia bellii	Sequencing in progress	n/a
Rickettsia canadensis	Sequencing in progress	n/a
Rickettsia montanensis	Sequencing in progress	n/a
Rickettsia conorii	NC_003103	1268755
Rickettsia felis URRWXCal2	NC_007109 NC_007110 NC_007111	1485148 62829 39263
Rickettsia prowazekii str. Madrid E	NC_000963	1111523
Rickettsia rickettsii	NZ_AADJ01000001	1257710
Rickettsia sibirica 246	NZ_AABW01000001	1250021
Rickettsia typhi str	NC_006142	1111496
Rickettsia akari str. Hartford	NZ_AAFE01000001	1231060

TABLE 2. Genomes stored at PATRIC

	Organism Expert (Affiliation)	Number of Genomes	Genome Size
Bacteria			
Brucella	Dr. Steven Boyle (Virginia Tech)	4	Ch1: 2.11 Mb Ch2: 1.17 Mb
Coxiella	Dr. Abdu Azad (University of Maryland)	2	1.5–2.1 Mb
Rickettsiae	Dr. Abdu Azad (University of Maryland)	10	1.1–1.6 Mb
Viruses			
Coronaviruses	Dr. Susan Baker (Loyola University of Chicago)	52	27–31 kb
Caliciviruses	Dr. Stephen Monroe (Centers for Disease Control and Prevention)	168	7.7–8.5 kb
Hepatitis A Viruses	Dr. Omana Nainan (Centers for Disease Control and Prevention)	17	7.4 kb
Hepatitis E Viruses	Dr. X. J. Meng (Virginia Tech)	42	7.2 kb
Rabies Viruses	Dr. Charles Rupprecht (Centers for Disease Control and Prevention)	10	11.9 kb

The three bacterial and five viral organisms are listed along with the organism expert for each organism, the number of genomes stored at PATRIC ([a] indicates as of July 2005) and the range of genome sizes for each organism.

Our approach to the annotation of *Rickettsial* and other genomes is a multi-level, comprehensive analysis (FIG. 1). We will identify and annotate the coding regions plus other non-coding features of the genomic sequence using a customized genome sequence annotation pipeline (GSAP). Curators will review automated analysis data and verify its correctness. Identified gene products will be analyzed further by an automated protein annotation pipeline (PAP) to characterize functional domain and motif structures as well as the protein function, where possible, using standardized conventions with regard to identifiers across all of the organisms annotated. An organism expert (OE), a scientist with several years of experience and a recognized authority in the field, has been selected for each of our organisms to ensure the quality of our curation effort (TABLE 2). Our annotation process utilizes the concept of reference genomes and associated genomes in which a representative genome serves as a model for related genomes. Reference genomes will be carefully curated and the annotations from the well-curated reference genome will be inherited by homologous genes of the associated genomes where applicable. A comprehensive reference gene set will be generated by pooling all the unique genes from the reference- and associated-genomes. For *Rickettsia*, *R. prowazekii* will be the reference genome. Metabolic pathways for each organism will be characterized once its proteome has been delineated.[1] Comparative genomics analysis will also be an integral component of our overall approach, identifying conserved, as well as non-syntenic, regions across species and strains. Additionally, experimental evidence derived from the literature will be carefully examined, cited, and included as it becomes available. All of the annotation, experimental data and curated information will be available to the researcher on our website using a suite of querying, visualization, and analysis tools.

USING THE PATRIC WEBSITE

Through careful and standardized annotation we aim to improve on the existing knowledge base for our eight pathogens, but this is only the first step to a much broader goal. Biological science, when compared with chemistry and physics, is not as capable of making predictions based on general principles. However, as the body of experimental data grows and our ability to interpret through bioinformatic methods increases, both our ability to represent the cellular milieu and to make predictions based on computational analyses with regard to the host-pathogen interactions will increase likewise. By using a systems biology approach to define and visualize the interactions that necessarily occur between the host and pathogen during the disease process, we will provide investigators with a comprehensive overview of the processes most likely to be targeted for therapeutic intervention. Gene expression and proteomics data superimposed onto graphical visualizations of this interaction will help to more fully illuminate this interaction. Additionally, comprehensive querying of our extensive database will allow the researcher to rapidly search across multiple *Rickettsial* species for similarities and differences in the proteomes to help identify those proteins that play a role in pathogenesis and that determine characteristics like vector specificity and symptom severity.

PATRIC exists to serve as a resource to the scientific research community and so it is critical to our goals that we receive feedback and advice as we move forward with our development. A review of the *Rickettsia* literature suggests numerous areas of research where PATRIC may be able to provide assistance. A few examples are presented below to illustrate this point. For *Rickettsial* background information, please refer to the following website (http://pathport.vbi.vt.edu/pathinfo/).

Rickettsia rickettsii has been shown to induce the activation of the ubiquitous transcription factor nuclear factor-κB (NF-κB) in endothelial cells in a biphasic pattern.[2] This activation, which may play an important role in the transcriptional responses of endothelial cells to *R. rickettsii* occurs outside of the normal signaling pathways.[3] The activation scenario involves amino-terminal serine phosphorylation, ubiquination and subsequent degradation by the 26S proteasome of NF-κB–associated inhibitory proteins,[4] which is triggered by the activation of IκB kinases (IKK).[5] Activation of NF-κB results in transcription of genes involved both in procoagulant and proinflammatory responses.[6] NF-κB–associated genes also play a role in the protection against infection-induced cell apoptosis by preventing the activation of caspase-mediated pathways.[7,8] Studies using anti-inflammatory IKK inhibitors suggest a possible therapeutic role for these compounds in blocking the early signaling mechanisms.[5] The bacterial component(s) that mediate IKK activation and subsequent NF-κB disinhibition are presently not known. However, delineation and representation of these host-pathogen interaction pathways, through the accumulation of expression and proteomic data, may further elucidate the mechanism. This, in turn, could lead to the development of additional efficacious therapeutic protocols to reduce vascular damage and human morbidity.

Another area that has received significant attention is the mechanism by which spotted fever group (SFG) *Rickettsiae* induce their uptake into host non-phagocytic cells. This uptake has been shown to involve a phospholipase activity as well as host cell actin polymerization, which also enables the bacteria to move within the endothelial cells and to spread to neighboring host cells.[9,10] The actin polymerization process has been shown to be induced by RickA in SFG *rickettsia*, through an interaction with the Arp2/3 complex in the host cell.[11–13] While the RickA protein has been shown to be highly expressed on the cell surface of SFG *Rickettsiae* in infected cells,[11] RickA doesn't display any signal sequence that could act as a membrane anchor. It is not known whether other *Rickettsial* proteins are involved in this process. Through the integration of protein interaction data, The PATRIC infrastructure will allow researchers to visualize and query for proteins known to interact with motility-related proteins. This ability may provide additional details on the pathways or complex formation within *Rickettsial* cells and host cells and thereby yield targets for therapeutic intervention.

Adherence to the target endothelial cells is critical for the successful establishment of infection. The putative adhesins rOmpA[14] and rOmpB[15] have been identified and described in SFG *Rickettsiae*. rOmpA has been shown to play an important role in the initial adhesion of *R. rickettsii* to the host cell,[14] although whether or not rOmpA is sufficient for internalization has not been fully elucidated. Identification of host receptor(s) and the bacterial surface proteins that mediate the adhesion process may provide insight into the development of therapeutics.[16] The ability to perform complex Boolean queries within the PATRIC website will allow researchers to search for cell surface proteins that are conserved among SFG species, and possess motifs involved in adhesion and cell entry. This ability may provide another means by which researchers may identify cell-entry mechanisms in SFG *Rickettsiae*.

SUMMARY

The information presented here reflects our immediate plans for basic genome annotation and our future goals to include analysis of metabolic and regulatory pathways, as well as host-pathogen interactions. Future incorporation of gene-expression and proteomics data highlights our aim to make this resource comprehensive. Our ultimate goal is to help the biomedical research community leverage information generated by high-throughput technologies to better understand the physiology of these organisms and their host interactions. In time this will lead to improved treatment and prophylaxis of disease caused by these potentially deadly organisms.

[*Competing interests statement:* The authors declare that they have no competing interests.]

REFERENCES

1. Karp, P.D., S. Paley & P. Romero. 2002. The Pathway Tools software. Bioinformatics **18:** S225–232.

2. SPORN, L.A. *et al.* 1997. Rickettsia rickettsii infection of cultured human endothelial cells induces NF-kappaB activation. Infect. Immun. **65:** 2786–2791.
3. SAHNI, S.K. *et al.* 1998.Proteasome-independent activation of nuclear factor kappaB in cytoplasmic extracts from human endothelial cells by *Rickettsia rickettsii.* Infect. Immun. **66:** 1827–1833.
4. GHOSH, S., M.J. MAY & E.B. KOPP. 1998. NF-kappa B and Rel proteins: evolutionarily conserved mediators of immune responses. Annu. Rev. Immunol. **16:** 225–260.
5. CLIFTON, D.R. *et al.* 2005. NF-kappaB activation during *Rickettsia rickettsii* infection of endothelial cells involves the activation of catalytic IkappaB kinases IKKalpha and IKKbeta and phosphorylation-proteolysis of the inhibitor protein IkappaBalpha. Infect. Immun. **73:** 155–165.
6. SHI, R.J. *et al.* 1998. Transcriptional regulation of endothelial cell tissue factor expression during *Rickettsia rickettsii* infection: involvement of the transcription factor NF-kappaB. Infect. Immun. **66:** 1070–1075.
7. CLIFTON, D.R. *et al.* 1998. NF-kappa B-dependent inhibition of apoptosis is essential for host cell survival during *Rickettsia rickettsii* infection. Proc. Natl. Acad. Sci. USA **95:** 4646–4651.
8. JOSHI, S.G. *et al.* 2003. Nuclear factor kappa B protects against host cell apoptosis during *Rickettsia rickettsii* infection by inhibiting activation of apical and effector caspases and maintaining mitochondrial integrity. Infect. Immun. **71:** 4127–4136.
9. SILVERMAN, D.J. *et al.* 1992. Penetration of host cells by *Rickettsia rickettsii* appears to be mediated by a phospholipase of rickettsial origin. Infect. Immun. **60:** 2733–2740.
10. WALKER, D.H., H.M. FENG & V.L. POPOV. 2001. Rickettsial phospholipase A2 as a pathogenic mechanism in a model of cell injury by typhus and spotted fever group rickettsiae. Am. J. Trop. Med. Hyg. **65:** 936–942.
11. GOUIN, E. *et al.* 2004. The RickA protein of *Rickettsia conorii* activates the Arp2/3 complex. Nature **427:** 457–461.
12. JENG, R.L. *et al.* 2004. A *Rickettsia* WASP-like protein activates the Arp2/3 complex and mediates actin-based motility. Cell. Microbiol. **6:** 761–769.
13. OGATA, H. *et al.* 2000. Selfish DNA in protein-coding genes of *Rickettsia.* Science **290:** 347–350.
14. LI, H. & D.H. WALKER. 1998. rOmpA is a critical protein for the adhesion of *Rickettsia rickettsii* to host cells. Microb. Pathog. **24:** 289–298.
15. UCHIYAMA, T. 2003. Adherence to and invasion of Vero cells by recombinant *Escherichia coli* expressing the outer membrane protein rOmpB of *Rickettsia japonica.* Ann. N.Y. Acad. Sci. **990:** 585–590.
16. MARTINEZ, J.J. & P. COSSART. 2004. Early signaling events involved in the entry of *Rickettsia conorii* into mammalian cells. J. Cell. Sci. **117:** 5097–5106.

Evaluation of Low Concentration Aerosol for Infecting Humans with the Q Fever Pathogen

EUGENE VOROBEYCHIKOV[a] ALEXANDER VASILENKO,[b]
NIKOLAY TOKAREVICH,[b] LUDMILA YAKOVLEVA,[a] AND BORIS NIKOLAEV[a]

[a]*State Research Center of Highly Pure Biopreparations, Saint Petersburg, Russia*

[b]*Saint Petersburg Pasteur Institute, Saint Petersburg, Russia*

KEYWORDS: ***Q fever;* modeling; aerosol; aspirating dose; infective dose**

INTRODUCTION

Conventional models describing accumulation of aspirating doses of pathogenic microorganisms in the respiratory organs are deterministic. They have been proven to be accurate when distribution concentration of the aerosol is high and have acceptable accuracy of an evaluation of aspirating dose of microorganisms (D). At low concentration, aerosol deterministic model roughly describes real accumulation of microorganisms into respiratory organs of the man that results in the overestimated evaluation of value (D) and reduction of critical exposition time (Δt).[1] On the basis of deterministic and probabilistic approaches one can calculate the comparative estimation of formation of infective aspiration dose of Q fever pathogen and critical exposition time for a person in the conditions of low-concentration aerosols.

DETERMINISTIC AND PROBABILISTIC APPROACHES

For the evaluation of value D the deterministic model[1,2] is usually employed:

$$D = CVK\Delta t \tag{1}$$

where D is the aspiration dose of microorganisms (count of cells); C is the microbial aerosol concentration (cells/L, cells/m^3); V is the volume of ventilation of the lungs or minute volume of pulmonary ventilation of the organism (L/min); K is the delay factor of microbial aerosol particles in the respiratory organs; and Δt is the time of exposure (min, hour). The model is based on the proposal, that at low or high constant values of parameter (C) and at the $\Delta t \to \infty$ the accumulation of microorganisms

Address for correspondence: Eugene Vorobeychikov, State Research Center of Highly Pure Biopreparations, Saint Petersburg, Russia.
evv@peterlink.ru

Ann. N.Y. Acad. Sci. 1063: 466–470 (2005). © 2005 New York Academy of Sciences.
doi: 10.1196/annals.1355.067

in respiratory organs occurs with the probability of 1. However, this scenario is not always conformed to, even with pathogenic microorganisms,[3] and more detail is required.

One of the parameters, which is connected with the formation of D value, is the penetration speed of microorganisms into the respiratory organs of a person (W, cells/min). At the known values of (C, V, K, Δt) the parameter (W) is determined from expression (1):

$$W = \frac{CVK}{1000} \tag{2}$$

Another way of evaluating parameter (W) is based on preliminary calculation of value D according the equation (1) and at the fixed time of exposure (Δt) the expression may be:

$$W = \frac{D}{\Delta t} \tag{3}$$

Preliminary analysis of these expressions demonstrates that at high concentrations of microbial aerosol, the value of parameter W is more than at low concentrations. Consequently, with the increase of parameter (C) the speed of microorganisms penetration also increases. This leads to quick formation of infecting aspiration doses of microorganisms and reveals the large infective efficacy of high aerosol concentrations. From the biological point of view equation (1) may be used for the accurate estimation of D, when high concentrations of aerosols act on respiratory organs. At the low concentrations of aerosol the value of W is less then at the high concentrations. This means that at the limited time of exposure (Δt) the slow formation of infective aspiration doses of microorganisms occurs. This leads to nonuniformity of aspiration dose accumulation and the probability of this dose is not equal to 1. At low concentrations of aerosol and limited time of exposure (Δt) evaluation of D on the base of expression (1) will be overestimated.

The analysis of expression (1) shows that the parameter V describes continuous mode of breath of the man. However the process of breath can be considered from the position of consistently repeating independent and non-uniformity of separate cycles consisting of one inhalation, a pause, and an exhalation. Thus the mode of human respiration is a discrete non-uniform process. In this case the probability of a quantity of particles getting into the respiratory organs does not depend on the number of particles inhaled in the previous respiratory cycles, i.e., the various variants of accumulation of particles in organs of breath are possible. Hence the probability accumulation of dose for each separate independent respiratory cycle cannot be equal to 1.

For estimation of D accumulation in human respiratory organs, we propose the probabilistic model.[6] This model takes into account nonuniformity of space-time distribution of microorganisms at low concentrations in the aerosol and non-similarity of respiratory cycles of the man. The following analysis of formation of most probable values of D is carrying out the estimation of W. The values (D), received on the base of probabilistic approach, are introduced into the equation (3).

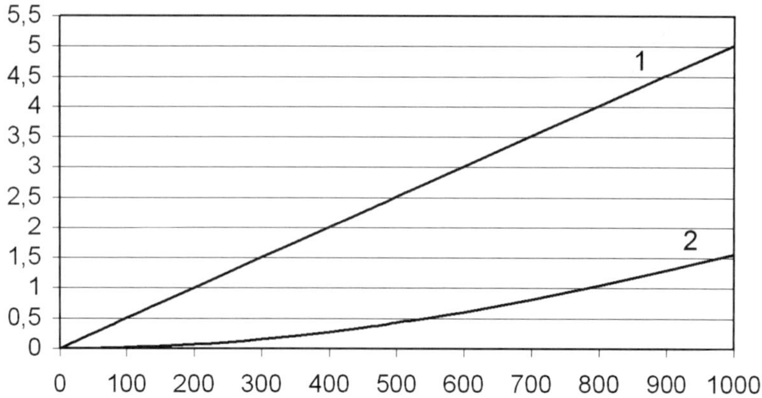

FIGURE 1. Dependence of the penetration speed of Q fever pathogen on aerosol concentration. *Abscissa* is the aerosols concentrations (C, cells/m^3). *Ordinate* is the penetration speed of microorganisms into the respiratory system (W, cells/min). Line 1, the calculation of value (W) is made on a basis of deterministic model. Line 2, the calculation of value (W) is made on a basis of probabilistic model. The fixed of exposure time ($\Delta t = 60$ min). Dispersity of particles –3.0 μ. Particles hold-up factor in the respiratory organs (K) – 0.67; respiratory of volume (V) – 0.5 L; lung ventilation of volume (V_v) – 7.5 L/min; number of respiratory cycles (N) for 1 h = 900.

RESULTS AND DISCUSSION

The data of aspiration doses of *Coxiella burnetii* for man, that are enough for infecting by penetrating into respiratory organs from individual cells up to ten-twenty cells of the microorganisms were used for calculation.[4,5] The results presented in FIGURE 1 describe the dependence of penetration speed (W) of microorganisms into the respiratory organs of man at respiration through the nose from aerosol concentration (C) and fixed time exposition ($\Delta t = 60$ min). Analysis of these dependencies demonstrates that the increase of parameter (C) is accompanied by the increase of W. It means that at high concentrations of the aerosol there is a prompt penetration of microorganisms that results in prompt formation of infecting aspiration doses. With increase of parameter (C) up to 1,500 cells/m^3, evaluations of parameter (W), calculated on the base of deterministic and probabilistic models differ twofold. From the biological point of view, such differences are very minimal. Therefore at high concentrations of an aerosol the evaluation of formation of infecting aspiration doses of microorganisms is possible on the basis of deterministic and probabilistic approaches.

At low concentrations of an aerosol the value of parameter (W), received on the basis of the probabilistic approach, testifies to the slow dynamics of penetration of microorganisms into human respiratory organs. Accordingly, the slow formation of infecting aspirating doses of microorganisms takes place. Thus, in range of aerosol concentrations less than 100–150 cells/m^3, parameter (W) has, practically, zero values. It testifies to very low opportunity of realization of the mechanism of aerosol infecting of the man by *C. burnetii.*

Further, the analysis of penetration of respiratory organs by *C. burnetii* is based on the definition of critical exposure time at which the infection occurs. Taking into account that the value (W) increases with augmentation of parameter (C), the evaluation of critical values (Δt) was done from formula (3):

$$\Delta t = \frac{D}{W} \tag{4}$$

where D is the fixed value of infecting aspiration dose of microorganisms (cells); W is the speed of penetrating of microorganisms into the respiratory organs (cells/min). At low concentrations of an aerosol the values of parameter (W) are introduced into expression (4), which was obtained earlier on the basis of the probabilistic approach. The infecting values (D) of *C. burnetii* for the man are known and in the expression (4) are set arbitrarily. The dependences of change of critical exposure time from the parameter of (C) and the fixed of value (D) are shown in FIGURE 2.

The analysis of dependences shows that with increase of aerosol concentration and known fixed values of infecting aspiration doses of microorganisms, there is a decrease of exposure time. So, for example, at the fixed values of infecting aspiration doses of *C. burnetii* for humans (D = 5, cells) and constant concentrations of microorganisms in aerosol (C = 200, 300, 400, 500, and 1000, cells/m^3) the dangerous exposure time will be accordingly: > 60 min, > 30 min, > 20 min, > 12 min and > 3 min. The formation of minimal infecting doses of *C. burnetii* for humans D = 1 cell)

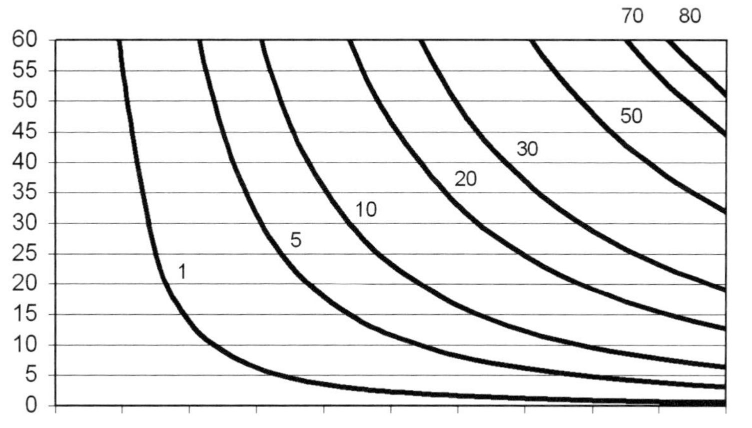

FIGURE 2. Dependence of the change of critical exposure time from an aerosol concentration and the fixed values of infecting doses of Q fever pathogen. *Abscissa* is the aerosols concentrations (C, cells/m^3). *Ordinates* is the critical time of exposure (Δt, min). Figures on lines (1, 5, 10 ...) are the fixed values (D, cells) Dispersity of particles – 3,0 μ. The calculation is made on a basis of probabilistic model.

can be realized at aerosol concentration 200 cells/m^3 and critical exposure time more than 20 min. Thus, to model of infective doses of Q fever pathogen and explain the opportunity for realization of aerosol infections of humans, it is necessary to take into account the following: the value of infecting dose of a definite microorganism, the concentrations and size of aerosol particles, the penetration speed of pathogens into respiratory organs, and critical time of exposure.[6]

CONCLUSIONS

The presented results make it possible to draw the following conclusions: (1) At low concentrations of aerosol (< 1000 cells/m^3) and limited exposure time (Δt =1 h) the probabilistic model has more objective description of the formation of infecting doses of Q fever pathogen for humans. This model takes into account the nonuniformity distribution of low aerosol concentration and the nonsimilarity of individual respiratory cycles. The deterministic model does not provide such an opportunity. (2) The concentrations of microbial aerosol less then 100–150 cells/m^3 and limited time (1 h) provide very limited opportunity to realize the mechanism of aerosol infecting of humans with *C. burnetii*. (3) The minimal infecting dose *C burnetii* for man (D = 1 cell) can be realized at aerosol concentration 200 cells/m^3 and critical exposure time more than 20 min.

ACKNOWLEDGMENT

The authors are grateful to Assistant Professor Boris Bershadsky (University of Minnesota, Division of Health Services Research & Policy, USA) and to Doctor Yuriy Lebedev (State Research Center of Highly Pure Biopreparations, Saint Petersburg, Russia) for helpful remarks and discussion.

[*Competing interests statement:* No competing interests statement was received.]

REFERENCES

1. VOROBEYCHIKOV, E. 2004, Accumulation aspirating doses of microorganisms at distribution of a low concentration aerosols. Presented at Eighth International Symposium on Protection Against Chemical and Biological Warfare Agents. Gothenburg, Sweden, June 2-6, 2004. p.117.
2. GAPOCHKO, K.G., O.P. MISNIKOV & K.K. RAYEVSKY 1985. Means and Methods of Microbial Aerosol Research. Medicine. (in Russian) .
3. OGARKOV, V.I. & K.G. GAPOCHKO. 1975. Aerogenic Infection. Medicine. (in Russian)
4. BELLAMY, R.J. & A.R. FREEDMAN. 2001. Bioterrorism. Q. J. Med. **94:** 227–224.
5. RAOULT, D., T. MARRIE & J. MEGE. 2005. Natural history and pathophysiology of Q fever. Lancet Infect. Dis. **5:** 219–226.
6. VOROBEYCHIKOV, E.V., G.M. KURTZER, A.Z. VASILENKO & O.P. MISNIKOV. 2003. Probabilistic evaluation of aspirating doses of Q fever pathogen. Ann. N.Y. Sci. **990:** 743–750.

Index of Contributors